B. Runnebaum T. Rabe L. Kiesel (Eds.)

Female Contraception

Update and Trends

With 83 Figures and 90 Tables

Springer-Verlag Berlin Heidelberg New York
London Paris Tokyo

Prof. Dr. med. Benno Runnebaum
PD Dr. med. Thomas Rabe
Dr. med. Ludwig Kiesel

Department of Obstetrics and Gynecology
Division of Gynecological Endocrinology
Women's Hospital, University of Heidelberg,
Voßstr. 9, D-6900 Heidelberg

ISBN-13: 978-3-642-73792-3 e-ISBN-13: 978-3-642-73790-9
DOI: 10.1007/978-3-642-73790-9

Library of Congress Cataloging-in-Publication Data.
Female contraception: update and trends / B. Runnebaum, T. Rabe, and L. Kiesel (eds.).
p. cm.
Includes index.
1. Contraception. 2. Contraceptives. I. Runnebaum, B. (Benno), 1933– . II. Rabe, T. (Thomas) III. Kiesel, L. [DNLM: 1. Contraception. 2. Contraception – trends. WP 630 F329] RG 136.F39 1988 613.9'4 – dc19 DNLM/DLC for Library of Congress 88-16069 CIP
ISBN 0-387-19396-0 (U.S.)

Softcover reprint of the hardcover 1st edition 1988

Typesetting: Brühlsche Universitätsdruckerei, Giessen
Offsetprinting: Saladruck, Berlin. Bookbinding: Lüderitz & Bauer, Berlin
2121/3030-543210 – Printed on acid-free paper

Preface

The Second International Symposium, held in Heidelberg on June 13–16, 1987, was concerned with the current state of knowledge and modern trends in female contraception. In evaluating different methods of female contraception, oral hormones continued to be a focus of attention. Most of the main presentations of the symposium are included in this book.

The side effects of oral contraceptives on metabolism, e.g., on lipids, carbohydrates, and blood clotting have been extensively analyzed. In general, low-dose oral contraceptives show a low impact on intermediate metabolism and are preferable to the high-dose formulations. It is difficult to determine and evaluate risk factors. Definite risk factors seem to be heavy smoking, especially at higher age. The importance of other often discussed risk factors cannot be clarified statistically. Furthermore, dosage is closely correlated to mortality and morbidity. Yet there are not only negative side effects; some effects are favorable to health, e.g., the lower incidence of inflammations of the fallopian tubes, of ovarian cysts, of rheumatoid arthritis, and of endometrial or ovarian carcinoma. These considerations are important when evaluating the risks and advantages before first use or during continued use of the pill. Thus, with regard to risk factors (such as smoking, hypertension, and others, which have to be excluded), there is no certain age after which women should not longer take the pill.

There were many discussions about the question whether the pill has a negative influence on metabolism, thereby increasing morbidity or even mortality. This question has not yet been answered, but it can be stated clearly that low-dose pills with the new gestagens (desogestrel, norgestimate, gestodene) show no negative impact on carbohydrate and lipid metabolism or on blood clotting.

Barrier methods might play a more important role in contraception in the future, because they considerably reduce the transmission of sexually transmitted diseases. In special cases these methods can be combined with oral contraceptives. Intrauterine devices will also gain in importance due to improvements in shape, structure, and medication.

In this respect highly promising new approaches in hormonal contraception are Norplant implantations with a permanent low release of gestagens, and the once-a-month injectable preparation. Furthermore, the practical application, both in the female and the male, of immunization techniques against pregnancy has been discussed.

Among the side effects of oral contraceptives that were analyzed were the carcinogenic aspects. Unfortunately, the paper dealing with oral contraception and the risk of breast cancer can not yet be published. The presentation dealing with sexual habits and the risks of transmission of AIDS also cannot be published in this book. We can only hope that these topics can be included in future publications.

Finally, the political and religious aspects of contraception were discussed, especially with a view to the problem of overpopulation. It is remarkable that the amount spent on family planning worldwide is only 2% of the defence budget. Meetings and books such as these will contribute to causing a gradual change in society's concern with such issues.

Heidelberg, July 1988

Benno Runnebaum
Thomas Rabe
Ludwig Kiesel

Contributors

Ackerman, S.
Alexander, N. J.
Anderson, D. J.
Anderson, R. A.
Assmann, G.
Audebert, A. J. M.

Bauer, L.
Beck, L. R.
Beier, S.
Benagiano, G.
Bergamaschi, M.
Bernstein, L.
Billings, J. J.
Bishop, C.
Bonnar, J.

Carroll, A.
Chalker, R.
Chillik, C. F.
Chwalisz, K.
Cleva, M.

Daly, L.
Danforth, D. R.
Demarest, K. T.
Diczfalusy, E.
Duesterberg, B.
Du Mingkun

Edelmann, A.
Elger, W.
Ellwanger, B.

Facchinetti, F.
Fähnrich, M.
Filshie, G. M.
Fotherby, K.

Gaur, A.
Genazzani, A. D.
Genazzani, A. R.
Gerhard, I.
Grunwald, K.
Gu Sujuan

Hahn, D. W.
Haimovici, F.
Haspels, A. A.
Helm, K.
Hill, J. A.
Hodgen, G. D.
Hoppe, G.
Huber, P. R.

Kaminski, J. M.
Keep, P. A. van
Kesserü, E.
Kiesel, L.
Kopera, H.
Kraft, H. G.

Laurent, H.
Lewis, D. H.
Loewit, K.

Mack, S. R.
Maier, C.
Mall-Haefeli, M.
McGuire, J. L.

Neumann, F.

Ortlieb, A.

Pasquale, S. A.
Perkin, G.
Petraglia, F.
Phillips, A.
Potts, M.

Quigg, J.

Rabe, T.
Rekers, H.
Roy, S.
Runnebaum, B.

Sabra, A.
Santoro, V.
Schenker, J. G.
Schulte, H.
Serfaty, D.
Shao-Quing, S.
Skouby, S. O.
Stanczyk, F. Z.

Talwar, G. P.
Thiery, M.
Tozzini, R.

Volpe, A.

Waller, D. P.
Wang Suhua
Werner-Zodrow, I.
Williams, R. F.
Wolfram, G.

Xu, C.
Xu Meifang

Yaneva, H.

Zaneveld, L. J. D.
Zatuchni, G. I.
Zhang Lingde

Contents

Epidemiology and AIDS in Contraception

The World Health Organization Special Programme

Introduction

Reproductive Behavior and Family Planning

M. Potts

Family Health International Research Triangle Park, NC 27709, USA

Darwin published *The Origin of Species* in 1859. Today, anyone who accepts the facts of Darwinian evolution is also, by definition, a sociobiologist – in the sense that we must also accept that our reproductive behavior, like the anatomy of our gait or the neurophysiology of our retina, has been finely tuned by natural selection to perform in a certain way. We test drugs on baboons, have a common blood group with rhesus monkeys and almost certainly caught HIV infection from some other primate. We smile in greeting and touch one another for reassurance. What can biology tell us about human reproductive behavior and family planning?

Patterns of Fertility. Biologically, human beings have an exceptionally late age of puberty; they are non-seasonal breeders that separate pregnancies by anovulation associated with lactation, and ovulation, when it occurs, is not marked by any external signs or changes in behavior in the female. Both sexes consistently cover up their genitals and copulate in the quietest part of the daily cycle; adults share the same nest at night; and females have a very distinct menopause. In all these ways we are a very remarkable ape!

We are probably the slowest breeding vertebrate that evolution has produced, and it is a paradox that we have come to dominate the globe and threaten the biosphere through our numbers. Whereas when experimented animals are put in crowded conditions the age of puberty rises, pregnancy intervals lengthen and infant mortality rises, among human beings the opposite is happening. The age at onset of the menarche has fallen substantially in the past 100 years and seems to have been even higher in preliterate societies. Among the hunter-gatherers, such as the contemporary Kalahari !Kung, whose lifestyle characterized most of human history, the menarche occurred very late in life. Among some of the clans in the highlands of New Guinea, such as the Gainj, who did not see a white person until 1954, the mean age at the onset of menstruation is 20.9 years [1]. The later a woman begins to menstruate, the more anovulatory cycles she is likely to enjoy, and Gainj women on average do not have their first child until they are about 25 years old.

Teenage sexuality and pregnancy is an unnatural product of civilized living, and it demands artificial solutions. Our hunter-gatherer ancestors (Fig. 1) had a late menarche and four to five live-born children in a fertile lifetime – probably half of whom died before they reached puberty. Historical societies and contem-

Originally published in W. Eicher/G. Kockott (eds): Sexology, Springer 1988.

Female Contraception
Eds.: B. Runnebaum, T. Rabe, L. Kiesel

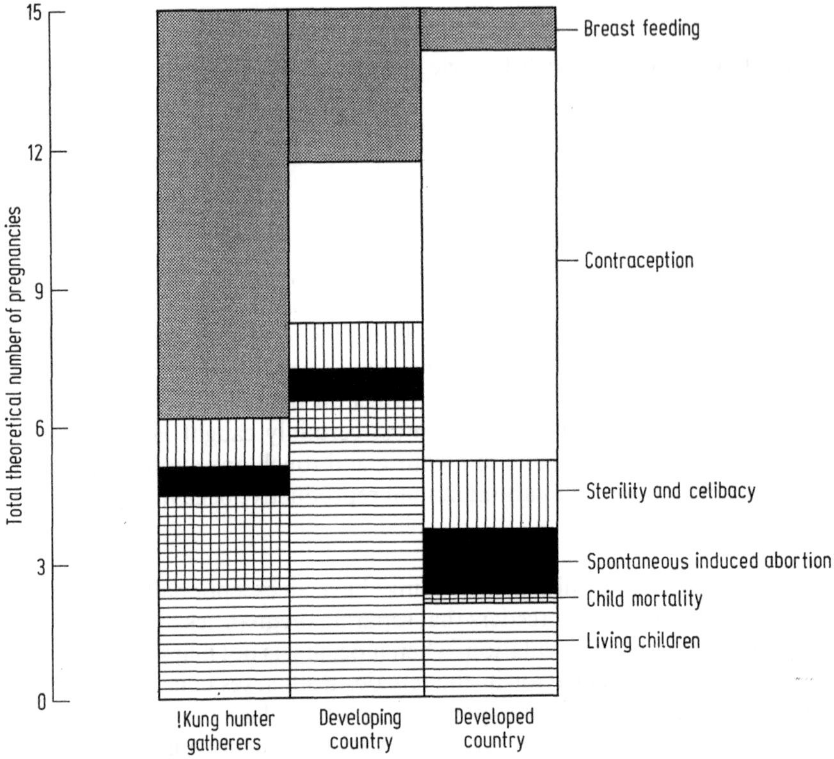

Fig. 1. Natural and artificial restraints on fertility. The figure assumes that in the absence of breast-feeding or any method of contraception a woman could have 15 pregnancies

porary agricultural and industrial societies have an earlier menarche and have abandoned or modified patterns of breast-feeding. If, like the Hutterites, one belongs to the modern world but rejects artificial contraception, one can expect on average to have ten or more live-born children in a lifetime. The problem is how to restore family size to the *natural* pattern of two children surviving into the next generation.

In contemporary developing countries, fertility is falling because the age of marriage has risen, and because the adoption of artificial contraception and abortion more than outweighs the fertility-enhancing effect of shorter intervals of breast-feeding (Fig. 2). The impact of lactation on pregnancy spacing depends on two factors. One is the duration of lactation and the other is the pattern of breast-feeding. There is a general relationship between the duration of breast-feeding and the duration of postpartum amenorrhoea. However, more detailed studies show that some patterns of breast-feeding appear to be more effective in suppressing ovulation than others. Again, to return to our hunter-gatherer ancestors, a !Kung woman breast-feeds her infant on average every 14 min [2]. Feeding on demand, the maintenance of the night feed and avoiding the artificially early introduction of supplementary food all prolong anovulation. In chimpanzees the birth

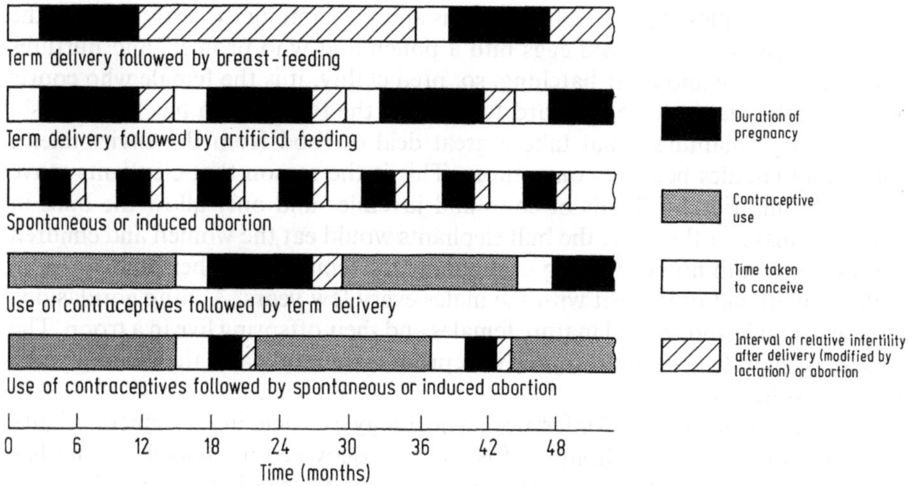

Fig. 2. Patterns of human reproduction

interval is 4.5–7.5 years [2]. Among the !Kung it averages 44 months. Chimpanzees do not use contraceptives and the !Kung have never seen a pill or condom.

Bottle-feeding is a *conceptive* human behavior, that is, it raises fertility. Those nations with the highest achieved fertility (e.g. 8 in Kenya) are using their reproductive systems much more intensively than nature intended.

Reproductive Strategies. Pregnancy and lactation demand a much greater investment from the female than sperm production and copulation takes from the male. In genuinely monogamous species the female, in order to adapt her to the strains of reproduction, is either the same size as the male, as in the marmoset monkey, or even larger than the male, as a blue whale or a beaver. In the struggle for existence the male, after all, is little more than a pair of testicles on legs. Among polygamous mammals, where males compete among themselves, as in the case of lions or elephant seals, the males are larger than the females. Biologically we are in indubitably polygamous species. One man, if sufficiently ruthless, can always father more children than one woman can bear in the same interval of time.

A culture may emphasize or negate biological differences, but I do not believe babies are a totally blank slate waiting for cultural messages to written upon them. We are dimorphic in our reproductive behavior, just as we are in our anatomy. As a woman puts such enormous physical and emotional effort into pregnancy, lactation and parenting to produce a single child, it is always in her interest to be sexually coy and to make a strong, lasting bond with one partner. Biology has given men two evolutionary strategies: they can invest in a close relationship with one woman and vastly increase the chances that her children will survive to pass on their father's genes, or, if the costs are low enough, a man can mate with any female, however worn out and hopeless, on the off-chance that he may father a child.

These principles apply to all viviparous animals: among the seahorses it is the *male* who takes the fertilized eggs into a pouch and who protects and nurtures the young before and after hatching, so, predictably, it is the female who courts the male, the male who plays hard to get, and the female who has the "penis". Among large mammals that take a great deal of food from the environment, males and females become competitors. This is the reason that elephants move around in matriarchal herds of cows and juveniles and only allow the bulls in briefly to mate – otherwise, the bull elephants would eat the women and children out of house and home. Among orangutans the females and their babies live in isolated pairs but only meet with the males every few years. Among gorillas one silverback male and several mature females and their offspring live in a troop. The female is the rate-limiting resource in reproductive terms and therefore sets the pace of evolution.

The 8th International Conference on Sexology was held in Heidelberg. Eighty years ago one of the first hominid fossils was discovered in Heidelberg and has now been assigned to the genus *Homo erectus* – a designation not based on our ancestors' sexual proclivities but on their posture. In reality since the female is the rate-limiting resource in reproductive terms, we really ought to speak about *Femina erecta* and *Femina sapiens*, and it is part of our blinkered approach to sex that there have been volumes of speculation about the brain size, tooth design, ability to walk upright and use of tools by our ancestors such as the owner of the Heidelberg jaw, while there has been little speculation about his or her reproductive behavior. What can we guess about Frau *Femina erecta heidelbergensis* is that she certainly menstruated; she had probably lost the vulval swellings that characterize ovulation in chimpanzees for the simple reason that she had already learned to walk upright on two legs. But did her breasts develop at puberty, as in *Homo sapiens*, or at the first pregnancy as in *Pan troglodytes*? She certainly breast-fed her infants for long intervals, but did she pair-bond with one male for some length of time? Did she gather tubers and share them with males who were beginning to specialize as hunters?

Chimpanzees, with whom we share 99% of our DNA, have an unusual social behavior where a number of related males defend a moderately large territory. Females mate promiscuously as they come into heat. Mothers and sons stay in the same troop throughout life, but at puberty females leave the troop of their birth and enter new troops. Sometimes the females are attacked by the older, more mature females in the troop [3]. We share much of this unusual pattern of social behavior. In most human societies the bride is "given away" by her family and enters her hunsband's troop, where quite often, like a young chimp, she may come into conflict with her mother-in-law. However, we do not regularly engage in chimpanzee-like "gang bangs", but establish defined polygamous, monogamous or serially monogamous sexual relationships. In the process we have acquired two biologically unique attributes – we share our food and the female conceals ovulation.

Although we are big animals that require a large range to supply our food, we can live in mixed-sex bands because men and women exploit somewhat different food supplies. Among the Kalahari bushpeople the women provide most of the family's calories from vegetable sources, and the men furnish most of the animal protein. Chimpanzees kill other monkeys and eat meat when a sort of tolerated scrounging may arise, but we are the only mammals that explicitly share food.

Ecologically, men and women are more like two different, partly non-competitive species, rather than like two sexes of the same species, eating the same type of food. Among the few other species to evolve the same tricks are certain hawks, which pair monogamously and where the male is smaller than the female and therefore more manoeuverable in flight and better adapted to prey on small birds then is the stockier female. In biological terms marriage is a compromise between the conflicting reproductive agendas of the two sexes, united by their complementarity in exploiting food supplies. A woman gives sex for love, a man gives love in order to obtain sex, and both give one another food. Different cultures at different times have promoted the sexual agenda of one sex at the expense of the other. What we see with homosexuality is each sex implementing its own biological drives without the need for compromise with the opposite sex. The "cruising" homosexual chooses his partners purely on physical grounds, often not knowing their names, seeking a high degree of eroticism and often having many sexual outlets in a single evening and persisting in this way of life for many years. Lesbian lovers tend to be consistently faithful over many years, to place companionship and human relations above erotic experience and to seek relatively infrequent sexual outlets [4].

Implications and Speculations. Biology does not tell us what to do, but it helps explain our behavior. As we cover up our genitals and usually copulate at night, one may predict that many human beings will be shy about acquiring contraceptives: for many people, it is easier to use a vending machine than to visit a family planning clinic.

As women naturally spend many years pregnant or lactating and for most of human prehistory rarely ovulated, we guess that methods which suppress menstruation will not necessarily make unpopular methods of contraception [5]. We

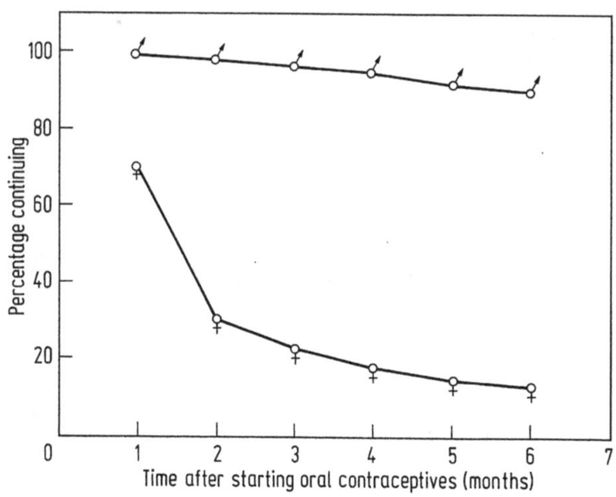

Fig. 3. Continuation rate for oral contraceptives distributed to Iranian women (♀) and to men (♂) to pass on to their wives (redrawn from Siassi 1972)

would expect the two sexes to have different attitudes towards contraception. In certain circumstances women will go to extreme lengths to postone or limit childbearing. However painful, however dangerous, however socially condemned, some women will always resort to abortion. Women accept sterilization more rapidly than men. It is, after all, only a fertility menopause without the hot flushes.

In Moslem culture Siassi (Fig. 3) has shown that if women are offered oral contraceptives, they have a high discontinuation rate whereas when the same method was given to men to pass on to their wives, more than 90% of women were still using the method after the first 6 months [6]. The change in the sociology of decision making is much greater than any alteration in acceptability brought about by differences in pharmacology or formulation. Men will accept vasectomy if it is offered in a male setting, but the rationale is probably different than for a woman's adoption of the operation. Deys has shown that role-dominant men commonly accept vasectomy before those who share their marital roles, and it may be that there is an element of male control over females in the way the operation is perceived [7]. Shanker has pointed out how Orthodox Jewish teaching forbids men to use condoms but permits women to use oral contraceptives and IUDs – a nice religious gloss on a biological drive!

Ultimately, male behavior evolved to pass as many genes as possible to the next generation, but in practice many aspects of both male and female behavior focus on proximate patterns of behavior. A biological model that attempts to explain the adoption of different methods of contraception, like a physiological or socioeconomic model, leaves many puzzles. Perhaps there are good reasons why this is so. We are a sexy animal programmed by evolution to use our sexuality in an infinite variety of ways in order to exploit many different types of environment. Biological determinism has made us, in large part, unpredictable. Perhaps the multivariant analyses so commonly performed to test hypotheses based on psychological or socioeconomic models of human behavior necessarily have their limitations.

Yet such a conclusion is not an empty one. Indeed, an evolutionary ability to be flexible in sexual behavior is exceptionally important. While it may be difficult to predict who will use an individual method of family planning, we can be certain that any one society needs the widest possible variety of birth control methods. Conversely, there is no "right" method of contraception. We may conclude that, when Japan forbids the pill, as indeed it does, or Egypt sterilization, or the USA fails to make IUDs available, they are each denying some couples, somewhere, of needed birth control choices.

Biology encourages us to look at reproduction over a lifetime rather than at a single menstrual cycle or at one pregnancy and its outcome. An early menarche, few children and little breast-feeding exposes the modern woman to numerous, repetitive menstrual cycles. This change, or some as yet unidentified part of it, carries in its train certain important pathologies: the more menstrual cycles a woman experiences, the greater her risk of ovarian cancer; uterine cancer also seems to follow a similar pattern. The later a woman bears her first child, the greater the risk of developing breast cancer [8] around and beyond the menopause (Fig. 4). The modern woman has an approximately 1 in 5000 lifetime risk of dying in childbirth, but a 1 in 11 risk of developing breast cancer and a 1 in 18 risk of dying

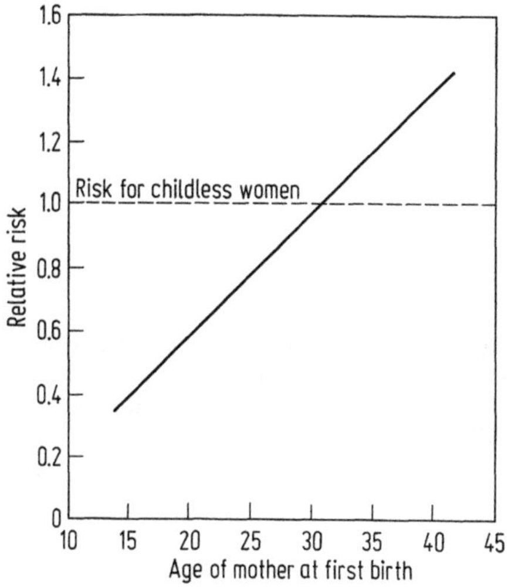

Fig. 4. Relative risk of developing cancer of the breast with age when first child born (after MacMahon et al. 1970)

of that difficult-to-treat malignancy. It seems we pay a very high price for deviating from reproductive behaviors bequeathed us by evolution.

In a fascinating way oral contraceptives partially reverse some of the adverse effects of modern living. The pill has been in human use for 30 years and is among the most intensively studied drugs in the pharmacopoeia. Indeed, there is so much information that it is difficult to put it together. A number of independent studies show that oral contraceptive use *reduces* the risk of dying of ovarian or endometrial cancers later in life. The longer a woman uses the pill the more marked the effect, and the effect persists after use – perhaps even a fertile lifetime – after discontinuing the pill. By contrast, the harmful effects of the pill on the cardiovascular system begin when a woman first takes the pill and end when she stops using it.

The problem is how to portray the risks and benefits of the pill in a single, grand, Einsteinian equation. One practical way is to ask what is the effect on the expectation of life if a woman uses the pill continuously for 5 years in a specified age group. Basically, the protective effects against cancer more than outweigh the adverse effects on the cardiovascular system. For a woman in the developing world, where the risks of pregnancy are greater, the beneficial effects are correspondingly larger (Fig. 5). Overall, both the risks and benefits of the pill are trivial in relation to other risks and benefits of life. Oral contraceptives increase the expectation of life by 12 days. The worst it can do to the expectation of life in older women is shorten life by 40–80 days. Smoking one packet of cigarettes a day decreases the users' expectation of life by an average of 4.6 years. (I stand by my aphorism of many years ago that cigarettes should be on prescription and pills in vending machines!) In a way, it is curious that the pill does not have an effect on breast cancer – neither a positive nor a negative one. One of the prime targets to research in the next decade should be how to tease out whether it is possible to formulate a combination of artificial steroids which reduces the risks of breast cancer in the same ways that they do endometrial and ovarian cancers.

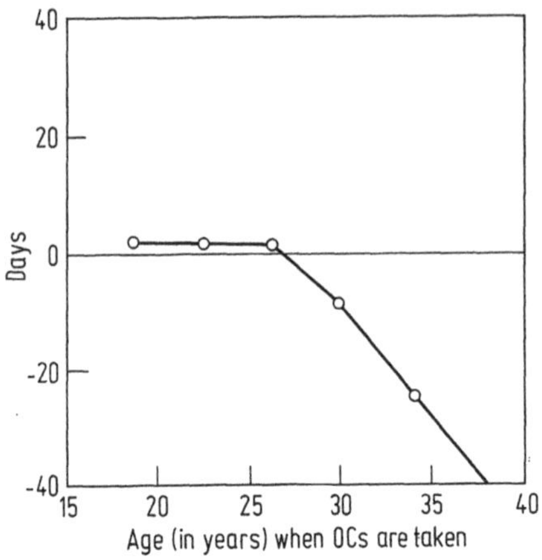

Fig. 5. Change in life expectancy attributable to 5 years of oral contraception in women aged 20–40 years, United States, 1978

It is not that the pill is a philosopher's stone which magically extends human life, but merely that it takes a woman one step nearer to the pattern which evolution intended her reproductive system to experience. Perhaps it should be a dream for the 21st century to so manipulate the dose and formulation of artificial steroids that they not only prevent pregnancy and reduce the risk of ovarian and endometrial cancers but also, eventually, reduce the risk of breast cancer.

Ethics. If biology tells us a little about contraceptive choices and throws up at least one startling clinical perspective, it also challenges us ethically.

Wet-nursing is surely a greater departure from nature than coitus interruptus – yet St. Augustine condemned the latter while taking the part of the former [9, 10]. To a biologist, a rubber nipple on a glass feeding bottle is more offensive than a rubber condom on an erect penis – one is a latex contraceptive and the other a lactose conceptive; while adults may consent to the use of contraception, infants have no choice as to what is put in their mouths.

In some parts of the world bottle-fed babies have up to 8 times the risk of infant mortality as those that are breast-fed. Somewhere in the world, one woman per minute dies in childbirth; 99% of these deaths takes place in the developing world, and half or more involve women who are either over 30 and/or have three or more children – the very groups who would plan their families were contraceptives more fully available. Infant mortality is 50% higher if the birth takes place within 1 year of a previous delivery rather than after a birth interval of 3–4 years [11]. In short, contraceptives save lives.

Ethics relates to the decisions we must take as our technology carries us further and further from the hunter-gatherer lifestyle in which we evolved. Biology cannot tell us how we ought to behave in the modern world, but it does provide an ethically relevant perspective. We come from a primate line that manifestly copulates for social reasons as well as for reasons of fertilization. Women are unique in that (a) they conceal ovulation and (b) accept the male at any time during the monthly cycle as well as during pregnancy and lactation. Natural family planning – while a valid and useful method of birth control – philosophically is an attempt to turn back the evolutionary clock and make evolution visible once again; it is an attempt to make women into chimpanzees. *Humanae Vitae* argues that every act of intercourse must be open to the possibility of procreation, which, to a biologist, must appear as an effort to turn women into rabbits.

Civilization has destroyed natural restraints on fertility. It has burdened women with a pandemic of reproductive cancers. We cannot return to a world where the menarche comes at 20 – would that we could – or where women breast-feed their babies four times an hour. But by looking at where we have come from we can ask sensible questions about where we want to go in relation to social behavior, family life, clinical care and all-important problems of ethics.

References

1. Wood JW, Lai D, Johnson PL, Campbewll KL, Maslar A (1985) Lactation and birth spacing in highland New Guinea. Breastfeeding and fertility. J Biosoc Sci [Suppl 9]:159–173
2. Konner M, Worthman C (1980) Nursing frequency, gonadal function and birth spacing among !Kung hunter-gatherers. Science 207:788
3. Jolly A (1985) The evolution of primate behavior. MacMillan, New York
4. Symonds D (1979) The evolution of human sexuality. Oxford, University Press, New York
5. Loudon NB, Foxwell M, Potts DM, Guild AL, Short RV (1977) Acceptability of an oral contraceptive that reduces the frequency of menstruation: the tri-cycle pill regimen. Br Med J [Clin Res] 2:487
6. Siassi I (1972) The psychiatrist's role in family planning. Am J Psychiatry 129:48–53
7. Deys CV, Potts DM (1972) Condoms and things. Adv Biosci 10:287–297
8. MacMahon B, Cole P, Lin TM, Lowe CR, Mirra AP, Ravhihar B, Salber EJ, Valaoras VG, Yuasa S (1970) Age at first birth and risk of breast cancer. WHO Bull 43:209–221
9. Noonan JT (1967) Contraception: a history of its treatment by catholic theologians and canonists. Harvard University Press, Cambridge, Massachusetts
10. Potts DM (1972) Coitus interruptus. In: Clinical proc. of the First International Planned Parenthood Federation S.E. Asia and Oceania Regional Medical and Scientific Congress. Aust N Z J Obstet Gynaegol 241–299
11. Thapa S, Short RV, Potts DM (1987) Breast-feedings, birth spacing and child survival. Family Health International, RTP, NC, USA (unpublished manuscript)

Trends in Contraception and Contraceptive Research

P. A. van Keep and H. Rekers
Organon International B.V., Kloosterstraat 6, 5340 BH Oss, The Netherlands

The years around 1960 were without doubt the most important in the history of contraception. These years brought us the discovery of the contraceptive pill and the re-discovery of the IUD. These two methods of contraception – both extremely reliable – have changed our world profoundly. Their availability may not have *caused* social changes, but it has at least allowed social changes to occur. They have changed the sexual behaviour of our generation and will probably have a similar influence on that of generations to come. A short history of these two methods of contraception may be useful.

Contraceptive Pill

It was in 1955 – now 32 years ago – that Pincus presented at the congress of the International Planned Parenthood Federation in Tokyo his paper on the effects of oral progestogens on ovarian function in women. According to the chairman of that session, Zuckermann, interviewed several years later, the audience was interested but clearly not aware of the historical significance of that moment. Only a posteriori was this moment seen to be the birth of the pill.

Today some 60 million women worldwide rely on the pill for their contraception. While an impressive figure, this must be seen against the total number of women in the world of fertile age (15–45 years of age): 1000 million. Against this backdrop the figure of 60 million looks less impressive.

Yet it all looked so simple in those early days of the pill. The pill was effective and induced regular cycles, both clear advantages over existing methods of contraception. The pill was easy to take, was hygienic and did not require touching one's genitals. There was no relation between taking the pill and the sex act. The daily ingestion of a small pill was an amulet against the consequences of intercourse. Side effects were minor and transient, and concern for health and future fertility hardly played a role. It is therefore surprising that it took so long for the pill to become as accepted as it now is. It took more than 25 years, thousands of studies, numerous campaigns, lectures and media coverage explaining the relative safety of oral contraception to reach the present degree of acceptance of the pill. It is a horrible thought that all these efforts could be made worthless by the publication of a single scare story and its subsequent waves of publicity in the lay press.

Originally published in W. Eichler/G. Kockott (eds.): Sexology, Springer 1988.

Female Contraception
Eds.: B. Runnebaum, T. Rabe, L. Kiesel

The curves showing acceptance of pill use in various countries are largely explained by such scare stories and their resulting publicity. Many such events have remained limited to one country or a group of countries sharing a language. Others, however, have had a global impact; these events have names comparable to those of battles in a world war. The 1967 papal encyclical *Humanae Vitae* had a global impact. So, too, did the Scowen Committee report in the United Kingdom in 1969, showing that pills with more than 50 μg estrogen were associated with a higher incidence of thromboembolism. The 1970 Nelson hearings in the United States on oral contraception led to a (fortunately) short-lived but massive abandonment of this method of contraception (and even to abandonment of all forms of contraception), leading to a sudden peak in birth statistics known as the "Nelson babies." The interim report of the Royal College of General Practitioners in 1977 expounded the cardiovascular risks of pill use, particularly in women over 35 years of age and in women who smoke. And the Pike Study in 1983 claimed an increased risk of mammary carcinoma in women who had used the pill before their first full-term pregnancy.

All these events have left troughs in the curves of pill use. In retrospect some of these events had little influence, such as *Humanae Vitae*, others were unjustified, such as the Nelson hearings, and others were only misleading, such as the Pike Study. Some events have been blessings in disguise because, although they temporarily hampered the acceptance of this form of contraception, they triggered developments which resulted in safer oral contraceptives. Two examples illustrate this. The Scowen report in 1969 caused the search for oral contraceptives with a lower estrogen content; first 50 μg, then 30 μg and now even 20 μg. This development has drastically lowered the incidence of thromboembolic disease in pill users. The report of the Royal College of GPs in the United Kingdom has also had interesting consequences. This triggered the search for pills with less progesterone, sometimes through ingenious dosage schemes such as the triphasics. These do indeed contain small quantities of hormones and consequently cause only minimal metabolic disturbances, but they are more complicated to take and may be less effective in suppressing ovarian activity. This report also triggered the search for better progestogens – not necessarily more potent but with an improved hormonal profile; these should have less affinity to androgen receptors in relation to their affinity to progesterone receptors. As a consequence they should have less effects on metabolism or even, in combination with an estrogen, have beneficial effects on metabolic parameters.

This then lead to the development of the so-called third-generation oral contraceptives. The first-generation progestogens were developed in the late 1950s and, with the exception of norethisterone and the structurally related lynestrenol, these disappeared when the second-generation progestogen, levonorgestrel, was introduced. This progestogen could be used in pills in a quantity of micrograms instead of milligrams. The third-generation progestogens, used in the third-generation oral contraceptives, came into use in the 1980s. The first introduced of this generation was Marvelon in 1981 by Organon, based on the progestogen, desogestrel; the second was Cilest, introduced in 1986 by Ortho-Cilag and based on norgestimate; and the third was Femovan, introduced in 1987 by Schering and based on gestoden. Although relatively little experience has been gained with the latter two, it seems that all three share one important quality: minimal impairment of the body's metabolism, in particular the lipid metabolism, and, by extrapolation, a virtual absence of cardiovascular risk.

This third-generation set of contraceptive pills is the result of many years of time- and money-consuming research, and only few companies are still willing to risk their research funds in research for new contraceptives, in particular medicamentous approaches. Consequently the development of new forms of contraception will by no means be as dramatic as that which we have observed in the past, in particular during the years 1957–1967. On the other hand, however, the third generation of pills is virtually perfect. We may predict the development of slightly different dosage schemes and, again, phasic preparations, but otherwise not much is likely to change in the field of oral contraception in the next decade. The third-generation oral contraceptives will be with us for the rest of this century.

Intrauterine Devices

The history of the intrauterine device (IUD) is infinitely longer than that of the pill. There are stories from ancient times of camels with a pebble in their uterus to prevent impregnation. Many more such stories also exist; they all have in common that they are difficult to substantiate. Modern IUD history begins in 1930 with von Gräfenberg, who inserted a ring into the uterus of women to obtain a contraceptive effect. His ideas were met with great enthusiasm until a few years later when they were (as he himself almost was) crushed by opponents inspired more by the political arguments of the Third Reich than by scientific arguments. Ohta, the Japanese investigator who developed a comparable device, suffered a similar fate. The IUD seemed to have been effectively killed. However, after World War II the notion of the IUD was still alive. A few enthusiasts used their own devices, but in 1962 – 7 years after the death of von Gräfenberg in New York City – the IUD was formally rehabilitated, now in the form of a plastic device. Since then many developments have taken place. Several different shapes were developed, as were long-acting medicated devices, treated with copper, copper and silver, or hormones. Optimal timing for insertion was also defined. We learned to determine indications and contra-indications for the safe and effective use of IUDs, and we learned how to identify serious complications, and how to prevent or minimize these.

Present-day IUDs are effective (and cost-effective) means of contraception. Yet they are denied to large portion of the world's population for a strange reason. Diczfalusy recently wrote, "Could Konrad Lorenz rewrite his book 'The eight mortal sins of civilized mankind' today, I am convinced that he would change the title from 8 to 9 mortal sins, in order to include: liability suits, American style." The excessive, even outrageous, claims that IUD manufacturers in the United States have had to fight has discouraged all but one company there from continuing sales of IUDs. As a consequence, Potts has observed that "an American woman, who cannot, for whatever reason use other forms of contraception than the IUD, has only two options: she can either enter into a convent or move across the border." One can only hope that the consequences of this development in the United States will not affect the availability of IUDs in the rest of the world.

What will be the future of IUD technology? New shapes, adaptable to the space that the uterine cavity has to offer? New medicated IUDs with antifertility compounds – spermatotoxic or embryotoxic? IUDs with antiseptic properties? IUDs with a progestogen are already in use, but these have not solved the problem of spotting and menorrhagia. Yet these are major problems of intrauterine contraception. Spotting is disquieting and embarrassing for many women, and menorrhagia and metrorrhagia decrease body iron stores, a health hazard particularly in developing countries. Will there be frameless, tailless but medicated IUDs anchored to the uterine wall? Or is the future, as Thiery proposed, for intracervical devices?

Time does not permit giving a similar review of other forms of contraception, quantitatively less important than the pill and the IUD but nevertheless essential in the 'contraceptive mix' that can be offered to today's couple asking for help. These include: (a) sterilisation, permanent or temporary; (b) natural family planning methods; (c) barrier methods, chemical or mechanical; (d) post-coital contraception; and (e) post-conception methods. These do have their place at present and will undergo developments in the future. We will return to this below.

Research in Contraception

Only few companies are still actively engaged in research in this field: three in Europe, one in the United States and none in Japan. The reasons for this are easy to understand. The financial commitment is enormous, and the chances of success are limited.

Djerassi wondered many years ago why governments participate financially in the development of new aircrafts but refuse to support the development of new contraceptives. The sums involved are comparable, but the impact of a new form of contraception on the future of mankind might be far greater than the impact of a new airplane, even if it is supersonic or able to transport 600 instead of 300 passengers.

It is industry – the pharmaceutical industry – which must decide whether it wants to risk its investments in this area. There is certainly a need for new approaches to contraception. There are leads which suggest that it is feasible to develop new approaches, and it may be economically attractive to do so. However, contraception – or, more precisely, the use of contraceptives – is certainly determined by developments in society, and it is these developments that will determine which forms of contraception will be acceptable or needed in the next decades. How will the fear of AIDS influence contraceptive needs? How will political and religious attitudes toward contraception and abortion develop? Regarding the latter question, for example, most present-day steroid-based contraception is aimed at the inhibition of ovulation. For most people this is ethically acceptable, but from a medical point of view it may be better to interfere later in the process of fertilization, for example just before or at the moment of nidation. Will this be acceptable for large groups of the population 10 or 15 years from now?

The United States Office of Technology Assessment published in 1982 a list of contraceptive technologies for the future. It may be an interesting exercise briefly to review this list now in 1987, only 5 years later. Those developments considered highly likely by 1990 include the following:

1. *Safer oral contraception.* This was not difficult to predict because the first of the third-generation progestogens (as discussed above) was introduced in 1981; this was desogestrel-based. Others followed in 1986 (norgestimate-based) and in 1987 (gestodene-based).
2. *Improved IUDs.* This was also easy to predict (see above).
3. *Improved barrier contraceptives for women.* Recent years have brought the sponge, now well accepted in some countries but not in others. The sponge is still based on the well-known spermicide nonoxynol-9. There are, however, more interesting spermicides available for study. The reasons why developments here have not been faster are, we think, to be found in the limited commercial attractiveness of this form of contraception and the problems in providing evidence for safety and effectiveness.
4. *Improved long-acting steroid injections.* We know of no major effort in this area. Of course, it is possible to develop a delivery system for such injections, but the dispute around the injection of medroxyprogesterone acetate (DMPA) will have had a discouraging effect on anyone who wants to develop such a contraceptive.
5. *Improved ovulation-detection methods for use with periodic abstinence.* Several devices have been developed, but their impact on the contraceptive scene remains limited. Such detection systems would narrow the period during which contraception is needed. Mechanical forms are being developed, but their acceptance is poor.
6. *Steroid implants.* These exist already, but they are certainly still open to improvement. Current research is aimed at easier application and at the use of third-generation progestogens.
7. *Vaginal rings.* This was also easy to predict in 1982. Rings are being developed to release both an estrogen and a progestogen. One may question, however, whether these will be available by 1990.
8. *Luteinizing hormone-releasing factor (LRF) analog contraceptives for women.* No practical applications are in sight.
9. *Prostaglandin analogues for self-administered induction of menses.* This idea has virtually disappeared from view.

Let us now look at the developments that were regarded as possible by 1990 but prospects of which were regarded as doubtful. As far as one can now see, none of these will be with us 1990. Only a few leads may find practical applications by the year 2000.

- *Vaccine against pregnancy.* There are two different approaches to this, a passive immunization, which gives protection for a number of months, and an active immunization, which will lead to life-long sterility.
- *Male contraception.* There are at present some 120 publications on efforts to use steroids for male contraception, involving a total of some 1100 men. Leads exist, but it requires optimism to believe that any practical application will be available before the next century.

– *Gossypol.* This Chinese approach to male contraception has been a major disappointment. Gossypol was probably the first chemical entity to be tried extensively in humans *before* it was tested in animals. It proved to be toxic for animals, and further research is far from promising.

We cannot comment here on a number of surgical techniques because in this area developments take place along different routes. It seems to us, however, unlikely that developments in this direction will have a significant impact on the worldwide contraceptive landscape in the near future.

The third part of the table produced by the Office of Technology Assessment in 1982 is now – only 5 years later – already completely unrealistic.

Contraception in 2001

In late 1986 we tried with a group of experts to fantasize about potential approaches to contraception in the distant future, taking the year 2001 after Clark's book, *2001 – A Space Odyssee*, as a metaphor for such a technological future. It proved difficult to detach ourselves from today's knowledge, and we produced hardly any ideas beyond an extrapolation of the approaches in vogue today.

One list of requirements for a contraceptive in the next century which is worth presenting stems from Klopper of Aberdeen. Among others, this list makes the following points: (a) The contraceptive must be constantly active, to be switched *off* rather than *on*; in other words, one must *do* something to be fecundable. (b) It must be under female control; this does not mean that the woman should *use* the method, although she is in control of it. (c)It should act before, rather than after, the beginning of pregnancy. For Klopper this latter point meant that the intervention should be just before or at nidation. Others have disagreed vehemently and insisted on interference before conception. This again confirms our earlier point: the type of contraception used in the next century will be determined by the norms and values of society itself at that time. The needs of society will determine the norms and values and hence developments in this field.

At this same meeting, Zeilmaker, an expert on in vitro fertilization presented an interesting option. The ovaries of a girl of 17 or so could be stimulated by gonadotrophins during one or two cycles until 7–10 egg cells can be harvested and then frozen; during harvesting she would be sterilized by closing both her tubes. Each time she wanted to be pregnant, she would present herself at her "egg bank" with a sperm sample of the man of her choice. A thawed egg cell would then be fertilized and implanted. All this could be done during her lunch break. She would never again need contraception.

One must be brave to live in that new world!

Side Effects of Oral Contraceptives

Analysis of Oral Contraceptive Risks

S. Roy [1], L. Bernstein [2] and F. Z. Stanczyk [1]

Departments of [1] Obstetrics and Gynecology and [2] Preventive Medicine, University of Southern California School of Medicine, Los Angeles, California, USA

Introduction

The important concern regarding cancer and pill use will be initially addressed with a special review of some of the important studies, focusing on their strengths and weaknesses, and suggesting that new concepts regarding pill use as, for example, "unmasking" rather than "inducing" certain cancers may be evolving. The formulation of the oral contraceptive has an important bearing on the production of metabolic effects; therefore, some observations about the composition, structure-function relationships, pharmacokinetic properties in terms of absorption, bioavailability, metabolism, and potency of the individual constituents of the currently and soon to be available pills will be made. A selected review will be presented of the clinical effects of reducing dosage and changing schedules (monophasic versus phasic), their corresponding metabolic effects on various important systems (notably, the cardiovascular system), the importance of smoking as a confounder in the analysis of data regarding cervical cancer, cardiovascular disease, and infertility, and the growing concern regarding the interaction with sexually transmitted diseases leading to cancer or to infertility.

Oral Contraceptives and the Risk of Cancer

Because of the increasing popularity of oral contraceptives as a birth control method assessment of the possible relationship between oral contraceptive use and cancer continues to be of great public health importance. There is now a substantial body of literature on the relationship between oral contraceptive use and cancers of the endometrium, ovary, breast, and cervix. Recently there have also been reports of a relationship between oral contraceptive use and cancer of the liver.

In examining the results of the epidemiologic studies presented here the following factors are considered: latent period, temporal changes in pill formulation, time of exposure (both in terms of the woman's age and in terms of her reproductive history), a woman's baseline risk for the particular cancer, and differences in study design.

The period of time between first exposure to a carcinogen and the development of overt malignant disease (the latent period) is generally long and is considered to be in the order of 15–30 years. In addition to time since first exposure, exposure intensity and exposure duration are important factors. Since widespread

Female Contraception
Eds.: B. Runnebaum, T. Rabe, L. Kiesel

use of oral contraceptives began in the middle 1960s (little more than 20 years ago), results of some epidemiologic studies may be premature, as few women will have had both prolonged exposure and extended follow-up. Rates of acceptance of oral contraceptives as a birth control method have varied geographically and by subgroups of women, so that these factors must be considered in the critical evaluation of epidemiologic studies of cancer risks. Early effects will be apparent, however, if oral contraceptives alter the rate of growth of occult tumors or act as late-stage carcinogens, promoting change from the premalignant to the malignant state.

There have been marked changes in pill composition over time. Sequential oral contraceptives were removed from sale in the United States in 1976. Also during the 1970s there was a shift to the use of combination formulations with lower steroidal content, and this trend has continued. The most recent data on prescription sales in the United States indicate that, as of March 1987, pills with less than 50 μg estrogen (including multiphasics) make up 78.6% of the market share, with 50-μg products comprising 19% of the market [1]. Only 2.4% of the prescriptions currently filled are for oral contraceptives with more than 50 μg of estrogen. Multiphasic pills continue to grow in popularity, as they now comprise 32% of all prescriptions in the United States [1]. There have been similar reductions in the progestogen content of the most popular pills. Because multiphasic preparations are so new, it is too early to assess the effects of these formulations on cancer risk.

Exposure to contraceptive steroids at particular ages or reproductive times of life, such as during adolescence, prior to first pregnancy, or in the perimenopausal period may be especially important. Initially the majority of oral contraceptive users were married women who used this method of contraception for spacing births after the first full-term pregnancy. The results of studies on cancer risk in such women will not be relevant to women who begin oral contraceptive use during adolescence. Age at first use has declined substantially, and oral contraceptives are now the contraceptive method of choice for sexually active teenage girls [2, 3].

Some women are at higher risk for a particular cancer than others. It is possible that oral contraceptives may have no effect on cancer risk for the general population of women but may have a striking effect on the risk in women with certain predisposing factors. As an example, for breast cancer women with a high risk would be those with a positive family history of breast cancer or those with a history of benign disease [4].

In addition to the timing of the study in relation to the availability of and prolonged use of different preparations, the study design, methods of data collection, and relevant characteristics of study subjects are important. Results are evaluated for both cohort studies and case-control studies. In either, the study population must be considered in drawing generalizations from study results. Furthermore, since these studies are all observational, potential sources of bias must be considered before interpreting the results.

Endometrial Cancer

After the association of prolonged use of estrogen-replacement therapy and endometrial cancer was established, case-series reports suggested a similar association between sequential oral contraceptives and endometrial cancer [5]. That sequential preparations have this effect is not surprising since they administer a constant, relatively high dose of estrogen without progestogen for the first 3 weeks of the cycle, followed by 5–6 days of estrogen with progestogen. Three of four case-control studies with data on the use of sequential oral contraceptives show a 2-fold increased risk for use of these preparations [6–8]. The one negative case-control study had only two cases who had ever used sequential preparations [9].

In contrast to the adverse effects on the endometrium of sequential oral contraceptives, use of combination oral contraceptives has been reported consistently in case-control studies to decrease the risk of endometrial cancer by about 50% (Table 1). The Walnut Creek Contraceptive Drug Study [12], a prospective cohort study, has demonstrated a similar decrease in risk. This protective effect of combination oral contraceptives is biologically plausible since the presence of the progestogen throughout the cycle reduces endometrial mitotic activity and causes differentiation of the endometrial cells to a secretory state.

In the large CASH study (Cancer and Steroid Hormone Study sponsored by the Centers for Disease Control and the National Institute of Child Health and Human Development) [6] there was no apparent difference in risk for use of oral contraceptives over short periods of time (<5 years) compared to longer use, although the most recent report [13] shows that very short term users (<1 year) are not so protected. Henderson et al. [7] observed a clear decrease in risk with increasing duration of use. In this study the relative risk for 5 or more years of use was 0.1. Certain subgroups of women were not protected, including those who were obese or of high parity (at least three live births).

Whether the protective effect persists with increasing duration of time since last use is an important question, and study results are mixed (Table 1). The CASH study [13] has found that the protective effect of pill use persisted for women who discontinued using oral contraceptives 15 years prior to participation in the study.

Table 1. Case-control studies of combination oral contraceptives and endometrial cancer

Reference	Age range	Relative risk	Number of cases using oral contraceptives	Length of protection after last use
Weiss and Sayvetz [8]	35–54	0.5	17	1–2 years
Kaufman et al. [9]	To 59	0.5	16	At least 5 years
Kelsey et al. [10]	45–74	0.6	6	Not stated
Hulka et al. [11]	To 59	0.4	5	Effect wanes
Centers for disease control (CASH) [6, 13]	20–54	0.6	70	At least 15 years
Henderson et al. [7]	To 45	0.5	43	Not stated

Table 2. Case-control studies of oral contraceptives and epithelial carcinoma of the ovary

Reference	Age range	Relative risk	Number of cases using oral contraceptives	Length of protection after last use
Newhouse et al. [14]	All ages	0.6	19	Not stated
McGowan et al. [15]	Mean, 52	0.7	Not stated	No data
Casagrande et al. [16]	25–49	0.8	41	Not stated
Hildreth et al. [17]	45–74	0.5	3	No data
Willett et al. [18]	30–55	0.8	13	Not stated
Franceschi et al. [19]	To 69	0.7	17	Not stated
Rosenberg et al. [20]	To 59	0.6	29	At least 10 years
Risch et al. [21]	34–75	0.4[a]	34	No data
Cramer et al. [22]	To 59	0.4	34	At least 10 years
Centers for disease control (CASH) [23]	20–54	0.6	90	At least 10 years

[a] Estimated.

Ovarian Cancer

More than ten case-control studies have examined the association between prior use of oral contraceptives and ovarian cancer (Table 2). Except for a small series of women in Utah reported by Risch et al. [21] all studies show a decreased risk among oral contraceptive users.

Because epithelial ovarian tumors are more common in less fertile women, this factor must be considered in interpreting results of studies, as it could lead to a spurious protective effect of pill use. Recent studies indicate that this is an unlikely explanation for the lower risk among oral contraceptive users. The risk of ovarian cancer clearly decreases with increasing duration of oral contraceptive use [16, 23], and the protection appears to be long-lasting. In the CASH study [23] women who first used oral contraceptives 10 or more years before participating in the study had about one-half the risk of nonusers (Table 2).

The risk of ovarian cancer is decreased by any pregnancy, whether complete or incomplete. Casagrande et al. [16] suggested that this protection as well as that provided by oral contraceptive use resulted from the suppression of ovulation. They combined periods of pregnancy and oral contraceptive use into a single measure of "protected time" in the analysis of their case-control study and demonstrated that risk of ovarian cancer decreased as protected time increased.

Breast Cancer

Numerous epidemiologic studies have examined the relationship between oral contraceptives and the risk of breast cancer. The majority of these were summarized by Kelsey and Hildreth [24]. Although results have now been published for seven cohort studies and 19 case-control studies, the possible relationship between oral contraceptive use and breast cancer continues to be a major source of

Table 3. Breast cancer risk and oral contraceptive use during the perimenopausal period

Reference	Type of study	Relative risk of current users compared to nonusers Age at Diagnosis	
		40–44	45–49
Vessey[a] et al. [28]	Case-control	0.7	1.5
Jick et al. [29]	Case-control within cohort	0.8	4.0
RCGP[b] [30]	Cohort	1.1	1.7
Brinton et al. [31]	Case-control within cohort	1.1	1.3
Lipnick[c] et al. [32]	Cohort	1.8	1.7

[a] For Vessey's study, age groups are 41–45, 46–50.
[b] Royal College of General Practitioners; study presents data for upper age group as 45+.
[c] Risk estimates presented for women who were current users in 1976.

controversy [25–27]. A number of the studies were begun in the late 1960s, less than 8 years after oral contraceptives became available for clinical use. Unlike the consistent protective effects of combination oral contraceptives on the risk of endometrial and ovarian cancer, there is no clear trend across studies for breast cancer.

Overall, breast cancer studies have provided no strong evidence that oral contraceptives either increase or decrease breast cancer risk when used during the middle reproductive years. However, use at two particular times during the reproductive years, the postmenarcheal period and the perimenopausal period, may substantially increase risk. Five studies have reported an elevated risk of breast cancer with use of oral contraceptives around the time of menopause [28–32], although the range of risk estimates is wide (Table 3). A probable explanation for this increased risk is that oral contraceptives produce a hormonal state approximating that of a normally menstruating woman, masking the onset of menopause by artificially prolonging menstrual life. The net effect of such use would be greater hormonal exposure to estrogens and progestogens than would have occurred naturally during the perimenopausal period.

The second group of oral contraceptive users who may be at increased risk of breast cancer are those women who use oral contraceptives for long periods of time early in menstrual life, particularly before their first full-term pregnancy. Because prolonged use by very young women is a recent phenomenon, only the most recently conducted studies would be able to measure such an effect. We review here the results of seven major case-control studies [4, 33–44] which have either examined specifically the breast cancer risk associated with early oral contraceptive use in young women (under age 40), or which have provided subgroup results for young women. These studies have produced conflicting results.

The design aspects of each of these studies are summarized in Table 4, and relevant results for "negative" studies and for "positive studies" are presented in Tables 5 and 6, respectively. One possible explanation for the discrepant results is that these studies have differed on design factors. They vary in terms of case source (population-based versus hospital-based), control source (population-

Table 4. Design aspects of seven case-control studies of oral contraceptives and breast cancer

Study and reference	Dates of diagnoses	Number of young women (cases/ controls)	Source of cases/controls	Age matched	Type of interview
CASH [33, 34]	12/80–12/82	2088/2065 <age 45	Population-based/ random digit dial	No	Face-to-face
Drug Epidemiology Unit [35, 36]	3/76– 9/83	521– 521 <age 45	Hospital/hospital	Yes[a]	Face-to-face
London/Oxford Phases 1–4 [37]	12/68– 9/80	1176/1176 <age 50	Hospital/hospital	Yes	Face-to-face
Phase 5 [38]	10/80–12/83	127/ 127 <age 40	Hospital/hospital	Yes	Face-to-face
Los Angeles [4, 39]	1/72– 5/82	314/ 314 <age 37	Population-based/ neighborhood	Yes	Telephone
New Zealand [40]	6/83– 6/85	433/ 897 <age 35	Population-based/ electoral rolls	No	Telephone
Sweden [41]	5/84– 5/85	195/ 195 <age 40	Population-based/ population register	Yes	Face-to-face

[a] Subgroup analysis presented in reference 36 is age matched.

Table 5. "Negative" case-control studies of the relationship between oral contraceptive use and risk of breast cancer

Study and reference	Age range	Subgroup	Duration of use	Relative risk
Cash [34]	20–44	Use before FFTP[a]	1–12 months	1.3
			13–48 months	1.1
			49+ months	1.2
Drug Epidemiology Unit [36]	<45	Use before FFTP[a]	1–11 months	0.7
			1–2 years	1.4
			3–4 years	0.8
			5–6 years	1.5
			7+ years	1.4
London/Oxford Phases 1–4 [37]	16–50	All use	1–12 months	0.8
			13–48 months	0.8
			49–96 months	1.6
			97+ months	1.0
New Zealand [40]	25–34	Any use	1 month–2 years	2.8
			2–5 years	1.6
			6–9 years	1.8
			≧10 years	4.6
	35–44	Any use	1 month–2 years	0.9
			2–9 years	0.9
			≧10 years	0.8

[a] First full-term pregnancy.

Table 6. "Positive" case-control studies of the relationship between oral contraceptive use and risk of breast cancer

Study and reference	Age range	Subgroup	Duration of use	Relative risk
London/Oxford Phase 5 [38]	16–34	Use before FFTP[a]	1–12 months	1.2
			13–48 months	1.7
			49+ months	3.1
Los Angeles [39]	<37	Use before age 25	1–24 months	1.3
			25–48 months	1.7
			49–72 months	2.0
			73+ months	4.9
Sweden [41]	<40	Any use	1 month–3 years	0.9
			4–7 years	1.4
			8–11 years	2.2
			12+ years	2.1
		Use before FFTP[a]	1 month–3 years	0.9
			4–7 years	1.5
			8+ years	4.4

[a] First full-term pregnancy.

based versus hospital-based), matching criteria used in selecting controls (none versus age, socioeconomic status, parity) and method of interview (face-to-face versus telephone). Hospital-based studies, which use as controls patients with diseases and conditions thought not to be related to oral contraceptive use, may produce biased estimates of relative risk. A survey conducted in the United States during the early 1970s showed that oral contraceptive users were 20%–40% more likely to be hospitalized for non-life-threatening conditions than were nonusers [42]. This could result in underestimates of the true strength of the association between oral contraceptive use and breast cancer in such studies. The degree of age matching also has varied widely, from matching on individual year of birth [41] to not matching on age at all [33–35, 40]. Close matching on age is critical because cohort trends in oral contraceptive use before age 25 and before first full-term pregnancy have been reported [43]. Face-to-face interviews with subjects are preferable to telephone interviews because the use of photographs of oral contraceptives and a calendar facilitates accurate recall of dates, brands, and doses of oral contraceptive used.

The largest of the negative studies is the CASH study [33, 34]. Stadel et al. [34] reported results for women under age 45 in this study, showing no increased risk with use prior to first full-term pregnancy. The Boston University Drug Epidemiology Unit study [35, 36] is also considered negative, although there was a significantly increased risk of breast cancer among women aged 30–39 who had more than 5 years of oral contraceptive use which started or ended many years prior to diagnosis. The estimated relative risk for such use beginning at least 15 years earlier was 2.6; the estimated relative risk for use ending at least 10 years earlier was 5.0. The later analysis is of a subset of cases less than 45 years of age, with controls selected from the larger control group and matched to cases by age, year of interview, and geographic area. In this subgroup the relative risk of breast cancer with oral contraceptive use was 1.0 among all women and among nulliparous women. Although there was some increased risk among long-term users, none of these risk estimates was large or statistically significant.

Results have been reported for five phases of the London/Oxford study of breast cancer and oral contraceptive use, a study restricted to married women. These results are largely negative for the first four phases of the study [37], but a recent report for phase 5 [38] shows significantly increased breast cancer risk for more than 4 years use prior to first full-term pregnancy.

Recently Paul et al. [40] have reported results of a national population-based case-control study conducted in New Zealand. Analysis of risk by duration of use, age at first use, and time since first use showed no increased risk, although one subgroup of women aged 25–34 did show an elevated relative risk of 2.2 for any use of oral contraceptives. In this subgroup of women, however, there was a U-shaped effect in the dose-response curve, with highest risk estimates for women who used oral contraceptives less than 2 years (relative risk, 2.8) or 10 or more years (relative risk, 4.6).

In a case-control study of women under age 33 living in Los Angeles County, California, Pike et al. [4] reported that the risk of breast cancer increased with increasing duration of oral contraceptive use before the first full-term pregnancy; a relative risk of 3.5 was observed for 8 or more years of use compared with nonuse. Recently, Pike et al. [39] updated their ongoing case-control study to include 317 breast cancer cases under age 37. Cases used oral contraceptives for an average of 49 months compared to 39 months for the controls and a large part (60%) of this difference in average duration of use was for use before age 23. For oral contraceptive use before age 25 the relative risk was 2.5 for 4 or more years of use, and the trend of increasing risk with increasing duration of use was statistically highly significant.

Swedish investigators [41] who matched their cases and controls on exact year of age and exact age at first full-term pregnancy subsequently reported a significant trend of increasing breast cancer risk with total duration of use and use before first full-term pregnancy. As noted above, further evidence that early long-term oral contraceptive use may increase breast cancer risk is provided by the latest phase of the London/Oxford study [38].

Early studies of oral contraceptive use and breast cancer risk generally were unable to test the hypothesis that early long-term oral contraceptive use increases breast cancer risk because oral contraceptive use before first pregnancy was uncommon in the 1960s, and even these more recent studies may be premature. Many early studies considered only married women whose major reason for taking oral contraceptives was family spacing, and all phases of the London/Oxford study maintained this restriction. Furthermore, a period of 10–20 years after exposure to oral contraceptives may be necessary before exposure-related increases in breast cancer risk are detectable. Patterns of use of oral contraceptives have varied with time in different countries. Early use was more common in the United Kingdom between 1970 and 1975 than in most of the United States [44].

Because both timing of menarche and timing of first full-term pregnancy are critical risk factors for breast cancer, exposure during the years between these two events may also be critical for establishing breast cancer risk. The period immediately after onset of menses is characterized by frequent anovular cycles [45], and even when ovulatory cycles occur in adolescent girls they are characterized by significantly lower levels of estradiol and progesterone than are those of adult fertile women [46]. For both reasons oral contraceptive use during the postmenarcheal years may expose young women to higher levels of estrogens and progestogens than would have occurred naturally, altering their subsequent risk of breast cancer. Logically, this would occur if a woman's average breast tissue mitotic activity when on oral contraceptives is greater than her average "normal" mitotic activity and could be due to either the estrogen or the progestogen component of the compound. Using a similar line of reasoning (in other words, measuring the effect of oral contraceptive use relative to the woman's "normal" hormonal state), one might expect that the more recently introduced low-dose oral contraceptives may protect against breast cancer in regularly ovulating women (for example, those who are past their first full-term pregnancy and/or between the ages of 24 and 35).

Cervical Cancer

The relationship between oral contraceptives and cervical neoplasia has also received considerable attention [47–54]. As with breast cancer, the nature of an association is unclear. Studies of such an association must control for subjects' sexual behaviors (e.g., age at first sexual intercourse and number of sexual partners) because these are not only identified risk factors for cervical cancer but also may be associated with the use of oral contraceptives [50]. Barrier methods of contraception are protective against cervical neoplasia, and this complicates the analysis of risk associated with oral contraceptive use. Another factor which complicates the assessment of cervical cancer risk is that a number of studies have focused on preinvasive abnormalities which are prone to pathologic classification difficulties [55], and which may, in fact, be easier to detect among pill users [56]. The majority of early studies of the possible relationship between oral contraceptive use and cancer of the cervix dealt with preinvasive lesions, dysplasia, or carcinoma in situ and did not control for sexual behavior as well or other important sources of confounding [50].

Cohort data from the Oxford Family Planning Association Contraceptive Study [57, 58] show that the incidence of biopsy-proven cervical neoplasia during a 10 year follow-up period was significantly elevated in oral contraceptive users. All 13 cases of invasive cervical cancer identified in this cohort occurred in women who were oral contraceptive users; nine of these women had used oral contraceptives for more than 6 years.

The World Health Organization has been conducting a hospital-based case-control study on oral contraceptives and the risk of gynecological, breast, and hepatic cancers primarily in developing countries. The preliminary report on cervical cancer showed a relative risk of 1.2 for users of oral contraceptives that was of borderline statistical significance [59]. Risk increased with duration of use, with more than 5 years of use associated with a relative risk of 1.5. Statistical analyses adjusted for potential confounding factors of the cervical cancer-oral contraceptive relationship including age, center, number of pregnancies, age at first sexual intercourse, number of sexual partners, history of vaginal discharge, and history of Papanicolaou (PAP) screening. In this study, the majority of cases had diagnoses of squamous cell carcinoma; 8% had been diagnosed with adenocarcinomas.

Brinton et al. [60] recently reported a relative risk of 1.5 overall for the risk of invasive cervical cancer associated with oral contraceptive use. In this study long-term users (5 or more years) had a 2-fold higher risk than nonusers. The association held for both squamous-cell carcinoma and adenocarcinoma of the cervix. Statistical analyses adjusted for potential confounders including age, ethnic origin, number of sexual partners, age at first sexual intercourse, education, history of genital infection or sore, and interval since last PAP smear.

Peters et al. [61] recently completed a case-control study of invasive squamous-cell carcinoma of the cervix among Latina and non-Latina women in Los Angeles County, California, which provided no evidence of an effect of oral contraceptive use. Significant risk factors for squamous-cell cervical cancer in this study were years since last PAP smear, years of education (protective), years of douching, pack-years of smoking, years of barrier contraceptive use (protective), number of sexual partners before age 20, and recognized episodes of genital warts.

Analytic studies involving oral contraceptive use have focused almost entirely on squamous-cell malignancies (with the exception of Brinton et al. [60], noted above); but the influence of oral contraceptives may well be greater on adenocarcinomas which originate from estrogen-responsive glandular cells. An increasing incidence of adenocarcinoma of the cervix has been reported among women under 35 years of age in Los Angeles County [62]. Among older women incidence remained essentially constant over the same period. It was hypothesized that the use of oral contraceptives during the teenage years might account for this trend, as oral contraceptives produce morphologic changes in the endocervix, characterized by stromal edema, excessive mucus production and glandular hyperplasia [63]; the extent of these histologic changes increases as continuous use of the contraceptive agents increases [64].

Liver Tumors

A causal association between the use of oral contraceptives and benign liver tumors, variously described as adenomas or focul nodular hyperplasia, is well documented [65, 66]. Experimental animal studies have shown that oral contraceptives can cause hepatocellular carcinomas in mice and are effective promoters of hepatocarcinogenesis in diethylnitrosamine-primed rats [67].

At least ten case reports of hepatocellular carcinoma arising in women taking oral contraceptives have been published. Recently, Henderson et al. [68] reported 11 more cases of rare malignant liver tumors in young women. Ten of the cases had used oral contraceptives for periods ranging from 6 to 168 months; the other patient had received multiple "hormone" shots of undetermined type for regulation of menstrual periods during the 9 months preceding diagnosis. Six of the 11 patients were taking hormones at the time of diagnosis. The average duration of use in the 11 cases was 65 months compared to 27 months in age-matched neighborhood controls, a difference which is statistically highly significant.

Two recent British studies have also addressed this issue. In the first study [69] oral contraceptive use by a series of 26 women under age 50 diagnosed with hepatocellular carcinoma was compared to the use of controls from the London/Oxford breast cancer case-control study described earlier [37, 38]. In this study short-term use of oral contraceptives was not associated with increased liver cancer risk; however, use for 8 or more years was associated with a significantly elevated relative risk of 4.4. When the case group was restricted to women without markers of hepatitis B infection, the relative risk remained significantly elevated (relative risk, 7.2) in users with 8 or more years exposure. The second study, a case-control study of young women (aged 20–44) who died of cancer of the liver showed that use of oral contraceptives was associated with a significantly elevated relative risk of hepatocellular carcinoma of 3.8, and that use for 8 or more years was associated with a significantly increased relative risk of 20.1 [70]. There was no apparent increase in risk for cholangiocarcinoma associated with oral contraceptive use in this study.

Estrogens

Structure-Function Relationships

Structural modification of the estradiol molecule by insertion of an ethinyl group at C-17 results in the formation of ethinylestradiol, a very potent estrogen with high oral activity (Fig. 1). This compound is widely used as a component in oral contraception. Modification of ethinylestradiol by attachment of a methyl group to the hydroxyl group at C-3 gives rise to mestranol (Fig. 1). This estrogen has been widely used as a component in oral contraceptives but is now utilized less frequently. It has been shown that the estrogen effect of mestranol is due to the fact that it is demethylated very rapidly in the liver, forming ethinylestradiol [71, 72]. Mestranol itself is not able to bind to the estrogen receptor in target tissues, whereas ethinylestradiol is very competitive with other estrogens for this receptor [73, 74].

Pharmacokinetic Properties

Absorption and Bioavailability. Following oral ingestion of commercial tablets of ethinylestradiol there is rapid gastric absorption of the steroid, and peak levels are usually attained within 1 h [75]. Ethinylestradiol undergoes first-pass metabolism, and its bioavailability is between 43% and 48% [76].

After an oral dose of mestranol the drug is absorbed very rapidly and maximum plasma levels are usually attained within 1–2 h [77]. However, peak circu-

Ethinylestrogens

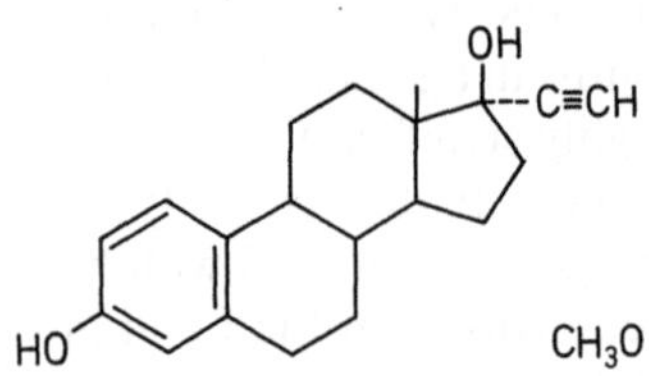

Ethinylestradiol

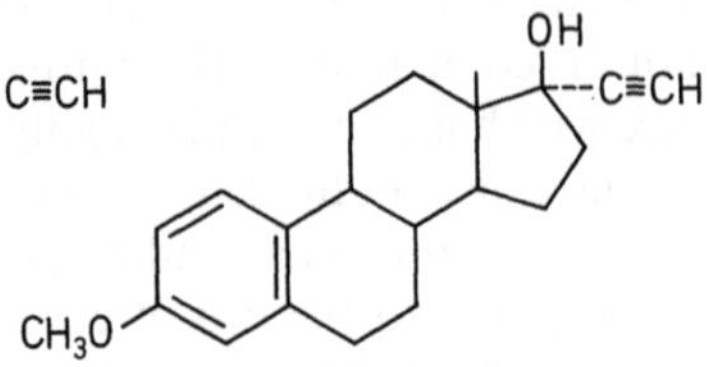

Mestranol

Progestogens structurally related to norethindrone

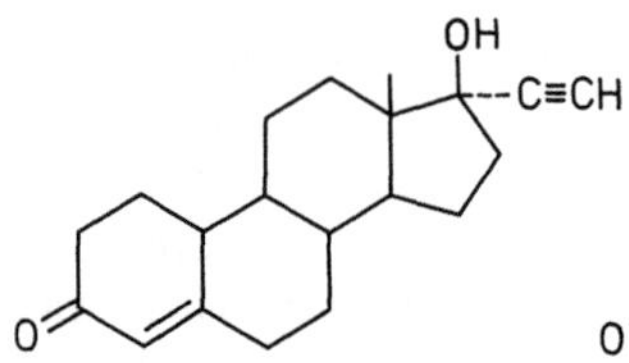

Norethindrone

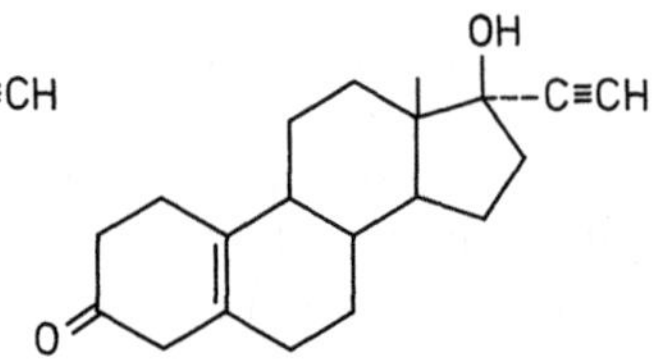

Norethynodrel

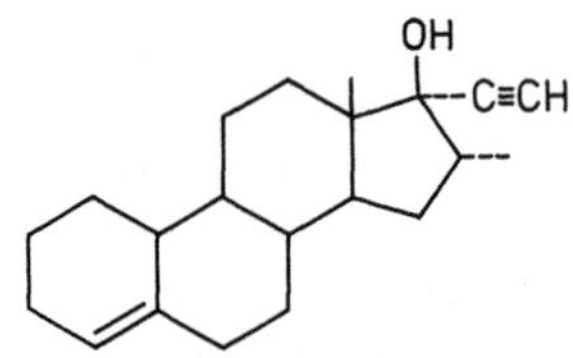

Lynestrenol

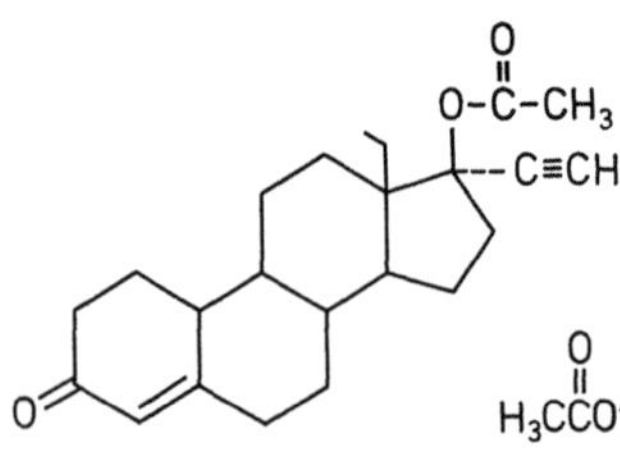

Norethindrone acetate

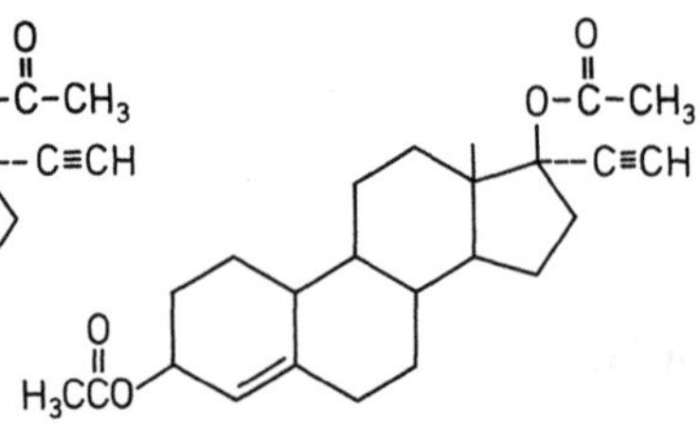

Ethynodiol diacetate

Progestogens structurally related to norgestrel

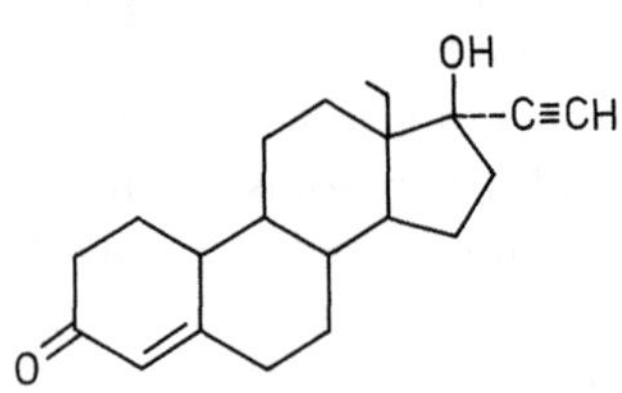

Norgestrel

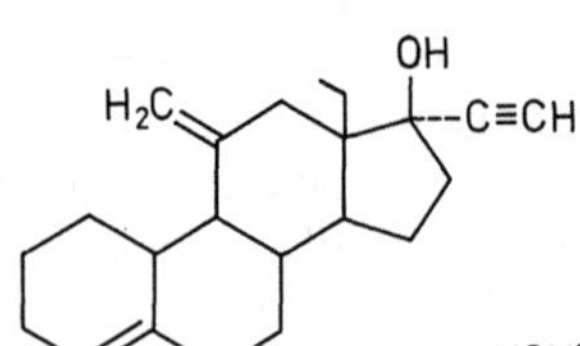

Desogestrel

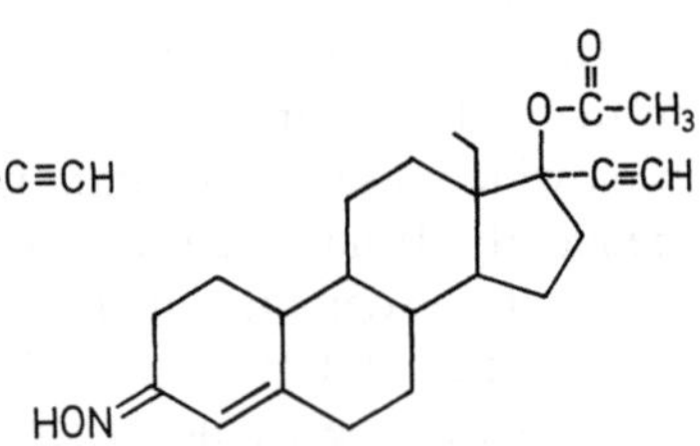

Norgestimate

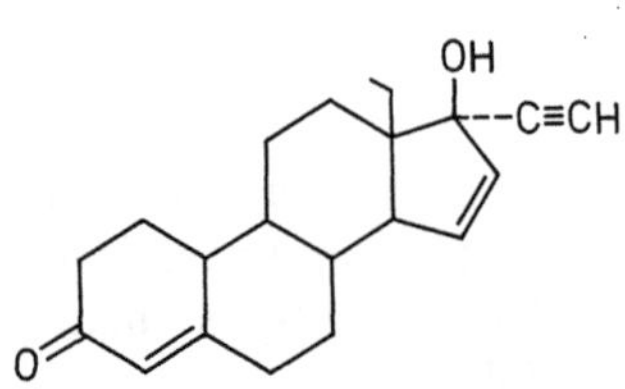

Gestodene

Fig. 1. Structures of some estrogens and progestogens

lating levels of ethinylestradiol are less and occur later following an oral dose of mestranol than after the same dose of ethinylestradiol [75, 78, 79]. This delay in peaking presumably reflects the fact that the circulating ethinylestradiol levels are dependent on the rate of demethylation of mestranol by the liver. The ratio of mestranol to ethinylestradiol in plasma was found to be 0.24 : 1 following the administration of ^{14}C-mestranol in women [80].

Metabolism. The metabolism of ethinylestradiol is similar to that of the natural estrogens [81–83]. Thus, ethinylestradiol undergoes extensive hydroxylation at the C-2, C-6, and C-16 positions of the molecule. The 2- and 3-methyl ethers of ethinylestradiol have also been identified as major metabolites. Both ethinylestradiol and its metabolites undergo extensive conjugation. Most of the conjugates in plasma and urine are found as glucuronides [84]. The principal circulating form of ethinylestradiol appears to be ethinylestradiol sulfate; the ratio of these compounds in plasma was found to be 1 : 6.5 following the administration of ^{3}H-ethinylestradiol in women [80].

The presence of significant amounts of de-ethinylated urinary metabolites of ethinylestradiol, such as estrone and estradiol, has been found after oral and intravenous administration of ^{3}H-ethinylestradiol [81, 85]. However, quantification is difficult from the reported data. In a similar study [86] neither ^{3}H-estrone nor ^{3}H-estradiol was found in blood. This finding does not rule out the possibility that other de-ethinylated metabolites of ethinylestradiol, for example, estrone sulfate, may be present in the circulation.

Relative Potency. As discussed earlier, the major metabolite of mestranol is ethinylestradiol. On the basis of the conversion ratio and metabolic clearance rates of mestranol and ethinylestradiol which were determined following intravenous injection of ^{3}H-mestranol into women it has been estimated that the transfer constant of conversion for the two compounds (MEE/PBB) is equal to approximately 0.20 [80, 87]. These findings imply that mestranol is only one-fifth as potent an estrogen as ethinylestradiol, assuming that mestranol must be converted to ethinylestradiol to exert its estrogenic effect. However, comparative studies of the differences in potency between mestranol and ethinylestradiol show a great deal of discrepancy. Although most studies using animal models show that mestranol is anywhere from 5% to 50% as potent as ethinylestradiol, other studies reveal little difference on the reproductive system in women, including endometrial response, antiovulatory potency, and effect on plasma gonadotropins [88].

Other metabolites of mestranol are similar to those described for ethinylestradiol. Like ethinylestradiol, mestranol also undergoes de-ethinylation in vivo. The extent of the de-ethinylation has been estimated to be 1%–2% of the administered dose of mestranol, based on measurement of derived urinary estrone, estradiol, estriol, and 2-hydroxyestrone [86, 89]. This conversion appears to be considerably less than that observed for ethinylestradiol, indicating that there is at least one major difference between the metabolism of mestranol and ethinylestradiol.

Progestogens

Structure-Function Relationships

Progestogens used for oral contraception are structurally related to testosterone (Fig. 1). Manipulation of the testosterone molecule alters its activity from androgenic to progestogenic. Of particular importance are changes at C-17 and C-10. When an ethinyl group is attached at C-17, there is a substantial loss of androgenicity, and progestational as well as oral activities are acquired. Further manipulation of the molecule by removal of the C-19 methyl group at C-10 results in enhanced oral progestational activity and deletion of most of the androgenic properties of the molecule. These two chemical alterations of the testosterone molecule produce norethindrone (17α-ethinyl-19-nortestosterone). Norethynodrel differs from norethindrone by having a double bond between C-5 and C-10 instead of C-4 and C-5. Other molecular manipulations of the norethindrone molecule include esterification (acetylation) of the oxygen functions at C-3, at both C-3 and C-17, or elimination of the oxygen function at C-3, resulting in the formation of norethindrone acetate, ethynodiol diacetate, and lynestrenol, respectively. Norgestrel differs from norethindrone by having an ethyl group, instead of a methyl group, attached at C-13. This difference leads to one of the most potent orally active 19-norsteroids. Norgestrel consists of a racemic mixture of the biologically active enantiomer, levonorgestrel, and the inactive enantiomer. It is only one-half as potent as levonorgestrel. Both norgestrel and levonorgestrel have potent progestational, androgenic, and antiestrogenic activities. Chemical alteration of the norgestrel molecule by formation of a double bond between C-15 and C-16, removal of the oxygenated function at C-3 and substitution of a methylene group at C-11, or formation of an oxime at C-3 and an acetate at C-17 give rise to gestoden, desogestrel and norgestimate, respectively. These three synthetic steroids are highly potent progestogens.

Pharmacokinetic Properties

Absorption and Bioavailability. All the progestogens shown in Fig. 1 are well absorbed, but their bioavailability varies. Norethindrone undergoes considerable first-pass metabolism. Its bioavailability is approximately 60% [90]. Although there is little information about the bioavailability of the progestogens structurally related to norethindrone (norethynodrel, ethynodiol diacetate, norethindrone acetate, and lynestrenol), it is known that they are rapidly converted to the parent compound. The available data indicate that the pharmacokinetics of these norethindrone derivatives are similar to those of norethindrone itself [83]. In contrast to norethindrone, levonorgestrel apparently is not subject to an appreciable first-pass effect. This observation is based on studies [91, 92] in which the systemic bioavailability of three different doses of orally administered levonorgestrel was determined in groups of 3 or 5 women. Although there was a large variation in the bioavailability between subjects (range 0.63–1.25; median, 0.93) in the small number of subjects studied, the data suggest that the bioavailability of levonorgestrel is greater than 80% in the majority of the subjects. With the exception of desogestrel little is known about the bioavailability of the progestogens that are structurally related to noregestrel. Studies show that the active metabolite of desogestrel is 3-ketodesogestrel [93, 94] and that there is a great deal of variation in the bioavailability of desogestrel between subjects [95].

Metabolism. The biotransformation of norethindrone and norgestrel occurs primarily by A-ring reduction, followed by conjugation with sulfuric and glucuronic acids [83]. Only minute amounts of norethindrone are converted to ethinylestradiol [82]. In addition to A-ring reduction, norgestrel also undergoes extensive hydroxylation. There is evidence that the metabolism of norgestrel is stereoselective, for example, the major metabolite of levonorgestrel is 1–3a,5B-tetrahydronorgestrel, whereas the predominant product of dextronorgestrel is d-16β-hydroxynorgestrel. In vitro studies show that there is insignificant metabolism of norgestrel by the gut wall [96]. This finding is consistent with the data showing that levonorgestrel is highly bioavailable [91, 92]. The large difference in bioavailability between norethindrone and levonorgestrel is surprising in view of their similar metabolic fate. Structurally the two molecules differ by one methyl group (levonorgestrel has an ethyl group instead of a methyl group at C-13). This structural difference appears to be sufficient to cause levonorgestrel to undergo a much slower metabolism in comparison to norethindrone.

There is little information about the metabolism of the progestogens structurally related to norethindrone and norgestrel. It appears that all the progestogens, with the exception of desogestrel, are first rapidly biotransformed to the parent compound by undergoing either oxidation, reduction, or hydrolysis [83]. Norgestimate is first metabolized to levonorgestrel-3-oxime and then more slowly to levonorgestrel [98, 99]. Desogestrel undergoes rapid and extensive oxidation to form 3-ketodesogestrel [93, 94]. Since the methylene group at C-11 appears to remain unaltered, desogestrel is not transformed to the parent compound, norgestrel.

Relative Potency. There is controversy about the relative potency of the synthetic progestogens used for oral contraception and whether the different formulations provide beneficial therapeutic alternatives. The disagreement arises from lack of reliable bioassays which can be used to establish the biological profile and relative potency of a synthetic progestogen. Most of our present information about the biological activity of progestogens is based on studies of the effects of high doses of the progestogens on animal models. These data may not be applicable to the clinical situation in the human. A variety of bioassays have been used to measure the activity of each progestogen, and different results have been obtained. The results are complicated by the fact that the progestogens possess different degrees of progestational, androgenic, and estrogenic activities. Furthermore, since progestogens are usually administered in combination with an estrogenic component, an additional complication may result from interaction between the estrogen and progestogen.

The response of a tissue to a progestogen is mediated via a specific cytoplasmic or nuclear receptor [100]. After crossing the cell membrane a steroid such as norethindrone binds to the receptor, forming a steroid-receptor complex which elicits a tissue-specific response attributed to that class of steroids (progestogens). The progestogens that are structurally related to 19-nortestosterone have high progestational activity. In addition, they are androgenic. There is evidence which suggests that in order to initiate their androgenic effects, progestogens require a functional androgen receptor [101]. The potency of the progestational and androgenic effects appear to be related to their affinity for the progesterone and androgen receptors, respectively [102].

The biological effects of progestogens vary. Although all of the progestogens commonly used in oral contraceptive preparations have potent progestational activity, not all of them bind significantly to the progesterone receptor, e.g., norethindrone acetate, ethynodiol diacetate, norethynodrel, and lynestrenol [103]. This suggests that these steroids exert their biological effects after metabolic conversion to norethindrone.

The biological effects of progestogens have been tested in both animals and humans. Although there are a number of tests of progestational activity, the most commonly used test in the laboratory is the Clauberg test, in which the effect of the progestogen is measured in estrogen-primed rabbits. Several clinical tests have also been used to measure the activity of progestational compounds, e.g., the delay of menses test. A striking difference in relative progestational potencies is observed between norethindrone and levonorgestrel [103]. The latter steroid is considerably more potent than the former.

Receptor binding and rat prostatic growth have been used as tests of androgenicity of progestogens. These tests show that levonorgestrel has considerably more androgenicity than norethindrone and some of its derivatives, e.g., ethynodiol diacetate and norethynodrel [103].

Estrogenic activity of progestogens has been measured on the basis of binding to the estrogen receptor and biological effects on vaginal epithelium in cervical mucus. It appears that only norethynodrel and ethynodiol diacetate have potent estrogenic activities [103].

An antiestrogenic effect has been attributed to some progestogens. Steroids that compete with estrogens for the binding site on the estrogen receptor are considered antiestrogenic. When estrogen and progestogen are administered simultaneously, the progestogen will alter the estrogenic effect on the vagina or uterus. A mouse vaginal smear assay has been used to measure antiestrogenic activity, but the clinical manifestation of this activity has not been well defined. Nevertheless it appears that with the exception of norethynodrel and ethynodiol diacetate most of the commonly used progestogens are antiestrogenic [103].

There is a paucity of data on the interaction of estrogens and progestogens when administered in a combined form. We cannot predict how the estrogenic, progestational, androgenic, antiestrogenic, and antiprogestational activities as well as synergistic interactions will be expressed. On the basis of the delay of menses test it has been shown that employment of mestranol in combination with norethynodrel or norgestrel can increase the potency of the progestogen approximately 4- and 30-fold, respectively [103].

Clinical Status

An effort will be made to review some of the more recent experience rather than to provide a comprehensive historical review of the developments associated with the low-dose preparations currently in use. The topics to be covered include efficacy, cardiovascular effects, effects on carbohydrate tolerance, coagulation effects, eicosanoid interaction, susceptibility for sexually transmitted diseases, infertility, pituitary tumors, and gallbladder disease.

Efficacy

While concern about metabolic effects has led to reduced doses of both the estrogen and progestogen constituents of the oral contraceptive pill, there is a minimum estrogen dosage consistent with clinical efficacy, about 30–35 µg, with formulations containing 20 µg estrogen having slightly less effectiveness [104]. The incidence of breakthrough bleeding or spotting is only slightly increased, while estrogen-mediated side effects such as nausea, breast tenderness, and fluid retention are reduced with these formulations. There have been recent reports that phasic preparations may be associated with a high rate of occurrence of ovarian cysts, which, at least for some physicians and their patients is unacceptable [105]. Interestingly, all of the new progestogen formulations (containing desogestrel, norgestimate, or gestoden) are being marketed as monophasic preparations. Therefore, the utility of phasic preparations is in question despite the argument for their use [106].

Cardiovascular Effects

Thromboembolism. Corresponding to the reduction of estrogen and progestogen in the combined oral contraceptive pill a reduction in the incidence of thromboembolism has been reported in Sweden: a drop in the incidence occurred in the early 1970s when 50-µg preparations became available, and a further drop occurred after 1975 when the 30- to 35-µg preparations began to be used [107]. In the United Kingdom a reduction in deaths for nonvenous and venous events as well as for stroke and ischemic heart disease corresponded to the use of 30-µg estrogen-containing preparations as compared to 50-µg preparations [108]. The 30-µg preparations altered clotting factors (VII, X, and fibrinogen) in an intermediate zone between nonusers and those using 50-µg preparations and was suggested to be the explanation for the observed vascular events. The Puget Sound study recently reported that a positive association existed between current oral contraceptive use and venous thromboembolism, similar to prior reports [109–111], and that it was diminished in association with a reduction in the estrogen dosage of the pills ingested [112].

Arterial Disease. A reanalysis of the Royal College of General Practitioner's (RCGP) Study in 1982 [113] demonstrated that while maintaining the estrogen content of the pill at 50 µg ethinylestradiol, a dose-response increase in arterial disease consisting of ischemic heart disease, cerebrovascular disease, and peripheral vascular disease – and additionally increased with smoking – corresponded to an increase of the progestogen norethindrone acetate from 1 to 3 to 4 mg. Similar findings were noted with two doses of levonorgestrel when matched with 30 μg ethinylestradiol. Of interest in this study was the inverse reduction in HDL-C (high-density lipoprotein cholesterol) with increasing progestogenic dose corresponding to the increasing arterial disease. Additionally, a parallel increase in hypertension was noted with increasing dose of norethindrone acetate [114] and with increasing dose of noregestrel [115]. No reported association with current oral contraceptive use and stroke was reported by the Puget Sound study [111, 112]. The Oxford Family Planning Association recently reported that women using oral contraceptives containing more than 50 μg estrogen had an association with nonhemorrhagic stroke while no strokes had yet been reported for women taking oral contraceptives containing less than 50 μg estrogen [116].

Effect on Lipids and Lipoproteins. Since the initial study of Bradley in 1978 [117] suggested that there may be a differing effect on HDL-C by dose and type of progestogen, Knopp et al. in 1981 [118] and Wahl et al. in 1983 [119] have reported on a variety of these formulations. The general conclusion of these studies was that use of oral contraceptives containing 50–100 μg estrogen with varying doses of progestins such as norgestrel was associated with a reduction of HDL-C while those containing norethindrone or ethynodiol diacetate did not affect HDL-C. Some of their data is consistent for the same oral contraceptive formulations between studies while some is not, largely because of small sample size in certain categories. Furthermore, since they pooled all doses of norethindrone-containing formulations, it is not possible to determine whether there is a consistent dose-response effect of this compound as has been suggested by one study [120] where a dose of 0.4 mg norethindrone with 35 μg EE_2 was associated with significant elevations of HDL-C while 1 mg norethindrone with 35 μg ethinylestradiol was not. Thus, the dose and type of progestogen, even the one usually thought to be least potent for this endpoint, may be important in affecting changes in potentially important lipids such as HDL-C. HDL-C has been reported in epidemiologic studies to correlate inversely with the risk of cardiovascular disease [121]. Whether alterations of this parameter in otherwise healthy women alters their risk for development of atherogenesis is at the present time not firmly established.

The measurement of LDL-C (low-density lipoprotein cholesterol) may be more strongly correlated with and predictive of the development of coronary artery disease than cholesterol, triglycerides, or HDL-C [122, 123]. Therefore the observation of Wahl et al. (1983) that formulations containing ethynodiol diacetate, norethindrone acetate, and norgestrel increased LDL-C significantly is a matter of concern. Since the former two products are metabolized to norethindrone in order to become active, and norethindrone does not appear to produce increases in LDL-C, why these products are associated with such increases is not understood. Another study reported similar increases in LDL-C with products containing ethynodiol diacetate and norgestrel [124].

The HDL_2 subfraction has been shown to correlate best with angiographically defined coronary artery disease [125] while apolipoprotein A-1, in addition to HDL-C, increased the discriminatory value in assessing angiographic evidence of coronary artery disease [126].

Preliminary studies with the triphasic product containing a reduced dosage of levonorgestrel and an increased dosage of ethinylestradiol demonstrates that lipids and lipoproteins may not be adversely affected [127], thereby suggesting that it may be possible to select appropriate dose and schedules of these progestogens, in combination with estrogens, in order to afford clinical utility while minimally affecting metabolic parameters. Similarly, the new compound desogestrel, when administered in a monophasic manner has been shown to produce favorable changes in lipids and lipoproteins [127], while other studies report that the triphasic levonorgestrel preparation affects lipids and lipoproteins in a manner not like the desogestrel monophasic preparation [128]. Data regarding formulations containing norgestimate and gestoden, the other two new progestogens in the new oral contraceptives, are only just becoming available. It is clear that pharmaceutical companies are sensitive to the effects of these progestogens on lipids, and each of these three new compounds are described as producing no deleterious effects, indeed, perhaps even favorable changes in lipids and lipoproteins.

Experience of Former Users. Historically, it is prudent to remember that a study in the United States has reported that former oral contraceptive users had a higher risk for developing subsequent myocardial infarction than nonusers [129]. Similarly, the RCGP study implicated former oral contraceptive use up to 6 years following discontinuation, with an increased risk of stroke as compared to the risk in nonusers [113]. While these studies are not consistent with others [130–133], it may be worthwhile for us to consider that they may tell us something important, namely, that small, consistent alterations in, for example, lipid parameters in a nonprotective direction for long periods of time, may lead to acceleration of atherogenesis in susceptible individuals.

Confounding Factors. In regard to lipids and lipoprotein effects of oral contraceptives, it is important to remember the potentially confounding effects of genetics, age, diet, exercise pattern, alcohol consumption, and smoking of the patients being studied. Some individuals are susceptible to oral contraceptive induced hypertriglyceridemia [134]. Typically, age alone may have an effect on the pattern of lipids and lipoproteins, and it is generally recommended that the oral contraceptive pill not be prescribed to women older than 40 years of age even if they do not smoke [135]. Diet may produce important changes in the pattern of lipids and lipoproteins according to whether vegetables or fish predominates, for example, as compared to a diet consisting of large quantities of egg and beef [136–143]. Extensive, consistent exercise is known to alter lipids and lipoproteins [144–146], and the bulk of evidence supports the view that even regular physical exercise may have a protective effect on developing coronary artery disease [134, 147]. Moderate alcohol consumption has been reported to have a positive association with HDL-C [148, 149]; this may mostly alter the pattern of HDL with an increase in the HDL_3 fraction, a fraction not believed to have a protective effect on the development of cardiovascular disease [150]. Smoking, of course, may produce important effects on the cardiovascular system independent of or in spite of oral contraceptive formulation and the other potentially confounding factors mentioned [113, 151]. All these parameters should be considered in clinical studies to evaluate the effects of oral contraceptives so as not to draw incorrect conclusions in regard to oral contraceptive effects which could more appropriately be ascribed to these confounding factors; nevertheless it is also possible that inherent genetic factors may predispose susceptible individuals to untoward events, while diet and exercise may permit others to induce cardioprotective changes that protect or ameliorate the effects of contraceptive steroids.

Effects on Carbohydrate Tolerance

Various studies have suggested that the estrogen component of contraceptive steroids when administered alone produces no deleterious effect on carbohydrate tolerance; indeed, they may improve carbohydrate metabolism [152], while the progestogenic constituent of the pill is responsible for altered glucose tolerance, probably by inducing relative insulin resistance [153]. Most studies have used oral glucose tolerance to assess carbohydrate tolerance [153, 154], and these have concluded that the dose and type of progestogen correlates with observed changes. Notably, none of the formulations studied, irrespective of the 19-norprogestins they contained (norethindrone, ethynodiol diacetate or norgestrel at standard doses), alter fasting glucose or insulin levels, although all cause a significant increase in the glucose or insulin curves with therapy [153, 154]. Among the progestogens available for use in United States the norgestrel has been reported to be more metabolically potent than the others [155]. A European report comparing seven low-dose formulations, some of which contained desogestrel and gestoden, reported no significant change with treatment with any of the formulations [156].

New Developments. Recently a tool to study glucose metabolism has been developed, the frequent-sample intravenous glucose tolerance test (FSIGT [157, 158]), which permits the investigator to determine various parameters of glucose metabolism such as glucose tolerance (K_g), insulin sensitivity (S_I), the two phases (phi 1 and phi 2) of pancreatic responsiveness to the glucose load, and the ability of glucose to be disposed by tissues in the presence of basal levels of insulin (S_g). Use of this tool in oral contraceptive users has led to preliminary reports [159] and ongoing studies [160] which suggest that the oral glucose tolerance test (OGTT) may not be as sensitive as the FSIGT in detecting glucose metabolism alterations. While the potential importance of these observations is not clearly established, it is important to remember that altered glucose metabolism is one of the important risk factors identified by epidemiologic studies on atherogenesis [161]. One explanation for this observation has been offered by Stout [162], who suggests that arterial walls are an insulin-sensitive tissue which, if exposed to chronic high concentration of insulin, results in proliferation of smooth muscle cells, inhibition of lipolysis, and increased synthesis of cholesterol, phospholipid, and triglyceride, leading to lipid-filled lesions similar to those of early atherosclerosis. Alternatively, as has been summarized by Wissler [163], atherogenesis is the culmination of a variety of processes, including stimulation of arterial smooth muscle cells, endothelial cells, and macrophages, with lipid accumulation (cholesterol ester, mediated by LDL receptors) and cell proliferation, all of which may be stimulated by factors which alter lipid and lipoprotein metabolism. The end result, however mediated, is the progressive development of atherogenic lesions.

Coagulation Effects

The majority of studies devoted to oral contraceptive usage and coagulation tendency have utilized measurement of individual clotting factors or groups thereof [164–166]. Whether such alterations in clotting factors are the sole effectors of clotting in vivo is debatable since the entire vessel environment may be critically important, including the vessel wall [166]. As described by Wissler [163], the atherosclerotic plaque has two major components. A fibrous cap, consisting primarily of smooth muscle cells, which with increasing size has a tendency to fracture or ulcerate, and a necrotic core, consisting of large amounts of cholesterol, cholesterol esters, and thromboplastic substances which may not adequately support the fibrous cap; this may lead to rupture of the cap with release from the necrotic core of thromboplastic substances into the circulation which, in turn, may promote thrombosis. In autopsy or angiographic studies a consistent pattern of thrombus formation and an inconsistent pattern of atheromatous changes are reported [167, 168]. While some subjects had thrombus formation in the absence of vessel wall disease as a result of suspected coronary artery spasm, the effects on former users reviewed earlier [113, 129] suggest that a progressive, persistent change in the vessel wall may be induced by oral contraceptive usage which may facilitate the development of coronary artery disease. In nonhuman primates, at least, the atherogenic process can be accelerated in the presence of hyperlipidemia, and it can be shown to regress with lowering of blood lipids [163]. Thus, the type and dosage of the oral contraceptives ingested for long periods of time may affect this process.

Eicosanoid Interaction

Another possible mechanism explaining the adverse effect of estrogen on the cardiovascular system is that of interaction with the eicosanoid system. The principal prostaglandin which has been shown to be vasodilatory and have important benefits for coronary heart disease is prostacyclin (PGI_2) [169–172]. PGI_2 may not only have a direct vasodilatory benefit function but also be beneficial because it opposes the proaggregatory effects of platelet-derived thromboxane A_2 (TXA_2). Platelet aggregation which occurs in vessels having "atherogenic" plaques may be offset by increasing concentrations of PGI_2 relative to TXA_2. Thus, PGI_2 and TXA_2 can be viewed as opponents, each having a powerful biological activity which counters or balances the other. Results from studies evaluating the effects of combined and progestogen-only oral contraceptives on PGI_2 and TXA_2 formation in women are variable, making it difficult to reach a definite conclusion [173–176]. Smoking and oral contraceptive usage, however, has been reported to be associated with a significantly reduced urinary PGI_2 stable metabolite, 6-keto-$PGF_{1\alpha}$, a significantly increased platelet aggregation using the endoperoxide/thromboxane A_2 analog N-46619, but not ADP [177]. Clearly, if this evidence is substantiated and clarified with respect to dose and type of estrogen and progestogen as well as to nicotine or some other constituent of smoke with which these observations are related, it will help to explain the mechanism by which smoking and oral contraceptive use leads to an increased myocardial infarction risk [151]. Studies with a large number of subjects, different estrogen and progestogen formulations and doses, and reliable prostanoid assays should be carried out to gain a better understanding of the interaction between prostanoids and contraceptive steroids administered orally.

Implications. The implications of this observation for oral contraceptive use and cardiovascular disease are multiple. First, measuring clotting factors and finding them not elevated may give us a false sense of security that thrombus formation may not occur. Second, subtle consistent changes in lipids/lipoproteins in a disadvantageous direction associated with oral contraceptive usage may be important determinants for subsequent atherosclerotic consequences if they accelerate the atherogenic process above the basal rate of this process inherent for the individual based on his age, hereditary tendency, diet, exercise pattern, alcohol consumption, or pattern of cigarette smoking. Third, effects of oral contraceptives on carbohydrate tolerance consistently show that, even with OGTT tests, a state of hyperinsulinemia is induced which independently may lead to atherogenic changes in arterial walls. Fourth, the interaction of eicosanoids with contraceptive estrogens, progestogens, and smoking may profoundly impact the atherogenic process, provoking a response such as myocardial infarction or stroke in susceptible individuals.

Susceptibility to Sexually Transmitted Diseases

On the basis of the Women's Health Survey [178] it was concluded that oral contraceptive users had a reduced likelihood of developing salpingitis. In part this observation carried forward the previous report that oral contraceptive users had less gonorrhoea [179]. In 1985 a review of 14 epidemiological studies showed that in 12 of them, oral contraceptive users had a 2- to 3-fold greater incidence of having *Chlamydia trachomatis* (CT) from cervical cultures than nonusers [180]. Similar conclusions were drawn from a recent Arizona study [181]. Since CT is considered to be the most prevalent sexually transmitted disease in certain parts of the world, notably in Scandinavia [182] and the United States [183], and since there has been concern that infections of the female genital tract with this organism may produce silent salpingitis leading to infertility [184–186], it is particularly important to consider studies that have tried to clarify the role of oral contraceptive usage and the development of upper genital tract infections and infertility.

Animal studies have concluded that progestogens may be necessary for initiation of infection with CT [187] while estrogens may be more important in its spread [188]. Thus, use of oral contraceptives could potentially influence the receptivity of cervical tissue to this or other infective organisms [189].

Upper Genital Tract Infections. In a Swedish study [190] patients hospitalized for presumed salpingitis had approximately twice the rate of CT as for *Neisseria gonorrhoeae* (NG) when cultures were obtained from the cervix, regardless of whether they were using oral contraceptives, the intrauterine contraceptive device, or were in the control group using either barrier methods or nothing. Following laparoscopy to make a firm diagnosis of salpingitis it was noted that, in fact, the oral contraceptive group had significantly less CT or NG than the two other groups, which had identical recoveries for these two organisms. A further report of this study [191] showed that the oral contraceptive group had less perihepatitis and a lower IgG antibody titer to CT, demonstrating less chronic infection with this organism and a trend to a milder degree of tubal inflammation as compared to the other two groups which did not significantly differ among these parameters.

Infertility

In a recent report [192] oral contraceptive usage and risk for tubal infertility was not significantly correlated with whether it was the method first used, longest used, or ever used; whether there was a history of pelvic inflammatory disease, gonorrhea infection, or hospitalized therapy. The risk with use of high-estrogen formulations had a p value of 0.06, while the risk in those using <50 µg with norethindrone acetate or ethynodial diacetate had a p value of 0.08, and the risk in those using <50 µg formulations with norethindrone or NG was not significant. The only significant finding of this study in regard to oral contraceptives concerned the first use of oral contraceptives other than those already mentioned or unknown preparations by females less than 20 years of age ($p=0.02$): younger users of >50 µg estrogen oral contraceptives were at a higher risk of subsequent tubal infertility.

Since these young oral contraceptive users are most susceptible to sexually transmitted diseases, and since they are more likely to use oral contraceptives, carefully performed additional studies are required before we can be comforted that oral contraceptives are protective against the development of sexually transmitted diseases.

Pathogenesis. It is important to determine whether use of oral contraceptives is more or less likely to be associated with infection of cervical tissues by the herpes or papilloma viruses [193]. One must remember here that the squamocolumnar junction of the immediately postmenarcheal female is generally on the ectocervix, demonstrating a process of ectopy, and has not undergone metaplasia with transformation and regression of this junction into the more protected endocervical canal [189]. Thus if a positive correlation is demonstrated, then early age at first sex, multiple sex partners, acquisition of CT, herpes or papilloma infections into the susceptible postmenarcheal cervical tissues may logically explain the associated higher likelihood of development of cervical dysplasia or cancer as well as the residual infectivity of CT for cervical tissues and the influence on development of upper genital tract infection.

Miscellaneous Factors

Pituitary Tumors. Oral contraceptive use has not been associated with the development of pituitary tumors [194] unless these formulations were prescribed to individuals with oligomenorrhea in order to regulate their cycles [195]. In the latter study it was noted that these individuals may have had a preexisting pituitary tumor causing the initial clinical presentation of oligomenorrhea.

Gallbladder Disease. A novel historical cohort study which was recently published appears to clarify some of the historically confusing reports on oral contraceptive use and gall bladder disease [196]. It was found that women 15–19 years of age had a significantly increased prevalence of gall bladder disease while each of the next older two 5-year age groups were also at significantly increased risk (albeit smaller); however, beyond 30 years of age there was no increased risk of developing gall bladder disease. Additionally, use of formulations containing less than 50 μg of estrogen demonstrated no age-adjusted association, while use of doses greater than or equal to 50 μg estrogen demonstrated an age-adjusted increase in the relative risk for the development of gallbladder disease.

Summary and Conclusions

In the quarter century since the introduction of the oral contraceptive pill numerous changes in the oral contraceptive dose, drug, and dosage schedule have evolved. Clinical observations relating thromboembolic disease to pill use led to epidemiological studies which implicated the estrogen dose as contributing to changes in clotting parameters responsible for thrombosis [197]. Further studies implicated the progestogen dose as leading to hypertensive and arterial disease [113, 114]. The important interaction between smoking and oral contraceptive use leading to cardiovascular disease was noted [151, 198]. The dosage of estrogens and progestogens in the combination oral contraceptive pill have been correspondingly reduced and special recommendations have been formulated that smokers should not take the pill beyond 35 years of age, and that in the absence of smoking pill use generally is not recommended beyond age 40 and only exceptionally beyond age 45 [198]. Absolute and relative contraindictions to pill use have been formulated (oral contraceptive package insert, Physician's Desk Reference, 1986, Medical Economics Company Inc., Oradell, NJ 07649, USA). Additionally, the woman who qualifies for pill use in the late 1980s is healthier and has available for choice oral contraceptive formulations which produce substantially fewer metabolic alterations than those when the pill was first introduced. Nonetheless, important health consequences of pill use still exist. Notable among these is the unresolved issue of impact on breast cancer, evidence of increasing cervical and liver cancer, and impact on cardiovascular disease, especially the interaction with smoking. In the case of breast cancer and cardiovascular disease we are soon likely to have sufficient numbers of individuals who have taken these formulations for sufficient durations of time to provide the basis for investigations. The information in the contribution by Kay in this book regarding the

RCGP study is provocative and illuminating, suggesting that the pill, if used at a certain vulnerable time in a woman's life, may "unmask" breast cancer in susceptible individuals even though longer pill use had no effect on "inducing" breast cancer.

Whether the pill facilitates the infectivity of CT in cervical tissues, as some have postulated [187, 188, 199], needs clarification. Whether oral contraceptive usage predisposes to herpes simplex or papilloma virus infections of cervical tissue, thereby explaining the increased incidence of cervical carcinoma, needs to be clarified [193]. And studies on the impact of pill use in potentially reducing the development of upper genital tract infection with known pathogens leading to infertility [190, 191] need to be extended.

Throughout this review smoking has been seen to be an important confounder, related to the development of cervical dysplasia and cancer (perhaps by suppressing the immune reaction, thereby facilitating infection by sexually transmitted diseases, which in turn lead to the development of these lesions [200]); associated with the development of cardiovascular disease, the mechanism only recently being elucidated [166, 177]; possibly associated with subsequent infertility [192, 201, 202]; and impairing the return of fertility in parous and in nulliparous women, especially if they smoke more than 20 cigarettes daily [203]. Clearly some of the putative effects of oral contraceptive usage on metabolic parameters can be more properly ascribed to smoking. Mechanisms for these associations require elucidation. Recent estimates by the United States Office of Smoking and Health show that 15.4 million women in the age group 20–33 smoke, and that this accounts for almost 60% of all women smokers [204]. Although oral contraceptive use varies among various age groups, it may be as high as 40% in the 18–29 age group [205]. Therefore there is an enormous number of women potentially susceptible to the health consequences that the independent or interaction effects of these two factors may engender.

It is important that new progestogens be developed and tested, and that new oral contraceptive formulations be subjected to investigations utilizing the best technology or tests that scientists have devised, regardless of whether they are required by regulatory agencies. The consumer deserves to know that new formulations have had the most careful scrutiny based on what we have learned from our quarter century of experience with this most popular and generally extremely safe method of contraception.

While this review has been focused on oral contraceptive risks, it should be recognized that this method of birth control in its current low-dose form is an extremely effective method, especially since women with high-risk conditions no longer have oral contraceptives prescribed [206]. There are ample areas for further investigation of existing preparations. Similar investigation should be performed on formulations containing new progestogenic compounds to determine whether the metabolic profile associated with their use will lead to a more favorable pattern than with the currently available formulations available for use. It is curious that all of the new pills which have been introduced in Europe use modifications of the levonorgestrel molecule as the 19-nortestosterone derivative (Fig. 1), use microgram quantities, and employ a monophasic formulation. Clarification of the first-pass effect of these progestogens is needed, especially as an understanding of their similarities and differences in producing metabolic effects is gained.

While some dispute the reduction in metabolic consequences paralleling a reduction in the estrogen content of the pill from 50 µg to 30–35 µg, with a concomitant reduction in the progestogen dosage, [207], and others deny any cardiovascular consequences of oral contraceptives on the basis of vital statistics [208], the information discussed in this review as well as specific critiques of the latter claim [206, 209, 210] all attest to these low-dose oral contraceptive formulations being effective and safe if prescribed to women selected carefully, preferably to those who do not smoke. Indeed, because of the noncontraceptive health benefits that accrue to those who use the now low-dose oral contraceptive formulations [211], it is reassuring that this popular method of birth control has spectra of safety and effectiveness. If the new progestogen formulations are associated with improved metabolic effects, the benefit/risk ratio, already increased with the new low-dose preparations will be further enhanced by their use.

References

1. IMS America (1987) National Prescription Audit. IMS America, Ambler
2. Russel-Briefel R, Ezzati T, Perlman J (1985) Prevalence and trends in oral contraceptive use in premenopausal females aged 12–54 years, United States 1971–1980. Am J Public Health 75:11713
3. Tyrer LB (1984) Oral contraception for the adolescent. J Reprod Med 29:551
4. Pike MC, Henderson BE, Casagrande JT, Rosario I, Gray GE (1981) Oral contraceptive use and early abortion as risk factors for breast cancer in young women. Br J Cancer 43:72
5. Silverberg SG, Makowski EL (1975) Endometrial carcinoma in young women taking oral contraceptive agents. Obstet Gynecol 46:503
6. Centers for Disease Control (1983) Oral contraceptive use and the risk of endometrial cancer. JAMA 249:1600
7. Henderson BE, Casagrande JT, Pike MC, Mack T, Rosario I, Duke A (1983) The epidemiology of endometrial cancer in young women. Br J Cancer 47:749
8. Weiss NS, Sayvetz TA (1980) Incidence of endometrial cancer in relation to the use of oral contraceptives. N Engl J Med 302:551
9. Kaufman DW, Shapiro S, Slone D, Rosenberg L, Miettinen OS, Stolley PD, Knapp RC et al. (1980) Decreased risk of endometrial cancer among oral contraceptive users. N Engl J Med 303:1045
10. Kelsey JL, Li Volsi VA, Holford TR, Fischer DB, Mostow ED, Schwartz PE, O'Connor T, White C (1982) A case-control study of cancer of the endometrium. Am J Epidemiol 116:333
11. Hulka BS, Chambless LE, Kaufman DG, Fowler WC, Greenberg BG (1982) Protection against endometrial carcinoma by combination-product oral contraceptives. JAMA 247:475
12. Ramcharan S, Pellegrin FA, Ray R, et al. (1981) In: The Walnut Creek Contraceptive Drug Study. A prospective study of the side effects of oral contraceptives. US Department of Health and Human Services, National Population Research, Bethesda (NIH publication 81–564, vol 3)
13. Centers for Disease Control (1987) Combination oral contraceptive use and the risk of endometrial cancer. JAMA 257:796
14. Newhouse ML, Pearson RM, Fullerton JM, Boesen EAM, Shannon HS (1972) A case control study of carcinoma of the ovary. Br J Prev Soc Med 31:148

15. McGowan L, Parent L, Lednar W, Norris HJ (1979) The woman at risk for developing ovarian cancer. Gynecol Oncol 7:325
16. Casagrande JT, Louie EW, Pike MC, Roy S, Ross RK, Henderson BE (1979) "Incessant ovulation" and ovarian cancer. Lancet 2:170
17. Hildreth NG, Kelsey JL, Li Volsi VA, Fischer DB, Holford TR, Mostow ED, Schwartz PE, White C (1981) An epidemiological study of epithelial carcinoma of the ovary. Am J Epidemiol 114:398
18. Willett WC, Bain C, Hennekens CH, Rosner B, Speizer FE (1981) Oral contraceptives and risk of ovarian cancer. Cancer 48:1684
19. Franceschi S, LaVecchia C, Helmrich SP, Mangioni C, Tognoni G (1982) Risk factors for epithelial ovarian cancer in Italy. AM J Epidemiol 115:714
20. Rosenberg L, Shapiro S, Slone D, Kaufman DW, Helmrich SP, Miettinen OS, Stolley PD, et al. (1982) Epithelial ovarian cancer and combination oral contraceptives. JAMA 247:3210
21. Risch HA, Weiss NS, Lyone JL, Daling JR, Liff JM (1983) Events of reproductive life and the incidence of epithelial ovarian cancer. Am J Epidemiol 177:128
22. Cramer DW, Hutchinson GB, Welch WR, Scully RE, Knapp RC (1982) Factors affecting the association of oral contraceptives and ovarian cancer. N Engl J Med 307:1047
23. Centers for Disease Control (1983) Oral contraceptive use and the risk of ovarian cancer. JAMA 249:1596
24. Kelsey JL, Hildreth NG (1983) Breast and gynecologic cancer epidemiology. CRC, Boca Raton
25. Editorial (1985) Another look at the pill and breast cancer. Lancet 2:985
26. Stadel BV, Rubin GL, Wingo PA, Schlesselman JJ (1986) Oral contraceptives and breast cancer in young women (letter). Lancet 1:436
27. McPherson K, Coope PA (1986) Early oral contraceptive use and breast cancer risk (letter). Lancet 1:685
28. Vessey MP, Doll R, Jones K, McPherson K, Yeates D (1979) An epidemiological study of oral contraceptives and breast cancer. Br Med J 1:1755
29. Jick H, Walker AM, Watkins RN, d'Ewart DC, Hunter JR, et al. (1980) Oral contraceptives and breast cancer. Am J Epidemiol 112:577
30. Royal College of General Practitioners (1981) Breast cancer and oral contraceptives. Findings in Royal College of General Practitioners' study. Br Med J 282:2089
31. Brinton LA, Hoover R, Szklo M, Fraumeni JF (1982) Oral contraceptives and breast cancer. Int J Epidemiol 11:316
32. Lipnick RJ, Buring JE, Hennekens CH, Rosner B, Willett W, et al. (1986) Oral contraceptives and breast cancer: a prospective cohort study. JAMA 255:58
33. Centers for Disease Control (1983) Long-term oral contraceptive use and the risk of breast cancer. JAMA 249:1591
34. Stadel BV, Webster LA, Rubin GL, Schlesselman JJ, Wingo PA (1985) Oral contraceptives and breast cancer in young women. Lancet 2:970
35. Rosenberg L, Miller DR, Kaufman DW, Helmrich SP, Stolley PD, et al. (1984) Breast cancer and oral contraceptive use. Am J Epidemiol 119:167
36. Miller DR, Rosenberg L, Kaufman DW, Schottenfeld D, Stolley PD, et al. (1986) Breast cancer risk in relation to early oral contraceptive use. Obstet Gynecol 68:863
37. Vessey MP, McPherson K, Yeates D, Doll R (1982) Oral contraceptive use and abortion before first term pregnancy in relation to breast cancer risk. Br J Cancer 45:327
38. McPherson K, Neil A, Vessey MP, Doll R (1983) Oral contraceptives and breast cancer (letter). Lancet 2:1414
39. Pike MC, Henderson BE, Krailo MD, Duke A, Roy S (1983) Breast cancer in young women and use of oral contraceptives: possible modifying effect of formulation and age at use. Lancet 2:916
40. Paul C, Skegg DCG, Spears GFS, Kaldor JM (1986) Oral contraceptives and breast cancer: a national study. Br Med J 293:723
41. Meirik O, Lund E, Adami HO, Bergstrom R, Christoffersen R, et al. (1986) Oral contraceptive use and breast cancer in young women. Lancet 2:650

41. Hoover R, Bain C, Cole P, MacMahon B (1978) Oral contraceptive use: association with frequency of hospitalization and chronic disease risk indicators. Am J Public Health 68:335
43. Le MG, Hill C, Kramer A, Moulton LH (1985) Possible cohort effects in studies of oral contraceptive use and breast cancer (letter). Br J Cancer 52:805
44. McPherson K, Drife JO (1986) The pill and breast cancer: why the uncertainty? Br Med J 293:709
45. Vihko R, Apter D (1984) Endocrine characteristics of adolescent menstrual cycles: impact of early menarche. J Steroid Biochem 20:231
46. Apter D, Raisanen I, Ylostalo P, Vihko R (1985) Ultrasonographic and hormonal patterns of adolescent menstrual cycles. 15th Acta Endocrinologica Congress, August, Helsinki
47. Thomas DB (1972) Relationship of oral contraceptives to cervical carcinogenesis. Obstet Gynecol 40:508
48. Boyce JG, Lu T, Nelson JH, Fruchter RG (1977) Oral contraceptives and cervical carcinoma. Am J Obstet Gynecol 128:761
49. Swan SH, Brown WL (1981) Oral contraceptive use, sexual activity and cervical carcinoma. Am J Obstet Gynecol 139:52
50. Swan SH, Pettiti DB (1982) A review of problems of bias and confounding in epidemiologic studies of cervical neoplasia and oral contraceptive use. Am J Epidemiol 115:10
51. Clarke EA, Hatcher J, McKeown-Eyssen GE, Lickrish GM (1985) Cervical dysplasia: association with sexual behavior, smoking and oral contraceptive use? Am J Obstet Gynecol 151:612
52. Ory HW, Conger SB, Naib Z, Tyler CW, Hatcher RA (1977) Preliminary analysis of oral contraceptive use and risk of developing premalignant lesions of the uterine cervix. In: Garratini S, Berendes HW (eds) Pharmacology of steroid contraceptive drugs. Raven, New York, pp 211–224
53. Harris RWC, Brinton LA, Cowdell RH, Skegg DCG, Smith PG, et al. (1980) Characteristics of women with dysplasia or carcinoma-in-situ of the cervix uteri. Br J Cancer 42:359
54. Stern E, Forsythe AB, Youkeles L, Coffelt CF (1977) Steroid contraceptive use and cervical dysplasia: increased risk of progression. Science 196:1460
55. Editorial (1975) Cervical epithelial dysplasia. Br Med J 1:294
56. Editorial (1977) Cervical neoplasia and the pill. Lancet 2:644
57. Vessey MP, Lawless M, McPherson K, Yeates D (1983) Neoplasia of the cervix uteri and contraception – a possible adverse effect of the pill. Lancet 2:930
58. Vessey MP, Lawless M, McPherson K, Yeates D (1983) Oral contraceptives and cervical cancer. Lancet 2:1358
59. WHO Collaborative Study of Neoplasia and Steroid Contraceptives (1985) Invasive cervical cancer and combined oral contraceptives. Br Med J 290:961
60. Brinton LA, Huggins GR, Lehman HF, Mallin K, et al. (1986) Long-term use of oral contraceptives and risk of invasive cervical cancer. Int J Cancer 38:339
61. Peters RK, Thomas DC, Hagan DG, Mack TM, Henderson BE (1986) Risk factors for invasive cervical cancer among Latinas and non-Latinas in Los Angeles County. JNCI 77:1063
62. Peters RK, Chao A, Mack TM, Thomas D, Bernstein L, et al. (1986) Increased frequency of adenocarcinomas of the uterine cervix in young women in Los Angeles County. JNCI 76:423
63. Minteot R, Fievez CL (1974) Endocervical changes with the use of synthetic steroids. Obstet Gynecol 44:53
64. Gall SA, Bourgeois CH, Maguire R (1969) The morphologic effects of oral contraceptive agents on the cervix. JAMA 202:2243
65. Edmondson HA, Henderson B, Benton B (1976) Liver cell adenomas associated with use of oral contraceptives. N Engl J Med 294:470
66. Rooks JB, Ory HW, Ishak KG, Strauss LT, Greenspan JR, et al. (1979) Epidemiology of hepatocellular adenoma. The role of oral contraceptive use. JAMA 242:644

67. Yager JD, Hager R (1980) Oral contraceptive steroids as promoters of hepatocarcinogenesis in female Sprague-Dawley rats. Cancer Res 30:3680
68. Henderson BE, Preston-Martin S, Edmondson HA, Peters RL, Pike MC (1983) Hepatocellular carcinoma and oral contraceptives. Br J Cancer 48:437
69. Neuberger J, Forman D, Doll R, Williams R (1986) Oral contraceptives and hepatocellular carcinoma. Br Med J 292:1355
70. Forman D, Vincent TJ, Doll R (1986) Cancer of the liver and the use of oral contraceptives. Br Med J 292:1357
71. Kappus H, Bolt HM, Remmer H (1972) Demethylation of mestranol to ethinyloestradiol in vitro and in vivo. Acta Endocrinol (Copenh) 71:374
72. Bolt HM, Bolt WH (1974) Pharmacokinetics of mestranol in man in relation to its estrogenic activity. Eur J Clin Pharmacol 7:295
73. Korenman SG (1969) Comparative binding affinity of estrogens and its relation to estrogenic potency. Steroids 13:163
74. Kappus H, Bolt HM, Remmer H (1973) Affinity of ethynylestradiol and mestranol for the uterine estrogen receptor and for the microsomal mixed function oxidase of the liver. J Steroid Biochem 4:121
75. De la Pena A, Chenault CB, Goldzieher JW (1975) Radioimmunoassay of unconjugated plasma ethynylestradiol in women given a single oral dose of ethynylestradiol or mestranol. Steroids 25:773
76. Newburger J, Goldzieher JW (1985) Pharmacokinetics of ethinylestradiol: a current view. Contraception 32:33
77. Goldzieher JW, Dozier TS, de la Pena A, Ojo OA, Lean TS, Chinnatamby S, Basnayake S, Koetsawang S (1980) Plasma levels and pharmacokinetics of ethynylestrogens in various populations. II. Mestranol. Contraception 21:17
78. Warren RJ, Fotherby K (1973) Plasma levels of ethynylestradiol after administration of ethynylestradiol or mestranol to human subjects. J Endocrinol 59:369
79. Brenner PF, Goebelsmann U, Stanczyk FZ, Mishell DR Jr (1980) Serum levels of ethinyloestradiol following its ingestion alone or in contraceptive formulations. Contraception 22:85
80. Bird CE, Clark AF (1973) Metabolic clearance rates and metabolism of mestranol and ethynylestradiol in normal young women. J Clin Endocrinol Metab 36:296
81. Helton ED, Goldzieher JW (1977) Metabolism of ethynyl estrogens. J Toxicol Environ Health 3:231
82. Breuer H (1977) Metabolic pathways of steroid contraceptive drugs. In: Garattini S, Berendes HW (eds) Pharmacology of steroid contraceptive drugs. Raven, New York
83. Orme ML'E, Back DJ, Breckenridge AM (1983) Clinical pharmacokinetics of oral contraceptive steroids. Clin Pharmacokinet 8:95
84. Goldzieher JW, Kraemer DC (1972) The metabolism and effects of contraceptive steroids in primates. Acta Endocrinol (Copenh) 71:389
85. Williams MC, Helton ED, Goldzieher JW (1975) The urinary metabolites of 17α-ethynylestradiol-9α,11 epsilon-^{3}H in women. Chromatographic profiling and identification of ethynyl and non-ethynyl compounds. Steroids 25:229
86. Longcope C, Williams KIH (1977) Estradiol and mestranol: Their pharmacodynamics and effects on natural estrogens. In: Garattini S, Berendes HW (eds) Pharmacology of steroid contraceptive drugs. Raven, New York
87. Longcope C, Williams KIH (1975) The metabolism of synthetic oestrogens in nonusers and users of oral contraceptives. Steroids 25:121
88. Goldzieher JW et al. (1975) Comparative studies of ethynyl estrogens used in oral contraceptives. I. Endometrial response. II. Antiovulatory potency. III. Effect on plasma gonadotropins. Am J Obstet Gynecol 122:615
89. Williams JG, Longcope C, Williams KIH (1975) Metabolism of 4-^{3}H- and 4-^{14}C-17α-ethinylestradiol 3-methyl ether (mestranol) by women. Steroids 25:343
90. Goebelsmann U (1986) Pharmacokinetics of contraceptive steroids in humans. In: Gregoire AT, Blye RT (eds) Contraceptive steroids: pharmacology and safety. Plenum, New York, p 67

91. Humpel M, Wendt H, Pommerenke G, Weiss C, Speck W (1978) Investigations of pharmacokinetics of levonorgestrel to specific consideration of a possible first pass effect in women. Contraception 17:207
92. Back DJ, Bates M, Breckenridge AM, Hall JM, MacIver M, Orme ML'E, Park BK, Rowe PH (1981) The pharmacokinetics of levonorgestrel and ethinylestradiol in women – studies with Ovran and Ovranette. Contraception 23:229–239
93. Viinikka L, Ylikorkala O, Vikko R, Wijnand HP, Booij M, van der Veen F (1979) Metabolism of a new synthetic progestogen, ORG 2969, in female volunteers. Pharmacokinetics after an oral dose. Eur J Clin Pharmacol 15:349
94. Viinikka L (1979) Metabolism of a new synthetic progestogen, OR 2969 by human lives in vitro. J Steroid Biochem 10:353
95. Hasenack HG, Bosch AMG, Kaar K (1986) Serum levels of 3-ketodesogestrel after oral administration of desogestrel and 3-ketodesogestrel. Contraception 33:991
96. Back DJ, Bates M, Breckenridge AM, Ellis A, MacIver M, Orme ML'E, Rowe PH (1981) The in vitro metabolism of ethinylestradiol, mestranol and levonorgestrel by human jejunal mucosa. Br J Clin Pharmacol 11:275
97. Weintraub HS, Adams LS, Patrick JW, McGuire JL (1978) Disposition of norgestimate in the presence and absence of ethinyloestradiol after oral administration to humans. J Pharm Sci 67:1406
98. Alton KB, Hetyel NS, Shaw C, Patrick JE (1984) Biotransformation of norgestimate in women. Contraception 29:19
99. Faber LE, Wakim NG, Duhring JL (1987) Evolving concepts in the mechanism of steroid action: current developments. Am J Obstet Gynecol 156:1449
100. Bullock LP, Barden CW, Sherman MR (1978) Androgenic, antiandrogenic, synandrogenic sections of progestins. Role of steric and allosteric interactions with androgen receptors. Endocrinology 103:1768
101. Bardin CW, Janne OA (1986) Steroids of one class can mimic, inhibit and potentiate the biological effects of other steroid classes when administered at high doses. In: Gregoire AT, Blye RT (eds) Contraceptive steroids: pharmacology and safety. Plenum, New York, p 123
102. Edgren RA (1986) Endocrine effects of systemic steroidal contraceptives. In: Gregoire AT, Blye RT (eds) Contraceptive steroids: pharmacology and safety. Plenum, New York, p 163
103. Swyer GIM, Little V (1968) Clinical assessment of relative potency of progestogens. J Reprod Fertil [Suppl] 5:63
104. Vessey MP, Lawless M, Yeates D (1982) Efficacy of different contraceptive methods. Lancet 1:841
105. Caillouette JC, Koehler AL (1987) Phasic contraceptive pills and functional ovarian cysts. Am J Obstet Gynecol 156:1538
106. Pasquale SA (1984) Rationale for a triphasic oral contraceptive. J Reprod Med [Suppl] 29:560
107. Bottiger LE, Boman G, Westerholm B (1980) Oral contraceptives and thromboembolic disease: effects of lowering estrogen content. Lancet 1(8178):1097
108. Meade TW, Greenberg G, Thompson SG (1980) Progestogens and cardiovascular reactions associated with oral contraceptives and a comparison of the safety of the 50 and 30 mcg estrogen preparations. Br Med J 280:1157
109. Petitti DB, Wingerd J, Pellegrin F, Ramcharan S (1979) Risk of vascular disease in women. JAMA 242:1150
110. Vessey MP (1980) Female hormones of vascular disease – An epidemiological overview. Br J Fam Plann [Suppl] 6:1
111. Porter JB, Hunter JR, Danielson DA (1982) Oral contraceptives and nonfatal vascular disease – recent experience. Obstet Gynecol 59:299
112. Porter JB, Hunter JR, Jick H, Stergachis A (1985) Oral contraceptives and nonfatal vascular disease. Obstet Gynecol 66(1):1
113. Layde PM, Ory HW, Beral V, Kay CR (1983) Incidence of arterial disease among oral contraceptive users. J R Coll Gen Pract 33:75

114. Royal College of General Practitioners (1977) Mortality among oral contraceptive users. J R Coll Gen Pract 2:727
115. Meade TW (1982) Effects of progestogens on the cardiovascular system. Am J Obstet Gynecol 142:776
116. Vessey MP, Lawless M, Yeates D (1984) Oral contraceptives and stroke: findings in a large prospective study. Br Med J 289:530
117. Bradley DD, Wingerd J, Petitti DB, Krauss RM, Rancharan (1978) Serum high density lipoprotein cholesterol in women using oral contraceptives. N Engl J Med 299(1):17
118. Knopp R, Walden C, et al. (1981) Oral contraceptive and postmenopausal estrogen effect on lipoprotein, triglyceride and cholesterol in an adult female population: relationships to estrogen and progestin potency. J Clin Endocrinol Metab 53:1123
119. Wahl P, Walden C, Knopp R, Hoover J, Wallace R, Heiss G, Rifkind B (1983) Effect of estrogen/progestin potency on lipid/lipoprotein cholesterol. N Engl J Med 308:862
120. Roy S, Krauss RM, Duda MJ, Mesen N (1985) Effects of three low-dose oral contraceptives on serum lipids and lipoproteins: differential changes in high-density lipoprotein subclasses (Abstr 317) 32nd Annual Meeting of the Society for Gynecologic Investigation, Arizona, March 20–23, Phoenix, p 183
121. Gordon T, Castelli WP, Hjortland M, Kannel WB, Dawber T (1977) High density lipoprotein as a protective factor against coronary artery disease: The Framington Study. Am J Med 62:707
122. Fredrickson DS, Levy R (1972) In: Stanbury JB, Wyngaarden JB, Fredrickson DS (eds) The metabolic basis of inherited disease, 3rd edn. McGraw-Hill, New York
123. Stone NJ, Levy RI, Fredrickson DS, Verter J (1974) Coronary artery disease in 116 kindred with familial type II hyperlipoproteinemia. Circulation 49:476
124. Lipson A, Stoy DB, LaRosa JC, Muesing RA, Cleary PA, Miller VT, Gilbert PR, Stadel B (1986) Progestins and oral contraceptive-induced lipoprotein changes: a prospective study. Contraception 34:121
125. Miller NE, Hammett F, Saltissi S, Rao S, van Zeller H, Coltart J, Lewis B (1981) Relation of angiographically defined coronary artery disease to plasma lipoprotein subfractions and apolipoprotein. Br Med J 282
126. Maciejko JJ, Holmes DR, Kottke BA, Ainsmeister AR, Dac, Dinh DM, Mao SJT (1983) Apolipoprotein A–I as a marker of angiographically assessed coronary-artery disease. N Engl J Med 309:385
127. Gaspard UJ, Buret J, Gillain D, Romus MA, Lambotte R (1985) Serum lipid and lipoprotein changes induced by new oral contraceptives containing ethinylestradiol plus levonorgestrel or desogestrel. Contraception 31:395
128. Kloosterboer HJ, van Wayjen RGA, van den Ende A (1986) Comparative effects of monophasic desogestrel plus ethinyloestradiol and triphasic levonorgestrel plus ethinyloestradiol on lipid metabolism. Contraception 34:135
129. Slone D, Shapiro S, Kaufman DW, Rosenberg L, Miettinen OS, Stolley PD (1981) Risk of myocardial infarction in relation to current and discontinued use of oral contraceptives. N Engl J Med 305:420
130. Collaborative Group for the Study of Stroke in Young Women (1973) Oral contraception and increased risk of cerebral ischemia or thrombosis. N Engl J Med 288:871
131. Petitti DB, Wingerd J (1978) Use of oral contraceptives, cigarette smoking and risk of subarachnoid haemorrhage. Lancet 2:234
132. Inman WHW (1979) Oral contraceptives and fatal subarachnoid haemorrhage. Br Med J 2:1468
133. Thorogood M, Adam SA, Mann JI (1981) Fatal subarachnoid haemorrhage in young women: role of oral contraceptives. Br Med J 283:762
134. Levy RI, Feinleib M (1984) Risk factors for coronary artery disease and their management. In: Braunwald E (ed) Heart disease: a textbook of cardiovascular medicine. Saunders, Philadelphia, p 1205

135. Ory HW (1983) Mortality associated with fertility and fertility control: 1983. Fam Plann Perspect 15:57
136. Phillips RL, Lemon FR, Beeson L, Kuzman JW (1978) Coronary heart disease mortality among Seventh-Day Adventists with differing dietary habits: a preliminary report. Am J Clin Nutr. 31:S191
137. The Framingham Study (1970) An epidemiological investigation of cardiovascular disease, sect. 23: The Framingham Diet Study: Diet and the regulation of serum cholesterol. US Government Printing Office, Washington
138. Nichols AB, Ravenscroft C, Lamphiear DE, Ostrander LD Jr (1976) Daily nutritional intake and serum lipid levels. The Tecumseh Study. Am J Clin Nutr 29:1384
139. Shekelle RB, Shryock AM, Paul O, Lepper M, Stamler J, Liu S, Raynor WJ (1981) Diet, serum cholesterol, and death from coronary heart disease. The Western Electric Study. N Engl J Med 304:65
140. Kromhout D, Bosschieter EB, de Lezenne, Coulander C (1985) The inverse relation between fish consumption and 20-year mortality from coronary heart disease. N Engl J Med 312:1205
141. Kushi LH, Lew RA, Stare FJ, Ellison CR, El Lozy M, Bourke G, Dalyl, et al. (1985) Diet and 20-year mortality from coronary heart disease: The Ireland-Boston Diet-Heart Study. N Engl J Med 312:811
142. Kahn HA, Phillips RL, Snowdon DA, Choi W (1984) Association between reported diet and all-cause mortality: Twenty-one year follow-up on 27,530 adult Seventh-Day Adventists. Am J Epidemiol 119:775
143. Phillipson BE, Rothrock DW, Connor WE, Harris WS, Illingworth DR (1985) Reduction of plasma lipids, lipoproteins, and apoproteins by dietary fish oils in patients with hypertriglyceridemia. N Engl J Med 312:1210
144. Morris JN, Everitt MG, Pollard R, Chave SPW, Semmence AM (1980) Vigorous exercise in leisure-time: protection against coronary heart disease. Lancet 2:1207
145. Gibbons LW, Blair SN, Cooper KH, Smith M (1983) Association between coronary heart disease risk factors and physical fitness in healthy adult women. Circulation 67:977
146. Hartung GH, Foreyt JP, Mitchell RE, Vlasek I, Gotto AM Jr (1980) Relation of diet to high-density-lipoprotein cholesterol in middle-aged marathon runners, joggers and inactive men. N Engl J Med 302:357
147. Merians DR, Haskell WL, Vranizan KM, Phelps J, Woods PD, Superko R (1984) Relationship of exercise, oral contraceptive use and body fat to concentrations of plasma lipids and lipoprotein cholesterol in young women. Am J Med 78:913
148. Castelli WP, Gordon T, Hjortland MC, Kagan A, Doyle JT, Hames CG, Hulley SB, Zukel WB (1977) Alcohol and blood lipids. The Cooperative Lipoprotein Phenotyping Study. Lancet 2:154
149. Gordon T, Ernst N, Fisher M, Rifkind BM (1981) Alcohol and high-density lipoprotein cholesterol. Circulation 64:111
150. Haskall WL, Camargo C Jr, Williams PT, Vranizan JM, Krauss RM, Lindgren FT, Wood PD (1984) The effect of cessation and resumption of moderate alcohol intake on serum high density lipoprotein subfraction: a controlled study. N Engl J Med 310:805
151. Jain AK (1976) Cigarette smoking, use of oral contraceptives and myocardial infarction. Am J Obstet Gynecol 126:301
152. Spellacy WN, Buhi WC, Birk SA (1972) The effect of estrogens on carbohydrate metabolism: glucose, insulin, and growth hormone studies on one hundred and seventy-one women ingesting premarin, mestranol and ethinyl estradiol for six months. Am J Obstet Gynecol 114:378
153. Spellacy WN (1982) Carbohydrate metabolism during treatment with estrogen, progestogen and low-dose oral contraceptives. Am J Obstet Gynecol 142:732
154. Wynn V (1982) Effect of duration of low-dose oral contraceptive administration on carbohydrate metabolism. Am J Obstet Gynecol 142:739
155. Perlman JA, Russell-Briefel R, Ezzati T, Liberknecht G (1985) Oral glucose tolerance and the potency of contraceptive progestins. J Chronic Dis 38:857

156. Van der Vange N, Kloosterboer HJ, Haspels AA (1987) Effect of seven low-dose combined oral contraceptive preparations on carbohydrate metabolism. Am J Obstet Gynecol 156:918
157. Bergman RN, Phillips LS, Cobelli C (1981) Physiologic evaluation of factors controlling glucose tolerance in man: measurement of insulin sensitivity and β-cell glucose sensitivity from the response to intravenous glucose. J Clin Invest 68:1456
158. Bergman RN, Finegood DT, Ader M (1985) Assessment of insulin sensitivity in vivo. Endocr Rev 6:45
159. Bergman RN, Roy S, Lobo RA (1984) Carbohydrate metabolism of normal women on levonorgestrel and norethindrone containing oral contraceptives (OC) (Abstr 213). 31st Annual Meeting of the Society for Gynecologic Investigation, March 21–24, San Francisco, p 127
160. Roy S (Personal Communication) NIH contract: measures of carbohydrate tolerance and lipid metabolism in users of norgestrel containing oral contraceptives
161. Rosenburg L, Miller DR, Kaufman DW, Helmrich SP, van de Carr S, Stolley PA, Shapiro S (1983) Myocardial infarction in women under 50 years of age. JAMA 250:2801
162. Stout RW (1985) Overview of the association between insulin and atherosclerosis. Metabolism 34:7
163. Wissler RW (1984) Principles of the pathogenesis of atherosclerosis. In: Braunwald E (ed) Heart disease: a textbook of cardiovascular medicine. Saunders, Philadelphia, p 1183
164. Meade TW (1982) Oral contraceptives, clotting factors, and thrombosis. Am J Obstet Gynecol 142:758
165. Notelovitz M, Levenson I, McKenzie L, Lane D, Kitchens CS (1985) The effects of low-dose oral contraceptives on coagulation and fibrinolysis in two high-risk populations: young female smokers and older premenopausal women. Am J Obstet Gynecol 152(8):995–1000
166. Mammen EF (1982) Oral contraceptives and blood coagulation: A critical review. Am J Obstet Gynecol 142:781
167. Jugdutt BI, Stevens GF, Zacks DJ, Lee SJK, Taylor RF (1983) Myocardial infarction, oral contraception, cigarette smoking and coronary artery spasm in young women. Am Heart J 4:757
168. Chilvers E, Rudge P (1986) Cerebral venous thrombosis and subarachnoid haemorrhage in users of oral contraceptives. Br Med J 292:524
169. Moncada S (1982) Prostacyclin and arterial wall biology. Arteriosclerosis 2:193
170. Pitt B, Shea MJ, Romson JL, Lucchesi BR (1983) Prostaglandins and prostaglandin inhibitors in ischemic heart disease. Ann Intern Med 99:83
171. FitzGerald GA, Pederson AK, Patrono C (1983) Analysis of prostacyclin and thromboxane biosynthesis in cardiovascular disease. Circulation 67:1174
172. Nadler J, Zipser RD, Coleman R, Horton R (1983) Stimulation of renal prostaglandins by pressor hormones in man: Comparison of prostaglandin E_2 and prostacyclin (6-keto prostaglandin $F_{1\alpha}$). J Clin Endocrinol Metab 56:1260
173. Schorer AE, Gerrard JM, White JG, Krivit W (1978) Oral contraceptive use alters the balance of platelet prostaglandin and thromboxane synthesis. Prostaglandins Med 1:5
174. Sinzinger H, Klein K, Kaliman A, Silberbauer K, Feigl W (1980) Enhanced prostaglandin formation in veins of women under chronic treatment with oral contraceptive drugs. Pharmacol Res Commun 12:515
175. Ylikorkala O, Puolakka A, Viinikka L (1981) Oestrogen-containing oral contraceptives decrease prostacyclin production. Lancet 1:48
176. Ylikorkala O, Puolakka A, Viinikka L (1982) The effect of oral contraceptives on antiaggregatory prostacyclin and proaggregatory thromboxane A_2 in humans. Am J Obstet Gynecol 142:573
177. Milekowsky GN, Roy S, Nadler J (1986) Effect of oral contraceptives and smoking on prostacyclin excretion and platelet function (Abstr 88). Society for Gynecologic Investigation, March 21, Toronto, p 70

178. Rubin GL, Ory HW, Layde PM (1982) Oral contraceptives and pelvic inflammatory disease. Am J Obstet Gynecol 144:630
179. Ryden G, Fahraeus L, Molin L, Ahman K (1979) Do contraceptives influence the incidence of acute pelvic inflammatory disease in women with gonorrhoea? Contraception 20:149
180. Washington AE, Gove S, Schachter J, Sweet RL (1985) Oral contraceptives, Chlamydia trachomatis infection and pelvic inflammatory disease: a word of caution about protection. JAMA 253:2246
181. Harrison HR, Phil D, Costin M, Meder JB, Bownds LM, Sim DA, Lewis M, Alexander ER (1985) Cervical Chlamydia trachomatis infection in university women: relationship to history, contraception, ectopy and cervicitis. Am J Obstet Gynecol 153:244
182. Ripa KT, Svensson L, Treharne JD, Westrom L, Mardh PA (1980) Chlamydia trachomatis infection in patients with laparoscopically verified acute salpingitis: results of isolation and antibody determinations. Am J Obstet Gynecol 138:960
183. Centers for Disease Control (1985) Sexually Transmitted Diseases Treatment Guidelines, 1985. MMWR [Suppl] 34:80
184. Henry-Suchet J, Catalan F, Loffredo V, Serfaty D, Siboulet A, Perel V, Sanson NJ, et al. (1980) Microbiology of specimens obtained by laparoscopy from controls and from patients with pelvic inflammatory disease or infertility with tubal obstruction: chlamydia trachomatis and Ureaplasma urealyticum. Am J Obstet Gynecol 138:1022
185. Henry-Suchet J, Catalan F, Loffredo V, Serfaty D, Samson NJ, DeBache C, Pigeau F, Coppin R (1981) Chlamydia trachomatis associated with chronic inflammation in abdominal specimens fro women selected for tuboplasty. Fertil Steril 36:599
186. Sweet RL, Schachter J, Robbie MO (1983) Failure of β-lactam antibiotics to eradicate Chlamydia trachomatis in the endometrium despite apparent clinical cure of acute salpingitis. JAMA 250:2641
187. Tuffrey M, Taylor-Robinson D (1981) Progesterone as a key factor in the development of a mouse model for genital tract infection with chlamydia trachomatis. FEMS Microbiol Lett 12:111
188. Rank RG, White HJ, Hough AJ Jr, Pasley JN, Baron AL (1982) Effect of estradiol on chlamydial genital infection of female guinea pigs. Infect Immun 38:699
189. Jordan JA, Singer A (1976) Effect of oral contraceptive steroids upon epithelium and mucus. In: Jordan JA, Singer A (eds) The cervix. Saunders, London, p 192
190. Wolner-Hanssen P, Svensson L, Mardh P-A, Westrom L (1985) Laparoscopic findings and contraceptive use in women with signs and symptoms suggestive of acute salpingitis. Obstet Gynecol 66:233
191. Wolner-Hanssen P (1986) Oral contraceptive use modifies the manifestations of pelvic inflammatory disease. Br J Obstet Gynaecol 93:619
192. Cramer DW, Goldman MB, Schiff I, Belisle S, Albrecht B, Stadel B, Gibson M, et al. (1987) The relationship of tubal infertility to barrier method and oral contraceptive use. JAMA 257:2446
193. Mitchell H, Drake M, Medley G (1986) Prospective evaluation of risk of cervical cancer after cytological evidence of human papillomavirus infection. Lancet 2:573
194. Maheux R, Jenicek M, Cleroux R, Beauregard H, de Muylder X, Gratton NM, van Campenhout J (1982) Oral contraceptives and prolactinomas: a case-control study. Am J Obstet Gynecol 143:134
195. Shy KK, McTiernan AM, Daling JR, Weiss NS (1983) Oral contraceptive use and the occurrence of pituitary prolactinoma. JAMA 249:2204
196. Strom BL, Tamragouri RN, Morse ML, Lazar EL, West SL, Stolley PD, Jones JK (1986) Oral contraceptives and other risk factors for gallbladder disease. Clin Pharmacol Ther 39:335
197. Royal College of General Practitioners (1967) Oral contraception and thromboembolic disease. JR Coll Gen Pract 13:267
198. Royal College of General Practitioners (1981) Further analyses of mortality in oral contraceptive users. Lancet 1:541

199. Sweet RL (1986) Pelvic inflammatory disease. Sex Transm Dis 13:192
200. Clarke EA, Hatcher J, McKeown-Eyssen GE, Lickrish GM (1985) Cervical dysplasia: association with sexual behavior, smoking and oral contraceptive use? Am J Obstet Gynecol 151:612
201. Daling JR, Weiss NS, Metch BJ, Chow WH, Soderstrom RM, Moore DE, Spadoni LR, Stadel BV (1985) Primary tubal infertility in relation to the use of an intrauterine device. N Engl J Med 312:937
202. Sherman KJ, Daling JR, Weiss NS (1987) Sexually transmitted diseases and tubal infertility. Sex Transm Dis 14:12–16
203. Howe G, Westhoff C, Vessey M, Yeates D (1985) Effects of age, cigarette smoking, and other factors on fertility: findings in a large prospective study. Br Med J 290:1697
204. US Government (1985) Current Population Report Series P-254, no 949. Statistical Abstract for the year 1983. US Government Printing Office, Washington
205. Vital and Health Statistics (1983) OC use in 1982. Series 23, no 10. US Government Printing Office, Washington
206. Vessey MP (1984) Comment on an article, "Absence of correlation between oral contraceptive usage and cardiovascular mortality." Int J Fertil 29:208
207. Russell M, Ramcharan S (1987) Oral contraceptive estrogen content and adverse effects: has a dose-response relationship been established? Can Fam Physician 33:445
208. Wiseman RA (1984) Absence of correlation between oral contraceptive usage and cardiovascular mortality. Int J Fertil 29:198
209. Chow LP (1984) Comment on an article, "Absence of correlation between oral contraceptive usage and cardiovascular mortality." Int J Fertil 29:210
210. Kay CR (1984) Response to the Paper by Richard Wiseman. Int J Fertil 29:211
211. Ory HW (1982) The noncontraceptive health benefits from oral contraceptives. Fam Plann Perspect 14:182

Effects of Oral Contraception on Blood Clotting

J. Bonnar, L. Daly, A. Sabra, and A. Carroll

Trinity College, Department of Obstetrics and Gynaecology, University of Dublin, St. James's Hospital, Dublin 8, Ireland

The major health hazard encountered in relation to fertility control with oral contraception is the occurrence of vascular complications. Epidemiological evidence from Europe and the United States has shown that estrogen/progestogen oral contraceptives increase the relative risk of thromboembolic complications. These hazards arise especially in association with older age of women, with smoking and also to some extent with prolonged usage of oral contraceptives containing 50 μg or more of estrogen. The main vascular complications are venous thromboembolic disease, myocardial infarction and both hemorrhagic and thrombotic stroke [1, 2]. These findings are from countries in which the incidence of vascular disease is high and may not be relevant to countries in which these diseases have a low incidence. Differences in coagulation tests are known to occur in different ethnic groups and geographic locations [3].

For any given dose of estrogen the available oral contraceptives have contained a wide range of types and doses of progestogen. Available evidence now suggests that venous thromboembolic complications are determined by the estrogen component while the thrombotic complications on the arterial side are due to both the estrogenic and the progestogenic components. This was suggested in the analysis of reports to the British Committee on Safety of Medicine, in which a significant positive association was found between the dose of norethisterone acetate and the incidence of ischaemic heart disease or stroke but not between the former and venous thrombotic events [4].

The increased incidence of venous thromboembolic episodes appears to be correlated with estrogen dosage, is limited to the period in which the oral contraceptive is taken and disappears within 4–6 weeks of stopping the pill. The increased incidence of coronary and cerebral episodes is not limited to the period of use of the oral contraceptive but persists over time and for about 10 years in women who have used oral contraceptives for 5 years or more. The pathogenic mechanisms involved in the arterial vascular complications arising in association with oral contraceptive use are much more complex than those responsible for venous thrombosis. Hypercoagulability and platelet aggregation are likely to be involved, but the other factors which predispose to the initiation of the atherosclerotic process in previously healthy vessels are clearly important, e.g. increase in arterial pressure and atherogenic modification in lipoprotein metabolism. Once an atherogenic lesion has developed in a vessel, the process is difficult to reverse because of self-maintaining mechanisms, and the lesions may therefore persist or take many years to disappear.

Female Contraception
Eds.: B. Runnebaum, T. Rabe, L. Kiesel

The Haemostatic System

The blood vessels, platelets, coagulation factors and the fibrinolytic system compose the haemostatic system. The physiological basis of the haemostatic system is to keep the blood flowing within an intact vascular tree. The system is finely balanced between coagulation and fibrinolysis. On the coagulation side a proteolytic enzyme, thrombin, is formed which converts fibrinogen to fibrin; likewise, on the fibrinolytic side a proteolytic enzyme, plasmin, is formed which dissolves the fibrin. In studies of the haemostatic system it is important that one investigates the balance between the two systems. Many studies emphasise one without looking at the response particularly between fibrinolysis and increased coagulation activity. The coagulation system operates like a biochemical amplifier, starting with picograms in initiating the process of activation of clotting and cascades downwards to produce grams of fibrin. The initial trigger may arise from within the blood (the intrinsic system) or from tissues (the extrinsic system). From either source the interaction of coagulation factors leads to the formation of either plasma thromboplastin or tissue thromboplastin which converts factor X to its activated form. The complex of activated factor X with factor V and calcium converts prothrombin to thrombin. Thrombin converts soluble fibrinogen into fibrin, which in the presence of factor XIII and calcium forms cross-linked fibrin.

Estrogen therapy is known to influence the clotting mechanism by increasing the levels of factors II, VII, VIII, IX and X, fibrinogen and soluble fibrin. The levels of antithrombin III and vessel wall fibrinolytic activator are also reported to decrease.

Comparison of 50- and 30-µg Estrogen Formulations

We have carried out serial studies comparing the effects of 50- and 30-µg estrogen pills on blood coagulation, fibrinolysis and platelets [5]. The estrogen/progestogen contraceptives which were studied initially were 50 µg mestranol with 1.0 mg norethindrone acetate, 30 µg ethinylestradiol in combination with 1.5 mg norethindrone acetate, and 30 µg ethinylestradiol combination with 0.15 mg levonorgestrel. The serial studies were carried out during a pre-treatment cycle, after 6, 12, 24, 36 and 48 weeks of treatment and 6 and 8 weeks following cessation of treatment.

Factor II activity increased significantly with all three preparations from the 6th week onwards and returned to the pre-treatment levels within 6–8 weeks of stopping the pill. The increase of factor II was significantly lower with the levonorgestrel combination from the 6th week of treatment onwards. Increases in the activity of factor VII were less in women taking the 30-µg preparations and were lower than those found with the 50-µg preparation. The increase in factor X activity was significantly lower with the levonorgestrel preparation.

A significant decrease of the coagulation inhibitor antithrombin III was found with the 50-µg pill and also with the 30-µg combination with norethindrone acetate. The group taking the levonorgestrel combination showed a decrease of antithrombin III at the 48th week. Fibrinolytic activity in the plasma was significantly increased with all three formulations. Similarly, fibrinolytic activity following venous occlusion showed a significant increase with all preparations. Spontaneous platelet aggregation was significantly reduced with all three preparations from the 6th week onwards.

These studies show that the effects of ethinylestradiol on coagulation, fibrinolysis and platelet function are dose-related, and that the 30-µg pills produce significantly less changes than those occurring with the 50-µg preparation. The results also show that the effects of the 30-µg pill are modified by the progestogen which is used in combination.

Levonorgestrel and Desogestrel Formulations

We have also studied the levonorgestrel triphasic pill, Trinordiol/Triquilar, and the monophasic formulation with desogestrel, Marvelon. A control group was included in this study.

Factor VII activity was increased by both preparations but more so in the women taking desogestrel. Factor X activity showed a similar increase with both preparations. The levels of fibrinogen and plasminogen were significantly increased with both preparations with no difference between the preparations. The triphasic levonorgestrel pill produced a significant increase in fibrinolytic activity, but the increase with desogestrel was less and did not reach statistical significance. Antithrombin III showed a significant decrease with desogestrel at 12 and 24 weeks, and a small decrease occurred with levonorgestrel at 48 weeks. Spontaneous platelet aggregation decreased significantly in women taking levonorgestrel compared to the control group, whereas no significant change was found with desogestrel.

Levonorgestrel and Gestoden Formulations

At present we are comparing low-dose estrogen in combination with levonorgestrel and in combination with gestoden. Our preliminary analysis shows that fibrinolytic activity is increased to a similar extent with both preparations. Factor VII is also slightly elevated by both preparations. An encouraging finding so far is that antithrombin III levels are depressed with neither the levonorgestrel nor the gestoden preparations.

Conclusions

These comparative serial studies have shown that the changes in coagulation activity, fibrinolysis and platelet function are related to the dosage of estrogen and progestogen. The new oral contraceptive formulations with low doses of estrogen and progestogen produce significantly less changes than occur with the 50-µg preparations. The absence of significant changes in antithrombin III with monophasic and triphasic levonorgestrel suggests that levonorgestrel counteracts the action of estrogen in depressing this coagulation inhibitor. The changes occurring in coagulation factors and inhibitors were less in women taking low-dose estrogen combined with levonorgestrel, indicating that the progestogen used in combination modifies the effect of the estrogen on the coagulation system. Fibrinolytic activity was also significantly increased with levonorgestrel preparations. The increase of coagulation activity may therefore be counter-balanced by the increased fibrinolytic activity and so protect the dynamic balance between coagulation and fibrinolysis.

Current research is aimed at finding the estrogen/progestogen combinations which produce the least changes in the blood clotting system and in other metabolic processes. The new preparations are a step forward and are likely to be associated with a further reduction of the relative risk of thrombotic complications. Since oral contraceptive formulations are used by many millions of healthy women, it is essential that both laboratory and epidemiological research continues, aimed at the increased safety of oral contraception.

References

1. Shapiro S (1986) Oral contraceptives – a time to take stock. N Engl J Med 315:450–451
2. Stadel BV (1981) Oral contraceptives and cardiovascular disease. N Engl J Med 305:612–618, 672–677
3. Bocaz JA, Barja P, Bonnar J et al. (1986) Differences in coagulation and haemostatic parameters in normal women of childbearing age from different ethnic groups and geographic locations. Task force on oral contraceptives – WHO programme of research, development and research training in human reproduction. Thromb Haemost 55(3):390–395
4. Meade TW, Haines AP, North WRS, Charkabarti R, Howarth DJ, Stirling Y (1977) Haemostatic, lipid and blood pressure profiles of women on oral contraceptives containing 50 mcg or 30 mcg estrogen. Lancet 2:948–951
5. Sabra A, Bonnar J (1983) Hemostatic system changes induced by 50 µg and 30 µg estrogen progestogen oral contraceptives. J Reprod Med 28:85–91

Effect of Oral Contraceptives on Carbohydrate Metabolism in Healthy Women*

S. O. Skouby

Diabetes Center, Department of Obstetrics and Gynecology;
Rigshospitalet, Department of Obstetrics and Gynecology,
Hvidovre Hospital Copenhagen and Hvidøre Hospital, Klampenborg, Denmark

Introduction

One of the earliest discovered metabolic effects following intake of oral contraceptives (OCs) was that upon glucose tolerance [1, 2]. Obviously any disturbance in glucose metabolism is of great interest because of possible clinical consequences. But the influence of steroid compounds on glucose metabolism is also of interest because glucose metabolism is closely integrated with lipid metabolism. Today a body of evidence substantiates that traditional brands of OCs with 50 µg estrogen or more and high progestational content decrease glucose tolerance and cause a rise in plasma insulin levels [3, 4]. Despite these findings no risk of developing clinical diabetes has been found in epidemiological studies [5].

The relative role of estrogens and progestogens for the impact on glucose metabolism has been a matter of discussion from the very beginning of the oral contraception era. The problem was first elucidated in the late 1960s and the early 1970s. Oral glucose tolerance tests (OGTT) were performed before and after 6 months' treatment with mestranol and ethinylestradiol, and no influence of the hormonal treatment was found [6]. The effect of the progestogens was later found to mimic the diabetogenic effect of the combined compounds [7].

Low-Dose Preparations and Glucose Tolerance

In the late 1960s and early 1970s OCs containing more than 50 µg estrogen were removed from the market and low-dose preparations with an estrogen concentration of 35 µg or less and with reduced and varied progestogen content were introduced. This happened after it became evident that both the steroid structure of the hormonal constituents and the amount of steroid were of significance in the undesired effects on glucose and lipid metabolism [8].

Only a limited number of studies have been published on the effect of low-dose OCs on glucose metabolism. Generally, two types of products have been investigated, both containing 30 µg or 35 µg estrogen combined with either an estrane (e.g., norethisterone) or a gonane (e.g., levonorgestrel). There has been conflicting evidence concerning the effects of these compounds. It has been postulated [9, 10] that products containing levonorgestrel are associated with more marked alter-

* Supported by The Danish Diabetes Association and a grant from Ove Villiam Buhl Olesen and Edith Buhl Olesen Memorial Foundation.

Female Contraception
Eds.: B. Runnebaum, T. Rabe, L. Kiesel

Table 1. Glucose areas (min × mmol/l) and insulin areas (min × nmol/l (mean ± SEM) calculated from glucose tolerance tests performed in normal women before and during intake of triphasic and monophasic oral contraceptives (ethinylestradiol and levonorgestrel)

Months	Glucose		Insulin	
	Monophasic	Triphasic	Monophasic	Triphasic
0	1038 ± 41	944 ± 44	53 ± 5	63 ± 17
2	999 ± 61	1071 ± 43	55 ± 8	58 ± 6
6	1039 ± 60	966 ± 44	65 ± 6[a]	63 + 5

[a] 0 versus 6 months, $p < 0.05$.

ations of glucose and/or insulin levels than products containing norethisterone, but not all investigations support these findings [11]. Using a monophasic preparation of 30 µg ethinylestradiol and 150 µg levonorgestrel we found in healthy nondiabetic women a slight decrease in fasting glucose values shortly after treatment was started [12]. No changes in fasting glucose, insulin or glucagon values or in glucose tolerance were observed after 2 and 6 months, although a significantly higher insulin response to the glucose load was seen during treatment [13].

More recently the triphasic ethinylestradiol/levonorgestrel preparations were introduced in an attempt to reduce the metabolic side effects of OCs by a lowering of the steroid dose. The progestogen is given in increments, 50 µg for the first 6 days, 75 µg for the next 5 days, and 125 µg for the last 10 days. The ethinylestradiol dose is 30 µg daily except during the middle 5 days when it is 40 µg. The ethinylestradiol ratio is 1.08 during one 3-week treatment period, whereas the levonorgestrel ratio is only 0.61 when compared to the most widely used low-dose monophasic ethinylestradiol/levonorgestrel combination. We have examined the influence of a triphasic compound on glucose tolerance [14]. After a 6-month treatment period the triphasic preparation resulted in a significantly lower insulin response to oral glucose in healthy, nondiabetic women than the low-dose monophasic estradiol/levonorgestrel preparation (Table 1).

Besides lowering the steroid dose, efforts have been made to develop new progestogens with less influence on metabolic functions. Several new drugs have been developed during recent years. Desogestrel and gestogen are among those which seem most promising. In a comparative study we found no change in glucose tolerance when these progestogens were used in low-dose combination with ethinylestradiol, although the insulin response to the glucose load increased during the hormonal treatment [15].

Mechanism of Action

The observed increase in plasma insulin during intake of low-dose OCs without a concomitant increase in plasma glucose points to a condition of insulin resistance. For these reasons it appears possible that the influence on glucose metabolism associated with the use of OCs may be mediated by a decrease in the binding of insulin to receptors in target tissues or perhaps by a postreceptor defect.

Insulin receptors are specific glycoproteins situated on the surface of the cell. The first direct demonstration of insulin receptors was performed 15 years ago [16], and further experiments established the relation between the binding reaction and the subsequent changes of intracellular metabolic pathways [17]. De Pirro et al. [18] reported cessation of the physiological cyclic variation of monocyte insulin receptor concentration and affinity during administration of traditional monophasic contraceptive compounds with 50 μg ethinylestradiol and a high progestogen content. Tsibris et al. [19] examined monocyte and erythrocyte insulin receptor binding in nonobese normal women. No differences in average affinity profiles and insulin receptor binding sites per cell were found between nonpregnant women in the follicular phase of the cycle and women taking either low-dose or traditional OCs. In a recent study [20] we have measured the influence of the triphasic estradiol/levonorgestrel compound on insulin receptor binding and found no direct relationship between intake of the hormonal contraceptive and change in insulin receptor binding to circulating erythrocytes or monocytes.

Measurements of insulin binding to blood cells in vitro do not necessarily reflect insulin action in vivo. Various other methods have therefore been used to assess insulin sensitivity in vivo. The euglycemic clamp technique is one of the best [21]. With this technique plasma insulin concentration is increased to a constant level by a primed continuous intravenous insulin infusion. Plasma glucose is maintained at euglycemic level by means of variable glucose infusion. After the initial insulin infusion a quasi steady state is reached in which total glucose turnover can either be quantified using a [^{3}H]3-glucose infusion or calculated from the unlabelled exogenous glucose infusion by a nonequilibrium equation [21]. We assessed in vivo insulin action using the euglycemic clamp technique before and during intake of a low-dose triphasic OC (ethinylestradiol and levonorgestrel) for 6 months and found the rates of glucose metabolised during the investigation decreased with 17% after hormonal intake for 6 months ($p=0.05$) [22].

Conclusion

The effects of combined OCs on glucose metabolism are dependent on the type of progestogen used and the estrogen/progestogen ratio. Use of low-dose monophasic or triphasic compounds seem to have no effect on glucose tolerance although a hyperinsulinemic response to oral glucose may be seen. The mechanism of action is most likely a decreased sensitivity towards insulin in target tissue due to decreased insulin receptor affinity or hormone-induced postreceptor defects.

References

1. Waine H, Frieden EH, Caplan HT, Colt T (1963) Metabolic effects of enovid in rheumatoid patients. Arthritis Rheum 6:796–797
2. Wynn W, Doar JWH (1966) Some effects of oral contraceptives on carbohydrate metabolism. Lancet 2:715–719

3. Kalkhoff RK (1975) Effects of oral contraceptive agents on carbohydrate metabolism. J Steroid Biochem 6:949–952
4. Spellacy WN (1976) Carbohydrate metabolism in male infertility and female fertility-control partients. Fertil Steril 27:1132–1141
5. Wingrave SJ, Kay CR, Vessy MP (1979) Oral contraceptives and diabetes mellitus. Br Med J 1:23–24
6. Spellacy WN, Buhi WC, Birk SA (1972) The effect of estrogens on carbohydrate metabolism: glucose, insulin and growth hormone studies on one hundred and seventy one women ingesting premarin, mestranol and ethinyl estradiol for six months. Am J Obstet Gynecol 114:378–384
7. Spellacy WN, Buhi WC, Birk SA (1976) Carbohydrate and lipid metabolic studies before and after one year of treatment with ethynodiol diacetate in "normal" women. Fertil Steril 27:900–905
8. Skouby SO (1986) Udate on metabolic effects of oral contraceptives. J Obstet Gynecol 6:104–109
9. Spellacy WN, Buhi WC, Birk SA (1979) Carbohydrate metabolism prospectively studied in women using a low-estrogen oral contraceptive for six months. Contraception 20:137–148
10. Wynn V, Adams PW, Godsland I, Niththyananthan R, Adams PW, Melrose J, Oakley NW, Seed M (1979) Comparison of different combined oral contraceptive formulations on carbohydrate and lipid metabolism. Lancet 1:1045–1049
11. Sadik W, Kovacs L, Pretnar-Darovec A, de Acosta M, Toddywalla VS, Ng CSA, Holck S, Belsey E, Pinol A, Hall P (1985) A randomized double-blind study of the effects of two low-dose combined oral contraceptives on biochemical aspects. Contraception 32:223–236
12. Skouby SO, Andersen O, Wagner HH (1983) The short term effects of a low dose oral contraceptive on glucose metabolism, plasma lipids and blood clotting factors. Contraception 28:411–420
13. Skouby SO, Mølsted-Pedersen L, Kuhl C (1982) Low dosage oral contraception in women with previous gestational diabetes. Obstet Gynecol 59:325–328
14. Skouby SO, Kuhl C, Mølsted-Pedersen L, Petersen K, Christensen MS (1985) Triphasic oral contraceptives: metabolic effects in normal women and those with previous gestational diabetes. Am J Obstet Gynecol 153:495–500
15. Petersen KR, Skouby SO, Dreisler A, Kuhl C, Svenstrup B (in press) Comparative trial of the effects on glucose tolerance and lipoprotein metabolism of two new oral contraceptives containing gestoden and desogestrel. Acta Obstet Gynecol Scand
16. Freychet P, Roth J, Neville DM (1971) Monoiodoinsulin: demonstration of its biological activity and binding to fat cells and liver membranes. Biochem Biophys Res Commun 43:400–408
17. Kahn CR (1985) Insulin receptors. Diab Ann 1:446–462
18. De Pirro R, Forte F, Bertoli A, Greco AV, Lauro R (1981) Changes in insulin receptors during oral contraception. J Clin Endocrinol Metab 52:29–33
19. Tsibris JCM, Raynor LO, Buhi C, Buggie J, Spellacy WN (1980) Insulin receptors in circulating erythrocytes and monocytes from women on oral contraceptives or pregnant women near term. J Clin Endocrinol Metab 51:711–717
20. Skouby SO, Kuhl C, Andersen O (1986) Oral contraceptives and insulin receptor binding in normal women and those with previous gestational diabetes. Am J Obstet Gynecol 155:802–807
21. DeFronzo RA, Tobin JD, Andres R (1979) Glucose clamp technique. A method for quantifying insulin secretion and resistance. Am J Physiol 237:E214–E223
22. Skouby SO, Andersen O, Saurbrey N, Kuhl C (1987) Oral contraception and insulin sensitivity: in vivo assessment in normal women and in subjects with previous gestational diabetes 1986d. J Clin Endocrinol Metab 64:519–523

Oral Contraceptives and Lipid Metabolism

T. Rabe, K. Grunwald, L. Kiesel, and B. Runnebaum

Department of Obstetrics and Gynecology, Division of Gynecological Endocrinology, Women's Hospital, University of Heidelberg, Voßstr. 9, 6900 Heidelberg, FRG

Introduction

The most important causes of higher mortality in users of oral contraceptives (OC) due to cardiovascular diseases such as thromboembolic insults, myocardial infarction and cerebral insults are related to changes in metabolism: changes in lipid metabolism with development of atherosclerosis, changes in carbohydrate metabolism with development of a chemical diabetes mellitus, and deterioration of the renin-angiotensin-aldosterone system leading to hypertension, changes in blood coagulation, fibrinolysis and morphological changes of blood vessels. These changes are caused predominantly by environmental factors (e.g., nutrition, physical activity, and standard of living) and less by genetic factors.

Large cohort studies in the United Kingdom and the United States have demonstrated for the white population a correlation between the dosage of contraceptive estrogen-progestin formulations and cardiovascular risk. According to these studies, estrogens are responsible for the development of venous thrombosis whereas progestins are responsible for the development of such arterial hazards as myocardial infarction, intracerebral bleedings and hypertension (Royal College of General Practitioners Oral Contraceptive Study 1981).

Atherosclerosis is the most frequent ethiological factor for cardiovascular mortality in the Federal Republic of Germany and in most other industrialized nations. The main risk factors are changes in the lipid metabolism (e.g., hypercholesterinemia), hypertension, and smoking. The detection of these risk factors and the determination of cholesterol and triglyceride levels are absolutely necessary for the prevention of diseases in women taking OC. If cholesterol and triglyceride levels are elevated, the low-density lipoprotein (LDL) and high-density lipoprotein (HDL) cholesterol levels must be determined.

Total cholesterol, triglycerides, and the cholesterol content of the lipoproteins LDL and HDL in the peripheral blood are prognostic factors for the development of atherosclerosis. Metabolic effects of serum cholesterol are modulated by the concentration of plasma lipoproteins. It is assumed that LDL channels cholesterol into the cell, whereas HDL removes excessive cholesterol from the cell. However, it is questionable whether lipoproteins of high density can be considered a protective physiological factor against coronary heart disease. Epidemiological studies revealing an inverse relationship between the incidence of coronary heart disease and the level of HDL-cholesterol have been performed in various countries with mixed groups of men and women in different age groups.

Female Contraception
Eds.: B. Runnebaum, T. Rabe, L. Kiesel

Therefore the epidemiological studies in the United States (e.g., Framingham study) can be applied only to a limited extent to OC-using women of reproductive age in the Federal Republic of Germany. Furthermore, the recent evaluation of the Tromsoe study in Norway showed that the incidence of coronary heart disease differs widely in different ethnic groups with identical HDL-cholesterol values. More recent data indicate that a possible protective effect of HDL cannot be evaluated in the presence of high LDL concentrations.

Epidemiological studies (Kannel et al. 1979; Hopkins and Williams 1981; Lewis 1983; Rifkind and Segal 1983; Grundy 1984) in which cholesterol, triglycerides, and lipoproteins have been measured show that LDL-cholesterol provides more specific and reliable information about the individual risk for coronary heart disease than any other parameter of the lipid metabolism. Additionally, the ratio LDL/HDL seems to be gaining in diagnostic value as far as coronary heart disease is concerned. It is assumed that the ratio of LDL/HDL (beta/alpha lipo-

Table 1. Composition of oral hormonal contraceptives used for metabolic studies

Progestin	German brand name	Formulation (no. tablets)		Dose (mg)
Norethisterone	TriNovum	7	Norethisterone	0.5
			Ethinylestradiol	0.035
		7	Norethisterone	0.75
			Ethinylestradiol	0.035
		7	Norethisterone	1.0
			Ethinylestradiol	0.035
Levonorgestrel	Microgynon		Levonorgestrel	0.150
			Ethinylestradiol	0.03
	Trinordiol 21	6	Levonorgestrel	0.05
	Triquilar		Ethinylestradiol	0.03
		5	Levonorgestrel	0.075
			Ethinylestradiol	0.04
		10	Levonorgestrel	0.125
			Ethinylestradiol	0.03
Desogestrel	Marvelon		Desogestrel	0.15
			Ethinylestradiol	0.03
	Oviol 22	7	Ethinylestradiol	0.05
		15	Ethinylestradiol	0.05
			Desogestrel	0.125
Gestoden	Femovan		Gestoden	0.075
			Ethinylestradiol	0.030
	Milvane[a]	6	Gestoden	0.05
			Ethinylestradiol	0.03
		5	Gestoden	0.07
			Ethinylestradiol	0.04
		10	Gestoden	0.1
			Ethinylestradiol	0.03
Norgestimate	Cilest		Norgestimate	0.250
			Ethinylestradiol	0.035

[a] German BGA approval claimed.

protein) gives more information concerning coronary heart disease than does total cholesterol alone. In control studies the LDL/HDL ratio was found to be 1.49 whereas in cases of coronary sclerosis, depending on severity, this ratio increased up to 2.75 (Stössel 1980). Nonetheless the basis of modern lipid analysis is still the determination of total serum cholesterol and triglycerides (Seidel et al. 1985).

Since only one-third of the cases at risk for cardiovascular disease can be detected by lipid analysis, other risk factors, such as disturbances of the carbohydrate metabolism, hypertension, smoking, way of living, and nutrition habits, must be taken into account particularly in young females using oral contraceptives. In this paper the influence of oral hormonal contraceptives on lipids, such as cholesterol, triglycerides, HDL- and LDL-cholesterol, and apolipoproteins is described. The formulation of oral hormonal contraceptives and the brand names in the Federal Republic of Germany as used in the various studies are summarized in Table 1.

Material and Methods

General Remarks

In this paper studies which are concerned with new synthetic progestins have been analyzed.

Observation Period. Metabolic studies during the use of oral contraceptives should be performed over a period of at least 6, preferrably 12–24 cycles, since many parameters need a long time to reach a steady state.

Types of Studies. A cohort study compares a parameter between a control group and a study group ("between-patient trial"). For this type of study larger numbers of probands and an exact selection of the control group is necessary. For metabolic tests a "within-patient trial" (longitudinal study) is generally chosen. In this type of study metabolic parameters during administration are compared to those before administration of oral contraceptives (pretreatment). The advantage of within-patient trials is the relatively small number of patients (minimum, $n=10$) required for statistical evaluation. Due to seasonal variations in the results of laboratory tests, values obtained in within-patient trials may give false positives or negatives if all probands are recruited at the same time; pretreatment values reflect the metabolic status at the respective time of year.

Data Analysis. For graphical display a boxplot analysis gives the most complete information for data analysis. Properties of the data distribution like 25th percentile (lower border of the box), 75th percentile (upper border of the box), median, mean, and outliers, are displayed simultaneously. For statistical analysis the individual metabolic data before and during use of oral contraceptives are related to each other. In respect to possible errors of measurement it is recommended for long-term studies to use two pretreatment cycles as a reference. Relative changes (percent of individual parameters) related to pretreatment values (100%) can also be displayed as boxplots. One advantage of this form of presentation is that results can be interpreted and compared to other reported data independently of the reference system, i.e., the normal range of respective laboratory parameters.

Analysis of the changes (as a percentage) of median metabolic parameters with one or two pretreatment cycles gives only weak information about the metabolic changes of individual probands. More accurate results can be obtained by, first, calculating the change in metabolic parameter of an individual as a percentage of pretreatment values and, secondly, calculating the median or boxplot for each cycle and the whole group. The studies considered here handle this problem variously.

Laboratory Tests. During the pretreatment cycle and during OC use laboratory tests should be performed during the highest steroid exposition in the blood. For steroids with short half-life this is identical with the day of administration of the highest steroid dose (in our studies days 20–22 of the menstrual cycle or OC cycle).

Clinical Trials

Clinical trials analyzing the influence of OCs on lipid and carbohydrate metabolism are summarized in Table 2. In the following, the individual clinical trials dealing with the metabolic effect of low-dose OCs are described. The studies are presented in order of the investigated progestins.

Formulations with Norethisterone

Rabe et al. (1984), Rabe and Runnebaum (1986c): within-patient trial with two pretreatment cycles and metabolic tests after 3, 6, 9, and 12 OC cylces during administration of a norethisterone triphasic pill (7 days, 0.5 mg norethisterone and 35 μg ethinylestradiol; 7 days, 0.75 mg norethisterone and 35 μg ethinylestradiol; 7 days, 1.0 mg norethisterone and 35 μg ethinylestradiol). Laboratory tests on days 20–22 at 8.00 a.m., fasting. Number of probands at beginning of study, 25; at end of study 12–15. In this study the influence of the norethisterone-containing triphasic on carbohydrate metabolism (oral glucose tolerance test with oligosaccharides corresponding to 100 g glucose; determination of serum glucose, insulin, and HbA_{1c}), lipid metabolism (total cholesterol, triglycerides, phospholipids, HDL-cholesterol, LDL-cholesterol, VLDL-cholesterol, and apolipoproteins A-I, A-II, and B), blood coagulation, liver enzymes, androgen metabolism, blood cell count, and electrolytes were analyzed.

Formulations with Levonorgestrel

Rabe and Runnebaum (1986b): randomized, comparative, within-patient trial of a levonorgestrel-containing, low-dose combined pill (150 μg levonorgestrel and 30 μg ethinylestradiol) and a gestoden-containing, low-dose combined pill. (For design of study see "Formulations with Gestoden.").

Table 2. Clinical OC studies on lipid metabolism

Gestagen, type of pill, FRG brand name	Author (year)	Number of subjects	Design of study	Blood sampling	Metabolism	Glucose metabolism
Norethisterone Triphasic pill TriNovum	Rabe et al. (1984, 1986c)	Start, 25; end, 14	Within-patient trial; 2 pretreatment cycles, 3, 6, 9, 12 OC cycles	8:00 a.m., fasting, 20th–22nd days of cycle	Lipids, carbohydrates	oGTT: 100 g
Levonorgestrel Combined pill Microgynon	Kuhl (1986), März et al. (1985)	Start, 11; end, 11	Within-patient trial with "switch-over"; pretreatment cycle, 3 OC cycles, 3 OC free cycles, 3 OC cycles (2nd OC)	8:00 a.m., fasting, pretreatment and 3rd OC cycle, 6th, 11th, 21st, 28th days of cycle	Lipids	Not investigated
	Rabe et al. (1986b, 1987a)	Start, 35; 6. OC, 22	Within-patient trial; 2 pretreatment cycles, 3, 6, 9, 12, 15, 18, 24 OC cycles, posttreatment cycle, interim analysis after 6 OC cycles	8:00 a.m., fasting, 20th–22nd days of cycle	Lipids, carbohydrates, hemostasis, hormones	oGTT: 100 g
Triphasic pill Triquilar Trinordiol	Gaspard et al. (1984a)	13	Within-patient trial; pretreatment cycle, 6 OC cycles	8:30 a.m., fasting, pretreatment cycle: 7 days before menstruation 6th OC: last 3 days of OC use	Lipids, carbohydrates	oGGT: 75 g
	Schijf et al. (1984)	11	Within-patient trial; pretreatment cycle 3, 6 OC cycles	9:00 a.m., fasting, pretreatment cycle: – early follicular phase – late luteal phase	Lipids	Not investigated

	Rabe et al. (1988b)	Start, 25; end, 12–15	Within-patient trial; 2 pretreatment cycles, 3, 6, 9, 12 OC cycles, posttreatment cycle	8:00 a.m., fasting, 20th–22nd days of cycle	Lipids, carbohydrates	oGGT: 100 g
Desogestrel Combined pill Marvelon	Schweppe (1983)	Start, 80; end, 40	Within-patient trial; pretreatment cycle, 1, 3, 6, 12 OC cycles, posttreatment cycle	Morning, fasting, on one of the last 7 OC days of the cycle	Lipids	Not investigated
	Gaspard et al. (1984a)	14	Comparative study: Triquilar and Oviol		Lipids, carbohydrates	oGGT: 75 g
	März et al. (1985), Kuhl (1986)	11	Within-patient trial; pretreatment cycles, 3 OC cycles, 3 OC free cycles, 3 OC cycles with, Triquilar	8:00 a.m., fasting, 3rd OC cycle, 6, 11, 21, 28 days of cycle	Lipids	Not investigated
		11	Reversed sequence comparative study desogestrel/levo-norgestrel		Lipids	Not investigated
Sequential pill Oviol	Gaspard et al. (1984b)	11	Comparative study: levonorgestrel (triphasic) desogestrel, see above		Lipids, carbohydrates	oGGT: 75 g
Gestoden Combined pill Femovan	Rabe et al. (1986b, 1987a)		Randomized comparative study with levonorgestrel-containing pill (Microgynon)		Lipids, carbohydrates, hemostasis, hormones	oGGT: 100 g
Triphasic pill Milvane	Gaspard et al. (1986a, b)	Start, 20; end, 13	Within-patient trial; 3, 6, 12 OC cycles	Not specified	Lipids, carbo-hydrates, hydrate	oGGT: 75 g

Table 2 (continued)

Gestagen, type of pill, FRG brand name	Author (year)	Number of subjects	Design of study	Blood sampling	Metabolism	Glucose metabolism
Norgestimate Combined pill Cilest	Anderson (1985)	Start, 603	Multicenter study; 1, 3, 6, 9, 12, 15, 18, 21, 24 OC cycles, interim analysis end of 1986	Not specified	Lipids carbohydrates	Fasting glucose
	Anderson (1985)	Start, 755	Multicenter study; 1, 3, 6, 9, 12, 15, 18, 21, 24 OC cycles interim analysis end of 1986	Not specified	Lipids, carbohydrates	Fasting glucose
	Kaiser et al. (1985)	Start, 21–22; end, 21–22	Within-patient trial; pretreatment cycle, 3, 6, OC cycles, posttreatment cycle	8:00 a.m., fasting, 20th–22nd days of cycle	Lipids, carbohydrates hemostasis	oGGT: 100 g

Gaspard et al. (1984a) performed a comparison trial with a desogestrel-containing pill (see "Formulations with Desogestrel") and a levonorgestrel-containing triphasic (days 1–6, 50 µg levonorgestrel and 30 µg ethinylestradiol; days 7–11, 75 µg levonorgestrel and 40 µg ethinylestradiol; days 12–21, 35 µg levonorgestrel and 30 µg ethinylestradiol) with 13 patients over six OC cycles.

Gaspard et al. (1986a, 1986b): randomized comparison trial with a levonorgestrel-containing triphasic and a gestoden-containing triphasic (see "Formulations with Gestoden"); 24 and 20 women, respectively, were observed over 1 year. A glucose tolerance test (75 g orally) was performed before OC use and after 6 and 12 OC cycles; serum glucose, insulin, glucagon, and insulin receptors on the erythrocytes were determined. Furthermore, serum lipids (total cholesterol, triglycerides, and HDL- and LDL-cholesterol) were measured.

Rabe et al. (1987d): within-patient trial with a levonorgestrel-containing triphasic with two pretreatment cycles, metabolic tests after 3, 6, and 12 OC cycles and 1 posttreatment cycle (part of all cases). Number of cases at start of study, 25; at end of study (12th OC cycle), 11–12; in the posttreatment cycle, 5. The study investigated the influence of an OC on the carbohydrate metabolism (oral glucose tolerance test with oligosaccharides corresponding to 100 g glucose; determination of serum glucose, insulin, and HbA_{1c}), lipid metabolism (total cholesterol, triglycerides, HDL- and LDL-cholesterol, and apolipoproteins AI, AII, and B), and blood coagulation. Blood sampling was performed between 8.00 a.m. and 9.00 a.m., fasting, on the days 20–22 of the menstrual cycle or OC cycle.

Formulations with Desogestrel

Schijf et al. (1984) performed a within-patient trial investigating 11 probands over six OC cycles with two types of OC: a desogestrel-containing, low-dose combined pill (150 µg desogestrel and 30 µg ethinylestradiol) or a levonorgestrel-containing pill (see "Formulations with Levonorgestrel"). Blood sampling and the oral glucose tolerance test were done at 9.00 a.m., and serum glucose and insulin were determined. In the pretreatment cycle metabolic tests were performed in the early follicular phase and the late luteal phase.

Gaspard et al. (1984a) compared the impact of a levonorgestrel-containing triphasic ($n=13$), a desogestrel-containing combined pill (see above), and a desogestrel-containing sequential pill (days 1–7, 50 µg ethinylestradiol; days 8–21, 125 µg desogestrel and 50 µg ethinylestradiol; $n=11$) before and after six cycles of OC use. Blood sampling was done at 8.30 a.m., 7 days before menstruation, during the pretreatment cycle, and during the last 3 days in the sixth OC cycle. Total cholesterol, triglycerides, HDL- and LDL-cholesterol, and apolipoproteins AI, AII, and B were determined. Furthermore, the carbohydrate metabolism was investigated by an oral glucose tolerance test (75 g glucose orally), and insulin receptors on the erythrocytes were assayed.

Schweppe (1983) investigated the effect of a desogestrel-containing combined pill (see above) on lipid metabolism (total cholesterol, triglycerides, and HDL- and LDL-cholesterol). Fasting values were determined (pretreatment, days 20–26 of the menstrual cycle; OC treatment, 1 of the last 7 days of OC use) after 1 ($n=80$), 3 ($n=78$), 6 ($n=75$), and 12 ($n=40$) cycles of OC use. Of 80 probands, 48 smoked more than 10 cigarettes per day, and of these 32 smoked more than 15 cigarettes per day.

März et al. (1985) and Kuhl (1986) investigated, in a randomized, comparative study with switch-over, 22 healthy volunteers (24–35 years of age) who had not taken OCs for the previous 3 months. A levonorgestrel-containing triphasic (see above; $n = 11$) and a desogestrel-containing combined pill (see above; $n = 11$) were compared. Blood sampling was performed during the pretreatment and OC cycles on days 6, 11, 21, and 28 at 8.00 a.m., fasting. Laboratory testing included parameters of lipid metabolism (total cholesterol; triglycerides; HDL-, HDL_2-, and HDL_3-cholesterol; LDL-cholesterol, -phospholipids, and -triglycerides; and apolipoproteins A-I, A-II, and B), testosterone, and SHBG. After the third OC cycle, OC use was interrupted for 3 months and resumed after switching the previously taken pill. Metabolic tests were performed as in the first part of the study.

Formulations with Gestoden

Rabe and Runnebaum (1986a, b) performed a within-patient comparison trial with a gestoden-containing combined pill (75 µg gestoden and 30 µg ethinylestradiol) and a levonorgestrel-containing pill (Microgynon; see above). Metabolic tests on days 20–22 of the menstrual cycle or OC cycle at 8.00 a.m. in two pretreatment cycles and after 3, 6, 12, 18, and 24 OC cycles and one cycle after end of OC use. Laboratory testing included carbohydrate metabolism (oral glucose tolerance test with 100 g glucose orally; determination of serum glucose, insulin, and HbA_{1c}), lipid metabolism (total cholesterol, triglycerides, phospholipids, HDL- and LDL-cholesterol, and apolipoproteins AI, AII, and B), blood coagulation, hormones, thyroid hormones, androgens, liver enzymes, blood cell count, and electrolytes. Number of subjects at start of study, 32. An interim analysis was performed after the sixth OC cycle ($n = 22$).

Gaspard et al. (1986a, b): randomized comparison study with a levonorgestrel-containing triphasic (see above; $n = 24$) and a gestoden-containing triphasic (days 1–6, 50 µg gestoden and 30 µg ethinylestradiol; days 7–11, 70 µg gestoden and 40 µg ethinylestradiol; days 12–21, 100 µg gestoden and 30 µg ethinylestradiol; $n = 20$). In total, 24 and 20 young healthy volunteers, respectively, were treated over 1 year. An oral glucose tolerance test was performed before OC use and after 6 and 12 OC cycles (determination of serum glucose and insulin and receptors on erythrocytes). Furthermore, investigation of the serum lipids (total cholesterol, triglycerides, and HDL- and LDL-cholesterol).

Formulations with Norgestimate

Kaiser et al. (1985; cited in Rabe et al. 1986) investigated the influence of a norgestimate-containing combined pill (250 µg norgestimate and 35 µg ethinylestradiol) on lipid and carbohydrate metabolism. Blood sampling was performed after one pretreatment cycle, after three and six OC cycles, and after one posttreatment cycle between days 18 and 22 of the menstrual cycle or OC cycle at 8.00 a.m., fasting. The following parameters were measured: total cholesterol, triglycerides, HDL- and LDL-cholesterol, and serum glucose, insulin, and HbA_{1c} before and after a glucose tolerance test (100 g glucose orally).

Anderson (1985): A comparison study with a norgestimate-containing combined pill (250 µg norgestimate and 35 µg ethinylestradiol) and a levonorgestrel-containing combined pill (300 µg levonorgestrel and 30 µg ethinylestradiol) was performed as a multicenter double-blind trial with 23 independent investigators in the United States. The observation period was 24 OC cycles (start of study, April 1981; interim analysis, January 1985). In all, 1196 women have participated in this study, of whom have 603 taken the norgestimate-containing pill over 5820 cycles, and 593 have taken the levonorgestrel-containing pill over 5928 cycles. All patients were evaluated for bleeding pattern, incidence of side effects, and contraceptive reliability. The majority of the women regularly underwent hematological and blood-chemical examinations. Glucose tolerance tests and ophthalmological examinations were performed by each investigator in 20%–30% of his probands. The probands of both groups had the same ethnic background, were approximately of the same age, height, weight, and blood pressure, and had an almost identical gynecological and obstetric history.

Anderson (1985): Investigation of the efficacy and side effects of a norgestimate-containing combined pill (see above) in a multicenter trial in which 23 independent investigators in the United States were involved. In all, 755 women were observed over 24 OC cycles (start of study, September 1983; interim analysis, January 1985); all were evaluated for bleeding pattern, incidence of side effects, and contraceptive efficacy. Hematological and blood-chemical examinations were performed at regular intervals. Each investigator performed a glucose tolerance test and an ophthalmological examination in 20%–30% of his probands.

Anderson (1985) also conducted another multicenter study with a norgestimate-containing pill, but details on this trial are not yet available. Two different groups of probands were evaluated: a combined group of women in which some of the probands had taken hormonal contraceptives until immediately before the trial (all subjects) and another in which none of the participants had taken any hormonal preparations for at least 3 months before entering the study (new subjects).

Influence of Hormonal Contraceptives on Lipid Metabolism

Total Cholesterol

Clinical Importance. Total serum cholesterol is an important factor correlating with development of atherosclerosis. The incidence of coronary heart disease seems to correlate with the serum level of total cholesterol (Carlson and Böttiger 1972; Assmann et al. 1981). The epidemiological relation between total cholesterol and coronary heart disease was shown by the Framingham study (Gordon et al. 1977) and the Primary Coronary Convention Trial (Lipid Research Clinics Program 1984 a, b). According to the latter, a decrease of 1% in serum cholesterol led to a 2% decrease in the risk of coronary heart disease. According to the Framingham study, a serum concentration of 260 mg/100 ml in the age group 30–49 multipled the relative risk by a factor of 7.6 when compared to a control group with a total cholesterol level of 200 mg/100 ml. In the age group 50–59 the same constellation led to an increase of relative risk by a factor of only 3.

The incidence of hypercholesteremia in the Federal Republic of Germany is below 5%. While the homozygous type with cholesterol concentrations between 700 and 800 mg/100 ml is fatal in many cases, the heterozygous type with cholesterol values between 300 and 400 mg/100 ml frequently cannot be recognized without adequate laboratory monitoring. This group of patients, in fact, has a higher risk through the use of OCs although only 25% of patients with cholesterol values above 300 mg/100 ml actually develop a coronary heart disease.

Oral Hormonal Contraceptives. Assmann (1986) showed an increase in total cholesterol of 15 mg/100 ml in the Procam study performed in the area of Münster (Federal Republic of Germany) with a group of 4500 females taking OCs.

Norethisterone. A norethisterone-containing triphasic pill led to a gradual increase in total cholesterol within 9–12 months of up to 13% (205 mg/100 ml) over initial values (Rabe and Runnebaum 1986a).

Desogestrel. A desogestrel-containing combined pill (150 µg desogestrel and 30 µg ethinylestradiol) did not change serum cholesterol values significantly during the first 12 OC cycles. No difference was found between a group of smokers and one of nonsmokers (Schweppe 1983). After three OC cycles an increase of 3% in total cholesterol was found in 11 probands (März et al. 1985; Kuhl 1986). In another study a 1.8% increase in total cholesterol was observed after six OC cycles ($n=11$; Gaspard et al. 1984a). Schijf et al. (1984) also found only minor changes (decrease of 1.1%) after six OC cycles ($n=11$). A desogestrel-containing sequential pill (0–125 µg desogestrel and 50 µg ethinylestradiol) caused a 9.6% increase of cholesterol after six OC cycles (Gaspard et al. 1984a).

Levonorgestrel. After three OC cycles a levonorgestrel-containing combined pill (150 µg levonorgestrel and 30 µg ethinylestradiol) decreased total cholesterol by 0.8%, and after six OC cycles by 2.4% (median, single values related to mean of the two pretreatment cycles = 100%; Rabe et al. 1987a). A levonorgestrel-containing triphasic (50–125 µg levonorgestrel and 30–40 µg ethinylestradiol) caused a 5% increase in total cholesterol after three OC cycles (März et al. 1985; Kuhl 1986). After six OC cycles Gaspard et al. (1984b) found a 4.6% increase in total cholesterol, whereas Schijf et al. (1984) reported a 12% decrease. In an unpublished study over 12 OC cycles Rabe et al. (1988d) found an increase in total cholesterol after three OC cycles of 2%, after six OC cycles one of 5%, and after 12 OC cycles one of 7% (median, single values related to mean of the two pretreatment cycles = 100%).

Gestoden. The gestoden-containing combined pill (75 µg gestoden and 30 µg ethinylestradiol) did not influence total cholesterol after three OC cycles (no change). six OC cycles (+2%) or twelve OC cycles (−2.2%) (median, single values related to mean of the two pretreatment cycles = 100%). No change of total cholesterol could be observed in a study with a gestoden-containing triphasic (50–100 μg gestoden and 30–40 μg ethinylestradiol) during 12 OC cycles (Gaspard et al. 1986a).

Norgestimate. Kaiser et al. (1985) analyzed the influence of a norgestimate-containing combined pill (250 μg norgestimate and 35 μg ethinylestradiol) on serum cholesterol in 21–22 probands. After three OC cycles a decrease in total cholesterol of 7% and after six OC cycles one of 3% was found; in the second posttreatment cycle total cholesterol levels were elevated by 5%. The impact of a norgestimate-containing combined pill (250 μg norgestimate and 35 μg ethinylestradiol) on lipid metabolism has been analyzed by Anderson (1985) in two studies in the United States. In the mixed group of switchers and new subjects total cholesterol increases ranged as follows: 3rd OC cycle, 0.5%; 6th OC cycle, 5.4%; 12th OC cycle, 4.2%; 24th OC cycle, 4.5%. For the group of new subjects (OC-free interval at least 3 months before beginning of the study) the following increases in total cholesterol could be found: 3rd OC cycle, 8.9%; 6th OC cycle, 9.6%; 12th OC cycle, 8.0%; 24th OC cycle, 8.1%. The higher relative increase of total cholesterol in the group of new subjects in comparison to the mixed group of new subjects and switchers is due to the use of other types of OC immediately prior to the study which had already caused elevated baseline values in the group of the switchers.

Summary. A review of the literature reveals that hormonal contraceptives cause variations between −10% and +15% of initial values (Fig. 1).

Triglycerides

Clinical Importance. Normal values of serum triglycerides are age dependent: under 40 years, below 120 mg/100 ml; between 40 and 60 years, below 150 mg/100 ml.

Triglycerides are components of lipoproteins and are potentially atherogenic, as has been shown by a prospective study in Stockholm performed by Carlson and Böttiger (1972), who found a positive correlation between the risk of cardiovascular disease and the serum triglyceride concentration. The atherogenic activity of serum triglycerides, as well as of VLDL and chylomicrons, and their catabolites has not been resolved satisfactorily and is presently controversial (Grundy 1984; Hopkins and Williams 1981; Kannel et al. 1979; Lewis 1983; Rifkind and Segal 1983). Hypertriglyceridemia, caused by an increase in VLDL of normal structure can be regarded as much less harmful than an increase caused by relatively small, abnormally structured particles of VLDL that contain high quantities of cholesterol. The role of plasma triglycerides, VLDL, chylomicrones, and their degradation products in atherogenesis has been discussed variously in the literature (Kannel et al. 1979; Hopkins and Williams 1981; Lewis 1983; Rifkind and Segal 1983; Grundy 1984). Since there are as yet no simple, routine methods to differentiate between the various forms of hypertriglyceridemia, there remains for clinical use only the determination of serum triglycerides, pre-β-lipoproteins and chylomicrons. With quantitative lipoprotein electrophoresis a method is available that has proven its value particularly in this respect.

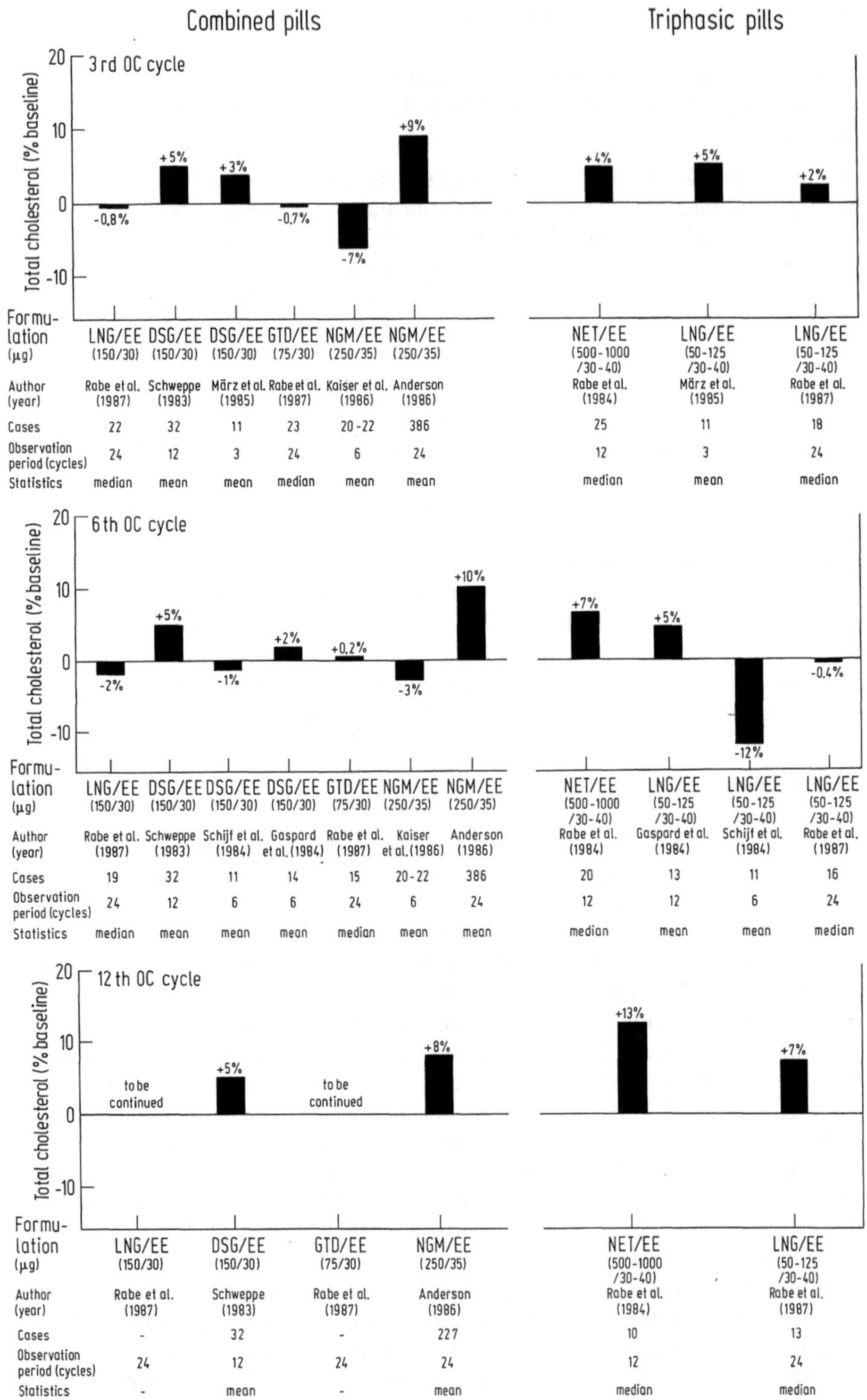

Fig. 1. Total cholesterol: changes related to pretreatment values in various studies after 3, 6, and 12 OC cycles. *LNG*, levonorgestrel; *DSG*, desogestrel; *GTD*, gestoden; *NGM*, norgestimate; *EE*, ethinylestradiol; *NET*, norethisterone

Hormonal Contraceptives. Contraceptives can increase triglycerides to up to 150% of baseline values (Wallace et al. 1977), particularly biphasic formulations and combined pills containing high doses of estrogens. The pathophysiological reason for these changes has been analyzed in oophorectomized patients; it could be demonstrated that triglycerides increase in oophorectomized patients after use of ethinylestradiol (Silferstolpe et al. 1982). Higher VLDL production is presumed to be responsible for this (Glueck et al. 1975). The effect of progestins on triglycerides seems to be dependent on their respective structure and dosage. Progesterone and norethisterone decreased the triglycerides by enhancing triglyceride catabolism via an induced VLDL catabolism (Glueck et al. 1975).

Norethisterone. Triglycerides were shown to have increased in the 3rd OC cycle by 26%, in the 6th OC cycle by 19%, in the 9th OC cycle by 41%, and in the 12th OC cycle by 19% (Rabe et al. 1984) in a group treated with a norethisterone-containing triphasic (0.5–1.0 mg norethisterone and 35 μg ethinylestradiol).

Desogestrel. Using a desogestrel-containing combined pill did not lead to a significant change in triglycerides during the first 12 OC cycles. No differences were found between smokers and nonsmokers (Schweppe 1983). In another study the desogestrel-containing combined pill lead to an increase in triglycerides of 25% after three OC cycles (März et al. 1985; Kuhl 1986). Gaspard et al. (1984a) found a 21% increase in triglycerides after six OC cycles ($n=14$). These results are similar to those of Schijf et al. (1984) who described a 27% increase of triglycerides after six OC cycles ($n=11$). A desogestrel-containing sequential pill (7 days, 50 μg ethinylestradiol; 15 days, 125 μg desogestrel and 50 μg ethinylestradiol; $n=11$) increased triglycerides by 90% after six OC cycles (Gaspard et al. 1984b).

Levonorgestrel. During the first six OC cycles of a levonorgestrel-containing combined pill (150 μg levonorgestrel and 30 μg ethinylestradiol) Rabe et al. (1987a) found after three OC cycles a 15% increase of triglycerides and after six OC cycles a 23% increase (median, single values related to mean of the two pretreatment cycles = 100%). Schijf et al. (1984) found in 11 probands that a levonorgestrel-containing triphasic (50–125 μg levonorgestrel and 30–40 μg ethinylestradiol) decreased serum triglycerides by 10% after six OC cycles. Gaspard et al. (1984a) found a 29% increase in triglycerides after six OC cycles ($n=13$). In an unpublished study over 12 OC cycles Rabe et al. (1987d) found a 33% increase of triglycerides in the 3rd OC cycle, a 28% increase in the 6th OC cycle, and a 28% increase in the 12th OC cycle (median, single values related to mean of the two pretreatment cycles = 100%).

Gestoden. In a study of Rabe et al. (1987a) the gestoden-containing combined pill 75 μg gestoden and 30 μg ethinylestradiol) led within the first three OC cycles to a 25% increase (third OC cycle), a 40% increase (sixth OC cycle) and a 49% increase (twelfth OC cycle) in triglycerides (median, single values related to the mean of the two pretreatment cycles). Testing a gestoden-containing triphasic (50–100 μg gestoden and 30–40 μg ethinylestradiol), an increase in triglycerides of about 35% could be observed after 6–12 OC cycles (Gaspard et al. 1986a).

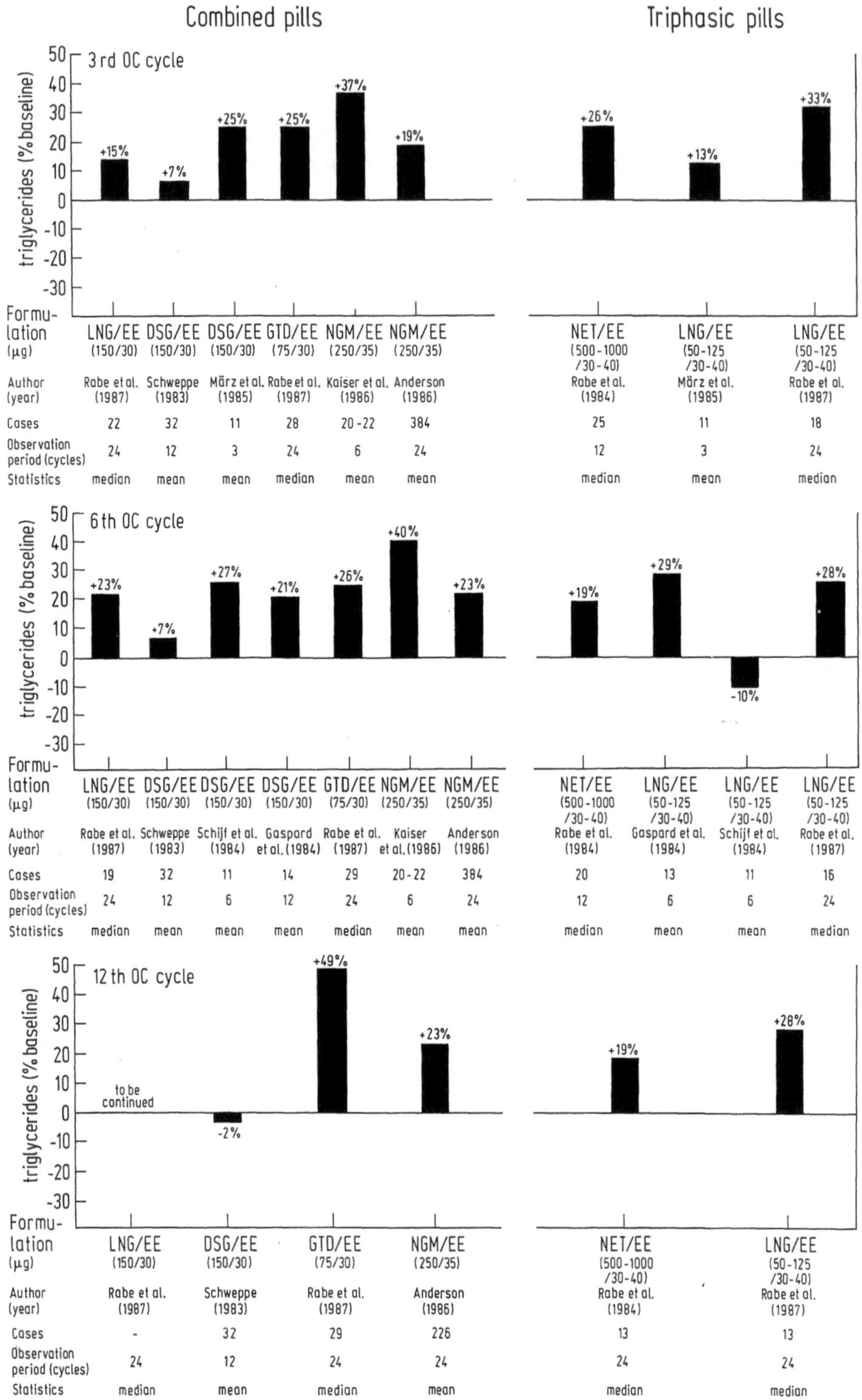

Fig. 2. Triglycerides: changes related to pretreatment values in various studies after 3, 6, and 12 OC cycles. *LNG*, levonorgestrel; *DSG*, desogestrel; *GTD*, gestoden; *NGM*, norgestimate; *EE*, ethinylestradiol; *NET*, norethisterone

Norgestimate. Kaiser et al. (1985) analyzed the influence of a norgestimate-containing combined pill (250 μg norgestimate and 35 μg ethinylestradiol) on serum triglycerides ($n = 21–22$). They found a 49% increase of triglycerides after three OC cycles and a 40% increase after six OC cycles. In a multicenter study in the United States the influence was examined of a norgestimate-containing combined pill (250 μg norgestimate and 30 μg ethinylestradiol) on triglycerides during 24 OC cycles (Anderson 1985). In the group of switchers and new subjects triglycerides increased as follows: 3rd OC cycle, 4.7%; 6th OC cycle, 6.7%; 12th OC cycle, 3.9%; 24th OC cycle, 2.3%. In the group of new subjects (OC-free interval before beginning of the study for at least 3 months) triglycerides increased as follows: 3rd OC cycle, 18%; 6th OC cycle, 23%; 12th OC cycle, 23%, 24th OC cycle, 9.3%. The changes in total triglycerides were statistically significant except the 2.3% increase after 24 OC cycles in the group of switchers and new subjects. The higher increase in total triglycerides in the group of new subjects is based on the fact that initial values of total triglycerides in the group of switchers and new subjects were increased by the previous use of other types of OC, and the relative increase consequently seems to be lower (see "Total Cholesterol").

Summary. Triglycerides under OC use stabilize after 8–12 OC cycles. During the use of low-dose oral contraceptives (combined pills or triphasic) triglycerides changed between −10% and +50% of pretreatment values (Fig. 2).

HDL-cholesterol

Various factors influence the HDL level in peripheral blood. Androgens are the most potent pharmacological agents which decrease serum HDL, specifically the HDL_2 fraction (Barr 1953, 1955).

Clinical Importance. The increase in the HDL fraction seems to be inversely correlated with the early occurrence of atherosclerotic lesions of blood vessels, an observation which had been mentioned by Gofman in 1951. In 1975 Glueck et al. reported in a study with 235 members of 18 families in which despite significant hypercholesterinemia only three cardiovascular deaths occurred. The observation that premenopausal women have a significantly lower risk of premature atherosclerosis than men can be explained by the fact that their mean HDL cholesterol is about 30% higher than that of men of corresponding ages. The best example of this new aspect in lipid research are the Eskimos in Greenland: their total cholesterol is as high as that of the population of Denmark, but atherosclerotic diseases have been registered considerably less frequently. This can be explained by their high HDL-cholesterol levels.

It is still unknown whether, as recently claimed, lipoproteins of high density are the only physiological protector against coronary heart disease. For instance, the recent evaluation of the Tromsö Heart Study in Norway (Miller et al. 1977) showed that the incidence of coronary heart disease in different ethnic groups with high HDL-cholesterol levels varied significantly. Recent data indicate that the possible protective influence of these lipoproteins is not effective in presence of high LDL concentrations. As early as 1951 it had already been shown that patients with low HDL levels had a higher risk of atherosclerosis (Barr 1953). Angiographic studies showed that the frequency of atherosclerosis correlated better with the HDL_2 fraction than with the total fraction of HDL (Miller et al. 1981). Assessment of HDL_3 provided no additional diagnostic and prognostic information (Wynn and Nithtyananthan 1982). An epidemiological correlation between HDL concentration and coronary heart disease risk could be shown for the first time by the prospective investigation of Rhoads et al. (1976) in a study of lipoproteins and coronary heart disease in Hawaii. This correlation was substantiated by the investigations of Gordon et al. (1977) and Miller et al. (1977). No relationship between HDL concentration and frequency of coronary heart disease could be shown by Bradley in The Walnut Creek Study in California (Bradley et al. 1978). If total cholesterol and triglycerides prove to be in the normal range in patients who suffer from coronary heart disease, HDL- and LDL-cholesterol need to be assessed for further analysis of risk factors.

Norethisterone. While pretreatment values of HDL-cholesterol were in the normal range (65 mg/100 ml), in patients taking a norethisterone-containing triphasic formulation (0.5–1.0 mg norethisterone and 35 μg ethinylestradiol) an increase in HDL-cholesterol of about 1% after 3 OC cycles, 7% after 6 OC cycles, 1% after 9 OC cycles, and 11% after 12 OC cycles could be seen (Kohlmeier et al. 1984; Rabe et al. 1986c).

Desogestrel. Schweppe (1983) analyzed the influence of a desogestrel-containing combined pill (150 μg desogestrel and 30 μg ethinylestradiol) on HDL-cholesterol in a group of healthy young females, some of whom were smokers. The pretreatment concentration of HDL-cholesterol in this study was in the lower range (45 mg/100 ml; pathological values lie below 45 mg/100 ml). During administration of the desogestrel-containing combined pill a normalization of HDL-cholesterol could be observed. During a longer treatment period (more than 12 OC cycles) a decrease of HDL-cholesterol to initial values occurred. In another study ($n=11$) OCs given over three cycles led to increases in HDL-cholesterol and HDL_3-cholesterol of 5.3% and 14%, respectively (März et al. 1985; Kuhl 1986). Gaspard et al. (1984a, b) found after six OC cycles an increase of HDL-cholesterol ($n=14$). Similar results have been found by Schijf et al. (1984), reporting a 6.8% increase after six OC cycles. A desogestrel-containing sequential formulation (125 μg desogestrel and 0–50 μg ethinylestradiol; $n=11$) in a study by Gaspard et al. (1984a, b) led to a 1.7% increase of HDL-cholesterol.

Levonorgestrel. During the first three OC cycles with a levonorgestrel-containing combined pill (150 μg levonorgestrel and 30 μg ethinylestradiol) Rabe et al. (1987a) found a 13% decrease of HDL-cholesterol. A levonorgestrel-containing triphasic (50–125 μg levonorgestrel and 30–40 μg ethinylestradiol) caused no change in total HDL-cholesterol after six OC cycles (Gaspard et al. 1984a). No significant change in HDL-cholesterol but a 6% increase of HDL_3-cholesterol was observed after three OC cycles by März et al. (1985) and Kuhl (1986). In a study by Schijf et al. (1984) no OC effect on HDL-cholesterol could be observed after six OC cycles ($n = 11$). In an unpublished study Rabe et al. (1988d) found a slight increase in HDL-cholesterol of 0.5% after 3 OC cycles but decreases of 10% after 6, 4.3% after 9, and 6.3% after 12 OC cycles (median, single values related to the mean value of the two pretreatment cycles = 100%).

Gestoden. A gestoden-containing combined pill (75 μg gestoden and 30 μg ethinylestradiol) caused a 2.1% increase in HDL-cholesterol after three OC cycles, no change after six OC cycles and a 11% increase after 12 OC cycles (median, single values related to the mean of the two pretreatment cycles = 100%) in studies by Rabe et al. (1986b, 1987a). The gestoden-containing triphasic (50–100 μg gestoden and 30–40 μg ethinylestradiol) has been investigated by Gaspard et al. (1986b). The investigators found a 9% increase of HDL-cholesterol after 12 OC cycles.

Norgestimate. Kaiser et al. (1985) analyzed the influence of a norgestimate-containing combined pill (250 μg norgestimate and 35 μg ethinylestradiol) on HDL-cholesterol. After six OC cycles they found a slight but statistically significant increase of 4% in HDL-cholesterol. In the second posttreatment cycle the HDL-cholesterol concentration was 3% above pretreatment values. During a multicenter study in the United States the influence of a norgestimate-containing combined pill (250 μg norgestimate and 35 μg ethinylestradiol) on HDL-cholesterol over 24 OC cycles was analyzed (Anderson 1985). In the combined group of switchers and new subjects (all subjects) HDL-cholesterol increased as follows: 3rd OC cycle, 6.6%; 6th OC cycle, 6.9%; 12th OC cycle, 6.9%; 24th OC cycle, 7.0%. In the group of new subjects (OC-free interval at least 3 months) HDL-cholesterol increased as follows: 3rd OC cycle, 4.7%; 6th OC cycle, 4.7%; 12th OC cycle, 3.9%; 24th OC cycle, 6.1%. These changes were statistically significant.

Comparison of Different Progestins. The influence of oral contraceptives on HDL-cholesterol depends on the type of progestin, its dosage, the dosage of estrogen, and the type of formulation (monophasic, sequential, or triphasic). The estrogenic, antiestrogenic, and androgenic partial actions of the different progestins seems to be important.

Summary. During use of low-dose OCs, combined pills, and triphasics, HDL-cholesterol ranged between −10% and +10% of pretreatment values (Fig. 3).

LDL-Cholesterol

Clinical Importance. LDL-cholesterol seems to play an important role in addition to that of HDL-cholesterol in the development of atherosclerosis. Circulating LDL-cholesterol complexes in the peripheral blood are channeled via a receptor-mediated process into the cells of target organs such as blood vessels and can subsequently accumulate there. Local inflammation or any process leading to damage of the endothelium, as occurs through nicotine, leads in the presence of high concentrations of circulating cholesterol to the development of subendothelial plaques. Therefore, LDL seems to be ineritably atherogenic. Possibly atherogenic

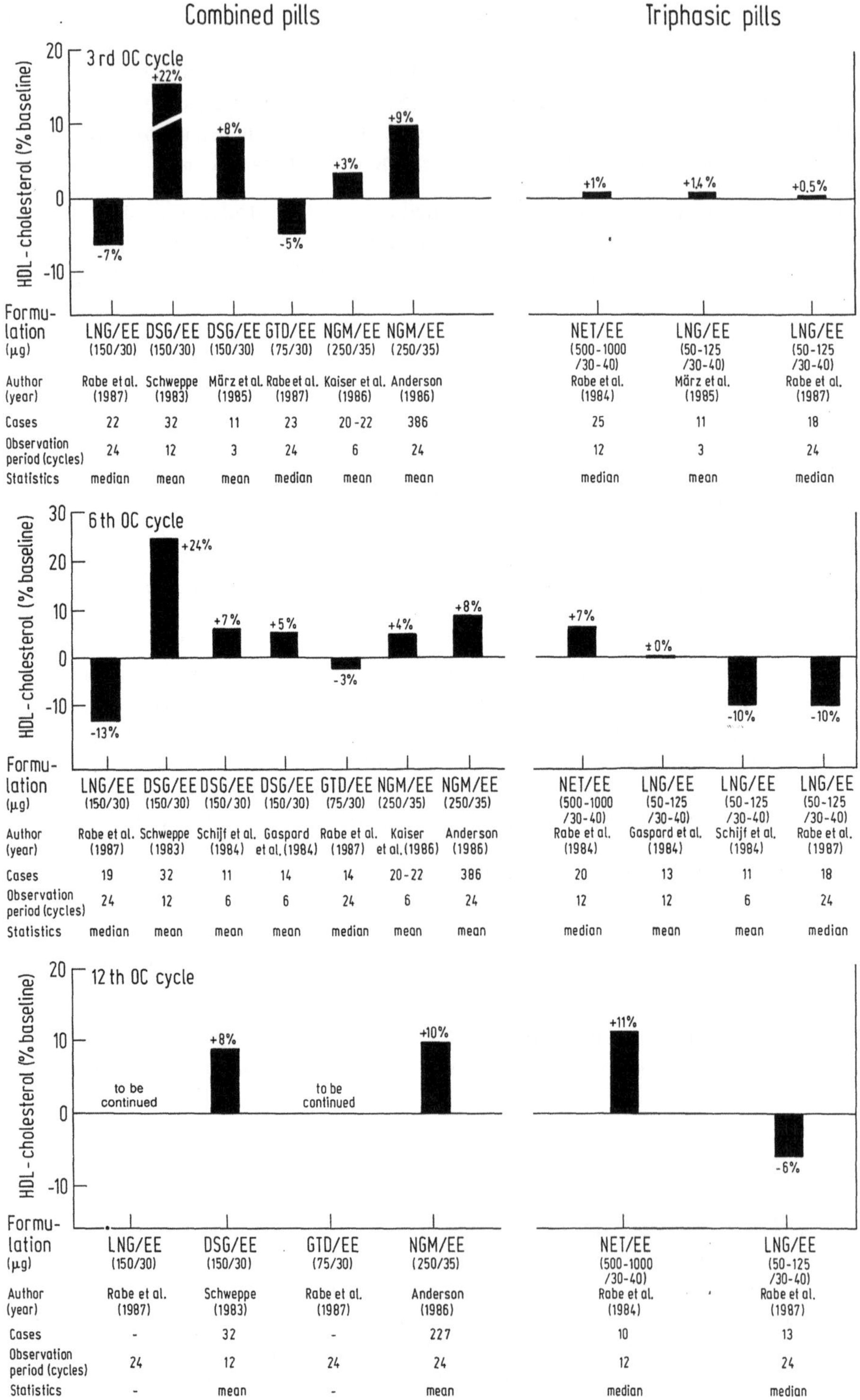

Fig. 3. High-density lipoprotein cholesterol: changes related to pretreatment values in various studies after 3, 6, and 12 OC cycles. *LNG*, levonorgestrel; *DSG* desogestrel; *GTD*, gestoden; *NGM*, norgestimate; *EE*, ethinylestradiol; *NET*, norethisterone

are VLDL and chylomicrons, whereas HDL exerts an antiatherogenic effect. The therapeutic aim of patients' taking steroid hormones consists of decreasing HDL-cholesterol and lowering the LDL-cholesterol fraction.

Norethisterone. In a study by Rabe et al. (1986c) pretreatment LDL-cholesterol levels were found to be 115 µg/100 ml. During administration of a norethisterone-containing triphasic (0.5–1 mg norethisterone and 35 µg ethinylestradiol) an increase of LDL-cholesterol up to 135 mg/100 ml (sixth to ninth OC cycle) could be observed. LDL-cholesterol increases (in relation to the two pretreatment cycles) could be specified as follows: 3 OC cycles, 2%; 6 OC cycles, 12%; 9 OC cycles, 9%; and 12 OC cycles, 3%.

Desogestrel. With a desogestrel-containing combined pill (150 µg desogestrel and 30 µg ethinylestradiol) a slight increase of LDL-cholesterol from 95 to 105 mg/100 ml was shown by Schweppe (1983). März et al. (1985) and Kuhl (1986) found an increase in LDL-phospholipids of 18% and an increase in LDL-triglycerides of 30% after three OC cycles. There was no significant increase in LDL-cholesterol ($n=11$). In a study by Gaspard et al. (1984a), OCs led after three OC cycles to a decrease in LDL-cholesterol of 5% ($n=14$). Gaspard et al. (1984a) reported that a desogestrel-containing sequential pill (0–125 µg desogestrel and 50 µg ethinylestradiol) led to a 3.6% increase of LDL-cholesterol after six OC cycles ($n=11$).

Levonorgestrel. During the first six OC cycles of a levonorgestrel-containing combined pill (150 µg levonorgestrel and 30 µg ethinylestradiol) Rabe et al. (1986b, 1987a) could show that the concentration of total cholesterol after three OC cycles decreased by 5% and increased after six OC cycles by 3.6% (median, single values related to the medium of the two pretreatment cycles = 100%). Using a levonorgestrel-containing triphasic pill (50–125 µg levonorgestrel and 30–40 µg ethinylestradiol), a 1% increase in LDL-cholesterol after six OC cycles was found (Gaspard et al. 1984a). März et al. (1985) and Kuhl (1986) found a 20% increase in LDL-phospholipids ($n=11$) and no changes in LDL-triglycerides ($n=11$) during three OC cycles. In an unpublished study by Rabe et al. (1988d) over a period of 12 OC cycles there was an increase in LDL-cholesterol of 7%, after 6 OC cycles 1%, and after 12 OC cycles 15%.

Gestoden. The gestoden-containing combined pill (75 µg gestoden and 30 µg ethinylestradiol) led in a study by Rabe et al. (1986b, 1987a) after three OC cycles to a decrease in LDL-cholesterol by 7%, while after six and twelve OC cycles LDL-cholesterol decreased by 6% and 9% respectively (median, individual values related to the medium of the two pretreatment cycles = 100%). A gestoden-containing triphasic pill (50–100 µg gestoden and 30–40 µg ethinylestradiol) was investigated by Gaspard et al. (1986b); after six OC cycles LDL-cholesterol decreased by 16% and after 12 OC cycles by 17%.

Norgestimate. Kaiser et al. (1985) investigated the impact of a norgestimate-containing combined pill (250 µg norgestimate and 35 µg ethinylestradiol) on LDL-

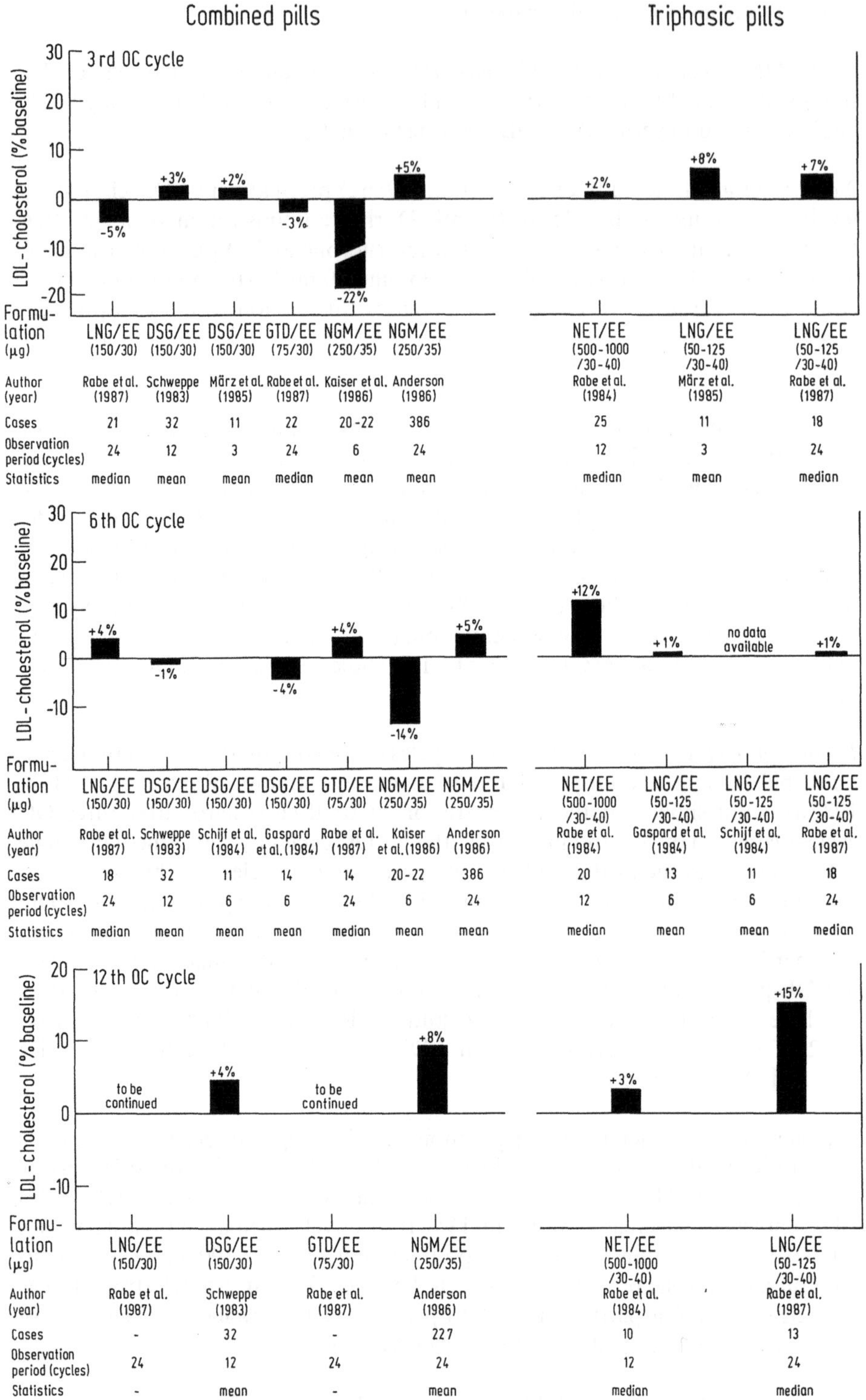

Fig. 4. Low-density lipoprotein cholesterol: changes related to pretreatment values in various studies after 3, 6, and 12 OC cycles. *LNG*, levonorgestrel; *DSG*, desogestrel; *GTD*, gestoden; *NGM*, norgestimate; *EE*, ethinylestradiol; *NET*, norethisterone

cholesterol. They could show a significant decrease in LDL-cholesterol of 22% after three OC cycles and 14% after six OC cycles. In the second posttreatment cycle no changes in relation to the pretreatment cycle could be shown. In a multicenter study in the United States Anderson (1985) investigated the impact of a norgestimate-containing combined pill (250 µg norgestimate and 35 µg ethinylestradiol) on LDL-cholesterol over a period of 24 cycles. Regarding all subjects together the concentration of LDL-cholesterol increased as follows: 3.4% after 3 OC cycles, 4.1% after 6 OC cycles, 2.4% after 12 OC cycles, and 5.9% after 24 OC cycles. In the group of new subjects (no OC use for at least 3 months) LDL-cholesterol increased as follows: 7.8% after 3 OC cycles, 8.2% after 6 OC cycles, 5.7% after 12 OC cycles, and 5.9% after 24 OC cycles. All changes of LDL-cholesterol were statistically significant. The relatively higher increase in the new subjects is based on the fact that the basal values in the combined group of volunteers (all subjects) are higher as a result of the previous OC treatment.

Summary. During the use of low-dose combined pills and triphasics the concentration of LDL-cholesterol varies between −20% and +15% of pretreatment values (Fig. 4).

LDL-/HDL-Cholesterol Ratio

The ratio of LDL-cholesterol to HDL-cholesterol is presumed to give more information concerning coronary heart disease than total cholesterol alone. In controls the LDL/HDL ratio was found to be 1.49, whereas in patients with coronary sclerosis a dose-dependent increase could be observed up to 2.75 (Stössel 1980). The results of recently published epidemiological studies (Grundy 1984; Hopkins and Williams 1981; Kannel et al. 1979; Lewis 1983; Rifkind and Segal 1983) in which lipids and lipoproteins have been measured show that LDL-cholesterol allows more specific and reliable evaluation of the individual risk of coronary heart disease than any other parameter of the lipid panel. Due to the fact that the LDL/HDL ratio has not been available in most of the studies cited in this paper or must be recalculated, no further details will be reported.

Apolipoproteins

Lipoproteins in the serum consist of a lipid and a protein component, the apolipoproteins. The lipid moiety of the molecule consists of phospholipids, cholesterol, and triglycerides; the protein moiety is composed of various apolipoproteins. Biochemical properties and molecular weight of at least eight different apolipoproteins have been determined to date. The amino acid sequence and biological function of a few of these are known. For a routine clinical diagnosis the most important apolipoproteins are A-I, A-II, and B.

Clinical Importance. In the literature the importance of apolipoproteins with regard to their evaluation for coronary heart disease has been controversially discussed. In patients with cardiovascular heart disease the concentration of apolipoproteins A-I and A-II is low, and the concentration of apolipoprotein B is highly increased. In patients with peripheral vessel diseases the concentration of apolipoproteins A-I and A-II is diminished and the concentration of B increased. In patients with cerebral vascular diseases the concentration of apolipoproteins A-I and A-II is strongly diminished and that of apolipoprotein B slightly diminished (nonsignificantly). It is assumed that the determination of apolipoprotein A-I and cholesterol allows a good prognosis as to whether patients with pectangious diseases will suffer a severe coronary stenosis or not. Significant differences of the apolipoprotein A-I concentration in patients with one-vessel, two-vessel, and multiple-vessel disease have been reported by Maciejko et al. (1983). The determination of HDL-cholesterol and total cholesterol allowed a discrimination between the groups with and without stenosis. The fact that normolipemic patients with coronary heart disease frequently showed normal LDL levels but increased apolipoprotein levels indicates the usefulness of an additional determination of apolipoprotein B.

Norethisterone. Changes in concentration of apolipoproteins A-I, A-II, and B under use of norethisterone-containing triphasic (0.5–1.0 mg norethisterone and 35 µg ethinylestradiol) has been analyzed by Kohlmeier et al. (1984) and Rabe et al. (1986c). An increase in concentration of apolipoprotein A-I by 3.8%, A-II by 6.9%, and B by 7.3% could be observed.

Desogestrel. The desogestrel-containing, low-dose combined pill (150 µg desogestrel and 30 µg ethinylestradiol) led to a 13% increase of apolipoprotein A; no changes of the apolipoprotein B level could be found ($n=11$; Schijf et al. 1984). In another study März et al. (1985) and Kuhl (1986) showed an increase of 27% in apolipoprotein A-I, an increase of 35% in apolipoprotein A-II, and no change of apolipoprotein B after three OC cycles.

Levonorgestrel. During the first six OC cycles of the levonorgestrel-containing combined pill (150 µg levonorgestrel and 30 µg ethinylestradiol) Rabe et al. (1986b, 1987a) could show that apolipoprotein A-I increased by 2.1%, A-II by 4.2%, and B by 15% ($n=19$). During three OC cycles with a levonorgestrel-containing triphasic pill (50–125 µg levonorgestrel and 30–40 µg ethinylestradiol) März et al. (1985) and Kuhl (1986) found that apolipoprotein A-I increased by 18% and apolipoprotein A-II by 22%, whereas apolipoprotein B did not change ($n=11$). In a group of 11 women taking OCs for three cycles März et al. (1984) found an increase in apolipoprotein A-I of 11% and apolipoprotein B of 7%. In an unpublished study over 12 OC cycles Rabe et al. (1987d) could show that apolipoprotein A-I increased after 3 OC cycles by 31%, after 6 OC cycles by 35%, after 9 OC cycles by 58%, and after 12 OC cycles by 30%. Apolipoprotein A-II increased after 3 OC cycles by 24%, after 6 OC cycles by 51%, after 9 OC cycles by 59%, and after 12 OC cycles by 42%. Apolipoprotein B did not change after 3 OC cycles, decreased after 6 OC cycles by 15%, after 9 OC cycles by 18%, and after 12 OC by 7% (median, single values related to the medium of the two pretreatment cycles = 100%; $n=13$–17).

Gestoden. The gestoden-containing combined pill (75 μg gestoden and 30 μg ethinylestradiol) led in the first six OC cycles in a study by Rabe et al. (1986b, 1987a) to an increase of apolipoprotein A-I by 7.5% ($n = 14$) and apolipoprotein A-II by 11.5% ($n = 14$), while apolipoprotein B did not change (median, single values related to the medium of the two pretreatment cycles = 100%; $n = 14$).

Norgestimate. No data are available about apolipoproteins under use of norgestimate-containing pills.

Summary. During OC use changes in apolipoprotein A-I have been observed between 0% and +60%, in apolipoprotein A-II between +4% and +60%, and in apolipoprotein B between −20% and +16%.

Conclusions

Atherosclerosis as the most frequent etiological factor for cardiovascular mortality is based mainly on a disturbed lipid metabolism. Therefore, with a view to preventing cardiovascular diseases, changes in lipids during use of OCs is of great interest.

In this paper it could be demonstrated that the difference between the various new low-dose oral contraceptives (combined pills and triphasics) in relation to formulation and duration of use lead to changes in total cholesterol between −10% and +15%, serum triglycerides between −10% and +50%, HDL-cholesterol between −10% and +10%, and LDL-cholesterol between −20% and +15%. Furthermore, variations of apolipoprotein A-I have been observed between 0% and +60%, apolipoprotein A-II between +4% and +60%, and apolipoprotein B between −20% and +15%.

It must be stressed that metabolic changes as discussed in this paper are expressed by mean and median values; this does not exclude that in an individual patient a strong deterioration of lipid metabolism may be observed.

As regards a negative impact of OCs on lipid metabolism, it seems important to measure total cholesterol and serum triglycerides before and after 12–24 cycles of OC use. In patients already taking OCs lipids should be determined, and if total cholesterol and serum triglycerides are in a normal range, no further lipid analysis is necessary since OCs can be regarded as a provocation test for lipid metabolism. In patients with pathological findings, HDL-cholesterol and LDL-cholesterol should be determined to detect any disturbance of lipid metabolism (e.g., hypercholesterinemia type II).

After exclusion of the risk factors of age, smoking, hypertension, diabetes mellitus, obesity, way of living, and nutrition habits, low-dose OCs (combined pills and triphasic) are considered to be safe and reliable methods for contraception in patients between 18 and 35 years of age. For patients between 35 and 45 years of age the use of OCs is possible when all risk factors are carefully excluded. No general suggestion can be made for patients between 40 and 50. Due to the fact that evidence of increased cardiovascular mortality in large-scale studies depends on only a small number of cases, the safety of the OCs in this age group has not been established.

References

Anderson FD (1985) Review of open phase-III clinical data on Cilest 250/35. Paper read at the XIth world congress of gynecology and obstretics, Berlin (West), September 15–20, 1985

Assmann G (1987) Oral contraceptives and lipids. 2nd International symposium: new aspects in female contraception – update and trends

Assmann G, Schettler G (1987) Die Prävention der koronaren Herzkrankheit. Deutsches Ärzteblatt – Ärztliche Mitteilungen 9:45–48

Assmann G, Schulte H (1986) Procam-Studie. Panscientia, Hedingen, Zürich

Assmann G, Schriewer H, Juchem KH (1981) Zur Rolle des HDL-Cholesterin bei der Präventivmedizin. Therapiewoche 31:5563–5574

Barr DP (1953) Some chemical factors in the pathogenesis of atherosclerosis. Circulation 8:641–654

Barr DP (1955) Influence of sex and sex hormones upon the development of atherosclerosis and upon the lipoproteins of plasma. J Chronic Dis 1:63–85

Bradley DD, Wingerd J, Petitti DB, Krauss RM, Ramcharan S (1978) Serum high-density-lipoprotein cholesterol in women using oral contraceptives, estrogens and progestins. N Engl J Med 299:17–20

Carlson LA, Böttiger LE (1972) Ischaemic heart-disease in relation to fasting values of plasma triglycerides and cholesterol. Stockholm prospective study. Lancet 1:865–868

Gaspard UJ, Romus MA, Gillain D (1984a) Comparative study of lipid metabolism and endocrine function in women receiving levonorgestrel- and desogestrel-containing oral contraceptives. In: Harrison RF, Bonnar J, Thompson (eds) Advances in fertility control and the treatment of sterility. MTP, Lancaster, pp 81–87

Gaspard UJ, Romus MA, Luyckx AS (1984b) Carbohydrate metabolism alterations with monophasic, sequential and triphasic oral contraceptives containing ethinyloestradiol plus levonorgestrel or desogestrel. In: Harrison RF, Bonnar J, Thompson (eds) Advances in fertility control and the treatment of sterility. MTP, Lancaster pp 107–111

Gaspard UJ, Lepot MR, Jaminet C, Jandrain B, Lefebvre PJ (1986a) Carbohydrate metabolism in women receiving two low-dose triphasic oral contraceptives, triquilar and trigestoden for one year. World congress of sterility and fertility, Singapur 1986, abstract, p 422

Gaspard UJ, Lepot MR, Gillain D, Sulon J, Buret J (1986b) Lipoprotein metabolism and carrier protein levels in women using two low-dose triphasic oral contraceptives (OCs), triquilar and trigestoden for one year. World congress of sterility and fertility, Singapur 1986, abstract, p 423

Glueck CJ, Fallat RW, Scheel D (1975) Effects of estrogenic compounds on triglyceride kinetics. Metabolism 24:537–545

Gordon T, Castelli WP, Hjortland MC, Kannel WB, Dawber TR (1977) High density lipoprotein as a protective factor against coronary heart disease. Am J Med 62:707–714

Grundy SM (1984) AHA special report: recommendations for the treatment of hyperlipidemia in adults. Atherosclerosis 4:445A–465A

Hopkins PN, Williams RR (1981) A survey of 246 suggested coronary risk factors. Atherosklerosis 40:1–52

Kaiser E, Panitz N, Groth (1985) Influence of cilest 250/35 on carbohydrate and lipid metabolism. XI World Congress on Obstetrics and Gynecology (unpublished data)

Kannel WB, Castelli WP, Gordon T (1979) Cholesterol in the prediction of atherosclerotic disease. Ann Intern Med 90:85–91

Kohlmeier M, Rabe T, Runnebaum B, Schlierf G (1984) Orale Kontrazeption und Lipidstoffwechsel. In: Runnebaum B, Rabe T (eds) Hormonale Kontrazeption. Steinkopff, Darmstadt, pp 58–62

Kuhl H (1986) Effekt von zwei oralen Kontrazeptiva mit abweichendem Gestagenanteil auf die Lipoproteinserumspiegel. In: Informed Institut für Medizinische Kommunikation (ed) 6. Internationales Gespräch, Münster/München 1986, Satelliten-Symposium: Hormonale Kontrazeption und Herzkreislauf pp 36–42

Lewis B (1983) The lipoproteins: predictors, protectors, pathogens. Br Med J [Clin Res] 287:1161–1164

Lipid Research Clinics Program (1984a) The lipid research clinics coronary primary prevention trial results. I. Reduction in incidence of coronary heart disease. JAMA 251:351–364

Lipid Research Clinics Program (1984b) The lipid research clinics coronary primary prevention trial results. II. The relationship of reduction in incidence of coronary heart disease to cholesterol lowering. JAMA 251:365–374

Maciejko J, Holmes D, Kottke B, Zinsmeister A, Dinh D, Mao S (1983) Apolipoprotein A-I as a marker of angiographically assessed coronary-artery disease. N Engl J Med 309:385–389

März W, Romberg G, Gahn G, Gross W, Kuhl H, Taubert H-D (1984) Effect of oral contraceptives upon serum lipoprotein pattern in healthy women. In: Rolland R (ed) Advances in fertility control and the treatment of sterility. MTP, Lancaster, pp 99–105

März W, Gross W, Gahn G, Romberg G, Taubert H-D, Kuhl H (1985) A randomized crossover comparison of two low-dose contraceptives: effects on serum lipids and lipoproteins. Am J Obstet Gynecol 153:287–293

Miller NE, Thelle DS, Forde OH, Mjos OD (1977) The tromsö-heart study: high-density lipoprotein and coronary heart-disease: a prospective case-control study. Lancet I:965–967

Miller NE, Hammett F, Saltissi S, Rao S, van Zeller H, Coltart Y, Lewis B (1981) Relation of angiographically defined coronary artery disease to plasma lipoprotein subfractions and apolipoproteins. Br Med J [Clin Res] 282:1741–1744

Rabe T, Runnebaum B (1986a) Progestins and carbohydrate metabolism. Int J Fertil [Suppl]:31–45

Rabe T, Runnebaum B (1986b) Arzneimittelprüfung von oralen Kontrazeptiva heute. In: Hammerstein J (ed) 25 Jahre hormonale Kontrazeptiva aus Berlin. Excerpta Medica, Amsterdam, pp 62–72

Rabe T, Grunwald K, Runnebaum B (1988a) Einfluß oraler hormonaler Kontrazeptiva auf den Lipidstoffwechsel; Teil 1: Lipidstoffwechsel, Cholesterin und Triglyzeride. Fertilität 4:35–51

Rabe T, Grunwald K, Runnebaum B (1988b) Einfluß oraler hormonaler Kontrazeptiva auf den Lipidstoffwechsel; Teil 2: Lipoproteine, Apoproteine. Fertilität (to be published)

Rabe T, Grunwald K, Runnebaum B (1988c) Pille und Kohlenhydratstoffwechsel. Fertilität 4:97–111

Rabe T, Runnebaum B, Weicker H (1984) Kohlenhydrat- und Androgenstoffwechsel unter oraler Kontrazeption mit einer norethisteronhaltigen Dreistufenpille (TriNovum). In: Runnebaum B, Rabe T (eds) Hormonale Kontrazeption. Steinkopff, Darmstadt, pp 40–57

Rabe T, Runnebaum B, Kohlmeyer M, Weicker H (1986) Lipid, carbohydrate, and androgen metabolism in women using a triphasic oral contraceptive containing norethindrone for one year. Int J Fertil 31:46–52

Rabe T, Runnebaum B, Unger R, Kohlmeier M, Harenberg J, Weicker H (1987a) Clinical and metabolic effects of two low dose combined pills for oral contraception containing gestodene (SHD 356C) or levonorgestrel (Microgynon). In: Genazzani AR, Volpe A, Facchinetti (eds) Research on gynecological endocrinology. Congress proceedings 1st World Congress of Gynecological Endocrinology, Madonna di Campiglio, Italien 1986, pp 503–516

Rabe T, Runnebaum B, Kaiser E, Anger H (1987b) Metabolic effects of a norgestimate containing low-dose pill (Cilest 250/35): on lipid and carbohydrate metabolism and blood clotting. In: Genazzani AR, Volpe A, Facchinetti (eds) Research on gynecological endocrinology. Congress proceedings 1st World Congress of Gynecological Endocrinology, Madonna di Campiglio, Italien 1986, pp 443–449

Rabe T, Grunwald K, Kiesel L, Runnebaum B (1988b) Einfluß einer levonorgestrelhaltigen Dreiphasenpille auf den Lipid- und Kohlenhydratstoffwechsel (to be published)

Rhoads GG, Gulbrandsen CL, Kagan A (1976) Serum lipoproteins and coronary heart disease in a population study of Hawaii Japanese men. N Engl J Med 294:293–298

Rifkind BM, Segal P (1983) Lipid research clinics programm reference values for hyperlipidemia and hypolipidemia. JAMA 250:1869–1872

Royal College of General Practitioners Oral Contraceptive Study (1981) Further analyses of mortality in oral contraceptive users. Lancet 1:541–546

Schijf CPT, Thomas CMG, Demacker PNM, Doesburg WH, Rolland R (1984) The influence of the triphasic pill and a desogestrel-containing combination pill on some physical, biochemical and hormonal parameters: a preliminary report. In: Harrison RF, Bonnar J, Thompson (eds) Advances in fertility control and the treatment of sterility. MTP Press, Lancaster, pp 61–69

Schweppe KW (1983) Erfahrung mit einem neuen Kontrazeptivum Marvelon unter besonderer Berücksichtigung des Fettstoffwechsels bei Raucherinnen und Nichtraucherinnen. In: Mall-Haefeli M (ed) Kongressband: Internationales Symposium des Sozialmedizinischen Dienstes der Univ. Frauenklinik Basel, 7./8. April 1983, Karger, Basel, pp 102–113

Seidel D, Cremer P, Thiery J (1985) Plasmalipoproteine und Atherosklerose. II. Lipoproteindiagnostik. Therapie der Fettstoffwechselstörungen. Int Welt 8:159–165

Silferstolpe G, Gustafson A, Samsioe G, Svanborg A (1982) Lipid and carbohydrate metabolism studies in oophorectomized women: effects produced by the addition of norethisterone acetate to two estrogen preparations. Arch Gynecol 231:279–287

Stössel J-P (1980) Wie entsteht Arteriosklerose? Med Klin 75:2–12

Wallace RB, Hoover J, Sandler D, Rifkind BM, Tyroler HA (1977) Altered plasma-lipids associated with oral contraceptive or oestrogen consumption. Lancet II:11–14

Wynn V, Nithtyananthan R (1982) The effect of progestins in combined oral contraceptives on serum lipids with special reference to high-density lipoproteins. Am J Obstet Gynecol 142:766–772

Oral Contraceptives and Lipid Metabolism: Interim Analysis of the PROCAM Trial*

G. Assmann and H. Schulte

Institute for Research of Atherosclerosis, University of Münster
Institute for Clinical Chemistry and Laboratory Medicine, Central Laboratory, Westfälische Wilhelms-Universität, Münster, FRG

Introduction

The Prospective Cardiovascular Münster Trial (PROCAM Trial) [1] was started at the beginning of 1979. The aim of the study was to establish the incidence of risk factors for myocardial infarction in the population, to investigate the relationship between the risk factors, and to improve prediction and early diagnosis of coronary heart disease. To this end employees from the public and private sectors were examined for risk factors for coronary heart disease and were surveyed to find new cases of lethal and nonlethal myocardial infarctions for comparison with already stored data. One main approach was to investigate the significance of a detailed diagnostic analysis of the lipid metabolism for the prediction of coronary heart disease. This investigation involved a physician using standardised questionnaires to put questions dealing with the history of the participant, the family history, nicotine and alcohol consumption, physical activities and – in women – the use of oral contraceptives. Additionally the blood pressure, the body height, and the body weight were measured and an electrocardiogram was done. Blood samples were taken after participants had fasted for 12 h, to assess more than 20 laboratory parameters. All results were communicated to the family doctor. The participant was informed whether the findings were normal or whether a check-up at the family doctor was necessary. This was the case in 25% of the women and in 40% of the men.

Results of the PROCAM Trial

By mid-1985 more than 18 000 employees from a total of 40 companies and public bodies had participated in the PROCAM Trial. One-third of the participants were women, two-thirds men and the age range was from 17 to 65 years of age.

In the PROCAM Trial 5322 women answered questions concerning the use of oral contraceptives. For the following evaluations 3630 premenopausal women participated, all of them between 20 and 49 years of age. They were not differentiated according to the specific oral contraceptives used.

* Supported by the Bundesministerium für Forschung und Technologie, Ministerium für Wissenschaft und Forschung NRW, Deutsche Forschungsgemeinschaft, and Landesversicherungsanstalt (LVA) Westfalen.

Female Contraception
Eds.: B. Runnebaum, T. Rabe, L. Kiesel

Table 1. The use of oral hormonal contraceptives related to age

Use of oral contraceptives	Age					
	20–29		30–39		40–49	
	(o)	(%)	(o)	(%)	(o)	(%)
Never	352	20.8	328	30.9	451	51.7
Formerly	527	31.1	430	40.5	272	31.2
At the moment	816	48.1	305	28.7	149	17.1
Total participants	1695		1063		872	

Table 2. Mean values of serum cholesterol level (mg/dl) and the proportion of participants with cholesterol concentrations of 260 mg/dl or more in relation to the use of oral contraceptives and age

Use of oral contraceptives	Age groups					
	20–29		30–39		40–49	
	Choles-terol	% 260 mg/dl or more	Choles-terol	% 260 mg/dl or more	Choles-terol	% 260 mg/dl or more
Never	174.6	0.9	189.2	3.1	207.6	5.8
Formerly	181.2	2.5	197.0	5.6	213.5	11.8
At the moment	188.9	1.8	201.3	8.5	215.1	10.1

One-third of the participants said they had never taken oral contraceptives (group I, 31.2%), one-third had formerly used the pill (group II, 33.8%) and one-third were using oral contraceptives at the time of the investigation (group III, 35.0%).

The frequency of the use of oral contraceptives in relation to age is given in Table 1. The proportion of the women who had never used oral contraceptives decreased with age; in the group of women who were 20–29 years old approximately one in two was using an oral hormonal contraceptive at the time of the study. The mean values of the total serum cholesterol level in the women who had formerly taken the pill were higher in all three age groups than in those who had never taken oral contraceptives, while the mean values in group III were even higher. The differences between the groups became smaller with increasing age. Differences in the mean values between present and former users of oral contraceptives were not due to an increase in pathological values (cholesterol level of 260 mg/dl or more), but to a slight shift in the distribution of the frequencies towards higher values, which, however, remain within the normal range.

The impact of oral contraceptives on the triglycerides (Table 3) was more marked than on the total cholesterol level. Although between the groups I and II only slight differences were found, the means of total triglyceride concentrations in group III were 20%–30% higher than in group I. In group III, triglyceride

Table 3. Mean values of serum triglyceride level (mg/dl) and the percentage of participants with triglyceride concentrations of 200 mg/dl or more (of 150 mg/dl in parenthesis) in relation to the use of oral contraceptives and age

Use of oral contraceptives	Age groups					
	20–29		30–39		40–49	
	Mean triglyceride	% ≧ 200 mg/dl (≧ 150 mg/dl)	Mean triglyceride	% ≧ 200 mg/dl (≧ 150 mg/dl)	Mean triglyceride	% ≧ 200 mg/dl (≧ 150 mg/dl)
Never	71.6	0.6 (2.9)	91.4	4.9 (8.9)	90.5	3.6 (10.3)
Formerly	74.2	1.1 (4.7)	84.8	2.6 (5.4)	93.3	3.7 (8.5)
At the moment	104.4	5.1 (12.6)	108.9	3.9 (16.0)	110.6	5.4 (16.9)
Total participants	1695		1063		872	

Table 4. Mean values of the HDL cholesterol level (mg/dl) and the percentage of participants with a HDL cholesterol value of ≦45 mg/dl in relation to the use of oral contraceptives and age

Use of oral contraceptives	Age groups					
	20–29		30–39		40–49	
	Mean HDL cholesterol level	% ≦ 45 mg/dl	Mean HDL cholesterol level	% ≦ 45 mg/dl	Mean HDL cholesterol level	% ≦ 45 mg/dl
Never	53.4	21.7	52.2	29.9	56.0	19.9
Formerly	56.9	17.1	57.0	20.0	59.2	14.7
At the moment	58.4	18.8	58.7	17.2	55.4	22.3
Total participants	1695		1063		872	

Table 5. Mean values of HDL apolipoprotein AI level (mg/dl) in relation to the use of oral contraceptives and age

Use of oral concentrations	Age groups					
	20–29		30–39		40–49	
	Mean HDL apo AI level	*n*	Mean HDL apo AI level	*n*	Mean HDL apo AI level	*n*
Never	140.0	150	137.7	142	146.6	165
Formerly	141.2	157	140.8	107	146.8	59
At the moment	150.8	168	156.2	85	146.8	51

values of 200 mg/dl were found only in those patients under 30 years of age, while in all older participants the differences in the mean values were caused by a more frequent incidence of values between 150 and 200 mg/dl.

The high density lipoprotein (HDL) cholesterol concentrations were higher in all age groups in group II than in group I (Table 4). In group III, only in women under 40 years of age are there mean values higher (by about 10%) than in group I. High density lipoprotein cholesterol concentrations markedly lower (45 mg/dl) than in group I were found only in the women between 30 and 39 years of age in group III.

High density lipoprotein apolipoprotein AI concentrations were only assessed in some of the participants ($n = 1084$). Between the subgroups of the women who had never and those who had formerly taken oral contraceptives no differences could be found. Like HDL cholesterol, the mean HDL apolipoprotein AI concentrations were 10% higher in those women who were using oral contraceptives at the time of investigation than in those women who were not using oral contraceptives (Table 5).

Low density lipoprotein (LDL) cholesterol values were calculated according to the Friedewald formula. No statistically significant differences could be found between the three age groups (Table 6).

Since the body weight correlates to lipid parameters we had to find out whether the observed differences between the lipid levels for groups I–III are explainable by differences in body weight. It was established that groups II and III had mean Broca indexes that were 5 to 10 points lower than in group I (Table 7). Consequently the differences in the serum concentrations of cholesterol and triglycerides would have been even greater if the body weight had been taken into account. The mean values of blood pressure did not reveal any differences between the three groups of the youngest age range (Table 8). A slightly higher incidence of increased blood pressure was found, increasing with age, in that group of women who were not taking oral contraceptives at the time of investigation.

The combination of smoking and the use of oral contraceptives increases atherogenic risk. It is thus highly relevant that the percentage of smokers among the 20–39-year-old women in groups II and III was significantly higher than in group I (Table 9).

Table 6. Mean values of the LDL cholesterol level (mg/dl) and the percentage of participants with increased values (of 150 mg/dl) in relation to the use of oral contraceptives and age

Use of oral contraceptives	Age groups					
	20–29		30–39		40–49	
	Mean LDL cholesterol	% (≧150 mg/dl)	Mean LDL cholesterol	% (≧150 mg/dl)	Mean LDL cholesterol	% (≧150 mg/dl)
Never	106.9	8.3	119.1	12.1	132.6	29.8
Formerly	109.4	8.9	123.1	19.1	136.0	28.7
At the moment	109.7	8.3	120.9	18.2	137.7	35.9

Table 7. Mean values of Broca-Index and proportion of overweight probands (Broca-Index >110/>120 in brackets) dependent on intake of oral anticonceptives and age

Intake of oral anticonceptives	Age		
	20–29	30–39	40–49
Never	96.6 17.6% (8.0%)	108.0 43.0% (25.3%)	109.0 40.7% (24.0%)
Formerly	92.3 9.3% (4.6%)	99.2 20.7% (11.0%)	102.1 26.3% (13.0%)
At the moment	91.0 6.1% (2.3%)	98.5 21.1% (10.2%)	104.1 31.8% (15.5%)

Table 8. Mean values of blood pressure (mmHg) and proportion of probands with values of 160/95 mmHg and more dependent on intake of oral anticonceptives and age

Intake of oral anticonceptives	Age		
	20–29	30–39	40–49
Never	117.2/76.4 (2.3%)	120.6/79.8 (6.4%)	127.7/84.1 (14.9%)
Formerly	116.1/75.3 (1.7%)	120.3/78.9 (5.1%)	125.8/83.1 (12.9%)
At the moment	118.2/76.0 (2.3%)	123.5/81.3 (7.6%)	132.8/86.7 (20.8%)

Table 9. Mean consumption of cigarettes and percentage of smokers in relation to the use of oral contraceptives and age

Use of oral contraceptives	Age of groups					
	20–29		30–39		40–49	
	Mean consumption	% Smokers	Mean consumption	% Smokers	Mean consumption	% Smokers
Never	13.5	30.4	14.5	28.0	13.8	21.3
Formerly	16.3	50.9	18.1	43.0	16.3	24.6
At the moment	17.0	48.2	17.4	39.7	17.6	24.8

In fact, 23.2% of *all* 20–29-year-old women and 11.4% of *all* 30–39-year-old women had both risk factors, while 15.8% of the youngest and 17.4% of the middle age group were smokers who were additionally using oral contraceptives. Thus in total almost 40% of all 20–29 year olds and 30% of all 30–39-year-old participants of the PROCAM Trial had been exposed at some time to this particular combination of atherogenic risks. The incidence of coronary heart disease is very rare in women in the age group investigated by the PROCAM Trial. For this reason no statistically proved statements about the significance of the risk factors in our study for predicting coronary heart disease in women – in contrast to men [2] – can be made. This is likely to be feasible in a few years time.

Oral Contraception and Ovarian Function

M. Mall-Haefeli, I. Werner-Zodrow, P. R. Huber, and A. Edelmann
Universitätsfrauenklinik, Kantonsspital, 4301 Basel, Switzerland

Introduction

Low-dose ovulation inhibitors are being used increasingly to reduce the adverse metabolic effects of oral contraceptives containing high doses of hormones. Both reduction and variation of dosage are applied during the individual treatment cycle. It has been observed that low-dose ovulation inhibitors are more likely to cause breakthrough bleeding and spotting in the first treatment cycles. Furthermore, mastodynia and mastopathy are frequently seen in women taking low-dose contraceptives. Functional ovarian cysts were detected by ultrasound in a high percentage of cases where lower abdominal pain persisted over a period of time [6]. Where ovarian cysts were not present, maturing follicles were found in some women. These clinical symptoms are often associated with elevated endogenous estrogen concentrations, an observation that has been confirmed by Spellacy et al. [9], Kuttenn et al. [3] and Gompel and Kuttenn [2].

Subjects and Methods

A total of 108 healthy young women took part in an extensive, controlled endocrinological study in order to determine whether ingestion of a low-dose hormonal contraceptive would lead to endogenous hyperestrogenicity as a result of inadequate suppression of the hypothalamic-pituitary-ovarian axis. Four groups of subjects were formed, and each group was given a differently combined contraceptive containing different doses of ethinylestradiol and desogestrel during six cycles. The composition of the four ovulation inhibitors used in the study can be seen in Table 1. The number of cases and age distribution within the individual groups are shown in Table 2.

Table 1. Composition of the preparations

CTR-10	21 tablets:	20 μg ethinylestradiol + 150 μg desogestrel
Marvelon	21 tablets:	30 μg ethinylestradiol + 150 μg desogestrel
CTR-14	7 tablets:	40 μg ethinylestradiol + 25 μg desogestrel
	+ 14 tablets:	30 μg ethinylestradiol + 125 μg desogestrel
Oviol	7 tablets:	50 μg ethinylestradiol
	+ 15 tablets:	50 μg ethinylestradiol + 125 μg desogestrel

Female Contraception
Eds.: B. Runnebaum, T. Rabe, L. Kiesel

Table 2. Age and number of subjects

	CTR-10	Marvelon	CTR-14	Oviol
Average age	22.76	20.33	24	25.6
Maximum age	38	28	34	33
Minimum age	15	15	19	17
Number of subjects	38	33	27	10

Age in years.
Study of the Department of Social Medicine, University Clinic of Obstetrics and Gynaecology, Basle 1986.

Table 3. Hormones tested, test system, manufacturer, literature

Hormone	Test system/Manufacturer/Literature
Luteinizing hormone (LH)	RIA, IRE (Institut National des Radioéléments, Fleurus, Belgium)
Follicle-stimulating hormone (FSH)	RIA, IRE (Institut National des Radioéléments, Fleurus, Belgium)
Prolactin	RIA, IRE (Institut National des Radioéléments, Fleurus, Belgium)
Progesterone	RIA, International CIS, France
Testosterone	RIA, International CIS, France
Estradiol	RIA, Hausmethode Frauenklinik, Kantonsspital, Basel, Switzerland
Sex hormone-binding globulin (SHBG)	Radioassay, Literature: [11]
Free testosterone	Wiest et al., Literature: [12]
DHEA-S	RIA, Eidg. Institut für Reaktorforschung (EIR), Würenlingen, Switzerland
DHEA	RIA, Diagnostic Products (DPC), USA
Androstendion (A 2)	RIA, Diagnostic Products (DPC), USA

An intravenous gonadotropin-releasing hormone (GnRH) test using 50 µg active substance was performed between the 21st and 23rd day of the pretreatment cycle, in the third and sixth cycles during treatment and in the first cycle after treatment. Parameters tested were the following: luteinizing hormone (LH), follicle-stimulating hormone (FSH), prolactin, estradiol (E_2), progesterone, sex hormone-binding globulin (SHBG), testosterone, free testosterone, and dehydroepiandrosterone-S (DHEA-S) (see Table 3).

Results

In the CTR-10 group the mean concentrations of basal and stimulated LH decreased significantly during treatment compared to pretreatment cycle levels. Posttreatment cycles showed a return to control values in basal LH levels and in

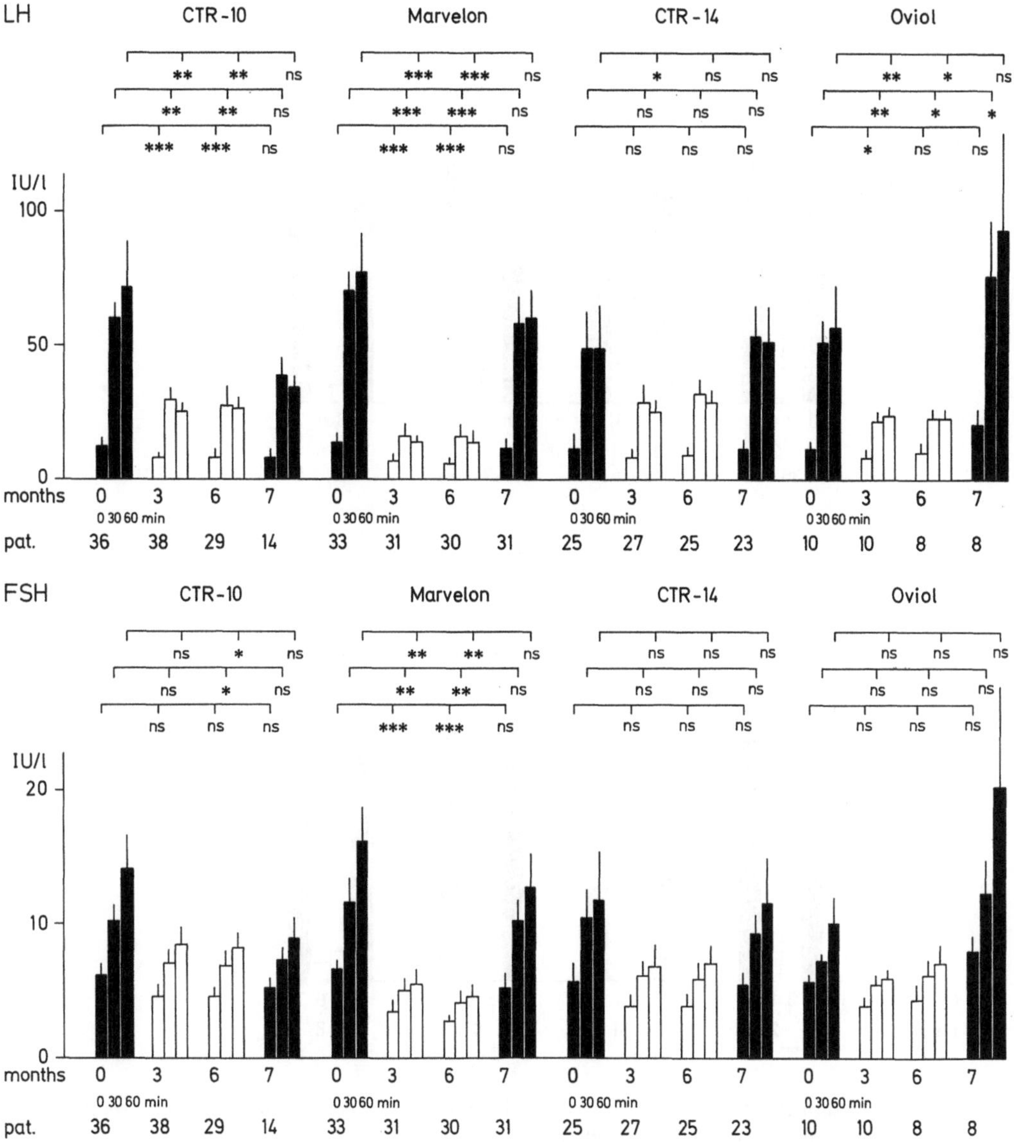

Fig. 1. Luteinizing hormone (*LH*) and follicle-stimulating hormone concentrations before and after stimulation with LH-RH. *Unshaded bars*, with medication; *shaded bars*, without medication; $^{*}p<0.05$; $^{**}p<0.01$; $^{***}p<0.001$

LH reserve. In the Marvelon group both basal and stimulated LH concentrations were significantly suppressed during treatment in comparison to the control cycles. The CTR-14 group showed no significant difference in basal LH values during the whole observation period of eight cycles. The standard error was, however, seen to be smaller in the posttreatment cycle. No variation was observed in the stimulated LH values, i.e., the reserve remained unchanged. In the Oviol

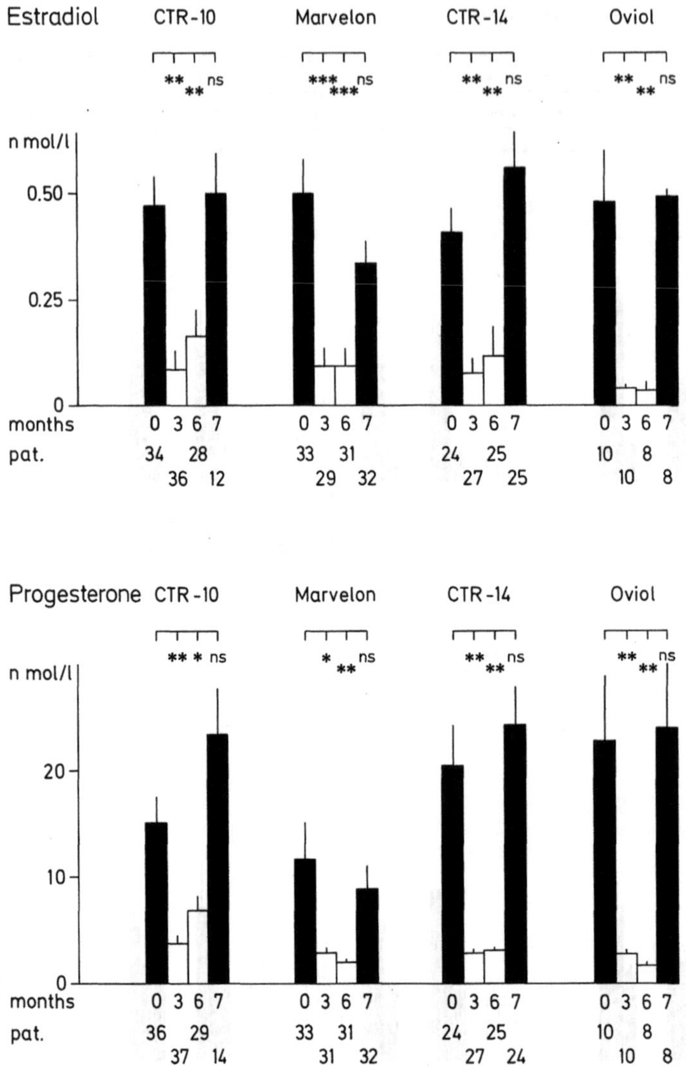

Fig. 2. Estradiol and progesterone concentrations. *Unshaded bars*, with medication; *shaded bars*, without medication; *p* values, see Fig. 1

Table 4. Ovarian suppression

Preparation	No suppression	Suppression	Total
CTR-10	10	21	31
CTR-14	4	21	25
Marvelon	2	31	33
Oviol	0	10	10

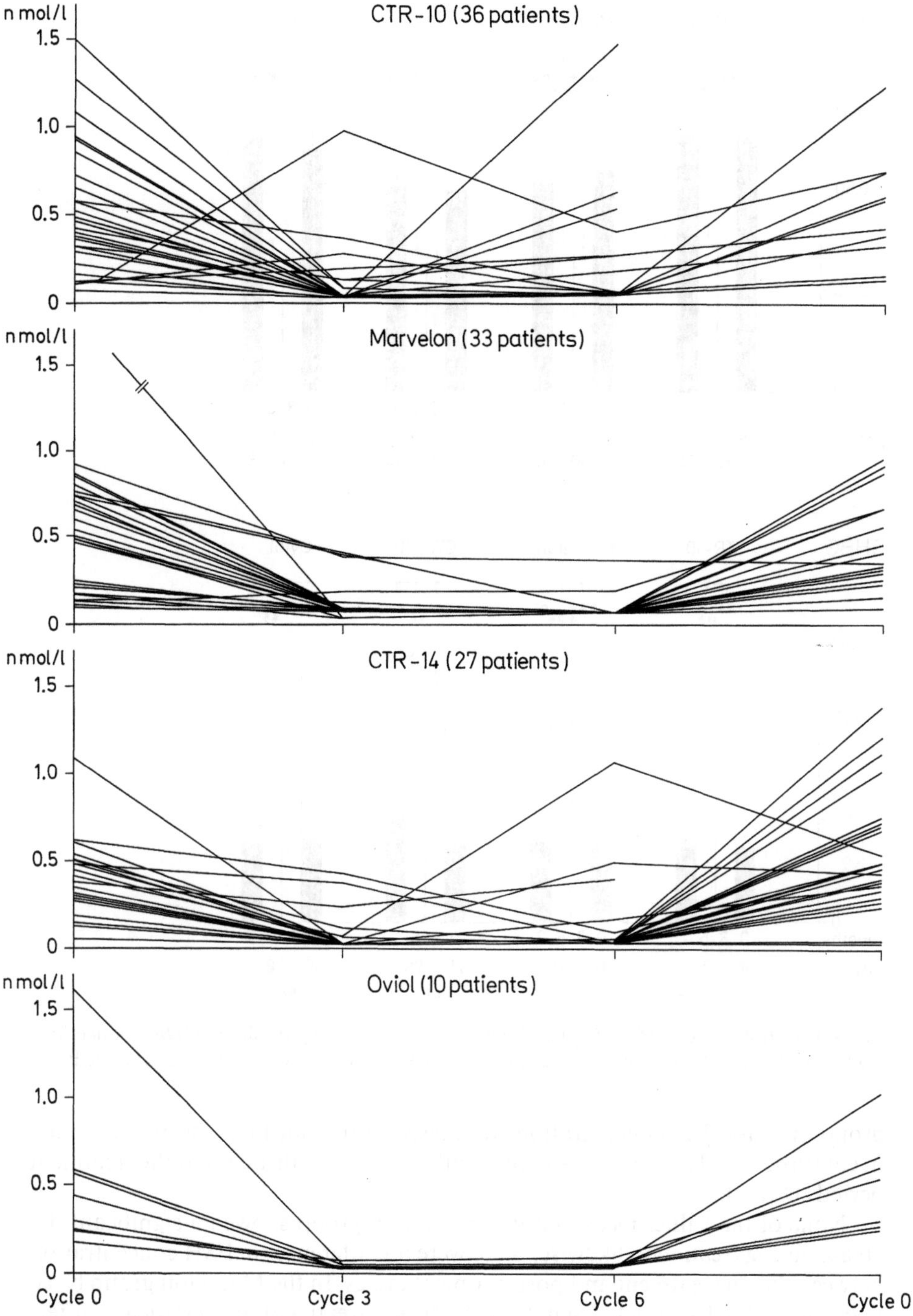

Fig. 3. Endogenous secretion of estradiol during treatment with different micropills

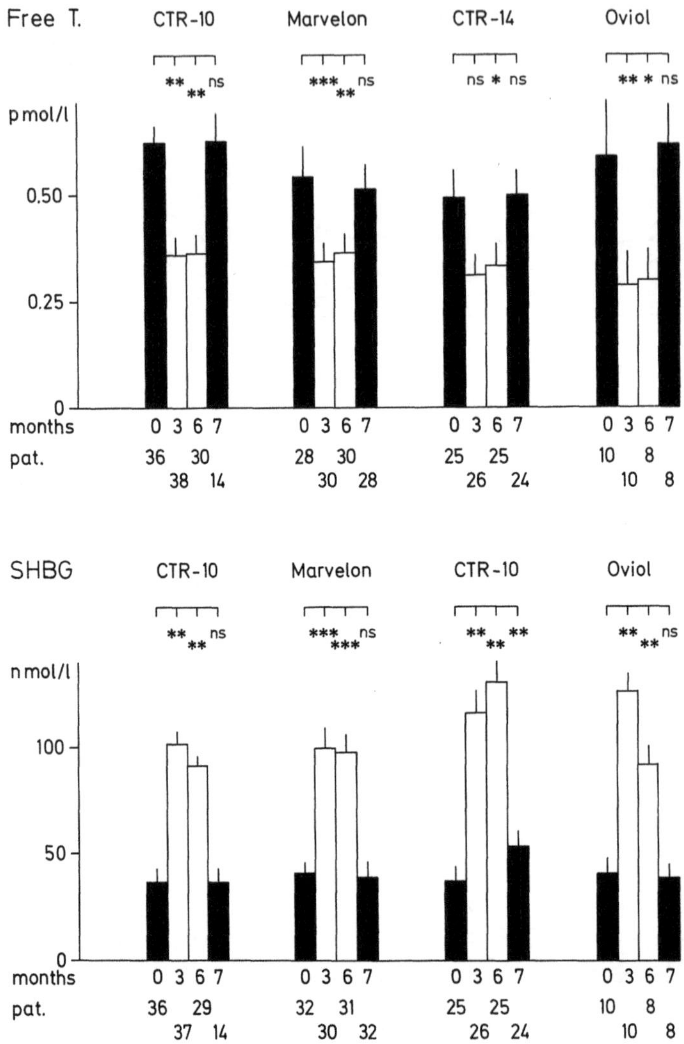

Fig. 4. Free testosterone (*FREE T*) and sex-hormone binding globuline (*SHBG*) concentrations. *Unshaded bars*, with medication; *shaded bars*, without medication; *p* values, see Fig. 1

group the basal LH concentrations decreased in the third treatment cycle only; in contrast, the LH reserve was significantly suppressed throughout the treatment periods (Fig. 1).

None of the values measured in the CTR-10 group showed a significant decrease during treatment; likewise, there were no differences in FSH concentration between the pretreatment and posttreatment cycles. In the Marvelon group basal and reserve FSH values fell significantly during treatment; no significant differences were observed in pretreatment compared to the posttreatment cycles. Neither basal nor reserve FSH concentrations in the CTR-14 group showed significant differences during treatment or posttreatment cycles. In the Oviol group there were no significant changes in FSH concentrations either during treatment or in the posttreatment cycles (Fig. 1).

Estradiol concentrations were significantly suppressed during treatment with all four preparations compared to pretreatment levels. Posttreatment cycles returned to baseline (Fig. 2).

There was a significant decrease of progesterone concentrations during treatment in all four groups of women. No differences were measured between the pretreatment and posttreatment cycles, but a wider standard error was seen for CTR-10 as compared to the other three preparations (Fig. 2).

Analysis of individual values for estradiol and progesterone indicated, however, that ten subjects in the CTR-10, two in the Marvelon and four in the CTR-14 group had elevated endogenous concentrations of both steroids (Table 4). This indicates inadequate ovarian suppression. Although there were no "stray" cases in the Oviol group, the small number of cases made it impossible to decide whether the correct degree of suppression had been obtained (Fig. 3).

None of the groups showed significant changes in prolactin concentrations during and after treatment. A slight increase was found after CTR-10 was discontinued.

There were no significant changes in the total testosterone concentrations. In contrast, free testosterone decreased significantly while SHBG increased significantly during treatment (Fig. 4).

Only two groups – the CTR-10 and the Marvelon – showed significant decrease of DHEA-S concentrations during treatment (Fig. 4).

Discussion

As we have reported previously [4], the central inhibitory effect of a contraceptive agent depends not only on the amount of estrogen which it contains but also on the structure and dose of the gestogen present in the preparation. Whereas estrogens alter the frequency of LH pulses and increase the pituitary reserve [10], gestogens presumably influence hypothalamic and hypophyseal release of LH and appear to modulate the secretion of FSH.

Since in three of the four preparations desogestrel was administered from the beginning of the cycle, suppression of FSH due to ethinylestradiol alone could not be demonstrated. However, treatment results with Oviol indicate that besides suppressing LH, suppression of FSH also occurs when ethinylestradiol alone is initially administered. A comparison of Marvelon and CTR-10 shows that the dose-dependent inhibitory effect of ethinylestradiol was exerted mainly on the basal and stimulated levels of FSH and to a lesser degree on the LH levels. The difference between the two preparations consists only in an ethinylestradiol dose of 10 μg. It appears that the FSH concentrations are less strongly suppressed below a critical ethinylestradiol dose.

It is remarkable that sequential preparations with a higher total estrogen content and a lower dose of gestogen do not have the same suppressive effect as monophasic preparations such as Marvelon, especially with regard to FSH. Both the critical estrogen dose and the desogestrel dose must be taken into account if adequate suppression is to be obtained; otherwise, so-called "stray" cases with follicular growth and even fully developed luteal phases may be found. Therefore, more pregnancies may be expected with very low-dose monophasic as well as with sequential preparations, particularly if such a preparation is not taken on a regular basis.

According to data published by Back and Orme [1] the reliability of ovulation inhibitors can also be influenced by environmental factors, concomitantly administered medication, diet, and gastrointestinal disorders. These effects may be more pronounced in the case of very low dose monophasic, biphasic, and triphasic preparations. The biochemical picture in peripheral blood which occurs when very low dose monophasic, biphasic, and triphasic preparations are administered is also seen during maturations of the cycle in adolescence. We have already pointed out the changes in the LH/FSH ratio in subjects taking ovulation inhibitors [8]. We have observed that a shift in this ratio in favor of FSH leads to follicular ripening and formation of ovarian cysts [6].

As we have shown earlier, even an increase of the estrogen dose does not protect the woman from the risk of inadequate ovarian suppression. However, such patients can be treated with a strongly suppressive gestogen. Administration of a strongly suppressive gestogen can prevent these undesirable occurrences. We know that preexisting irregular cycles show their former patterns to a more pronounced extent after discontinuation of oral contraceptives. These manifestations include the oversuppression syndrome previously mentioned in the literature.

The very low dose monophasic and biphasic preparations do not evoke these changes. It seems that they are more suitable for antiovulatory prophylaxis of immature cycles in adolescents, despite the side effects mentioned. Cycle disturbances following ingestion of oral contraceptives have not been observed with these preparations. Based on our experience we prescribe very low dose monophasic, biphasic, or triphasic preparations for adolescents with maturing cycles. Here too, the gestogen plays a crucial role [5]. If abdominal discomfort, spotting or breast symptoms occur, we give the patient monophasic preparations containing a more strongly suppressive gestogen.

Several authors (Rey, personal communication) pointed to the greater flexibility of the juvenile endocrine system. This flexibility may eventually be traced back to the lower dosage and to the modified composition of the contraceptives used today and not represent a property per se.

Summary

The degree of suppression of the gonadal axis was investigated using four hormonal contraceptive agents containing the same steroids with different dosage schedules. In comparison to the conventional low-dose preparations, very low dose monophasic as well as bi- and triphasic contraceptives lowered FSH serum concentrations to a significantly lesser degree. These findings indicate a possible reversal of the physiological LH/FSH ratio which in turn can lead to endogenous estrogen secretion with its well-known clinical symptoms. The observed hormonal behavior shows similarities to events described for the maturing cycle.

References

1. Back DJ, Orme MLE (1977) Drug interactions with oral contraceptive steroids. Prescribers' Journal 17:6
2. Gompel A, Kuttenn F (1983) Minipilules estroprogestatives et hyperestrogénie. Gynécologie 34:21
3. Kuttenn F, Detoeuf M, De Lignières B (1980) Contraceptifs oraux. Rev Prat 30:4025
4. Mall-Haefeli M, Werner-Zodrow I, Huber PR, Darragh A, Lambe R (1983) Effects of various combined oral contraceptives on sex steroids, gonadotropins and SHBG. Ir Med J 76, 6:266
5. Mall-Haefeli M, Werner-Zodrow I, Huber PR (1984) Der kontrazeptive Effekt niedrig dosierter Ovulationshemmer mit verschiedenen Gestagenen. Geburtshilfe Frauenheilkd 44:177–179
6. Mall-Haefeli M, Werner-Zodrow I, Birkhäuser M, Huber PR (1985) Advantages and disadvantages of low-dose hormonal contraceptive agents. In: Runnebaum B, Rabe T, Kiesel L (eds) Future aspects in contraception, proceedings of an International Symposium held in Heidelberg, 5–8 September 1984, Part 2. Female contraception. MTP, Boston
8. Mall-Haefeli M (1988) Empfängnisverhütung bei Jugendlichen und bei prämenopausalen Frauen. Wien Med Wochenschr (to be published)
9. Spellacy WN, Kalra PS, Buhi WC, Birk SA (1980) Pituitary and ovarian responsiveness to a graded gonadotropin releasing factor stimulation test in women using a low-estrogen or a regular type of oral contraceptive. Am J Obstet Gynecol 137:109
10. Yen SSC, Lein A (1976) The apparent paradox of the negative and positive feedback control system on gonadotropin secretion. Am J Obstet Gynecol 126:942
11. Mickelson KE, Petra PH (1974) A filter assay for the sex steroid binding protein (SBP) of human serum. FEBS Lett 44:34–36
12. Wiest WG, Paulson JD, Keller DW, Warren JC (1978) Free testosterone concentrations in serum: a method for determination. Am J Obstet Gynecol 130:321–328

Development of New Progestagens

Trends in Hormonal Contraception

B. Runnebaum, T. Rabe, and L. Kiesel

Department of Obstetrics and Gynecology, Division of Gynecological Endocrinology, Women's Hospital, University of Heidelberg, Voßstr. 9, 6900 Heidelberg, FRG

Introduction

Oral hormonal contraceptives have been available since the early 1960s when Pincus and Rock found that norethynodrel (9.65 mg) in combination with mestranol (150 μg) inhibited ovulation and provided sufficient control of the menstrual cycle. Since then, different approaches to contraception have been pursued. Hormonal steroids can either act as ovulation inhibitors or prevent conception by altering the cervical mucus.

In this paper a brief survey about the present stage of and future developments in the field of hormonal contraception will be presented. In the use of hormonal oral contraceptives today health aspects play a decisive role, and this will be even more important in the future. On the other hand, the pill of today is expected to provide high contraceptive reliability. In the present paper we will try to see whether the modern low-dose pills can be further improved with regards to their effects on health and metabolic neutrality. In addition, other hormonal contraceptives such as injectables, implants, vaginal rings, postcoital pills, and different delivery systems will be discussed.

Oral Hormonal Contraception

Synthetic Gestagens. In the last 25 years, research has been focused on the development of (pro)gestagens with a similar pharmacological profile to progesterone, but with long half lives and high antiovulatory potencies (Fig. 1). All synthetic gestagens are derived either from 17-hydroxyprogesterone or from 19-nortestosterone. This paper focuses on the 19-nortestosterone derivatives which can be divided according to their structure into the estranes and the biologically more effective gonanes. The new gestagens (e.g., desogestrel, noregestimate, gestodene) in oral contraceptives belong to the group of gonanes. The estranes are chemically characterized by a lack of the methyl group between rings A and B and by an ethinyl group in position C-17 alpha. Due to these substitutions their inactivation in the liver is delayed and the androgenic effects are greatly reduced. Among the gonanes, which are also characterized by an ethyl group in position C-13, can be found the most effective synthetic gestagens such as levonorgestrel, desogestrel, norgestimate, and gestodene. This presentation mainly deals with these new gestagens.

Female Contraception
Eds.: B. Runnebaum, T. Rabe, L. Kiesel

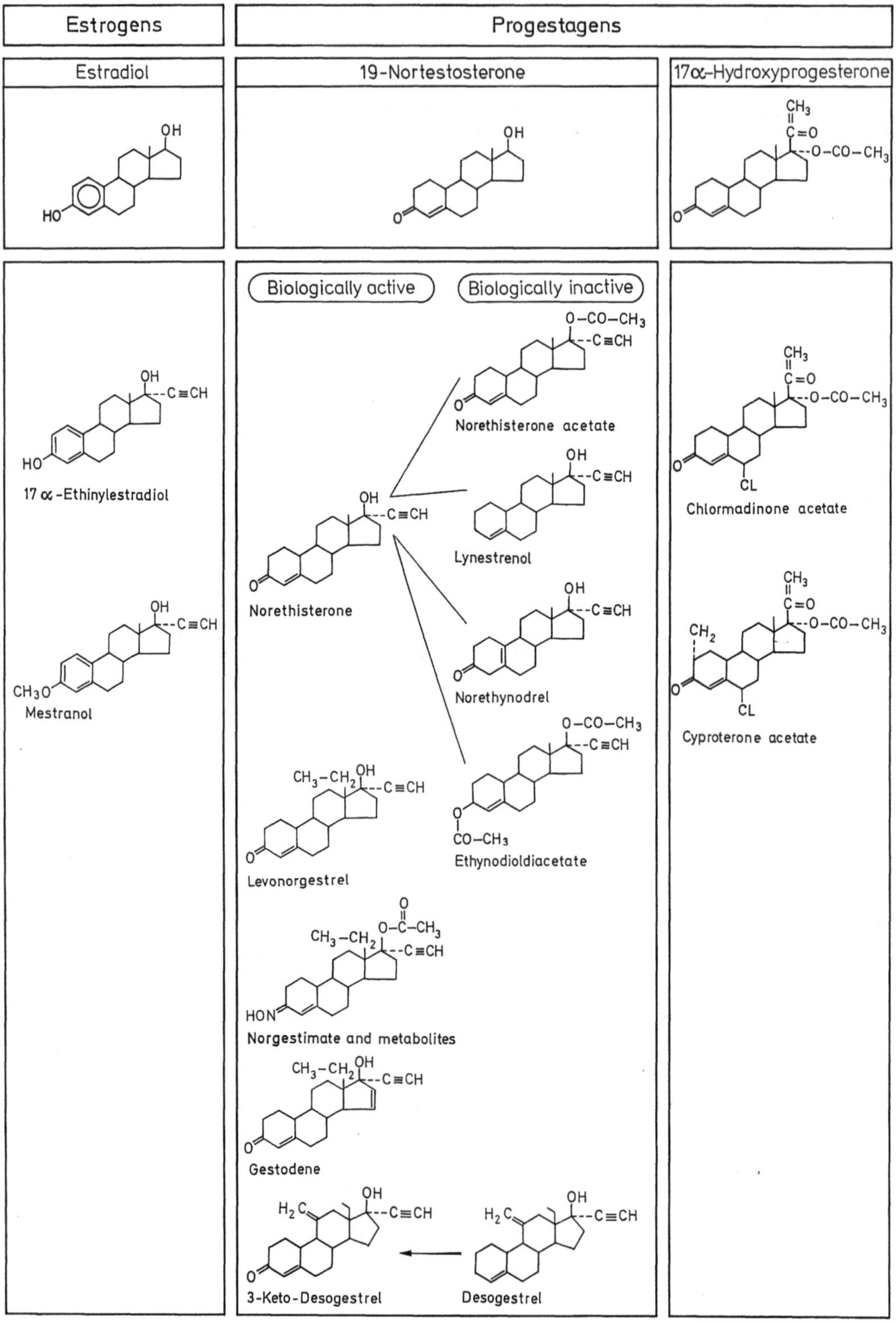

Fig. 1. Synthetic estrogens and progestagens used for oral contraception

The different synthetic gestagens are differently reabsorbed in the gastrointestinal tract and partially metabolized, i.e., activated, inactivated, or transformed into metabolites with other partial effects. This occurs to a large degree in the liver. The individual structure of the gestagens not only determines the binding affinity to the receptor, but also the affinity to various enzymes in the whole organism. At the same time, enzyme inductions do occur. In addition, the biological effect of the gestagens depends on their ability to bind to a serum protein, on the distribution and storage in the organism, and on the metabolism of the target tissue itself. Furthermore, receptor concentration and receptor affinity play an important role in the biological effect. The activity of many enzymes can be competitively or noncompetitively inhibited by gestagens, so other metabolic pathways in the target organ, for example the liver, can be altered in this way. Finally, the effect of the gestagens depends on the synergic influence of the estrogens, for two reasons: on the one hand, estrogens induce the synthesis of progesterone receptors and thus create the basis for the action of the gestagen, and, on the other hand, they determine the amount of existing receptors and to a certain extent the potency of the particular gestagen.

The large number of effects of gestagens, partly created synergistically with estrogens, makes it very difficult to characterize a particular gestagen. A number of properties of the synthetic gestagens (gestagenic, estrogenic, antiestrogenic, androgenic, or antiandrogenic), with emphasis on the newer ones, are summarized in Table 1. Furthermore, the clinical effects of the new gestagens in combination with estrogens must be analyzed. This analysis has shown that the new gestagens have strong gestagenic effects in relation to ovulation inhibition, effects on the endometrium, binding affinity to the progesterone receptor, and pregnancy maintenance. The new, third generation of gestagens such as desogestrel, norgestimate,

Table 1. Characteristics of synthetic progestogens used for oral contraception

	Norethisterone	Levonorgestrel	Desogestrel	Norgestimate	Gestodene
Ovulation inhibition (mg/day)	0.5	0.05–0.1	0.06	0.25	0.04
Transformation dosage (mg/cycle)	100–150	5–6	0.4–2.5	~5–10	2–3
Menstrual delay test (mg/day)	10–15	0.25–1.0	~0.25	5	~0.2
Binding affinity[a] to the progesterone receptor (%)	305	628	11 ~628[b]	400–500	?
Maintenance of pregnancy	(+)	+	+	+	+
Estrogenic effects	+	0	0	0	0
Antiestrogenic effects	(+)	+	+	(+)	+
Androgenic effects	+	+	(+)	(+)	(+)
Antiandrogenic effects	0	0	0	0	0

Some data were obtained from the pharmaceutical companies.
[a] Relative binding affinity to cytosol of human uterine tissue; progesterone = 100%.
[b] 3-Ketodesogestrel.

and gestodene are real gestagens with pregnancy-maintenance effects like those of levonorgestrel. They possess no estrogenic effect but clear antiestrogenic effects. The androgenic effects of new gestagens in the low-dose formulations appear to be of no clinical relevance and no antiandrogenic effects have been found.

At present, it seems that no oral contraceptive with a new gestagen will come on the market in the near future.

Estrogens. In recent years, no new long-acting synthetic estrogen has been developed. Besides mestranol, which is the 3-methylester of ethinylestradiol and ethinylestradiol itself, no other compound with high antiovulatory potency and giving good control of the menstrual cycle has been developed. In several experiments the efficacy of natural estrogens with regards contraception and control of the menstrual cycle and metabolic effects has been analyzed. Percutaneous administration of estradiol (3 mg/day) had no measurable effect on renin substrate, very low density lipoprotein levels, sex hormone binding globulin, or antithrombin activity (De Ligniers et al. 1986). Luteinizing hormone (LH) and follicle-stimulating hormone (FSH) were sufficiently suppressed.

Other delivery systems with natural estrogens that bypass the gastrointestinal tract such as intravaginal polysiloxane rings (Stumpf et al. 1982; Elkik et al. 1986), transdermal skin patches (Laufer et al. 1983), or subdermal pellets (Lobo et al. 1980) also showed no negative effects in terms of increasing the risk of hypercoagulopathy, hypertension, or metabolic changes. Combinations with natural estrogens and micronized crystalline progesterone have been used in women for different purposes (Holst et al. 1983). The problems with using natural steroids for contraception are mainly cycle control and contraceptive safety.

Dose Reduction. As a result of the large-scale clinical studies in England and thereafter in many other countries, it became evident that venous thrombosis is closely related with the estrogen dose in the oral contraceptive. After reduction of the estrogen dose from 100 µg to 50 µg, the incidence of venous thrombosis was reduced. In the middle of the 1970s, clinical trials in England revealed that the gestagens harmfully affect the arterial vessel system. There were even indications that the gestagens caused heart attacks, strokes, and hypertension. The number of women with hypertension was clearly related to the gestagen dosage of the oral contraceptive. Even with treatment with the "minipill" cases of hypertension occurred. The exact mechanism of the induction of hypertension by gestagens remains unknown.

Because of this, the doses of estrogens and gestagens have been reduced markedly. Low-dose formulations contain ethinylestradiol at between 20 and 37.5 µg and have a low gestagen content. In addition to dose reduction, various estrogen/gestagen combinations have been developed, for example biphasic and triphasic oral contraceptives. The lowest amount of steroids per menstrual cycle is administered with the triphasic regimen.

Risk Factors. It has been demonstrated in developed countries that the use of oral contraceptives increases the risk of cardiovascular diseases (cerebral stroke, myocardial infarction, pulmonary embolism), whereas in developing countries this has not yet been observed. Therefore, a WHO study in 20 countries focused on this problem both in developing and in developed countries. Until now, the following risk factors have been proved to be closely related to cardiovascular disease in oral contraceptive users: smoking, age, hypertension, diabetes mellitus, hypercholesterinemia, and preexisting obesity and cardiovascular diseases.

Lipid Metabolism. Large-scale studies in the USA demonstrated a close relationship between serum cholesterol and coronary heart diseases (Hahn et al. 1984). A reduction of total cholesterol by 1% leads to a 2% reduction of the risk of coronary heart disease. Various effects of synthetic gestagens alone and progestogen/estrogen combinations on lipid metabolism have been observed (Fig. 2). Generally, a low impact of new low-dose combined pills and triphasics was found in clinical studies over 6–12 cycles. Long-term clinical trials are necessary for evaluating the specific effects in detail. Cholesterol and triglycerides should be determined before and during use of oral contraceptives to prevent hazards caused by a previously unknown deterioration of lipid metabolism (e.g., hypercholesterinemia type II) in users which might be responsible for cardiovascular morbidity and mortality.

The impact of different low-dose combined and triphasic oral contraceptives on total cholesterol, triglycerides, high density lipoprotein (HDL) cholesterol, and low density lipoprotein (LDL) cholesterol is summarized in Fig. 2.

Carbohydrate Metabolism. The question of whether oral contraceptives might be responsible for the development of clinical diabetes mellitus has been studied for several years. Most of the low-dose oral contraceptives have only a small effect on carbohydrate metabolism, low insulin resistance, and slight glucose intolerance. According to recent data diabetes mellitus has not been induced by using the pill (Skouby 1987).

Blood Coagulation. As yet, no clinical and biochemical measurers are available for routine analysis of an increased risk of cardiovascular diseases. For research purposes metabolites of fibrinogen such as fibrinopeptides A and B can be measured. Analysis of antithrombin III allows the detection of the very rare antithrombin III deficiency (1 : 8000) which is an absolute contraindication for oral contraception; due to its low incidence an assessment of antithrombin III cannot be recommended for screening purposes.

Advantages (Positive Side Effects). The positive effects of oral contraceptives (found only for those containing 50 μg ethinylestradiol or more) consist of the prevention of diseases or unfavorable symptoms such as benign mammary cysts, ovarian cysts and ovarian carcinoma, endometrial carcinoma, salpingitis, ectopic pregnancy, dysfunctional bleedings, anemia, premenstrual tension, dysmenorrhea, acne, seborrhea, and rheumatoid arthritis.

Disadvantages (Negative Side Effects). Negative effects are cardiovascular diseases, hypertension, thrombosis, the influence on metabolism, and the influence

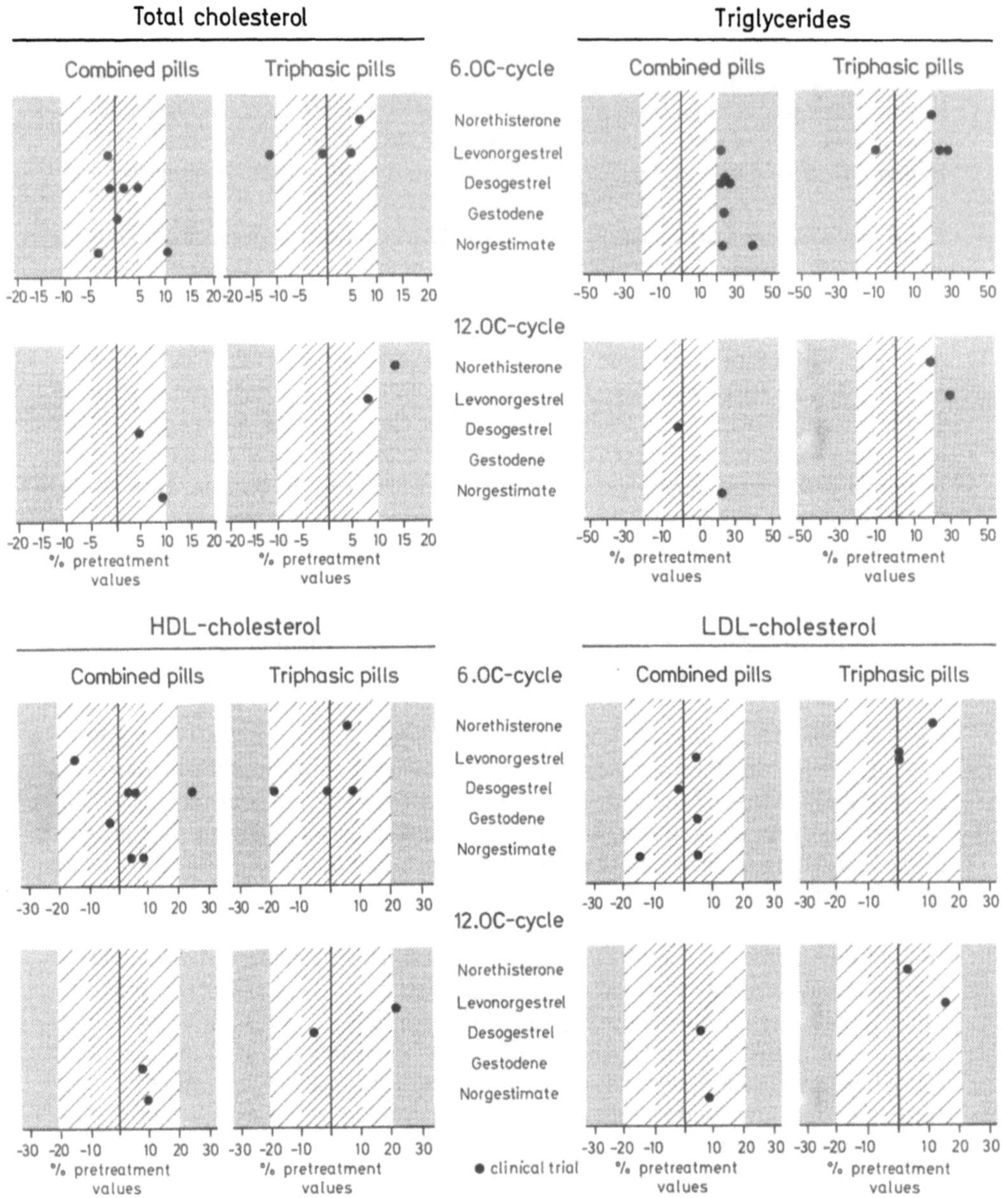

Fig. 2. Total cholesterol, triglycerides, and HDL- and LDL-cholesterol during use of low-dose combined pills and triphasics in various clinical trials

on the development of liver tumors. In patients using oral contraceptives, preventive measures should include measurement of blood pressure, cancer screening, and blood examination for glucose and lipids. Health care systems can also save money, e.g., by preventing undesired pregnancies and many diseases.

Ambivalence between Contraceptive Safety and Natural Contraception. The effect of the contraceptive method on the natural body feeling (e.g., breast tension, psychological changes during the menstrual cycle), i.e., the sexuality, must be considered in the choice of contraception; on the other hand, the lower contraceptive efficacy of natural contraceptive methods must be realized.

In recent years, the attitudes of women towards safe methods of avoiding pregnancy and the less safe but more natural methods of contraception have been ambivalent. Women, particularly those between 20 and 30 years of age, often want a natural form of contraception which involves both partners. It is important for many women that they have a natural body feeling during the menstrual cycle. Couples preferring a natural contraceptive method often do not realize that the contraceptive safety of many of these methods is low.

Psychological Acceptance. The psychological acceptance of a particular contraceptive method is important and depends on the individual situations of a partnership or the partners. Furthermore, it is also influenced by the users' knowledge of contraceptive methods. Finally, the users should be in a position to decide by themselves which contraceptive method is the best for them. A consultation with the advising physician on the appropriate method should take place and thus preventive measures can be planned in case of any risks. It is a great task for medical and national institutions to guarantee broad education of the youth about contraceptive methods. One achievement has been the significant reduction in the number of abortions. In industrialized countries of today, profound education on contraceptive methods is needed. In developing countries, as is well known, there are many problems concerning the availability, the distribution, and the application of these methods, as well as religious aspects.

Delivery Systems. To avoid peaks of steroid hormone levels in the peripheral blood and thereby hazardous steroid effects on the metabolism and the cardiovascular system, various attempts have been made to maintain a constant release of steroids (e.g., micronised steroids) by use of specific delivery systems (e.g., microcapsules, liposomes, rods, implantables).

Gestagen-Only Pills

In the Federal Republic of Germany, only 40000 women use gestagen-only pills for contraception. The low acceptance may be due to a need for very regular ingestion of the contraceptive (daily ±3 h) and the high rate (30%–40%) of disturbances of the menstrual bleeding pattern. Gestagen-only pills are a second possible method of contraception in patients with contraindications for or who are intolerant of oral contraceptives or intrauterine devices, and they are specially indicated for breast-feeding patients. Due to the relatively high failure rate and the poor control of the menstrual cycle the gestagen-only pill cannot be generally recommended.

Injectables

General Remarks. Major side effects of injectables are high rate of menstrual disturbances (breakthrough bleedings) during the first months of treatment and the occurrence of amenorrhea during long-time use.

Monthly Injectable. Recent research has focused on the development of monthly injectables. For this reason, different chemical modifications of progestins (e.g., esters) and the combination of gestagens with estrogens are being studied worldwide. Some 1.5 million women in China and Latin America already use monthly injectables. Two new monthly injectables with either norethisterone enanthate or Depo-medroxyprogesterone acetate may be available in the early 1990s.

Pharmacokinetic and pharmacodynamic studies with cyclobutylcarboxylate (HRP 001) and butanoate (HRP 002) have been performed in the following dosages: 12.5, 25, and 50 mg. As a result of these studies, 12.5 mg HRP 002 has been selected for further investigations in a phase II clinical trial with norethisterone enanthate (200 m every 2 months).

Various injectable steroid contraceptives with a duration of action ranging from 1 to 6 months have been analyzed. Some new steroid formulations providing contraceptive protection for more than 2 months are in an early phase of development, and two once-a-month injectables with HRP 102 and HRP 112 have been studied intensively. Recent results indicate that the dosages of the two once-a-month injectables (HRP 102 and HRP 112), which are now in phase III of clinical trials (50 mg norethisterone enanthate and 5 mg estradiol valerate in HRP 102; 35 mg Depo-medroxyprogesterone acetate and 5 mg estradiol cypionate in HRP 112), seem to be optimal.

Earlier results from the phase III clinical trial in 17 centres covered more than 2300 patients. The withdrawal rate due to disturbed menstrual bleeding after 12 months was 6.4% for HRP 112 and 7.4% for HRP 102 (compared to 14%–15% in patients treated with Depo-medroxyprogesterone acetate and norethisterone enanthate).

The once-a-month injectable has advantages as far as unpredictable bleedings and amenorrhea is concerned. A disadvantage is that a monthly visit to a health centre for injections is needed.

Three-Monthly Injectable. Injectables releasing steroid hormones from intramuscular depots have been available since 20 years. The most favored injectables are Depo-Provera, releasing medroxyprogesterone acetate, and Noristerat, releasing norethisterone enanthate.

Preclinical studies in primates with a microcapsule delivery system containing 25–50 mg norgestimate indicate that in women 75 mg may be the right dosage, lasting for 6 months (Hahn et al. 1984).

The cancer risk in patients using medroxyprogesterone acetate or norethisterone enanthate is not increased with respect to breast, cervical, ovarian, endometrial, and liver cancer.

Implants

General Remarks. Implants release gestagens either from a nonbiodegradable delivery system (Norplant) or a biodegradable carrier (e.g., Capronor). There are two types of biodegradable implants: Capronor, a single capsule containing levonorgestrel; and three or four pellets of the hormone norethindrone combined with small amounts of cholesterol. Capronor is expected to prevent pregnancy for at least 18 months, the pellets for at least 12 months. They may be available by the middle of the 1990s.

Norplants II and VI. The implants Norplant VI (six rods containing levonorgestrel) and Norplant II (two silastic implants with levonorgestrel), which were introduced more recently, have excited great interest (Fig. 3). Contraceptive efficacy is provided for a period of up to 5 years. Major hazards are disturbances of the menstrual cycle in 20%–30% of all women leading to a removal of the implants in 20% of all cases. The remaining 80% of patients benefit from the long-time contraception without any severe side effects.

Norplant implants have been approved and introduced in Finland, Sweden, Ecuador, the Dominican Republic, Indonesia, Thailand, and Columbia. Further applications are pending in other countries. Already about 75000 Indonesian women have used Norplant (Population Reports 1987).

Indications for the use of Norplants are oral contraceptive or intrauterine device intolerance or contraindications, or when long-term (more than 2 years) contraception is required. There are some data that Norplant loses efficacy in severly obese patients.

Capronor. The National Institute of Child Health and Human Development, Bethesda, Maryland, USA, has finished a 2-year study on the toxicology of Capronor implants (levonorgestrel-releasing polymer, epsilon caprolacton) in rats and monkeys. The Task Force has now started a phase II clinical trial analyzing the efficacy and side effects of 2.5 and 4.0 cm long rods over a period of 1 year.

Microspheres and Microcapsules. Injectable microspheres and microcapsules suspended in a solution are administered via a hypodermic needle. The tiny particles are of different sizes and consist of a polymer carrying the hormone, they dissolve and release the hormone at various rates providing a nearly constant dose that prevents pregnancy for 1–6 months. The first microsphere contraceptive may be available in some countries in the early 1990s.

Midcycle Contraception

General Remarks. Midcycle contraception would provide high contraceptive efficacy in patients by using contraceptives only during the periovulatory phase. For this reason low steroid impact on the menstrual cycle and metabolism would be expected. Problems are irregularity of the menstrual cycle and unpredictable ovu-

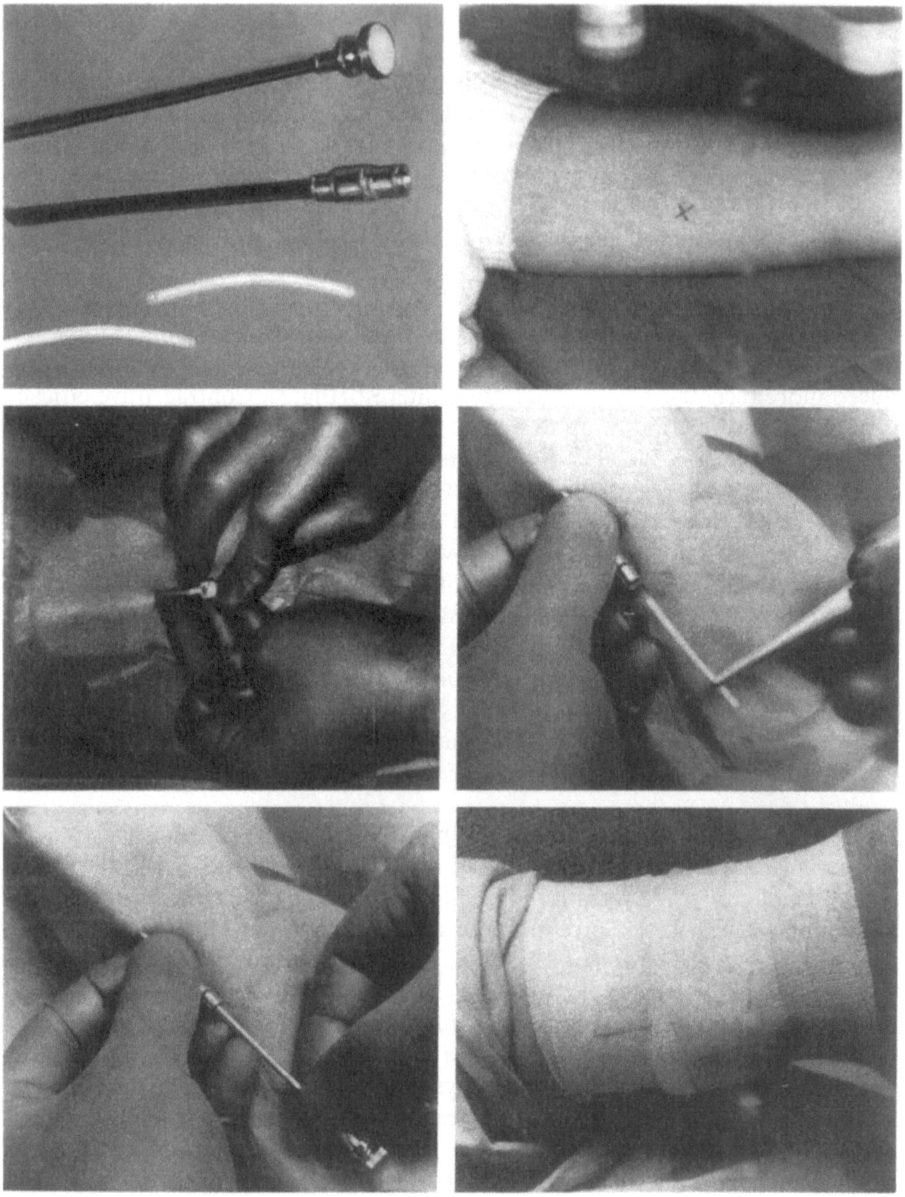

Fig. 3. Implantation of Norplant II as a female contraceptive. *Upper row: left*, Norplant II rods, trocar and mandrin; *right*, place of implantation. After local anesthesia (2–5 ml 1% Meaverin) skin incision (3 mm) at the inner side of the left upper arm approx. 10 cm above the elbow joint. *Middle row: left*, insertion of the trocar and the mandrin. *right*, insertion of Norplant capsules. *Lower row: left*, insertion of Norplant capsules through the trocar by use of mandrin. *right*, wound dressing by pressure bandage for 24 h

lation. Two different approaches are possible. One is the application of antigestagens, especially RU 486. This compound can be used either alone or in combination with prostaglandins. The second approach is to use levonorgestrel, even in the periovulatory phase.

Levonorgestrel. A multicenter clinical trial analyzed the efficacy of levonorgestrel during the periovulatory phase of the menstrual cycle. The failure rate was found to be 0.8%, which is similar to the failure rate of 1%–2% using an estrogen/progestin (500 µg levonorgestrel, 50 µg ethinylestradiol) combined pill for postcoital interception (two within 48 h after coitus and two 24 h later; (Juzpe 1984).

Norethisterone. In Shanghai, China, the pharmacokinetics and pharmacodynamics of the "visitor" pill, which contains 5 mg norethisterone, have been compared with the same preparation in a 3-mg dose. With regards the suppression of ovarian function, the 3-mg pill is not as effective as the higher-dose one and causes, rarely, systemic side effects.

Antigestagens. Periovulatory contraception with antigestagens or in combination with prostaglandins will become important in the future (van Santen 1987). Studies with RU 486 given at a dosage of 100 mg/day from day 10 to day 16 of the menstrual cycle blocked the LH/FSH surge (Shoupe et al. 1986). A combination with prostaglandin E_2 has been tested but these studies clearly showed that sequential treatment with RU 486 and oral prostaglandin E_2 was no more effective than treatment with RU 486 alone.

Vaginal Rings

General Remarks. Vaginal rings releasing either synthetic gestagens alone or estrogen/gestagen mixtures have recently been developed by the WHO (Fig. 4). This ring can be inserted by the women herself and is worn for 3 weeks to be then removed for 1 week. This method is quite practicable, but metabolic advantages in comparison with oral contraceptives must be examined. A 3-month levonorges-

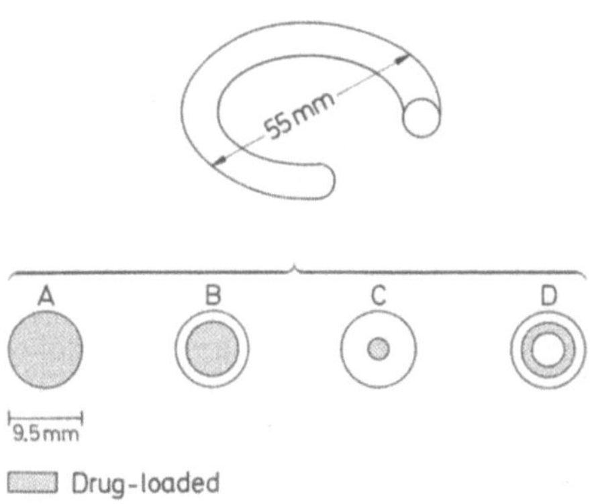

Fig. 4 A–D. Different types of vaginal rings

trel-containing ring may be available in some countries by 1988. A 3-month progesterone-containing ring is being developed.

Levonorgestrel Ring. A WHO trial (phase III) is analyzing the efficacy and side effects of a levonorgestrel-releasing vaginal ring over a period of 2 years in 12 different countries.

Progesterone Ring. A progesterone-releasing vaginal ring developed by the Population Council in new York has a release rate of 10–20 mg progesterone daily. Another progesterone-containing ring releasing 4–5 mg has been developed by the WHO. Clinical studies are in progress testing the ring in breast-feeding women.

Future Developments

It can be assumed that the use of low-dose pills will increase worldwide. Low-dose oral contraceptive pills with new gestagens will be further analyzed with regards their cardiovascular and metabolic risks. Until the year 2000 no new synthetic gestagen will be available on the market due to extended periods of clinical trials. Furthermore, risk factors for oral contraceptive use will be better characterized and the risk of carcinoma of the breast and the cervix has to be ruled out. Before the year 2000 implantables and vaginal rings for family planning will be available all over the world. They should be very effective, convenient to use, and long-acting – from 1 month to 5 years. The implants Norplant II and VI, consisting of small silastic rods releasing levonorgestrel, are among them. In the meantime Norplant implants have already been approved in seven countries. Modern delivery systems such as the implants (Norplant and Capronor), injectables, and vaginal rings will be intensively investigated and should gain popularity. Other new methods are in various stages of development and testing. The new methods share one obvious disadvantage: to varying degrees, all change the menstrual bleeding patterns. If women accept this and know it is not harmful, many will be willing to use them. Vaginal rings and intrauterine devices medicated with hormones which have no significant effect on metabolism will gain in importance in the future. Further trials with natural steroids such as estradiol and progesterone will be undertaken. Monthly injectables will be advantageous if new formulations provide good control of menstrual cycle and contraceptive efficacy at the same time.

Antigestagens (e.g., RU 486) might be available for use in the near future for unprotected intercourse in women using behavioral methods. There has still been no final evaluation of antigestagens (in combination with prostaglandins) for broad application as a periovulatory contraceptive method or for induction of an early abortion. Midcycle contraception may be of interest for couples where intercourse only occurs a few times each month.

In general, the aims of future developments in family planning are to improve patients' health and to diminish the risk of side effects of all contraceptive methods, thus allowing couples worldwide to make their choice from a broad selection of contraceptive methods and promoting responsible parenthood.

References

De Ligniers B, Basdevant A, Thomas G et al. (1986) Biological effect of estradiol 17β in postmenopausal women: oral versus percutaneous administration. J Clin Endocrinol Metab 62:536

Elkik F, Basdevant A, Jackanicz TM, Guy-Brand B, Mercier-Bodard C, Conard J, Bardin CW, Corvol P (1986) Contraception in hypertensive women using a vaginal ring delivering estradiol and levonorgestrel. J Clin Endocrinol Metab 63:29

Hahn DW, McGuire JL, Cohn RM, Beck LR, Tice TR, Lewis DH (1984) Development of microencapsulated norgestimate as a long-acting contraceptive. In: Zatuchni GI, Mishell DR, Shoupe D, Goldsmith A, Shelton JD, Sciarra JJ (eds) Long-acting contraceptive delivery systems. Harper and Row, Philadelphia, pp 96–112

Holst J, Cajander S, Carlstrom K, Damber MG, von Schoulz B (1983) Percutaneous oestrogen therapy opposed by lunestrenol or natural progesterone – effects on circulating oestrogens, FSH, sex hormone binding globulin and pregnancy zone protein. Maturitas 5:1–8

Juzpe AA (1984) Postcoital contraception. Clin Obstet and Gynaecol 11:787–797

Laufer LR, De Fazzio JL, Lu JKH et al. (1983) Estrogen replacement therapy by transdermal estradiol administration. Am J Obstet Gynecol 146:533

Rifkind BM, Segal P (1983) Lipid research clinics programm reference values for hyperlipidemia and hypolipidemia. J Am Med Ass 250:1869–1872

Lobo RA, March CM, Goebelsmann U et al. (1980) Subdermal estradiol pellets following hysterectomy and oophorectomy. Am J Obstet Gynecol 138:714

Population Reports (1987) Injectables and implants. Popul Rep 3

Shoupe D, Spitz I, Osborn C, Page MA, Mishell DR Jr, Lobo RA (1986) Effects of progesterone (P) antagonists on gonadotropins at midcycle and during the luteal phase. In: Society for gynecologic investigation, Toronto, Ontario, Canada, 19–22 March 1986, abstract 40

Skouby SO (1987) Oral contraceptives and diabetes mellitus. Gynecol Endocrinol (Suppl) 2:30

Stumpf PG, Maruca J, Santen RJ et al. (1982) Development of a vaginal ring for achieving physiologic levels of 17β estradiol in hypoestrogenic women. J Clin Endocrinol Metab 54:298

Van Santen MR (1987) Postcoital interception and contragestion. Elinkwijk, Utrecht

Clinical Pharmacology of Gestagens

K. Fotherby

Royal Postgraduate Medical School, Hammersmith Hospital, Ducane Road, London, W12 OHS, UK

Introduction

Differences between the gestagens in their biological activities when tested in experimental animals have been known for a considerable time, and the screening of new compounds in animals is widely used to decide which merit further development. However the validity of extrapolating the results to give an indication of the activity of the gestagens in humans is questionable. Only one such animal test, the Clauberg-McPhail test measuring uterine development in the rabbit, appears to show any correlation with the activity of the gestagens in humans. The important question is whether significant differences between the gestagens exist in humans when they are administered in the doses used for contraception. This topic has assumed importance since the demonstration that some of the adverse side effects experienced by women using combined oral contraceptives are due not only to oestrogen but to a combined action of the oestrogen and gestagen.

Two gestagens, norethisterone (NET) and levonorgestrel (LNG), have been used for many years in oral contraception, and recently new gestagens have been developed. The formulae for these compounds are shown in Fig. 1. Little information has been published on norgestimate, and it will therefore not be considered here. Only preliminary information is available for gestoden (GES). The pharma-

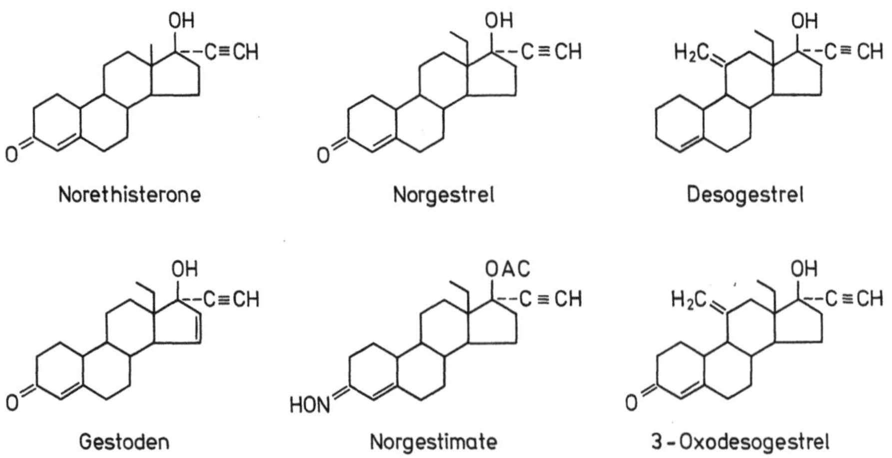

Fig. 1. Structural formulae of the gestagens

Female Contraception
Eds.: B. Runnebaum, T. Rabe, L. Kiesel

cokinetic properties of the four gestagens NET, LNG, GES and desogestrel (DSG) will be compared, and aspects of the clinical pharmacology of the formulations of these gestagens as oral contraceptives will be considered. DSG is converted in vivo to its active metabolite 3-oxo DSG and the data presented in this paper refers to this.

The oral contraceptive formulations (in combination with ethinyloestradiol, EE) considered are: 30 μg EE, 150 μg LNG; 30 μg EE, 150 μg DSG; 35 μg EE, 1000 μg NET; triphasic LNG (6 tablets 30 μg EE, 50 μg LNG; 5 tablets 40 μg EE, 75 μg LNG; and 10 tablets 30 μg EE, 125 μg LNG); 30 μg EE, 75 μg GES; and triphasic GES (6 tablets 30 μg EE, 50 μg GES; 5 tablets 40 μg EE, 70 μg GES; and 10 tablets 30 μg EE, 1000 μg GES).

More details of the clinical pharmacology of the gestagens are found in a recent review [1].

Pharmacokinetics of the Gestagens

Since the recognition that the steroid hormones usually exert their biological activity by interaction with cellular receptors, measurements of the relative binding affinity (or some other kinetic parameter) of the gestagens to receptor proteins in vitro has been widely used in comparing different gestagens. Some representative results are shown in Table 1. In all studies NET binds more weakly to the progesterone receptor than LNG, which binds less strongly than 3-oxo DSG, whereas for the androgen receptor, or sex hormone-binding globulin (SHBG), NET and 3-oxo DSG show a similar degree of binding, which is lower than that of LNG or GES. However this type of study has limitations, and the values obtained must not be taken too literally. There is a wide variation between different investigations, and values depend on the cell preparation used and on the temper-

Table 1. Binding of gestagens to various receptors

	NET	LNG	3-oxo DSG	GES
Progesterone receptor				
Uterine cytosol, human, 4 °C	55	101	117	NA
Uterine cytosol, rabbit, 4 °C	50	113	123	NA
Uterine cytosol, rat, 4 °C	8	29	67	NA
Uterine cytosol, human, 30 °C	45	120	200	NA
MCF, 7 cells, 37 °C	41	91	180	NA
Uterine endometrial cytosol, human, 30 °C	38	80	178	NA
Androgen receptor				
Rat prostate	15	27	16	27
MCF, 7 cells, 37 °C	7	18	9	NA
Sex hormone-binding globulin	11	60	19	50

Values are relative binding affinity in terms of appropriate standard; values mainly from Bergink et al. [2].
NET, norethisterone; LNG, levonorgestrel; DSG, desogestrel; GES, gestoden.

Table 2. Some pharmacokinetic parameters in humans.

	NET	LNG	3-oxo DSG	GES
First-pass effect (%)	40	0	0	0
Half-life of elimination (h)	5–12	11–20	15–21 [a]	18 [a]
Binding in plasma (%):				
Albumin	61.0	47.5	99 [a]	NA
Sex-hormone binding globulin	35.5	50.0	0 [a]	NA
Unbound	3.5	2.5	1 [a]	5 [a]

[a] Values are approximations and more information is required.
NET, norethisterone; LNG, levonorgestrel; DSG, desogestrel; GES, gestoden.

ature at which the binding is measured; for technical reasons most studies are performed at temperatures below 37 °C, the most relevant temperature. These in vitro binding studies may therefore have little relevance to physiological conditions.

In addition, only initial binding to cytosol receptors is usually measured, but subsequent events, such as transformation of the steroid-receptor complex and nuclear binding and dissociation, are also important. The chemical structure of the gestagens and the variable specificity of some of the cellular receptors lead to the gestagens interacting not only with the receptors for progestational activity but also to varying extents with receptors for other biological activities; this type of interaction may be responsible for some of the side effects produced by the gestagens. The demonstration that under artificial in vitro conditions a gestagen binds to a particular receptor does not mean that it will do so in vivo, since the amount of the gestagen reaching the tissues and other pharmacokinetic factors as well as competition with endogenous steroids determine the availability of the steroid to the receptors.

Pharmacokinetic differences between the gestagens were first demonstrated over 20 years ago (for review of early work see [3]) and some important pharmacokinetic parameters for the four gestagens under consideration are shown in Table 2. Values for the pharmacokinetic parameters differ depending on whether the gestagen is administered alone or with EE. Whilst much information is available for NET and LNG, less is available for DSG and particularly for GES, so that the values for the latter two compounds should be accepted with caution. There is a wide (3- to 5-fold) variation between subjects in their metabolism of NET and a number of other contraceptive steroids [4], and there is no reason to expect that similar variations will not occur with the other gestagens.

The data in Tables 1 and 2 indicate that quite minor variations in the chemical structure of the four gestagens lead to marked differences in their interaction with body tissues. Table 2 shows a marked difference in metabolism in the intestine and liver during absorption (first-pass effect) and rate of metabolism (elimination half-life) between NET and the other three gestagens. Almost half of orally administered NET is not bioavailable as a result of the first-pass effect, and the remainder is rapidly metabolised, whereas LNG, DSG and GES are almost 100%

bioavailable and are metabolised at only half the rate of NET. These major differences in pharmacokinetics undoubtedly account for the lower potency of NET. Marked variations occur in binding to plasma proteins. NET is known to interact less strongly than LNG with SHBG. Preliminary results suggest that the proportion of NET present in the circulation in the unbound, biologically active form is slightly higher than that of LNG, and less is bound to SHBG. Almost no information is available regarding the binding of GES, although a preliminary report suggests that as much as 5% may be unbound. Preliminary data for DSG suggests that, interestingly, binding to SHBG is not important, with almost all bound to albumin and about 1% unbound. Confirmation of these provisional and surprising results is awaited.

Pharmacodynamics of the Gestagens

Various procedures for estimating the relative potency of the gestagens in humans have been described. These include inhibition of ovulation, histological or biochemical changes in the oestrogen-stimulated uterus [5, 6] and the delay of menstruation [7]. Results obtained from the first two of these procedures must be accepted with caution since the total number of subjects studied at each dose level of the gestagen is very small, and the end point is often indistinct. For example, inhibition of ovulation may be based, by assessment of ovarian hormone production, on complete suppression of follicular and luteal function or suppression only of the latter, and there may be marked variations in the sensitivity of the response from cycle to cycle. Approximate daily doses for suppression of ovulation are: NET, 300–500 μg; LNG, 50–60 μg; DSG, 30–50 μg; GES, 30–40 μg. In the delay-of-menses test the gestagens administered alone have only weak activity and need to be given with EE. None of the above procedures would satisfy the criteria for a reliable assay.

Of the four gestagens only NET and LNG are currently used by a small proportion of women as progestogen-only pills and – however interesting the comparison of the gestagens given alone might be – what is of more interest and importance is the extent of the difference between the gestagens when they are combined with EE at the dose levels used in the formulations marketed as oral contraceptives. Combination of the gestagen with EE markedly alters the activity of both compounds, and the two may exert independent effects or act synergistically or antagonistically. For many of the responses investigated, the differences between the four gestagens combined with EE may be very small and insignificant (e.g. glucose tolerance [8]) or show a wide variability (e.g. coagulation factors [9]), or the data from various investigations may not have been obtained and analysed in a standardised manner (e.g. break-through bleeding). For these and other reasons, valid comparisons between the different oral contraceptives across a wide range of responses are not possible. It must also be emphasised that the order of relative potencies of the oral contraceptives for one response cannot be extrapolated to another response.

In two areas of metabolism, lipids and serum proteins, enough reliable information is available to provide a comparison of the five oral contraception for-

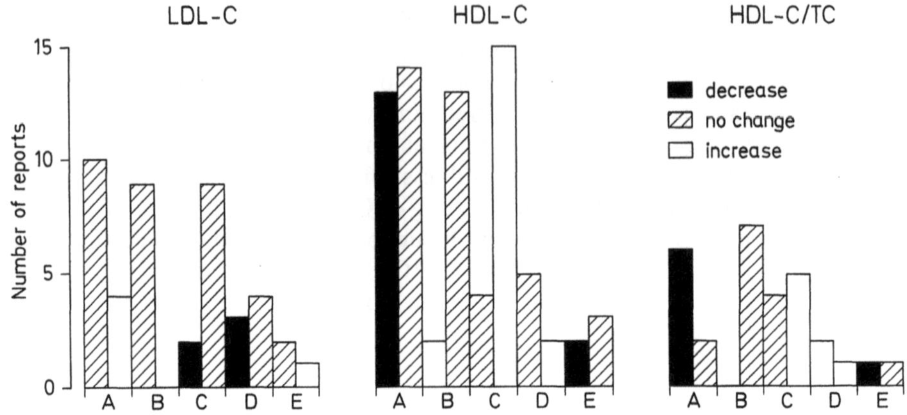

Fig. 2. Effect of oral contraceptives on serum low-density lipoprotein cholesterol (*LDL-C*), high-density lipoprotein cholesterol (*HDL-C*) and the HDL-C/LDL-C ratio (*HDL-C/TC*). *Columns* show number of published reports claiming an increase, decrease or no change in comparison with pretreatment values. *A*, 30 µg EE, 150 µg LNG; *B*, LNG triphasic; *C*, 30 µg EE, 150 µg DSG; *D*, 30 µg EE, 75 µg GES, and GES triphasic; *E*, 35 µg EE, 500–1000 µg NET

mulations. Figure 2 shows a compilation from all the published reports of their effects on serum low-density lipoprotein cholesterol (LDL-C) and high-density lipoprotein cholesterol (HDL-C) and the ratio of these two measurements, which is considered to be a good indicator of the risk of developing cardiovascular disease. Clear differences exist between the formulations. Monophasic LNG (column A, Fig. 2) and EE-NET (column E) tend to raise LDL-C and to lower HDL-C and hence reduce the HDL-C:LDL-C ratio. The triphasic LNG preparation (column B) does not affect either lipoprotein. EE-DSG (column C) does not change LDL-C but increases HDL-C so that there is an increase in the ratio; EE-GES (column D) has a similar but less pronounced effect. Thus EE-DSG, and to a lesser extent EE-GES, tend to have a presumably beneficial effect, increasing HDL-C with a tendency to decrease LDL-C. Two points need to be emphasised concerning the results shown in Fig. 2. Firstly, they refer only to the direction of change (increase or decrease) and not to the magnitude of change. Secondly, due to the paucity of information for gestoden, results from trials of the monophasic and triphasic formulations have been combined, although it is likely that differences between the two formulations will be apparent when more results are available (see results for the monophasic and triphasic formulations of levonorgestrel).

Figure 3, based upon a consensus of a number of published reports, shows the effect of the formulations on serum SHBG in comparison to the effect of 30 µg EE alone. It is clear that the formulations containing DSG and GES do not antagonise the EE-induced increase, that the NET and triphasic LNG formulations reduce the EE-induced increase by about half, and that the monophasic LNG formulation completely antagonises the increase.

In order to provide a clearer comparison between the SHBG data and the lipid data shown in Fig. 2, the latter in respect of LDL-C and HDL-C has been

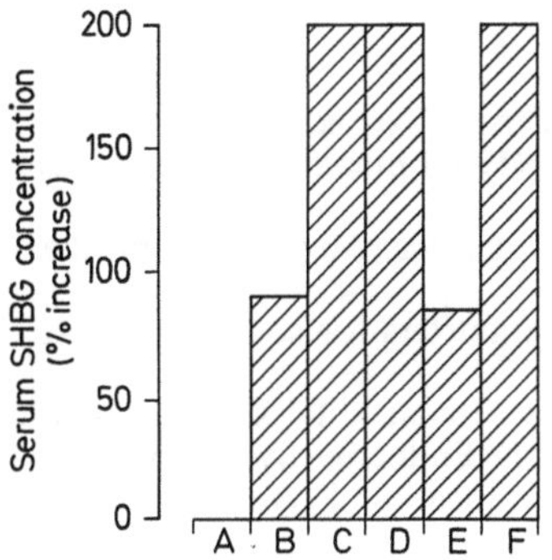

Fig. 3. Effect of oral contraceptives on serum sex hormone-binding globulin (SHBG) concentrations. *Columns* show percentage increases compared to pretreatment values. *A–D*, as in Fig. 2; *E*, 35 µg EE, 1000 µg NET; *F*, 30 µg EE

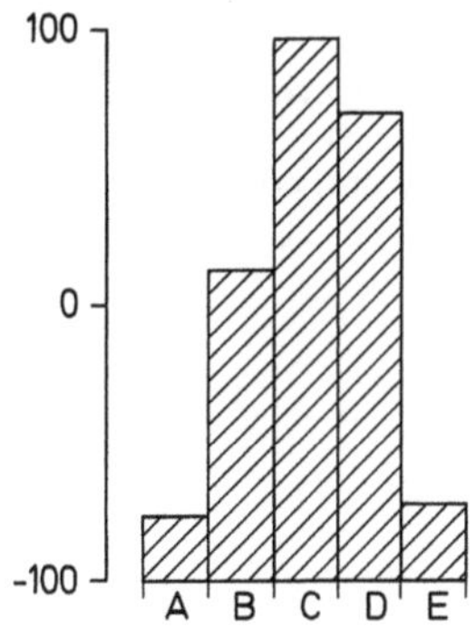

Fig. 4. Effect of oral contraceptives on serum low-density lipoprotein cholesterol (LDL-C) and high-density lipoprotein cholesterol (HDL-C) derived from data shown in Fig. 2. *Columns* show percentage of total reports for each oral contraceptive indicating a change in LDL-C or HDL-C. Negative score given for decrease in HDL-C or increase in LDL-C; positive score given for increase in HDL-C or decrease in LDL-C. *A–D*, as in Fig. 2; *E*, 35 µg EE, 1000 µg NET

"scored" on an arbitrary points system, and the values are shown in Fig. 4. The higher the value in Fig. 4, the more "beneficial" (increase in HDL-C and decrease in LDL-C) is the change in the lipoproteins. A comparison of Figs. 3 and 4 clearly shows the differential effects of the oral contraceptives on the two responses.

Thus, for some pharmacological responses sufficient information is available to show differences between oral contraceptive formulations. The demonstration that the various gestagens, in combination with a similar dose of EE, show differential effects is important in the development of an effective and acceptable oral contraceptive. Many of the responses can be modified by adjusting the relative doses of the components, but the specificity of the gestagen is important in producing a "balanced" contraceptive which has a high efficacy, a low incidence of break-through bleeding and does not produce any adverse metabolic effects. No information is available which would indicate whether there is any difference between the low-dose oral contraceptives in inducing serious clinical side effects. The low incidence of such side effects in oral contraceptive users implies that it will probably be many years before sufficient epidemiological data is available to answer this question. In the meantime more detailed and extensive metabolic investigations of the oral contraceptives should be performed, preferably on a comparative basis, so that the relative merits of the formulations can be assessed. At the present time it would appear prudent to use a low-dose contraceptive which is associated with minimal adverse metabolic changes.

References

1. Fotherby K (1984) A new look at progestogens. Clin Obstet Gynaecol 11:701–722
2. Bergink EW, van Meel F, Turpin EW, van der Vies J (1983) Binding of progestogens to receptor proteins. J Steroid Biochem 19:1563–1570
3. Fotherby K, James F (1972) Metabolism of synthetic steroids. Adv Steroid Biochem 3:67–165
4. Fotherby K (1983) Variability of pharmacokinetic parameters for contraceptive steroids. J Steroid Biochem 19:817–820
5. Ferin J (1972) Orally active progestational compounds. Human studies: effects on the uterovaginal tract. In: Tausk M (ed) Pharmacology of the Endocrine System, vol 2. International Enzyclopedia of Pharmacology and Therapeutics. Pergamon, Oxford, p 245
6. King RJB, Withehead MI (1986) Assessment of the potency of orally administered progestins. Fertil Steril 46:1062–1066
7. Swyer GIM (1984) The development of potency tests. J Obstet Gynaecol 4 [Suppl 2]:S110–S113
8. van der Vange N (1986) Low dose oral contraceptives and their influence on metabolic pathways. Thesis presented to University of Utrecht, pp 53–62
9. Sabra A, Bonnar J (1983) Haemostatic system changes induced by oral contraceptives. J Reprod Med 28:85–91

Development of Progestogens

F. Neumann, B. Duesterberg, and H. Laurent

Research Laboratories of Schering AG, Berlin (West)-Bergkamen, FRG

The development of progestogens is one of the most fascinating chapters in the history of steroid chemistry and biology. When in 1934 the structure of progesterone was elucidated [1], no one could have guessed just how important progestogens would later become as a component of hormonal contraceptives. It is truly amazing what has been achieved in this field in the relatively short period of just over 50 years. The goal from the very start was the development of orally active progestogens and depot preparations. Progesterone, the natural substance, is inactive on oral administration; we shall return to this later (Fig. 1).

The first orally active oestrogen was discovered in 1938 with the synthesis of ethinylestradiol [2]. It was thought at that time that it would be possible to extrapolate this principle to the testosterone molecule, that is, to obtain an orally active androgen by introducing an ethinyl group in the C_{17} position (testosterone itself is also metabolised too quickly) (Fig. 2).

Although ethinyl testosterone displayed some androgenetic activity on oral administration, much more surprising and completely unexpected was the finding that the compound had progestational properties even after oral administration [2]. The ethinyl group can also be written into the steroid skeleton in a slightly

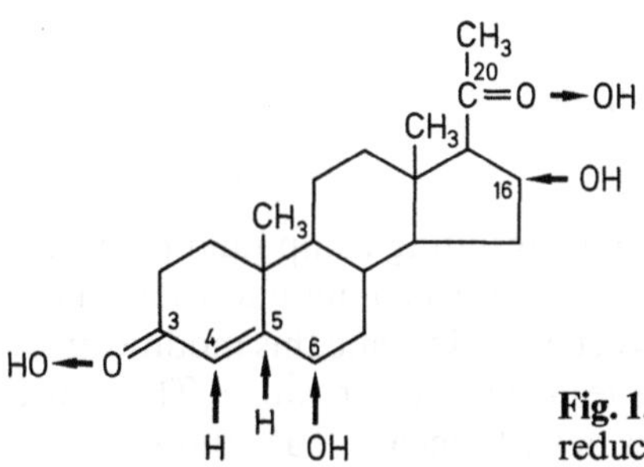

Fig. 1. Metabolism and inactivation of progesterone by reductases, hydroxylases and dehydrogenases

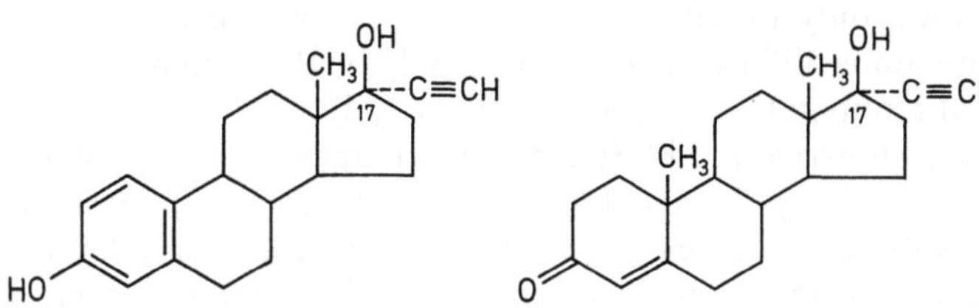

Fig. 2. 17-α-Ethinylestradiol (*left*) and 17-α-ethinyl testosterone (ethisterone) (*right*)

Female Contraception
Eds.: B. Runnebaum, T. Rabe, L. Kiesel

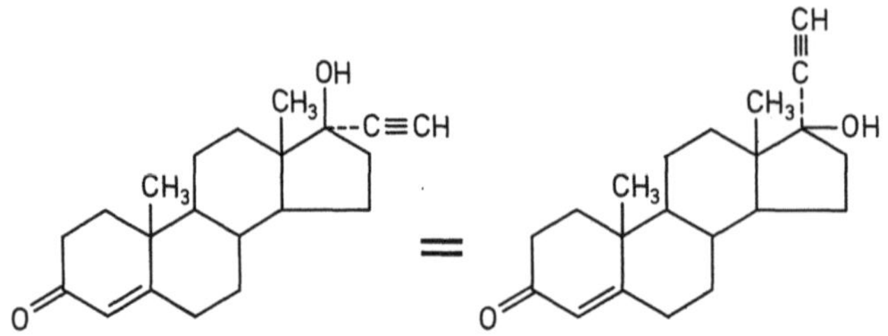

Fig. 3. Ethisterone (*left*) and pregneninolone (pregnen-yn-ol-on) (*right*)

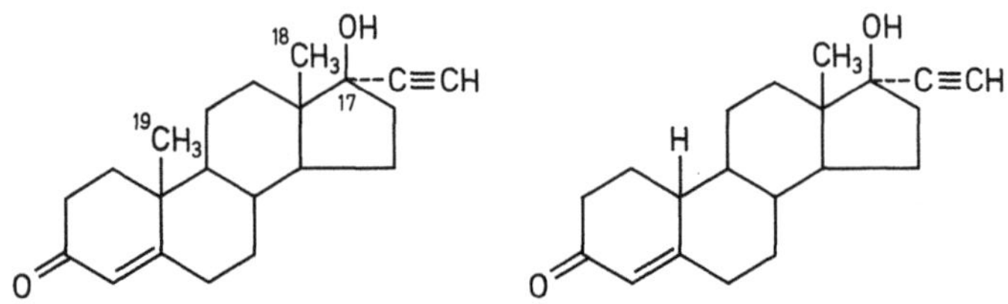

Fig. 4. Ethisterone (*left*) and norethisterone (17-α-ethinyl-19-nortestosterone) (*right*)

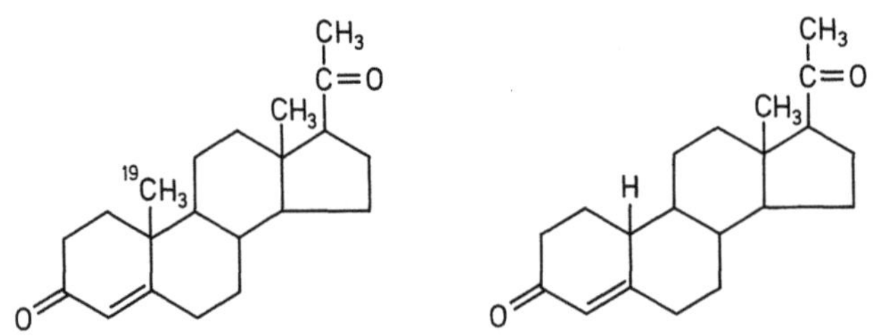

Fig. 5. Progesterone (*left*) and 19-norprogesterone (*right*)

different way; the chemists did this and called the resulting compound pregneninolone (Fig. 3). Their obvious intention was to produce a compound which more closely resembled progesterone, which is a C_{21} steroid. Despite this modification, however, the substance naturally remained a testosterone derivative. This was a highly innovative development even if its low activity meant that ethinyl testosterone was out of the question as a progestational component for an oral contraceptive. However, it was only a small step from ethinyl testosterone to norethisterone. The two compounds differ from each other only by the presence or absence of a single methyl group in the C_{19} position (Figs. 4, 5).

But how did the chemists arrive at this? Scientists working in the United States in the 1950s found that removing the angular methyl group in the C_{19} position of progesterone led to substantial increase of activity on subcutaneous administration [3]. The correct conclusions were drawn from this, and the same principle was applied to ethinyl testosterone in the hope and intention of obtaining an orally more potent progestogen. This hope was fulfilled with the synthesis of ethinyl-19-nortestosterone, or norethisterone [4]. Norethisterone became the parent

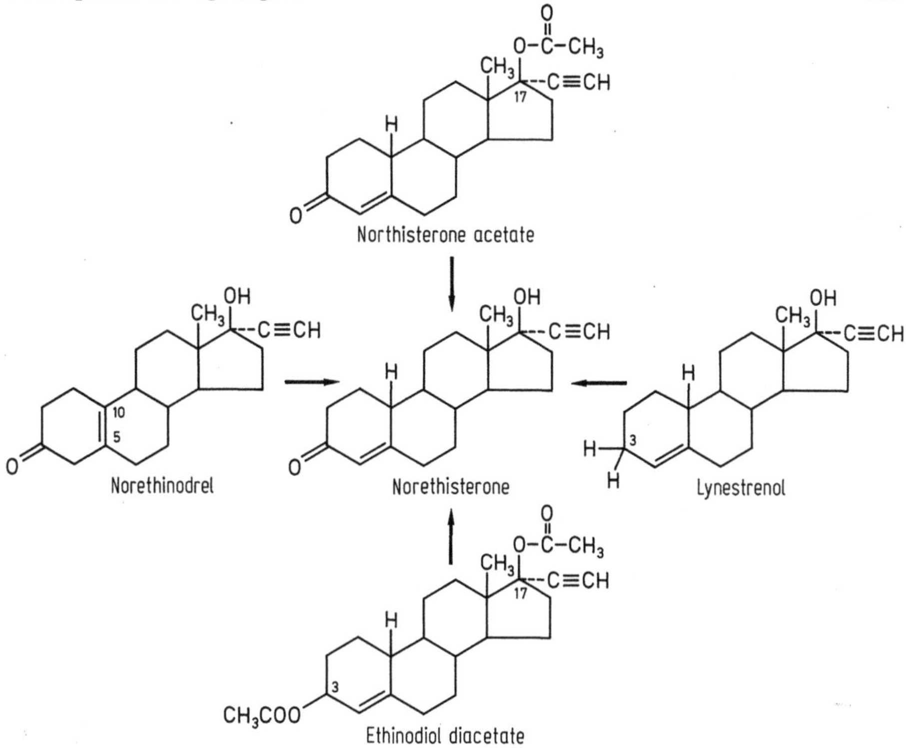

Fig. 6. Norethisterone as the parent substance for a series of progestogens

substance for a whole series of progestogens which are still being used in oral contraceptives (Fig. 6).

Norethisterone itself is, of course, one of these, and it is worth noting that all derivatives of norethisterone are metabolised to the parent substance [5]. To this extent, they hardly represent an advance in that the biologically active steroid is norethisterone itself. It might also be mentioned that an ester of norethisterone – norethisterone oenanthate – was introduced in 1978 as a 3-month depot contraceptive. A 1-month injectable consisting of norethisterone oenanthate and oestradiol valerate is being developed by the WHO and will probably be available in the foreseeable future (Fig. 7).

In the 1960s Smith substituted ethyl for the methyl group at C atom 18 [6]. The result was norgestrel, initially a racemate. Further development later led to the selective synthesis of the biologically active form of norgestrel, levonorgestrel [7]. This was a major advance, since norgestrel was not only considerably more potent – enabling it to be administered at much lower doses – but also differed positively from ethinyl-19-nortestosterone as regards its spectrum of action, at least as far as the pharmacology was concerned. Levonorgestrel is still in use today as the progestational component in most, or the most frequently prescribed, oral contraceptives. The youngest generation of progestogens developed for hormonal contraception includes desogestrel [8], norgestimate [9] and, as the most recent development, gestoden [10]. The strucutral formulas are shown in Fig. 8

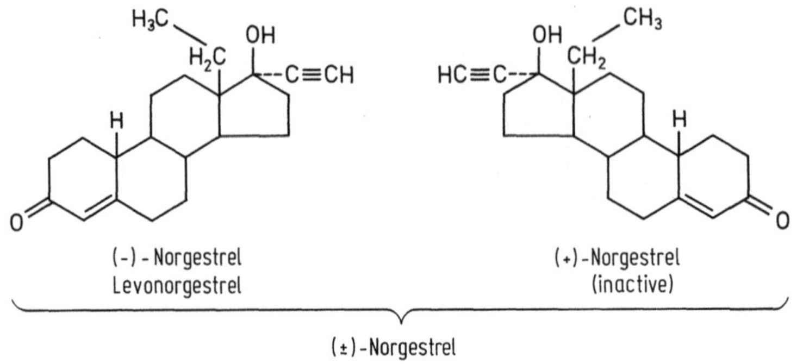

Fig. 7. Norgestrel isomers

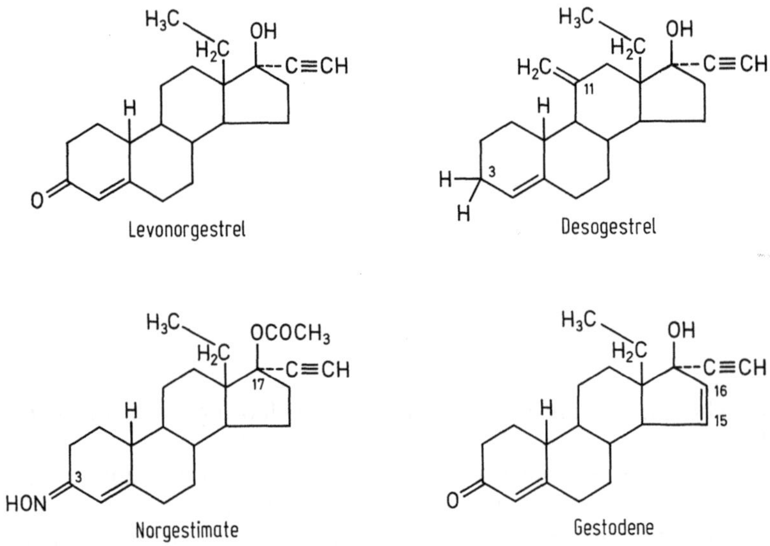

Fig. 8. The latest generation of progestogens

and the particular properties of these progestogens will be dealt with in later presentations.

Attempts have, of course, also been made to synthesise orally active derivatives of progesterone. Progesterone is virtually ineffective on oral administration; it is completely broken down into biologically inactive metabolites, at the latest on passing through the liver.

Figure 1 represents a simplified diagram of the metabolism and inactivation of progesterone by enzymes such as reductases, hydroxylases and dehydrogenases in positions 3, 4, 5, 6, 16 and 20. Reduction of the 20-keto group alone leads to 20-hydroxy compounds with only a very weak progestational effect.

This led to attempts to block the reduction of the 20-keto group by the introduction of a space-filling substituent into the neighbouring 17 position. The compound synthesised as a result of this, 17-α-acetoxyprogesterone (see Fig. 9), dis-

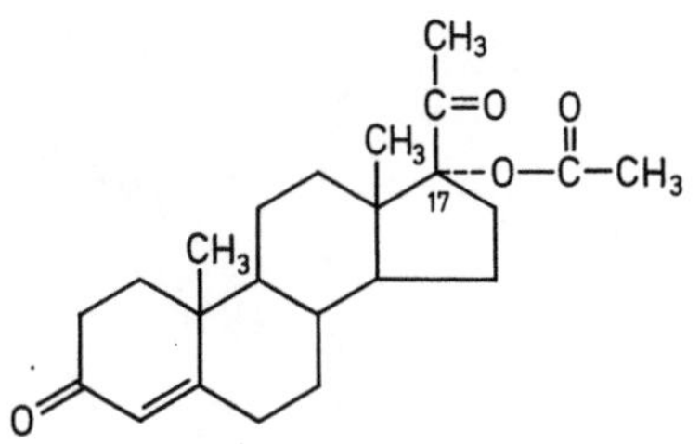

Fig. 9. 17-α-Hydroprogesterone acetate

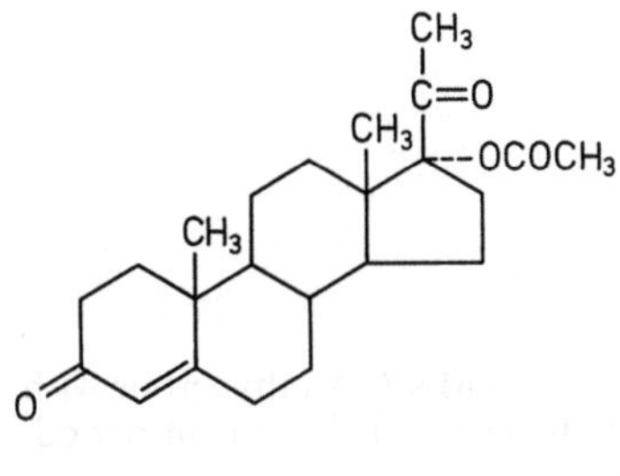

17α -Hydroprogesterone acetate
A

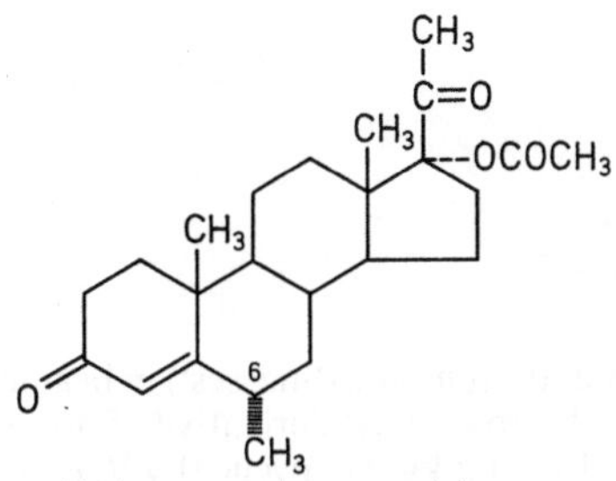

Medroxyprogesterone acetate
B

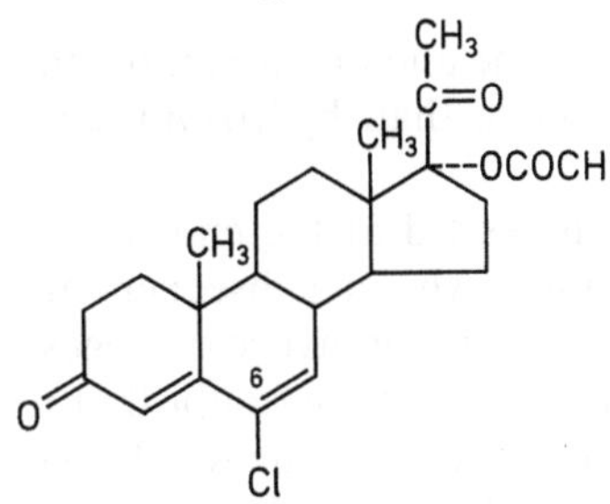

Chlormadinone acetate
C

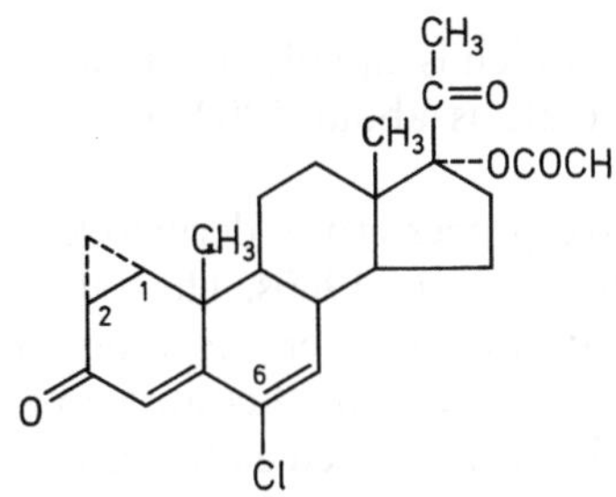

Cyproterone acetate
D

Fig. 10 A–D. Progestogens of the hydroxyprogesterone series. Relative oral progestational activities: **A** 1, **B** 100, **C** 400, **D** 1200

played remarkable oral efficacy [11]. 17-α-Acetoxyprogesterone became the parent substance for an entire substance class. It can be seen in Fig. 1 that a biological metabolic reaction of progesterone takes place via hydroxylation in position 6. To block this metabolic step as well, acetoxyprogesterones were synthesised with an alkyl or halogen group (e.g. methyl or chlorine) and with an additional double bond in position C_6. The results were potent progestogens, such as chlormadinone acetate [12] (double bond in C_6 + chlorine atom) and medroxyprogesterone acetate [13]. The chemical structure of these progestogens from the hydroxyprogesterone series is illustrated in Fig. 10.

Some of these compounds were remarkably potent progestogens even on oral administration. Compound B, for example, was about 100 times stronger than the parent substance, 17-α-acetoxyprogesterone. Steroid C was even 400 times stronger. The strongest of the 17-α-hydroxyprogesterone derivatives is cyproter-

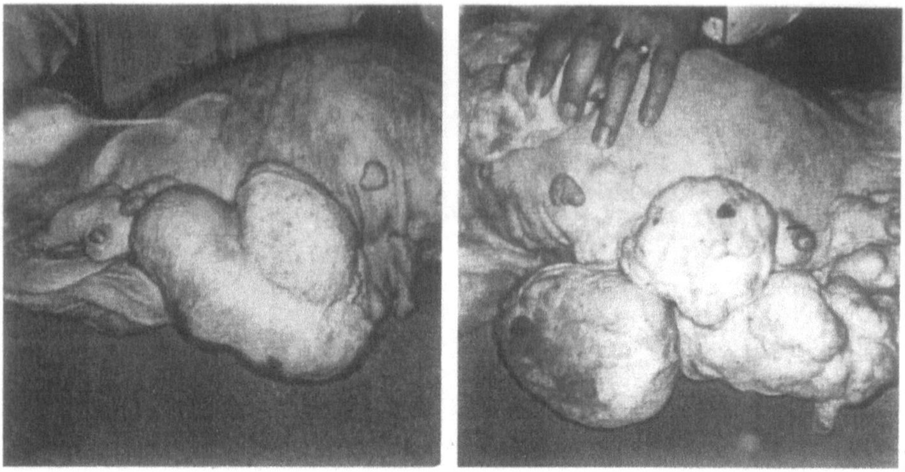

a b

Fig. 11 a, b. Mammary tumours ('masses') in beagles treated by **a** MK 665, ethynerone with mestranol; **b** the chloro-ethynyl derivative of norgestrel with nestranol. Treatment period, 4 years; Dosage, 1.05 mg/kg/day cyclic (by V. R. Berliner)

one acetate [14], which is equally potent as a progesterone and an antiandrogen. Cyproterone acetate is about 1200 times more effective than hydroxyprogesterone acetate.

All 17-hydroxyprogesterone derivatives were synthesised at the end of the 1950s and beginning of the 1960s. The natural question is why no subsequent attempts were made to find even more potent or more suitable hydroxyprogesterone derivatives for hormonal contraception. There can be little doubt that it was the beagle dog which acted as the brake in the truest sense of the word. The photo shown in Fig. 11 went round the world in 1970. It shows mammary tumours weighing several kilograms in a beagle dog treated with a progestogen for several years as part of the obligatory toxicity studies. Several hydroxyprogesterone derivatives in particular – including chlormadinone acetate and medroxyprogesterone acetate – came under suspicion in this respect. It was thought by some at that time that the mammary tumor-inducing effect was a particular (negative) property of progestogens. We now know that this was wide of the truth when extrapolated to man and other animal species. The mammary tumour-inducing effect correlates with the progestogenicity, and hydroxyprogesterone derivatives in particular display extremely high bioavailability and a long duration of action in the dog. We are now also aware of the mechanisms on which this phenomenon is based. It is primarily a positive feedback between progesterone and the secretion of growth hormone which is specific to the dog. Canine growth hormone is highly mammotropic, and the mammary tumours develop on the basis of chronic overstimulation of the mammary glands (for review see [15, 16]). This is further supported by the fact that dogs treated over several years with high doses of progestogen develop the symptoms of acromegaly and diabetes (Figs. 12, 13). It is a generally known fact that growth hormone displays insulin-antagonistic properties.

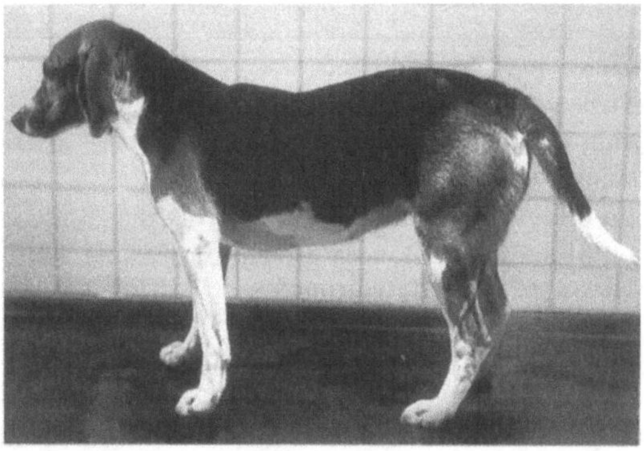

Fig. 12. Normal beagle dog

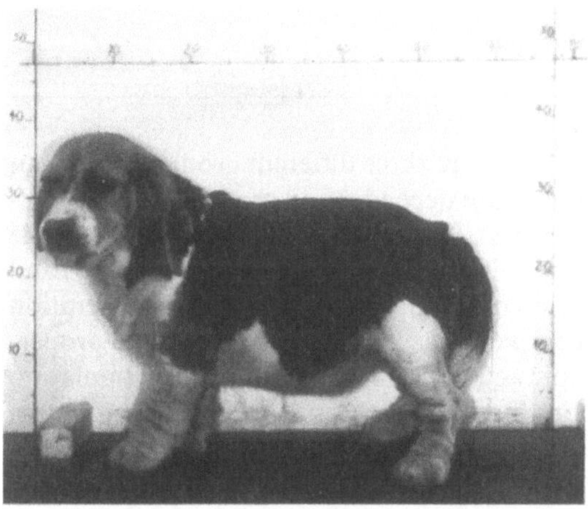

Fig. 13. Beagle dog after many years' treatment with a progestogen. Note the symptoms of acromegaly (paws, face) and diabetes (trunk)

Although we now know that these findings cannot be extrapolated to women, some authorities still stubbornly refuse to accept this. Medroxyprogesterone acetate has still not been approved in the United States for contraception for instance, although it has been – paradoxically – for the indication metastatic mammary carcinoma. There can be no doubt that these findings brought hydroxyprogesterone derivatives into disrepute and also caused great damage to developments in this field.

We shall now deal briefly with the biology of progestogens. The term 'progestogen' is sometimes no more than a convenient partial description, since there are some synthetic progestogens which, at least on the basis of their properties and effects in many animal species, could just as easily be classed as androgens or oestrogens. The individual synthetic progestogens have varying spectra of effects, none of which corresponds exactly with that of progesterone. A number of possible effects of progestogens are listed in Table 1. Table 2 presents the effects of a number of synthetic progestogens and of progesterone. This very simplified table [9, 17, 18] ignores the relative potencies of the individual compounds.

Table 1. Possible activities of progestogens

Progestational	e.g.	Transformation of the endometrium
Oestrogenic	e.g.	Positive Allen-Doisy assay
Androgenic	e.g.	Stimulation of prostate and seminal vesicle growth in castrated rodents
Anti-oestrogenic	e.g.	Inhibition of oestrogen-induced uterine growth
Anti-androgenic	e.g.	Inhibition of androgen-induced growth of prostate and seminal vesicle in castrated rodents
Antigonadotrophic	e.g.	Inhibition of ovulation
Glucocorticoid-like activity	e.g.	Inhibition of ACTH secretion and adrenal atrophy
ACTH stimulation	e.g.	Increased glucocorticoid secretion, increase of transcortin
Virilisation of female foetuses		(Androgenic)
Feminisation of male foetuses		(Anti-androgenic)

As regards the chemical structure there are three different groups, and it can be seen at a glance that particular effects are dependent on certain structures, although there are exceptions to these 'rules'. For instance, all 19-*nor*-testosterone derivatives have androgenic properties (with the exception of norethynodrel) and oestrogenic activities (with the exception of levonorgestrel and the last generation of compounds). None of these progestogens has any glucocorticoid-like properties. The progestogens with oestrogenic activity lead rather to ACTH stimulation (again, with the exception of levonorgestrel and last generation of compounds). In the case of norethynodrel the oestrogenic properties are so pronounced that this compound could almost be classed as an oestrogen. This oestrogenic activity is also seen in humans, e.g. by an increase of transcortin [19].

The alkylating or halogenated acetoxyprogesterone derivatives are distinguished by the absence of androgenic and oestrogenic effects. Megestrol acetate, chlormadinone acetate and cyproterone acetate have antiandrogenic properties, which are most pronounced in the case of cyproterone acetate [20].

All the progestogens of this group listed here also have certain glucocorticoid-like effects, which can become manifest clinically at extremely high dosage [21–25]. Because of their antiandrogenic effects, chlormadinone acetate, megestrol acetate and cyproterone acetate all have the potential of feminising male foetuses [20, 26]. Medroxyprogesterone acetate, on the other hand, has virilising properties, although it is not androgenic in the classical tests [27].

The clinical use is determined largely by the spectrum of effects of the individual progestogens. A substance with strong antigonadotrophic and strong anti-oestrogenic effects is to be preferred as the progestogen component for a hormonal contraceptive. Such a compound is said to contribute to the inhibition of ovulation and to induce the known changes in the cervical mucus that render sperm ascent difficult (minipill effect).

An oral contraceptive containing cyproterone acetate or chlormadinone acetate is to be preferred for women predisposed to acne, seborrhoea or mild hirsutism, since the antiandrogenic effect represents an advantage in such cases.

Table 2. Activity spectrum of some progestogens

	Endometrial transformation	Antigonadotrophic	Antioestrogenic	Oestrogenic	Androgenic/anabolic	Antiandrogenic	Glucocorticoid-like activity	Antimineralocorticoid	Virilisation	Feminisation
Progesterone	+	+	+	−	−	− (±)	+[a]	+	−	−
Norethisterone	+	+	+	+	+	−	−	−	+	−
Lynestrenol	+	+	+	+	+	−	−	−	+	−
Norethynodrel	+	+	±	+	±	−	−	−	?	?
Levonorgestrel	+	+	+	−	+	−	−	−	+	−
3-keto-desogestrel	+	+	+	−	+	−	?	−	+	−
Gestodene	+	+	+	−	+	−	+[a]	+	+	−
Chlormadinone acetate	+	+	+	−	−	+	+	−	−	+
Cyproterone acetate	+	+	+	−	−	+	+	−	−	+

[a] In non-relevant doses.

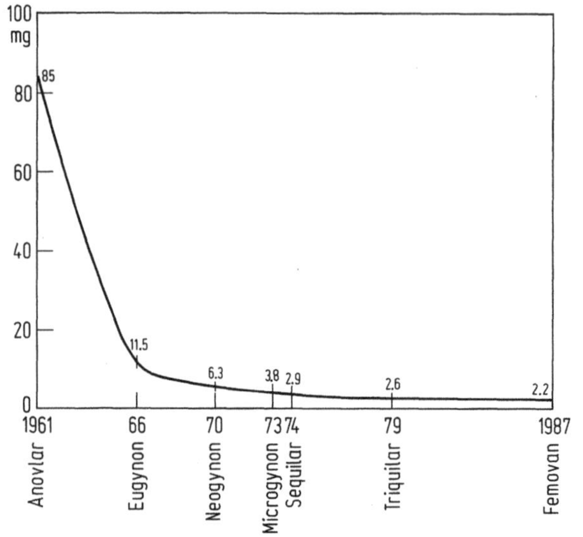

Fig. 14. Oral contraceptives. Reduction of total hormone doses (Schering AG)

Only so-called "pure" progestogens, which have no androgenic or oestrogenic effects, can be considered for use in disturbances of pregnancy. Clinical experience indicates that progestogens with androgenic effects – in combination with an oestrogen – achieve particularly favourable results in the therapy of the female climacteric. Women with depression are said to respond especially well to such progestogens.

These few examples are sufficient to show that the indication is dependent on the spectrum of activities and that selective use of progestogens is not always simple for the physician.

To conclude, we should like to make a prediction regarding further developments in this field and as to whether there will ever be a still better progestogen for oral contraception. Important criteria for an oral contraceptive are contraceptive reliability, good cycle control and a further reduction of the side effects potential. This can be done either by reducing the dose or by developing new substances which differ positively from other progestogens as regards their spectrum of action and the presence or absence of certain partial effects.

As Fig. 14 illustrates, a further reduction of the dose is hardly conceivable. Today's modern micropreparations contain only a fraction of the amount of hormones contained in the old "pills." The second criterion – good cycle control – has also been achieved to all intents and purposes. As regards the third criterion, all modern preparations are marked by extremely good tolerance and no longer have any adverse influence on lipid and carbohydrate metabolism or on clotting parameters. For all these reasons, no new progestogen will be developed in the foreseeable future. If any further progress is at all conceivable, this will perhaps be in the class of the somewhat neglected hydroxyprogesterone derivatives. At present, however, there is no sign of any new developments here, either.

References

1. Butenandt A, Westphal U, Hohlweg W (1934) Über das Hormon des Corpus luteum. Hoppe-Seylers Z Physiol Chem 227:84–98
2. Inhoffen HH, Hohlweg W (1938) Neue per os wirksame weibliche Keimdrüsenhormonderivate: 17-Aethinyl-oestradiol und Pregnen-in-on-3-ol-17. Naturwissenschaften 26:96
3. Miramontes L, Rosenkranz G, Djerassi C (1951) The synthesis of 19-norprogesterone. J Am Chem Soc 73:3540
4. Djerassi C, Miramontes L, Rosenkranz G, Sandheimer F (1954) Synthesis of 19-nor-17alpha-ethyltestosterone and 19-nor-17alpha-methyltestosterone. J Am Chem Soc 76:4092
5. Fotherby K (1974) Metabolism of synthetic steroids by animals and man. Acta Endocrinol (Copenh) 185:119–147
6. Smith H, Hughes GA, Douglas GH, Wendth GR, Buzby GC jun, Edgren RA, Fisher J, Foell T, Gadsby B, Hartley D, Herbst D, Jansen ABA, Ledig K, McLoughlin BJ, McMenamin J, Pattison TW, Phillips PC, Rees R, Siddall J, Siuda J, Smith LL, Tokolics J, Watson DHP (1964) Totally synthetic steroid hormones. Part II: 13β-alkylgona-1.3 5(10)-trienes,13β-alkylgon-4-en-3-ones, and related compounds. J Chem Soc 4:4472–4479
7. Rufer C, Kosmol H, Schröder E, Kieslich K, Gibian H (1967) Totalsynthese optisch aktiver Steroide. III. Totalsynthese von optisch aktiven 13-Äthylgonan-derivaten. Liebigs Ann Chem 702:141
8. van den Broek AJ, van Bokhoven C, Hobbelen PMJ, Leemhuis J (1975) 11-Alkylidene steroids in the 19-nor series. Recl Trav Chim Paus Bas Belg 94:35
9. Hahn DW, Allen GO, McGuire JL (1977) The pharmacological profile of norgestimate, a new orally active progestin. Contraception 16:541
10. Hofmeister, Annen K, Laurent H, Petzoldt K, Wiechert R (1986) Synthesen von Gestoden. Arzneimittelforschung 36:781
11. Junkmann K (1954) Über protrahiert wirksame Gestagene. Naunyn Schmiedebergs Arch Exp Pathol Pharmakol 223:244
12. Brückner K, Hampel B, Johnsen U (1961) Darstellung und Eigenschaften monohalogenierter 3-Keto-4.6-diensteroide. Chem Ber 94:1225
13. Babcock JC, Gutsell ES, Herr ME, Hogg JA, Stucki JC, Barnes LE, Dulin WE (1958) 6Alpha-methyl-17alpha-hydroxyprogesterone-17-acylates; a new class of potent progestines. J Am Chem Soc 80:2904
14. Wiechert R, Neumann R (1965) Gestagene Wirksamkeit von 1-Methyl- und 1.2Alpha-Methylen-Steroiden. Arzneimittelforschung 15:244
15. Beier S, Düsterberg B, El Etreby MF, Elger W, Neumann F, Nishino Y (1983) Endocrine effects of contraceptive steroids given in excessive doses. In: Benagiano G, Diczfalusy E (eds) Endocrine mechanisms in fertility regulation. Raven, New York
16. Neumann F, Elger W, El Etreby MF (1986) Experimental endocrinology and pathology of mammogenesis. In: Bässler R, Hübner K (eds) Pathology of neoplastic and endocrine induced diseases of the breast. Fischer, Stuttgart
17. Neumann F (1986) Grundlagen der hormonalen Kontrazeption. In: Hammerstein J (ed) 25 Jahre hormonale Kontrazeption. Excerpta Medica, Amsterdam, p 18
18. Pasquale SA et al. (1976) Preclinical studies with norgestimate (ORF 10131), a new orally active progestin. Abstracts of the 8th World Congress of Gyncecology and Obstetrics, Mexico 1976. Excerpta Medica Int Congr Series No 396, p 186
19. Schwarzt U, Hammerstein J (1974) The oestrogenic potency of various contraceptive steroids as determined by their effects on transcortin-binding capacity. Acta Endocrinol (Copenh) 76:159
20. Neumann F, Steinbeck H (1974) Antiandrogens. In: Eichler O, Farah A, Herken H, Welch AD (eds) Handbook of Experimental Pharmacology, vol 35/2. Springer, Berlin Heidelberg New York, p 235
21. Camanni F, Massara F, Molinatti GM (1963) The cortisone-like effect of 6alpha-methyl-17alpha-acetoxy-progesterone in the adrenalectomized man. Acta Endocrinol (Copenh) 43:477

22. Girard J, Baumann JB (1975) Hemmung des CRF ACTH Nebennierenrindensystems durch Cyproteronacetat. Klin Wochenschr 53:933
23. von Mühlendahl KE (1977) Cyproteronacetat and adrenocortical function. Lancet I:1160
24. Mathews JH, Abrams CAL, Morishima A (1970) Pituitaryadrenal function in ten patients receiving medroxyprogesterone acetate for true precocious puberty. J Clin Endocrinol Metab 30:653
25. Sadeghi-Nejad A, Kaplan SL, Grumbach MM (1971) The effect of medroxyprogesterone acetate on adrenocortical function in children with precocious puberty. J Pediatr 78:616
26. Neumann F, von Berswordt-Wallrabe, Elger W, Steinbeck H, Hahn JD, Kramer M (1970) Aspects of androgen-dependent events as studied by antiandrogens. Rec Prog Horm Res 26:337
27. Neumann F, Gräf KJ, Elger W (1974) Hormone-induced disturbances in sexual differentiation. In: Raspe G (ed) Hormones and embryonic development. Advances in the biosciences 13. Pergamon, Oxford, p 71

Review of the Preclinical Pharmacology and Clinical Studies of the Norgestimate-containing Oral Contraceptive, Cilest

Samuel A. Pasquale

Robert Wood Johnson Medical School, 1 Robert Wood Johnson Place, New Brunswick, NJ 08903-0019, USA

Introduction

When oral contraceptives (OCs) first became available in the early 1960s, hormonal contraception represented an entirely new approach to the prevention of pregnancy. Consequently, attention was focused on the ability of an OC to prevent pregnancy and maintain good cycle control.

In common with the OCs of today, the earliest pills contained various types of synthetic estrogens and/or progestogens. The first estrogen used was mestranol, which was soon replaced in large part by ethinyl estradiol. Various progestogens of the 19-nortestosterone derivation were consistently used as the progestogen component of the pill. As with our current OCs, the earliest pills were combination products taken once a day for 21 days of each menstrual cycle. However, these early forms differ from today's OCs in that they contain relatively high doses of progestogen and/or estrogen.

Patients' experiences with the early OCs confirmed that this was the most effective and convenient contraceptive method available. However, contraceptive efficacy was achieved at some cost in terms of unwanted effects. As clinical experience with high-dose OC formulations accumulated, some potentially serious and annoying side effects were reported. Subsequent research indicated that some of the serious unwanted effects of OCs were associated with their high steroid dosages and activity.

Until recent years, it was reported that estrogen was responsible for most of the serious side effects of combination OCs [1–4]. Today, it is widely recognized that the progestogenic component of the preparation may also be associated with important adverse effects [5–8]. The higher the dose of progestogen, the greater the probability of increased low-density lipoprotein (LDL) cholesterol levels, decreased high-density lipoprotein (HDL) cholesterol levels, and decreased glucose tolerance.

Recent research has focused on the development of new OCs that contain the lowest possible doses of both the estrogen and progestogen while maintaining contraceptive efficacy and good menstrual cycle control. This is in keeping with the recommendations of the World Health Organization (WHO), which issued a statement in 1978 advising that the lowest-dose OCs should be used to reduce the incidence of metabolic and hemostatic side effects.

It was against this background that norgestimate was developed in 1979. Norgestimate demonstrates significant qualitative differences from other progestogens currently used in OCs. It demonstrates high progestational activity, yet it

Female Contraception
Eds.: B. Runnebaum, T. Rabe, L. Kiesel

is virtually devoid of androgenic activity, and hence is a highly specific progestogenic agent. Evidence of the efficacy of norgestimate and of its advantages over other progestogens has led to its use in several OC preparations, one of which is currently marketed in several European countries.

This review describes the preclinical endocrine profile of norgestimate.

Preclinical Pharmacology of Norgestimate

Norgestimate, a new progestogen with an oximo at position 3 and an 18-methyl group (Fig. 1), is the result of a research program whose goal was the development of a potent, but selective, progestogen that could be utilized in a new, lower-dose

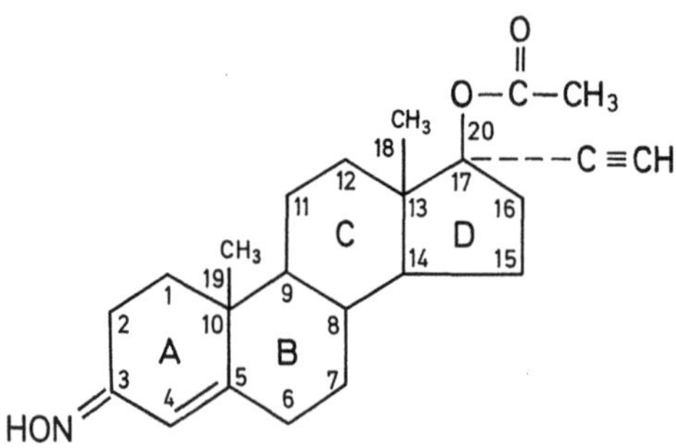

Fig. 1. Chemical structure of norgestimate

OC. The foremost requirements for this new agent were that it: (a) be an effective suppressor of ovulation; (b) have antiestrogenic activity; (c) demonstrate minimal androgenicity; and (d) maintain normal endometrial morphology.

Antiovulatory Activity

An extensive preclinical evaluation of norgestimate was conducted in several animal models to determine its endocrine activities in various bioassay systems. The results of these investigations demonstrated that norgestimate is a very effective progestogen which inhibits ovulation by inhibiting luteinizing hormone (LH) and stimulates endometrial transformation.

Norgestimate's binding to the progestational receptors was demonstrated by its displacement of tritiated progesterone from these sites (Fig. 2). Its IC_{50} is about 5×10^{-8} *M*.

In common with other progestogens, the site of norgestimate's antiovulatory activity is the hypothalamic-pituitary axis. The results of controlled preclinical studies in rats showed that norgestimate 1 mg/kg suppresses ovulation in all animals. This inhibition correlates with the suppression of the preovulatory LH surge, as demonstrated by control animals continuing to have a surge of LH on the day of proestrus, whereas norgestimate-treated animals demonstrate no such surge.

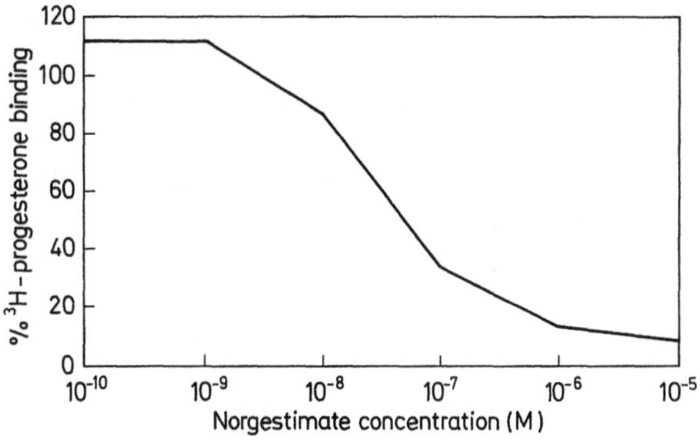

Fig. 2. Binding of norgestimate to rabbit uterine progesterone receptor

The ability of luteinizing hormone-releasing hormone (LH-RH) to reverse the antiovulatory activity of norgestimate was further evidence that its site of antiovulatory activity is on the hypothalamic-pituitary axis. Ovulation data in the rat show that norgestimate inhibits ovulation but that this can be reversed by the administration of LH-RH.

A semiquantitative assay was used to measure the degree of uterine proliferation in the rabbit after administration of norgestimate. McPhail units were used to grade the degree of endometrial proliferation, with 0 being equivalent to "no response" and 4 being equivalent to "maximal response." Norgestimate produced the maximal degree of proliferation of the endometrium in the rabbit uterus, with a McPhail index of 4.

Norgestimate also stimulates endometrial proliferation when applied *locally* to the uterus. Studies were performed in rabbits in which a section of one uterine horn was tied off and norgestimate injected between the ligatures. That segment was later removed, prepared histologically, and graded using the McPhail index. Local application of norgestimate caused endometrial proliferation, whereas the contralateral horn of the test animal showed a McPhail index of 0.

Antiestrogenic Activity

The antiovulatory activity of a progestogen is believed to be closely linked to its antiestrogenic activity. To measure this effect, an experimental model has been devised in which adult rats are ovariectomized and administered estrogen to produce cornified vaginal cells. A progestogen is then coadministered with the estrogen. If the progestogen exerts an antiestrogenic effect, the cells become leukocytic. Norgestimate is very effective in inhibiting the action of estrogen in this assay system. When the inhibition of estrogen-induced vaginal cornification in ovariectomized rats was measured, it was found that response was positive.

Androgenic Activity

Androgenic side effects of OCs can be quite disturbing and may be cause for discontinuation of drug. Untoward androgenic effects include acne, oily skin, weight gain, amenorrhea, and other lipoprotein changes. Research has revealed that different derivatives of testosterone have varying levels of androgenicity. Thus, one goal of OC development is to find as effective as possible a progestin with as little as possible androgenic activity.

A series of preclinical studies was conducted to evaluate norgestimate's androgenic activity. One very simple, but sensitive, indicator of androgenic activity is a progestogen's effect on ventral prostate weight. With testosterone propionate used as the standard, a series of progestogens – including norgestimate and levonorgestrel – was tested in immature rats using this model. Levonorgestrel was almost identical to testosterone propionate in its ability to induce ventral prostate weight increases (Fig. 3). In contrast, norgestimate, medroxyprogesterone acetate (MPA), and progestogen caused only slight and insignificant degrees of prostate weight increase.

These findings were confirmed by in vitro androgen receptor-binding studies. In this test, levonorgestrel was found to be equivalent to MPA and just slightly less potent than testosterone propionate in binding to the androgen receptors. Both norgestimate and progesterone showed a similarly low and nonspecific degree of receptor binding.

The ability of norgestimate to displace testosterone from sex hormone binding globulin (SHBG) was also studied. Both testosterone and 17β-estradiol demonstrated a high affinity for binding to SHBG. Norgestimate was the only steroid studied to show no competitive displacement of ^{3}H-labeled testosterone from human SHBG.

In vivo studies in rabbits comparing plasma concentrations of SHBG before and after steroid administration clearly demonstrated that norgestimate was not

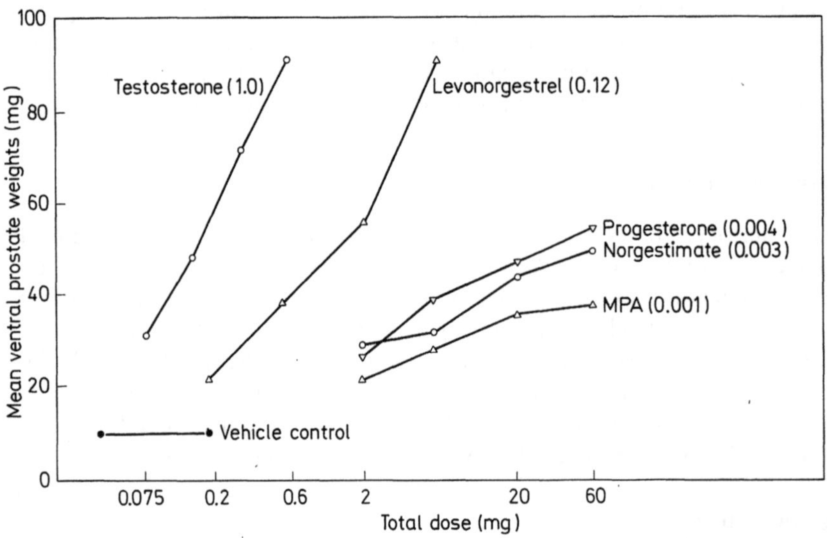

Fig. 3. Androgenic activity: stimulation of ventral prostate weights in immature rats, subcutaneous administration

different from control in its effects on SHBG concentrations. In comparison, levonorgestrel produced a mean increase in SHBG plasma levels of 55%.

These data indicate that levonorgestrel is the most potent androgen among progestational agents. In comparison, the androgenicity of norgestimate appears to be less than or comparable to that of progesterone, which essentially lacks any androgenic activity.

Effects on Endometrial Morphology

A variety of techniques have been used to assess the effects of norgestimate on the normal endometrium including histochemistry, light microscopy, transmission electron microscopy (TEM), and S-scanning election microscopy (SEM). Using these techniques, biopsied specimens from both humans and baboons have been examined.

Norgestimate produced no adverse endometrial changes. Despite its strong progestational effect, endometrial tissue recovers rapidly. As demonstrated by the absence of bleeding, micropolyps, blood clots, metaplasia, extreme epithelial regression, or significant structural defects in the endometrium wave seen with other progestogens norgestimate appears to have a unique effect.

Cilest – Clinical Efficacy

The results of preclinical studies indicated that norgestimate was a potent but highly selective progestogen. Accordingly, norgestimate was formulated in a monophasic combination OC containing 250 µg norgestimate and 35 µg ethinyl estradiol, made available in Cilest. Cilest appears to be a safe and effective low-dose combination OC. Preclinical studies indicate that norgestimate achieves its antiovulatory effect without producing androgenic side effects or disrupting the normal endometrial morphology. Norgestimate's potent but highly selective mechanism of action is reflected in the favorable clinical profile of Cilest.

The results of three large-scale, multicenter studies of Cilest were consistent with those of other lose-dose combination OCs. In particular, Cilest is as effective in suppressing ovulation as other products. Changes in bleeding patterns were minimal and decreased rapidly after cycle 1. There were no instances of amenorrhea among women taking Cilest.

The incidence and type of adverse experiences associated with the use of Cilest were typical of those observed with other low-dose combination OCs. In addition, few clinically significant changes in laboratory parameters were noted. Of particular interest is the statistically significant increase in HDL cholesterol levels seen in subjects treated with Cilest. This desirable trait of Cilest may recommend its use over other OCs whose contraceptive efficacy and side effect profile are otherwise comparable.

References

1. Vessy MP, Doll R (1969) Investigation of relation between use of oral contraceptives and thromboembolic disease: a further report. Br Med J 2:651–657
2. Inman WH, Vessey MP, Westerholm B et al. (1970) Thromboembolic disease and steroidal content of oral contraceptives. Br Med J 2:203–209
3. Bottinger LE, Boman G, Eklund G et al. (1980) Oral contraceptives and thromboembolic disease: effects of lowering estrogen content. Lancet I:1097–1101
4. Meade TW (1982) Oral contraceptives, clotting factors, and thrombosis. Am J Obstet Gynecol 142:758–761
5. Bradley DD, Wingerd J, Petitti DB et al. (1978) Serum high density lipoprotein cholesterol in women using oral contraceptives, estrogens, and progestins. N Engl J Med 299:17–20
6. Kay CR (1982) Progestogens and arterial disease: evidence from the Royal College of General Practitioners' study. Am J Obstet Gynecol 142:762–776
7. Wingrave SJ (1982) Progestogen effects and their relationship to lipoprotein changes. Acta Obstet Gynecol Scand 105 (Suppl):33–36
8. Wahl P, Walden C, Knopp R et al. (1983) Effect of estrogen/progestin potency on lipid/lipoprotein cholesterol. N Engl J Med 308:862–867

Gestoden: An Innovative Progestogen

G. Hoppe
Berlimed, Philippine Cop., PO Box 331, MCC, 1299 Makapi, Metro, Manila, Philippines

Introduction

Case reports and epidemiological retrospective case control studies suggested an increased cardiovascular risk associated with the oral contraceptive pill (OC) soon after its introduction. These findings prompted the initiation of three large epidemiological prospective cohort studies: in the United Kingdom those of the Royal College of General Practitioners (RCGP) and the Oxford Family Planning Association and in the United States the Walnut Creek Contraceptive Study. All started in 1968, at a time when older high-dose preparations were those commonly used [1, 2, 3].

Only one of these studies, that of the RCGP found a statistically significant increase in cardiovascular mortality due to myocardial infarction and subarachnoid haemorrhage in two subgroups of women, those over 45 years of age and those older than 35 who smoke cigarettes. It probably was this finding on myocardial infarction that prompted the subsequent publications on the pill and HDL-cholesterol which assumed an atherosclerotic aetiology.

Were the deaths in the RCGP study due to coronary atherosclerosis? If indeed atherosclerosis was the cause of the significantly increased mortality, there should have been a time lag between the start of pill use and the increase in mortality. Furthermore, there should be a significant association between duration of pill use and mortality rate, considering the gradual development of atherosclerosis over many years. Neither is evident in the RCGP study. The remaining plausible explanation for a myocardial risk in certain subgroups of women taking the pill therefore would be that of a thromboembolic event.

This assumption is further supported by a notable absence in literature of a significantly increased incidence of angina pectoris, the clinical manifestation of coronary atherosclerosis, among OC users. Moreover, a study among 53 women taking the pill and suffering from angiographically confirmed myocardial infarction showed that 66% of them did not show any atherosclerotic changes on coronary angiography [4]. This confirms the finding of case reports and post-mortem examinations suggesting that myocardial infarction attributable to current OC use is more likely to be thrombotic than arteriosclerotic in origin [4, 5], as outlined in a previous review [6].

A more recent analysis of the Oxford Family Planning Association cohort study on pill users revealed that the association with venous thromboembolism is limited to current users, unrelated to duration of use, and lower with pills containing less oestrogen ($< 50\ \mu g$) [7]. The association with non-haemorrhagic

Female Contraception
Eds.: B. Runnebaum, T. Rabe, L. Kiesel

stroke was not significant, and the association with thromboembolic stroke was significant only for pills with a higher oestrogen dose (≧50 μg) and, again, limited to current users and unrelated to duration of use [8].

A different, more recent, large prospective study confirmed an increased association with thromboembolism in pill users but no increased risk of stroke or myocardial infarction [9, 10]. The authors speculate that this discrepancy with older findings may be because their study population mainly used the modern, lower dose pills which are commonly used today. Apart from these thromboembolic events an increased association of pill use with hypertension was recently confirmed again [11].

One can conclude from these recent epidemiological studies that the aetiology of pill-associated thromboembolic events or hypertension can best be explained by pill-induced adverse changes of the coagulation and fibrinolytic systems and of the renin-angiotensin-aldosterone (RAA) mechanism. The synthetic ethinylestradiol (EE) most commonly used in OCs has a much stronger effect on liver metabolism than do natural oestrogens, thereby inducing greater metabolic and haemostatic changes [12, 13]. Such oestrogen-sensitive changes are found regarding SHBG (sex hormone binding globulin); plasma lipids and lipoproteins, e.g. increase of high-density lipoprotein (HDL) cholesterol and triglycerides; and adverse interference with coagulation and fibrinolytic factors and with the RAA system. The extent of SHBG increase induced by a pill formulation can be used as an indicator of its inherent oestrogenicity [14, 15].

EE-induced changes of lipids and lipoproteins, e.g. an increase of HDL-cholesterol, are probably clinically rather irrelevant as there is no evidence so far of pill-associated arteriosclerosis or coronary sclerosis. Clinically more relevant ap-

Table 1. Non-progestogenic effects of synthetic progestogens: the pregnan group

Progestational agent	Transformation dose (mg)	Comparative effect/action						
		Oesterogenic	Androgenic	Anabolic	Glucocorticoid	Antiandrogenic	Antioestrogenic	Aldosterone-antagonistic
Progesterone	200 IM	(−)	(−)	(−)	(−)	(−)	+	+
Pregnan group								
Medroxyprogesterone acetate	120	(−)	(+)[a]	(−)	+	(−)	+	(−)
Megestrol acetate	35	(−)	(−)	(−)	ND	(+)	+	(−)
Chlormadinone acetate	30	(−)	(−)	(−)	(+)	(+)	(+)	(−)
Cyproterone acetate	20	(−)	(−)	(−)	(+)	+	(+)	(−)

ND, no data.
[a] Not in the classical tests; only in the Foetus.

pear to be the EE-induced adverse changes of the coagulation and fibrinolytic systems and of the RAA mechanism. In order to reverse or minimize such EE-induced adverse changes the progestogen component of OCs therefore should have a strong anti-oestrogenic (or better, anti-EE) effect, stronger than that of natural progesterone, and an aldosterone-antagonistic effect, similar to that of natural progesterone.

Other non-progestogenic hormonal effects of progestogens are usually undesired, with the exception of the pronounced anti-androgenic effect of cyproterone acetate, which is useful for women with signs of androgenization. Tables 1–3

Table 2. Non-progestogenic effects of synthetic progestogens: the oestran group

Progestational agent	Trans-formation dose (mg)	Comparative effect/action						
		Oestero-genic	Andro-genic	Ana-bolic	Gluco-corti-coid	Anti-andro-genic	Anti-oestro-genic	Aldos-terone-anta-gonis-tic
Progesterone	200 IM	(−)	(−)	(−)	(−)	(−)	+	+
Oestran group								
Norethisterone	120	+	+	+	(−)	(−)	+	(−)
Norethynodrel	100	++	(+)	(−)	(−)	(−)	(−)	(−)
Lynestrenol	80	+	+	+	(−)	(−)	+	(−)
Norethisterone acetate	60	+	+	+	(−)	(−)	+	(−)
Ethynodiol diacetate	10	(+)	+	+	(−)	(−)	+	(−)

Table 3. Non-progestogenic effects of synthetic progestogens: the gonan group

Progestational agent	Trans-formation dose (mg)	Comparative effect/action						
		Oestero-genic	Andro-genic	Ana-bolic	Gluco-corti-coid	Anti-andro-genic	Anti-oestro-genic	Aldos-terone-anta-gonis-tic
Progesterone	200 IM	(−)	(−)	(−)	(−)	(−)	+	+
Gonan group								
Norgestimate[a]	5–6	(−)	+	(+)	ND	(−)	+	(−)
Levonorgestrel	5–6	(−)	+	(+)	(−)	(−)	++	(−)
3-Keto-desogestrel	2,5	(−)	+	(+)	ND	(−)	+	(−)
Gestoden	2–3	(−)	(+)	(+)	(−)	(−)	++	+

ND, no data.
[a] The main metabolite is levonorgestrel.

summarize the non-progestogenic hormonal effects of the three groups of progestogens.

Gestoden is a new synthetic progestogen from the gonan class with a strong anti-oestrogenic effect. Furthermore, it is the first and so far only progestogen with an aldosterone-antagonistic activity, which is about 60% that of natural progesterone [16]. Gestoden also has the highest biological progestogenic activity, allowing for the lowest hormonal content among OCs available today. Unlike other progestogens from the gonan class, such as desogestrel and norgestimate, gestoden is biologically active on its own and does not require hepatic transformation into active metabolites.

Material and Methods

A fixed combination contains only 75 μg gestoden, which is half the progestational content of the otherwise lowest fixed-dose pills today, together with 30 μg EE. The total gestoden dose per cycle is only 1.575 mg and the EE dose 0.630 mg, resulting in a gestoden : EE ratio of 2.5. Results will be presented here from clinical phase II and phase III trials in 1095 women taking the pill for up to 24 cycles, comprising a total of 14281 cycles.

Results

In this study 970 women completed 6 cycles, 668 women 12 cycles, 353 women 18, and 269 women 24 cycles. Despite errors of tablet taking in 329 cycles (2.3% of all cycles) no pregnancies occurred. The amenorrhoea rate was only 0.5% of cycles.

The length of the menstrual cycle during the trial is shown in Table 4. During pill administration the occurrence of long cycles (>30 days) was reduced whereas short cycles (<26 days) occurred more frequently. The duration of bleeding (Table 5) as well as the amount of bleeding (Table 6) were reduced during pill intake. Table 7 shows the occurrence of intermenstrual bleeding as a percentage of all women, including those with tablet intake error and those with a history of intermenstrual bleeding

In the first treatment cycle the incidence of spottings was only 6.7%, of breakthrough bleeding 0.4%, and of spottings and breakthrough bleeding 1.3%. In-

Table 4. Length of menstrual cycle; figures are percentages of women in the study group

	Amenorrhoea	<26 Days	26–30 Days	>30Days
Pre-treatment	0.8	6.5	82.3	10.4
Cycle 1	0.4	11.0	83.9	4.7
Cycle 6	0.5	8.2	88.7	2.6
Cycle 12	0	9.0	89.4	1.6
Cycle 24	0	15.3	84.0	0.7

Table 5. Duration of menstrual bleeding; figures are percentages of women in the study group

	Amenorrhoea	<4 Days	4–7 Days	>7 Days
Pre-treatment	0.8	26.0	71.6	1.6
Cycle 1	0.4	34.4	64.1	1.1
Cycle 6	0.5	42.9	55.9	0.7
Cycle 12	0	53.3	46.5	0.2
Cycle 24	0	66.5	33.5	0

Table 6. Amount of menstrual bleeding; figures are percentages of women in the study group

	Light	Normal	Heavy
Pre-treatment	16.5	75.8	7.7
Cycle 1	19.6	77.6	2.8
Cycle 6	27.7	70.8	1.5
Cycle 12	34.0	65.3	0.7
Cycle 24	51.7	48.0	0.3

Table 7. Intermenstrual bleeding by cycles; figures are percentages of women in the study group

% of women[a]	Spottings	BTB	Spottings and BTB
Pre-treatment	3.1	0.4	1.3
Cycle 1	6.7	1.2	0.8
Cycle 6	4.1	0.9	0.9
Cycle 12	4.0	0.6	0.4
Cycle 24	3.7	0	0

BTB, breakthrough bleeding.
[a] Includes those with intake error and those with history of intermenstrual bleeding.

Table 8. Intermenstrual bleeding by background; figures are percentages of total number of cycles

	Spottings	BTB	Spottings and BTB
All cycles	5.0	0.7	0.5
Cycles without intake error	4.7	0.6	0.5
Cycles without intake error and without history of intermenstrual bleeding	3.9	0.4	0.5

BTB, breakthrough bleeding.

Table 9. Body weight

After cycle	% of women unchanged (± 2 kg)
3	96.1
6	88.2
12	83.5
24	73.8

Table 10. Blood pressure

	% of women	
	<140 mm Hg systolic	<90 mm Hg diastolic
Pre-treatment	98.0	94.0
After cycle:		
3	97.7	94.0
6	97.2	93.0
12	98.1	94.4
24	97.3	93.8

creased intermenstrual bleedings during the first treatment cycles are often a problem with low-dose OCs. Therefore these figures obtained with the even lower dosed gestoden pill appear very favourable. As expected, the incidence of intermenstrual bleedings decreased in subsequent cycles and by the sixth cycle was virtually the same as before treatment. Table 8 demonstrates the incidence of intermenstrual bleeding in percentage of cycles. As expected, this was lower when cycles with tablet intake error and a history of intermenstrual bleeding were excluded.

Body weight was unchanged (± 2 kg) in about 85% of women after 12 cycles and in about 75% after 24 cycles (Table 9). Blood pressure remained virtually unchanged during the trial (Table 10). In more than 50% of the women with an elevated diastolic blood pressure (>90 mm HG) before treatment, blood pressure normalized during treatment (Table 11).

The incidence of subjective complaints was very low, as seen in Table 12. Whereas some were slightly increased during the first treatment cycle only (nausea and breast tension), others decreased (compared to pre-treatment) already in the first cycles (e.g. mild and severe dysmenorrhoea).

Objective side effects are shown in Table 13. The incidence of acne decreased from 4.3% of women before treatment to 1.2% after 12 cycles. The percentage of women with oedema decreased from 1.3% before to 0.3% after 24 cycles.

The cumulative drop-out rate because of side-effects was 10.3% after 12 cycles and only 11.2% after 24 cycles (Table 14). Some of the clinical trials had a predetermined duration of less than 24 cycles or were cut off earlier for evaluation of trial results.

Table 11. Normalization of blood pressure among women with pre-treatment diastolic pressure of <90 mm Hg (6% of subjects)

After cycle	% of women
3	57.8
6	71.7
12	66.7
24	55.6

Table 12. Subjective complaints; figures are percentages of women in the study group

	Pre-treatment	Cycles 1–3	Cycles 4–12	Cycles 13–24
Dysmenorrhoea				
Mild	17.9	9.0	4.3	3.2
Severe	4.5	0	0.1	0.2
Nausea	2.3	6.6	1.9	0.9
Vomiting	0.2	0.2	0	0
Dizziness	2.9	2.2	1.7	2.4
Breast tension	6.9	8.1	6.5	7.5
Headache	7.8	8.3	7.6	6.6
Migrainous	0.6	0.6	0.9	0.5
Nervousness	7.1	7.7	6.0	6.6
Depression	1.9	2.0	1.5	1.5
Libido increase	0.4	1.3	0.9	0.5
Libido decrease	1.2	2.0	2.6	4.9
Varicose complaints	1.8	1.8	2.3	1.5

Table 13. Objective side effects; figures are percentages of women in the study group

	Pre-treatment	Cycle 1	Cycle 6	Cycle 12	Cycle 24
Acne	4.3	3.7	2.8	1.2	1.1
Chloasma	3.9	3.9	4.2	5.5	1.5
Oedema	1.3	1.1	0.5	0.7	0.3
Other[a]	0.5	1.5	1.5	1.5	0.7

[a] Includes vaginal discharge, tiredness, sleep disorders, etc. (One patient had a light superficial thrombophlebitis in the third cycle which disappeared despite continuation of pill intake.)

Table 14. Drop-out rate (%)

	Because of side effects	Because of other reasons
After cycle: 1	0.8	1.5
6	7.0	16.6
12	10.3	39.8
24	11.2	48.5

Figures are cumulative.

Discussion

The results of multicentre clinical trials with a combination of 75 μg gestoden plus 30 μg EE in 1095 women over 14281 treatment cycles demonstrate reliable contraceptive efficacy combined with excellent cycle control and general tolerance. The very low incidence of intermenstrual bleedings compares very favourably with other low-dose OCs, where increased frequency of spotting and breakthrough bleeding in the first cycles of administration often result in premature discontinuation. The cumulative drop-out rate because of side effects with the gestoden pill hence was only 10.3% after 12 cycles and 11.2% after 24 cycles of use. The percentage of women with oedema decreased during pill intake, and in the majority of those with elevated diastolic blood pressure (>90 mmHg) before treatment this was normalized during pill administration.

Wambach [17] recently demonstrated the disturbance of the RAA balance among OC users compared to non-users. In the normal ovulatory menstrual cycle oestrogens stimulated the RAA meachanism. This stimulation is, however, counteracted by the natural aldosterone-antagonistic progesterone. In women taking OCs the situation is quite different. EE compared to natural oestrogens stimulates the RAA mechanism much more strongly, leading to increased plasma aldosterone levels compared to non-users. At the same time, the natural aldosterone-antagonistic progesterone is suppressed by OC, leading to a disturbance of this delicate balance, with resulting aldosterone predominance. Wambach therefore concluded that progestogens in OCs should have an aldosterone-antagonistic effect resembling natural progesterone in order to reduce the incidence of pill-induced hypertension and its cardiovascular implications.

Gestoden so far is the only progestogen used in OCs with such an aldosterone-antagonistic effect, although in the dosage used it is probably rather weak. But the added strong anti-oestrogenic (or better anti-EE) effect may help to counteract the otherwise undesired strong EE-induced stimulation of the RAA mechanism, with resulting increased plasma aldosterone levels.

A number of metabolic studies are being performed. Preliminary results suggest that this gestoden formulation is well balanced and devoid of an undesirable oestrogenic dominance. Although it produces an increase of SHBG and HDL plasma levels, it appears to be without the adverse effect on the coagulation and fibrinolytic system of other too oestrogen-dominant OC formulations [18].

In conclusion, gestoden is a new progestogen with a unique pharmacological profile. In an OC pill formulation with the lowest hormonal content available to date, it was shown to provide reliable contraceptive efficacy combined with excellent cycle control, tolerance and a reassuring metabolic and haemostatic profile.

References

1. Layde P, Beral V (1981) Further analyses of mortality in oral contraceptive users. Lancet 1(8219):541–546
2. Petitti DB et al. (1979) Risk of vascular disease in women smoking, oral contraceptives, noncontraceptive estrogens, and other factors. JAMA 242 11:1150–1154

3. Vessey MP, McPherson K, Yeaytes D (1981) Mortality in oral contraceptive users. Lancet 1 (8219):549–550
4. Engel HJ, Engel E, Lichtlen P (1985) Koronarsklerose und Herzinfarkt bei jungen Frauen. Muench Med Wochenschr 127, 16:415–417
5. Mann JI, Inman WHW (1975) Oral contraceptives and death from myocardial infarction. Br Med J [Clin Res] 2:245–248
6. Hoppe G (1986) The pill, the heart and HDL: facts and fictions. Adv Contracept 2, 3:405–411
7. Vessey M et al. (1986) Oral contraceptives and venous thromboembolism: findings in a large prospective study. Br Med J [Clin Res] 292, 6519:526
8. Vessey MP, Lawless M, Yeates D (1984) Oral contraceptives and stroke: findings in a large prospective study. Br Med J [Clin Res] 289 (6444):530–531
9. Porter JB, Hunter JR, Danillson DA, Jick H, Stergachis A (1982) Oral contraceptives and nonfatal vascular disease – recent experience. Obstet Gynecol 59:299–302
10. Porter JB, Hunter JR, Jick H, Stergachis A (1985) Oral contraceptives and nonfatal vascular disease. Obstet Gynecol 66, 1:1–4
11. Khaw Kay-Tee, Peart WS (1982) St. Mary's Hospital Medical School, London, U.K. Blood pressure and contraceptive use. Br Med J [Clin Res] 285:403–407
12. Ottossen U-B (1984) Oral progesterone and estrogen-progestogen therapy. Acta Obstet Gynecol Scand [Suppl] 127:1–37
13. Varma TR (1983) Effect of oestrogen replacement therapy on blood coagulation factors in postmenopausal women. Int J Gynaecol Obstet 4, 21:291–296
14. Larsson-Cohn U, Fahraens L, Wallentin L, Zador G (1981) Lipoprotein changes may be minimized by proper composition of a combined oral contraceptive. Fertil Steril 35, 2:172–179
15. Cullberg G, Dovre P, Lindstedt G, Steffensen K (1982) On the use of plasma proteins as indicators of the metabolic effects of combined oral contraceptives. Acta Obstet Gynecol Scand [Suppl] 111:47–54
16. Losert W, Casals-Stenzel J, Buse M (1985) Progestogens with antimineralocorticoid activity. Arzneimittelforschung 35 (1), 2:459–471
17. Wambach G (1986) Wie beeinflussen Gestagene den Natriumhaushalt? Fortschr Med 104, 29:37–40
18. Bruni V et al. (1986) Proceedings 1st International Congress on Gynecology and Endocrinology Madonna di Campiglio.

Desogestrel: Review of Pharmacology and Clinical Trials

H. Kopera

Department of Experimental and Clinical Pharmacology,
Karl-Franzens-University Graz, Graz, Austria

Introduction

In recent years it has been increasingly realized that not only estrogens but also progestogens [4] can be responsible for a variety of both favorable and adverse side effects of oral contraceptives, and that their metabolic effects belong to the potentially serious ones. The fact that some untoward effects of progestogens seem to be structure-related encouraged chemical and pharmaceutical research to look for new substances with properties which might better meet medical requirements. As a result many new compounds were synthesized and three of the so-called new-generation progestogens have been subjected to extensive trials: norgestimate (Ortho), gestoden (Schering) and desogestrel (Organon).

Desogestrel is not only the one most intensively studied and extensively used in clinical practice, but it is also the first and until very recently the only compound available worldwide. As active constituent of a third-generation oral contraceptive it seems to live up excellently to the expectations of modern medicine (for extensive literature documentation see [5, 6]).

Chemistry

The compound with the generic name desogestrel (code name Org 2969) is a 13-ethyl-11-methylene-18,19-dinor-17α-pregn-4-en-20-yn-17-ol (Fig. 1). It was synthesized in the laboratories of Organon International, Oss, The Netherlands. Desogestrel was selected for further development from a series of compounds prepared after discovery that 11-β as well as 11-alkylidene substitution in 17α-ethinyl-19-nortestosterone enhances the biological activity of parent compounds. Desogestrel is bioactivated by means of hydroxylation at carbon 3, followed by oxidation to 3-keto-desogestrel (Fig. 2), the active compound at the cellular level; both compounds can be determined by radioimmunoassay.

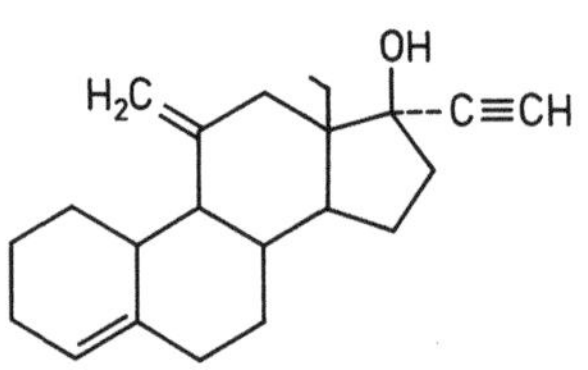

Fig. 1. Formula of desogestrel

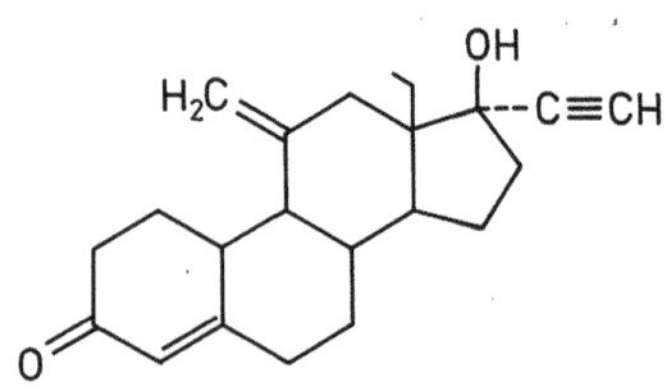

Fig. 2. Formula of 3-keto-desogestrel

Female Contraception
Eds.: B. Runnebaum, T. Rabe, L. Kiesel

Safety Studies

Safety Studies in Animals

Acute and Chronic Toxicity in Animals. Oral administration to rats and dogs for 52 weeks of 165, 200 and 300 times the human dose produced the expected powerful hormonal effects but no chronic toxicity. Likewise, all effects observed in the 1-year studies in rats an dogs with desogestrel plus ethinylestradiol could be expected on the basis of the estrogenic and progestational activities of the test compounds; in all safety studies the combination of desogestrel with ethinylestradiol was given in the ratio 125:50.

Acute toxicity is very low. The LD_{50} value (after 1 and 7 days) in mice and rats is more than 2000 mg/kg after oral and more than 500 mg/kg after intraperitoneal administration.

Reproductive Toxicity in Animals. Studies on reproductive toxicity were carried out in rats and rabbits. In examining effects on fertility desogestrel alone or in combination with ethinylestradiol in ovulation-inhibiting doses induced no serious adverse after-effects either on the reproductive processes of the F_0 generation or on the development to maturity and fertility of the F_1 offsprings. Experiments were performed on embryotoxicity with doses up to 1600 times the human dose. Desogestrel did not affect pregnancy rates, litter parameters, embryonic or fetal development, nor did it increase the postimplantation loss in rats. Some embryolethal activity was observed in the Dutch rabbit with 2 and 4 mg/kg. Teratogenic effects were not found in any of the desogestrel dosage groups in rats and rabbits or in tests with desogestrel plus ethinylestradiol in New Zealand white rabbits.

Desogestrel alone or in combination with ethinylestradiol tested in vivo in the micronucleus test and in vitro in the Ames test was found not to be mutagenic. The potential to produce tumors was tested in mice (81 weeks) and rats (2 years). Studies with desogestrel have shown that the overall incidence, types and distribution of benign and malignant tumors were not influenced. In combination with ethinylestradiol the expected effects of estrogens were observed.

Safety Studies in Humans

Administration to healthy women of increasing or continuous high doses for 3 weeks of 60, 125 or 750 µg desogestrel per day, alone or in combination with 50 µg ethinylestradiol showed no untoward effects on blood pressure, body weight or glucose tolerance or on the function of the thyroid, adrenal, liver or kidney, on triglycerides, cholesterol, total protein, inorganic ions, or on hematological parameters; no subjective side effects have been reported in these studies.

Pharmacology

Pharmacokinetic Studies

Intravenous administration of radioactive desogestrel to rats showed that the radioactivity is quickly distributed throughout the animal. After oral administration desogestrel is readily (absorption half-life 0.2 h) and completely absorbed, most probably in the duodenum. It is rapidly metabolized in vitro and in vivo.

In man the highest plasma concentrations of desogestrel are reached after 0.8–1.3 h (t_{max}) and these of the major metabolite 3-keto-desogestrel as soon as 1–3 h following ingestion of desogestrel. The serum levels of desogestrel decrease very rapidly, the half-life being 1.3–1.5 h. A two-compartment open-body model describes the kinetics of 3-keto-desogestrel, which has a mean half-life of elimination of 21 h. Pretreatment with ethinylestradiol does not affect the kinetics of desogestrel directly but it increases the concentration of SHBG (sex hormone binding globulin), which modifies the area under the curve of 3-keto-desogestrel due to a significantly reduced apparent volume of distribution as a consequence of an increased number of serum protein-binding sites. There is also the possibility of an increased metabolism of desogestrel to its 3-keto-metabolite. Both processes are involved in the production of a steady-state level of 3-keto-desogestrel, which is achieved within the first 10 days of daily administration of ethinylestradiol and desogestrel.

No correlation has been found between the duration of treatment (up to 26 cycles) and serum levels of 3-keto-desogestrel, indicating the absence of enzyme induction during long-term administration. The minimum serum levels of 3-keto-desogestrel, prior to the subsequent dose, vary from 0.4% to 1.3% (equimolar) dose/l.

In human plasma 99% of desogestrel is bound with low affinity to albumin; 3-keto-desogestrel is bound to two different binding sites to an extent of 98%.

Elimination of desogestrel is due only to biotransformation (in the liver) and not to excretion; no parent compound or 3-keto-desogestrel is found in the urine. After an oral dose of labelled desogestrel 85% of radioactivity can be recovered as biotransformation products in 6–8 days: 50% in the urine and 35% in the feces. In mother milk 0.3% of radioactivity dose is secreted over a period of 24 h after intake.

Interaction with Receptor Proteins. Desogestrel and 3-keto-desogestrel do not compete with estradiol-17β for estrogen receptors; at most they have an undetectable low affinity to it.

The binding affinity to the progesterone receptor of 3-keto-desogestrel at 4 °C is equal to that of levonorgestrel and about 6 times greater than that of progesterone; it is also greater than that of desogestrel and its metabolites. At 30 °C the binding affinity of 3-keto-desogestrel is about twice that of levonorgestrel and 25 times that of progesterone in both rabbit and man.

The affinity of desogestrel to the androgen receptor in rat prostate is extremely low, that of 3-keto-desogestrel is higher but is less than that of levonorgestrel. The binding to human SHBG of levonorgestrel has been found to be about 120 times stronger than that of desogestrel and about 3 times stronger than that of 3-keto-desogestrel. This is of importance insofar as the androgenicity of some progestogens is attributed to the competitive displacement of testosterone from SHBG.

Studies at body temperature (37 °C) in MCF-7 cells from a human breast tumor containing progesterone, estrogen and androgen receptors confirmed the above results: no binding to the estrogen receptor for 3-keto-desogestrel. 3-keto-desogestrel binds more strongly than levonorgestrel to the progesterone receptor. Norethisterone and 3-keto-desogestrel have the same affinity to the androgen receptor, although less than levonorgestrel.

The ratio of affinity to the progesterone and the androgen receptor – an expression of the selectivity of the steroid – is similar for norethisterone and levonorgestrel but 3–4 times higher for 3-keto-desogestrel. This indicates a preference of 3-keto-desogestrel for the progesterone rather than for the androgen receptor.

The results of these receptor-interaction studies make it unlikely that desogestrel could display significant androgenic effects in the human because it is a weak competitor of endogenous testosterone for binding to androgen receptor protein and to SHBG. It will, furthermore, be devoid of estrogenic effects. Desogestrel thus appears to be a more selective and purer progestational compound in women than other progestogens currently used in oral contraceptives.

Pharmacodynamic Studies

Animal Experiments. Desogestrel has been extensively studied in animal experiments. The pharmacodynamic profile is characterized by the following findings:

1. Strong progestational activity after oral and subcutaneous administration (twice as potent as norgestrel, 8–16 times as potent as norethisterone in the rat, mouse and rabbit)
2. Strong anti-estrogenic activity (8–16 times as potent as norethisterone in the rat, mouse and rabbit)
3. No estrogenic activity
4. Very weak androgenic and anabolic activities (in the same order as those of norethisterone)
5. No acceleration of the transport of fertilized ova
6. No inhibiting effect on nidation
7. Inhibition of cervical function (64 times as potent as norethisterone on cervical mucus in the rabbit)
8. Inhibition of ovulation; in the rabbit 4 times and in the rat 8 times as strong as levonorgestrel
9. No corticoid activities
10. No effect on platelet aggregation
11. No cardiovascular effects

Clinical trials have been initiated after establishing that desogestrel is:

1. A very potent progestational compound
2. A safe progestogen as based upon general toxicology, reproductive and tumorgenicity studies
3. A more selective progestogen

Clinical Pharmacological Studies. Desogestrel is certainly one of the most potent progestogens available. Data indicate that the active progestogenic moiety of desogestrel at the cellular level is for the greater part mediated via bioactivation to 3-oxo-desogestrel

Clear progestational effects on vagina and cervical function are achieved with daily doses of 60 µg. Desogestrel produces secretory transformation of the endometrium in daily doses of 30–60 µg. Inhibition of ovulation, as judged from suppression of gonadotropin release, the midcyclic follicle-stimulating hormone (FSH) and luteinizing hormone (LH) peaks, and the estrogen and progesterone plasma concentrations, is obtained with (30–) 60 µg/day desogestrel, both alone and when it is used in combination with an estrogen. The suppressive effect of 3-keto-desogestrel on ovulation is similar. In most cases studied the first posttreatment cycle was ovulatory. No substantial effect of desogestrel has been found on prolactin nor on diurnal cortisol secretion.

The increase of plasma renin activity during treatment with desogestrel plus ethinylestradiol is perhaps more an effect of the estrogen than of the progestogen; the same explanation might also hold true for the observed rise in growth hormone; however, it is uncertain whether the recorded elevation of immunoreactive insulin is caused by the estrogen or by desogestrel.

Clinical Studies for Efficacy and Side Effects

Preparations

Based on these encouraging toxicological and pharmacological data, 13 different combinations of desogestrel with ethinylestradiol were clinically tested for their suitability as contraceptives. Data were collected of more than 16000 women treated during more than 190000 cycles. Finally two preparations were selected for marketing in 1981: (a) a monophasic preparation with 21 tablets, each containing 0.150 mg desogestrel plus 0.030 mg ethinylestradiol; and (b) a normophasic preparation with 21 tablets, the first 7 tablets containing 0.05 mg ethinylestradiol and the 15 tablets to be taken subsequently containing 0.05 mg ethinylestradiol plus 0.125 mg desogestrel each.

Results

Both preparations lived up to the expectations of modern low-dose oral contraceptives [1]. Optimal effectiveness and acceptance were established in meticulously planned and carefully analyzed trials as well as in large-scale clinical use [2, 6]. They had no significant untoward effect on liver function or on blood pressure [3, 6].

The two formulations do not differ significantly from other comparable contraceptives as far as most unintended adverse effects are concerned, with the exception of influences on metabolism.

Metabolic Effects

Effects on Carbohydrate Metabolism. Recent data suggest that some diabetogenic effects of oral contraceptives might depend on the dose and on the structure of the progestogen. No significant diabetogenic effects were found with desogestrel [7].

Effects on Protein Metabolism. Desogestrel interferes significantly neither with the synthesis-increasing effect of the estrogen on corticosteroid-binding globulin or on ceruloplasmin nor on SHBG, i.e., it has no antiestrogenic or androgenic effect. This is in concert with the finding that in women treated with desogestrel the serum level of total testosterone usually is reduced and those of free testosterone and of free 5α-dihydrotestosterone are always significantly reduced (there is more SHBG available for binding and biological inactivation of the androgen). Accordingly, desogestrel-containing contraceptives lack androgenic side effects and are beneficial in women with symptoms of increased androgenicity.

Desogestrel in low-dose pills has very little effect on body weight, except in young women who gain weight because of physiological growth; this can be concluded from preliminary results after 2 years treatment in a multicenter study with 10000 women [3].

Effects on Lipid Metabolism. In studies on high-density (HDL) and low-density (LDL) lipoprotein cholesterol desogestrel elevated HDL-cholesterol in more than half the studies and never caused a decrease of HDL- or HDL_2-cholesterol; it either did not affect or lowered LDL-cholesterol, so that atherogenic indices such as the ratio of HDL-cholesterol to total cholesterol or that of HDL-cholesterol to LDL-cholesterol were increased. Desogestrel caused an elevation of apolipoprotein A-1 and had no, or in some studies even a significantly lowering, effect on apolipoprotein B with the consequence of a favorable increase of the A-1/B ratio, a situation which has been encountered with no other progestin so far.

Conclusions

The presented data indicate that desogestrel is a very safe and potent progestogen, excellently suitable for contraceptive preparations. It differs favorable from most other progestogens in that:

1. It is hardly bound to either estrogen or androgen receptors and thus can be expected to lack estrogenic (proliferative), peripheral androgenic (virilizing), or anabolic (body weight increasing) effects.
2. It lacks intrinsic androgenicity and therefore does not interfere with the capacity of estrogen to increase SHGB. Consequently, desogestrel-estrogen combinations increase the binding capacity for androgens and cause a substantial decrease in biologically active free testosterone and free 5α-dihydrotestosterone.
3. It has no influence on liver function.
4. It has no clinically relevant influence on blood pressure.

5. Most importantly, desogestrel does not affect lipoproteins in such a way that atherogenic indices are influenced negatively. If the established inverse correlation of the levels of HDL-cholesterol and apolipoprotein A and the direct correlation of LDL-cholesterol and apolipoprotein B with the risk of cardiovascular disease can be extrapolated to changes produced in women using oral contraceptives, the desogestrel-containing preparations are the only ones presently available which cause beneficial changes in the lipoproteins. This means they will most probably not only fail to increase the risk of cardiovascular disease but might even exert some protective antiatherogenic effects.

The development of desogestrel must be regarded as an important advance towards efficacious oral contraceptive preparations with minimal adverse side and aftereffects.

Summary

Desogestrel (Org 2969, a 13-ethyl-11-methylene-18,19-dinor-17α-pregn-4-en-20-yn-17-ol) is readily converted to 3-keto-desogestrel, the active moiety at the cellular level. Safety studies showed very low acute and chronic toxicity, no adverse aftereffects on fertility, no embryotoxicity, mutagenicity or carcinogenicity, and excellent tolerance in safety studies in humans.

Pharmacokinetics. Oral desogestrel is completely absorbed (absorption half-life 0.2 h) and maximum plasma concentration is reached after 1–3 h; plasma half-life 1.3–1.5 h; half-life of elimination of 3-keto-desogestrel is 21 h; elimination via biotransformation in the liver. No enzyme induction. No binding to estrogen receptors, low binding to androgen receptors, very high binding to progesteron receptors (selective progestogen).

Pharmacodynamics. In animals: potent progestational, antiestrogenic, ovulation and cervical function inhibiting activity; no estrogenic, corticoid, very weak androgenic activities, no cardiovascular effects. In humans: potent progestational and ovulation-inhibiting effect, no disturbance of carbohydrate metabolism, no inhibition of estrogen-induced SHBG synthesis, no untoward effects on lipoproteins.

Clinical trials. The clinical use of mono- and normophasic preparations containing desogestrel and ethinylestradiol for 7 years has established excellent contraceptive efficacy and good cycle control. It has confirmed the lack of estrogenic, androgenic, and anabolic effects, as expected from pharmacological data, and has revealed no influence on liver function, blood pressure, or body weight. An antiandrogenic activity due to lowering of plasma levels of free testosterone and 5α-dihydrotestosterone as well as the lack of an atherogenic influence on the lipid profile, and in some trials even an anti-atherogenic shift of lipoprotein fractions, are important advantages of desogestrel in contraceptive preparations.

References

1. Bettendorf G et al. (1987) Hormonelle Empfängnisverhütung. Dtsch Ärztezeitung 6, 57:23
2. Geißler KH (1983) Hormonelle Kontrazeption mit Marvelon, Erfahrungen mit Marvelon in der gynäkologischen Praxis – Multicenter-Studie bei 265 Gynäkologen und über 26000 Frauen. Fortschr Med 101:1060–1064
3. Geißler KH (1986) Long term study of the effect on body weight and blood pressure of a desogestrel containing micropill. 12th World Congress on Fertility and Sterility, Singapore, Okt. 26–31.
4. Kopera H (1985) Unbeabsichtigte Wirkungen der oralen Kontrazeptiva. II. Progestagen-bedingte Effekte, Wechselwirkungen mit Arzneimitteln. Wien Med Wochenschr 135:415–419
5. Kopera H (1986) Efectos metabolicos de los contraceptivos orales. Med Int 2, 2:76–92
6. Kopera H, Weijers MJ (1983) Desogestrel: a new progestogen. In: van Keep PA, Kopera H (eds) Oral contraceptives and lipoproteins. Workshop Conference in Hawaii, pp 64–84
7. Luyckx AS, Gaspard UJ, Romus MA, Grigorescu F, de Meyts P, Lefèbre PJ (1986) Carbohydrate metabolism in women who used oral contraceptives containing levonorgestrel or desogestrel: a 6-month prospective study. Fertil Steril 45:635–642

References

1. Bettendorf G et al. (1987) Hormonelle Empfängnisverhütung. Dtsch Ärzteblatt [illegible] 3723
2. Gräfke KH (1983) Hormonelle Kontrazeption mit Marvelon. Erfahrungen [illegible] aus der gynäkologischen Praxis [illegible] und Ethinylestradiol [illegible] Fortschr Med 101: 1060–1064
3. [illegible] (1986) Long term study on the effect on body weight and blood pressure of a [illegible] containing [illegible]
4. [illegible]
5. [illegible]
6. [illegible]
7. [illegible]
8. [illegible]

Steroids and Brain

Progesterone and Progestins Modulate Hypothalamic and Pituitary β-Endorphin*

A. R. Genazzani, F. Petraglia, M. Bergamaschi, A. D. Genazzani, F. Facchinetti, M. Cleva, V. Santoro, and A. Volpe

Department of Obstetrics and Gynecology, University of Modena, Italy

Gonadal steroids and neuropeptides interact in the central nervous system in some mechanisms regulating reproductive functions. The activity of luteinizing hormone-releasing hormone (LH-RH) and of peptidergic neurons is influenced by the hormonal signals originating in the gonads. β-Endorphin (β-EP) is an endogenous opioid peptide synthesized in the hypothalamus and with morphine-like effects [1]. Indeed, β-EP decreases circulating LH levels by inhibiting LH-RH secretion [2] and decreases sexual activity [3]. β-EP is present in plasma and is secreted from the pituitary. Interestingly, chronic estradiol benzoate (EB) treatment increases hypothalamic, pituitary, and circulating β-EP levels in ovariectomized rats [4, 5, 6].

Because during the estrous cycle hypothalamic [7], pituitary and plasma [8] β-EP levels show significant changes, we evaluated the possible effect of progesterone on these parameters and the possible interaction between estrogens and progesterone. Moreover, because several new progestin-derived compounds interestingly show positive effects on the mood of postmenopausal patients [9], the effect of these was also studied. In the present study we evaluated the effects of chronic treatment with progesterone or various progestins – medroxyprogesterone acetate (MAP), norethisterone acetate (NET), and desogestrel (DES) – on the hypothalamic and pituitary β-EP-like immunoreactivity (β-EP-LI) in ovariectomized rats. These effects were also evaluated in the presence of a concomitant treatment with EB.

Material and Methods

Animals. Female Sprague-Dawley rats (200–220 g; supplied by Morini, S. Polo d'Enza, Italy) were used in all assays. They were housed in a climate-controlled room on a light-dark cycle of 12:12 (lights on at 0700 hours) with food and water freely available. Bilateral ovariectomy was performed under ethyl ether anesthesia. Treatments were started 3 weeks after surgery.

Drugs. All steroids were supplied by Organon (Oss, Netherlands). They were dissolved in sesame oil and were injected subcutaneously every day for 2 weeks. Groups of six rats each received either vehicle, progesterone (1 mg/day), MAP

* This study was supported in part by the Consiglio Nazionale delle Ricerche, P.F. MPR, SP8.

Female Contraception
Eds.: B. Runnebaum, T. Rabe, L. Kiesel

(500 µg/day), NET (500 µg/day), or DES (10 µg/day). EB (2 µg/day), alone or combined with progesterone or the various progestins, was administered in a second set of experiments.

Tissues. Rats were killed by decapitation. After removal of the brain from the skull the mediobasal hypothalamus was dissected, and the pituitary was removed and divided into the anterior lobe and neurointermediate lobe. Tissues were placed in a bath at 100 °C for 15 min, homogenized and processed as previously described [4].

β-EP Assays. B-EP-LI in tissue extracts was measured by radioimmunoassays. Camel β-EP was used to prepare the standard curve and the tracer. Anti-camel β-EP serum (kindly donated by Dr. E. Panerai, Milan, Italy) was used as previously described [4]. The inter- and intra-assay coefficients of variation were 6.5% and 3.5%, respectively. Assay sensitivity was 5 pg/tube. Results were expressed as ng/mg protein for the mediobasal hypothalamus and the anterior lobe and as ng/lobe for the neurointermediate lobe.

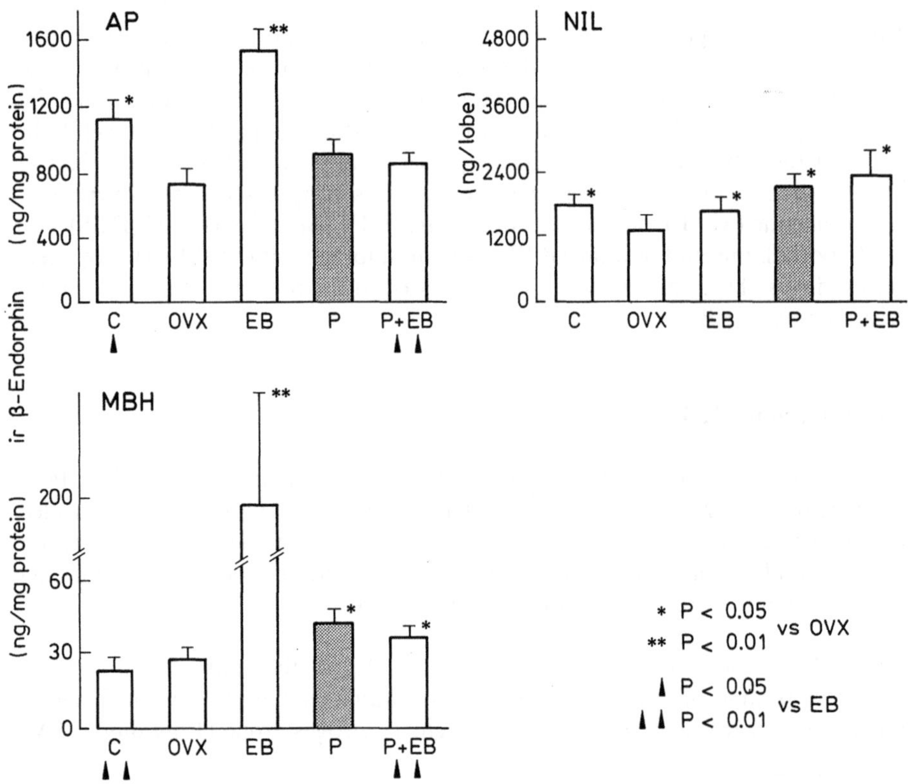

Fig. 1. β-Endorphin-like immunoreactivity in anterior pituitary (*AP*), neurointermediate lobe (*NIL*), and mediobasal hypothalamus (*MBH*) of control (*C*) and ovariectomized (*OVX*) rats following 2 weeks' treatment with estradiol benzoate (*EB*), progesterone (*P*), or progesterone plus estradiol benzoate (*P*+*EB*)

Results

In the mediobasal hypothalamus ovariectomized rats showed β-EP-LI concentrations similar to those found in controls. DEG and MAP were inactive. Rats treated with progesterone, NET, and EB showed β-EP-LI contents in the mediobasal hypothalamus higher than in controls. Progesterone and progestins reduced the effect of EB (Figs. 1–4).

In the anterior pituitary lobe of ovariectomized rats showed β-EP-LI levels significantly lower than controls. β-EP-LI content of the anterior lobe was unaffected by progesterone, MAP, and NET, while they were significantly increased by DEG and EB. Progesterone and progestins significantly reduced the EB-induced increase of β-EP-LI in the anterior pituitary.

Ovariectomized rats showed lower β-EP-LI concentrations in the neurointermediate lobe than controls. The treatment with progesterone, DEG, MAP, and EB significantly increased β-EP-LI content of the neurointermediate lobe, while

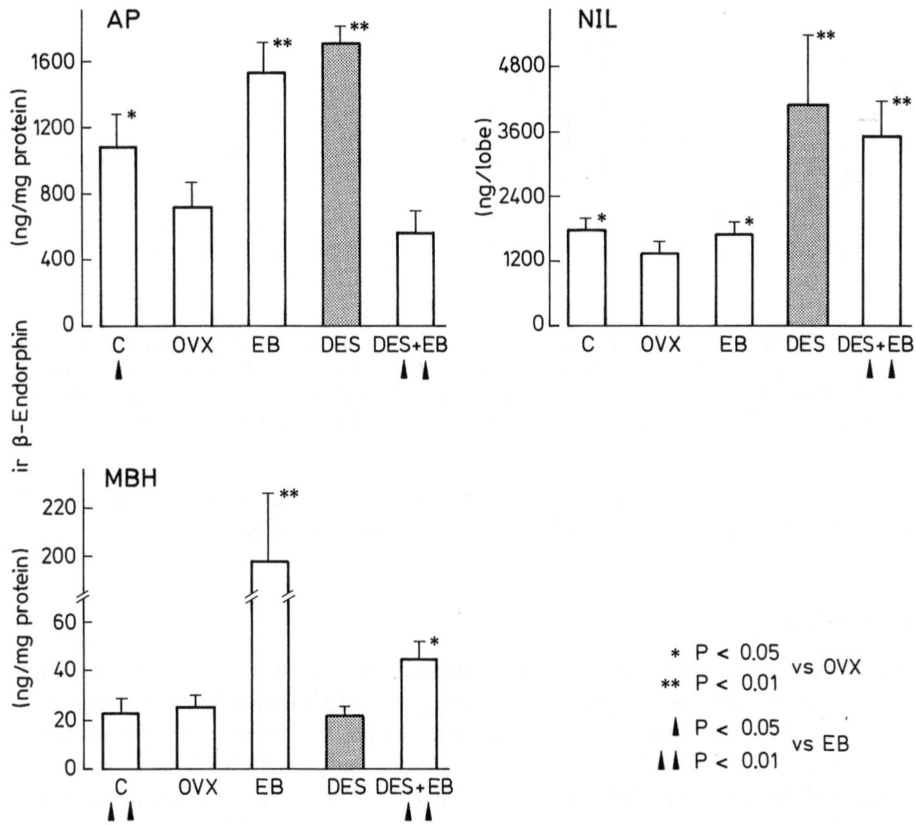

Fig. 2. β-Endorphin-like immunoreactivity in anterior pituitary (*AP*), neurointermediate lobe (*NIL*), and mediobasal hypothalamus (*MBH*) of control (*C*) and ovariectomized (*OVX*) rats following 2 weeks' treatment with estradiol benzoate (*EB*), desogestrel (*DES*), or desogestrel plus estradiol benzoate (*DES+EB*)

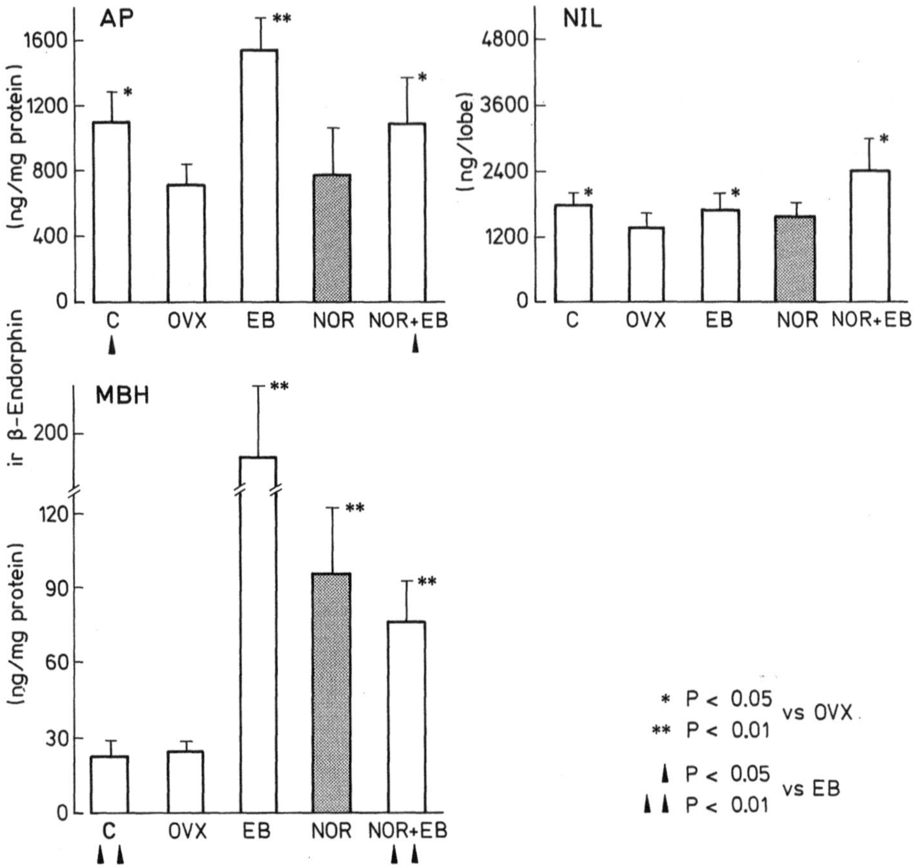

Fig. 3. *β*-Endorphin-like immunoreactivity in anterior pituitary (*AP*), neurointermediate lobe (*NIL*), and mediobasal hypothalamus (*MBH*) of control (*C*) and ovariectomized (*OVX*) rats following 2 weeks' treatment with estradiol benzoate (*EB*), norethisterone oenanthate (*NET*) or norethisterone oenanthate plus estradiol benzoate (*NET+EB*)

NET was inactive. In ovariectomized rats treated with EB the progesterone and progestin treatments were not affected by EB administration.

Discussion

The present results indicate that the various progestins have different effects on pituitary and mediobasal hypothalamus. Progestins do not modify the content of β-EP-LI in the anterior lobe of ovariectomized rats, but increase the neurointermediate lobe content. However, it must be observed that DEG is inactive in the anterior lobe, and that NET fails to change β-EP-LI in the neurointermediate lobe. These results suggest a lower sensitivity of corticotrophs to progesterone and progestins in comparison with the neurointermediate lobe. It seems interesting that DEG, which displayed some estrogenic effects [9], mimics the effect of EB on anterior lobe β-EP-LI contents.

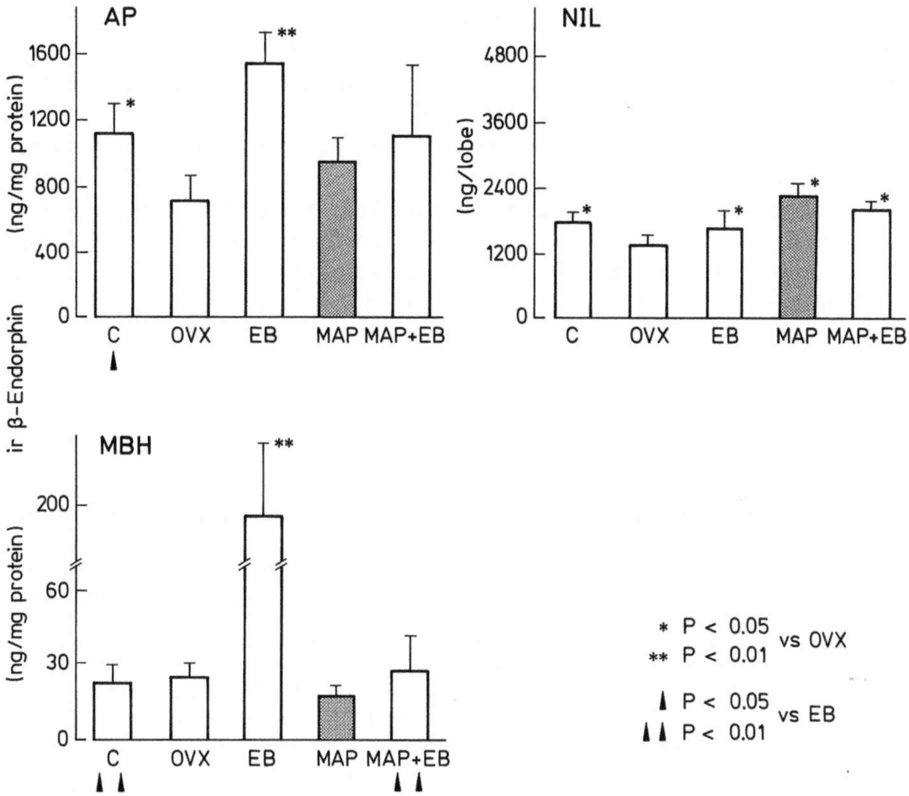

Fig. 4. β-Endorphin-like immunoreactivity in anterior pituitary (*AP*), neurointermediate lobe (*NIL*), and mediobasal hypothalamus (*MBH*) of control (*C*) and ovariectomized (*OVX*) rats following 2 weeks' treatment with estradiol benzoate (*EB*), medroxyprogesterone (*MAP*) or medroxyprogesterone plus estradiol benzoate (*MAP+EB*)

The positive effect of progesterone and NET on the mediobasal hypothalamus β-EP-LI content in ovariectomized rats agrees with previous reports [10]. These results may be related to the observation that circulating progesterone (during the luteal phase of the menstrual cycle) [11] or chronic MAP treatment in postmenopausal women [12] has a positive effect on the central opioid system, as shown by the resumption of LH response to naloxone challenge. Moreover, the observation that progesterone and other progestins significantly reduce the effect of the pharmacological dose of EB on β-EP concentration in the anterior pituitary lobe and the mediobasal hypothalamus suggests a possible modulatory effect of gonadal steroids. Conversely, the concomitant administration of the progestins does not seem to interfere with the positive effects of EB on β-EP contents in the neurointermediate lobe.

The different results observed in the neurointermediate lobe might be explained by the different regulation of β-EP secretion at this level [13]. Indeed, β-EP synthesis and secretion from the neurointermediate lobe in rats is under direct dopamine inhibitory control [14]. The observation is of great interest that progesterone and progestins commonly used for oral contraception (DEG and NET) endometrial hyperplasia (NET and MAP), endometriosis (MAP) and luteal supplementation in chronic anovulation are all able to modulate the pituitary and hypothalamic β-EP content. In fact, opioid peptides play an important role in the control of several neuro-endocrine axes [15] and are involved in behavioral and mood disorders.

In conclusion, the present results indicate that progestins, other than glucocorticoid, estradiol, and testosterone, can affect the central and pituitary concentrations of β-EP, modulating the effect of the other steroids. This may play a role in the changes of peripheral and central opioids in the female reproductive cycle.

References

1. Clement-Jones V, Besser GM (1984) Opioid peptides in humans and their clinical significance. In: Udenfriend S, Meienhofer J (eds) The peptides. Academic, New York, pp 323–390
2. Rasmussen DD, Liu JH, Wolf PL, Yen SSC (1983) Endogenous opioid regulation of gonadotropin-realing hormone from the human hypothalamus in vitro. J Clin Endocrinol Metab 57:881
3. Gessa GL, Paglietti E (1979) Induction of copulatory behaviour in sexually inactive rats by naloxone. Science 204:203–205
4. Petraglia F, Penalva A, Locatelli V, Cocchi D, Panerai AE, Genazzani AR, Muller EE (1982) Effects of gonadectomy and gonadal steroids replacement on pituitary and plasma B-EP levels in the rat. Endocrinology 111:1224–1229
5. Wardlaw SL, Wehrenberg WS, Ferin N, Antunes JL, Frantz AG (1982) Effect of sex steroids on B-endorphin hypophysial portal blood. J Clin Endocrinol Metab 55:877
6. Forman FG, Sonntag WS, Hylka VW, Meites J (1985) Mediation by gonadal steroids of plasma B-endorphin and LH in castrated female and male rats. Peptides 6:835–839
7. Barden N, Merand Y, Rouleau D, Garon M, Dupon A (1981) Changes in the B-endorphin content of discrete hypothalamic nuclei during the estrous cycle of the rat. Brain Res 204:441
8. Ishizuka B, Wilkes MM, Stewart RD, Rasmussen DD, Yen SSC (1982) Increase of B-endorphin concentration in the plasma and pituitary neurointermediate lobe of the rat on the afternoon of proestrous. Life Sci 31:2113
9. Volpe A, Facchinetti F, Grasso A, Petraglia F, Campanini D, Genazzani AR (1987) Benefits and risk of different hormonal replacement therapies in post-menopausal women. Maturitas (in press)
10. Tejwani GA, Vaswani KK, Barbacci JC (1985) Effect of oral contraceptives on the rat brain and pituitary opioid peptides. Peptides 6:555–561
11. Petraglia F, Porro C, Facchinetti F, Cicoli C, Bertellini E, Volpe A, Barbieri GC, Genazzani AR (1986) Opioid control of LH secretion in humans: menstrual cycle, menopause and aging reduce effect of naloxone but not of morphine. Life Sci 38:2103
12. Casper RF, Rubillovitz SA (1985). Progestins increase endogenous opioid peptide activity in postmenopausal women. J Clin Endocrinol Metab 60:34–36
13. Petraglia F, Locatelli V, Penalva A, Cella SG, Genazzani AR, Cocchi D (1984) Autonomous secretion from the pituitary neurointermediate lobe: in vivo studies. Life Sci 34:1605–1611
14. Przewlocki R, Hollt V, Voigt KH, Herz A (1979) Modulation of in vitro release of B-endorphin from the separate lobes of the rat pituitary. Life Sci 24:1601
15. Grossman A, Rees LH (1983) The neuroendocrinology of opioid peptides. Br Med Bull 39:83–88

Contraceptive Potential of GnRH Antagonists

D. W. Hahn[1], K. T. Demarest[1], A. Phillips[1], C. Bishop[1], J. L. McGuire[1], D. R. Danforth[2], C. F. Chillik[2], and G. D. Hodgen[2]

[1] Research Laboratories, Ortho Pharmaceutical Corp., Raritan, New Jersey 08869, USA.
[2] Jones Institute for Reproductive Medicine, Eastern Virginia Medical School, Norfolk, Virginia 23507, USA

Introduction

Following elucidation of the structure of gonadotropin-releasing hormones (GnRH) by the laboratories of Schally [1] and Guilleman [2] in 1971, hundreds of analogs, both agonists and antagonists of GnRH, were synthesized and tested. Early success in increasing the potency of agonists and recognition of the ability of GnRH agonists paradoxically to inhibit the pituitary-gonadal axis quickly brought GnRH agonists to the forefront of investigation. It is now known that chronic administration of GnRH agonists effectively inhibits the reproductive/endocrine systems and is useful in the treatment of conditions such as precocious puberty, prostatic carcinoma and uterine fibroids.

Upon initiation of treatment with GnRH agonists, however, an acute stimulatory phase occurs during which gonadotropins and gonadal hormone levels increase, and there is concern that this may exacerbate symptoms of these disease-states. Competitive GnRH antagonists, on the other hand, suppress the reproductive system without an initial stimulatory phase and may thus provide more effective therapy. Thus, interest in the development of GnRH antagonists has been growing, and more potent antagonists have recently been successfully synthesized in several laboratories [3]. Substitution with arginine at position 6 yields some of the most potent antagonists [4, 5], one of which, [*N*-Ac-D-Nal(2)^{1}D-*p*H-Phe^2,D-Trp^3,D-Arg^6]LHRH, was proposed for clinical studies. However, during toxicity studies with this peptide, Schmidt and coworkers [6] observed vascular permeability changes in rodents treated with this compound, and clinical plans for the compound were suspended. General concerns about GnRH antagonists also arose as a result of this finding.

We initiated studies in our laboratories to characterize the nature of these vascular permeability changes and to look for potent GnRH antagonists lacking this side-effect liability. Our studies suggested that these reactions were identical to a cutaneous anaphylactoid-like reaction, possibly as a result of the direct action of the GnRH antagonist on mast cell mediator release. In the process of analyzing a full series of analogs for this anaphylactoid-like activity, we have demonstrated several analogs which possess potent GnRH antagonist activity while being devoid of significant cutaneous anaphylactoid-like activity [7, 8].

We describe here studies which demonstrate that (a) the antiovulatory activity of GnRH antagonists can be separated from their cutaneous anaphylactoid activity, (b) GnRH antagonists can inhibit gonadotropin secretion and ovulation, and (c) intermittent GnRH antagonist administration can be utilized to inhibit ovulation without induction of a pronounced estrogen deficiency.

Female Contraception
Eds.: B. Runnebaum, T. Rabe, L. Kiesel

Separation of Antiovulatory and Anaphylactoid Activities of GnRH Antagonists

Initial toxicity studies with [*N*-Ac-D-Nal(2)[1]D-*p*H-Phe[2],D-Trp[3],D-Arg[6]]LHRH revealed that upon local injection increased vascular permeability changes occurred [7]. Reported here are results obtained with two GnRH antagonists studied in our laboratories, ORF 18260 and ORF 21243 (Table 1). Both ORF 18260 and ORF 21243 are potent GnRH antagonists; however, the former possesses marked anaphylactoid activity while the latter peptide is devoid of significant anaphylactoid activity, demonstrating that GnRH antagonist activity and anaphylactoid activity need not be directly related.

A comparison of the antiovulatory and anaphylactoid-like activities of ORF 18260 and ORF 21243 are presented in Table 2. Cutaneous vascular permeability activity was analyzed in an in vivo rat model. In this model, activity was measured in female Wistar rats by injecting Evan's blue dye intravenously into the tail vein. Evan's blue is a standard dye which binds to serum proteins after intravenous administration. Increases in vascular permeability can then be visualized as serum proteins diffuse into the interstitium carrying the dye, which, in turn, stains the connective tissue. Immediately following dye injections, various dilutions of GnRH antagonists were injected intradermally into a shaved section on the back of the rat. Fifteen minutes after the intradermal injection, the rats were killed, the dorsal skin reflected, and the area of wheal was estimated using the mean of the longest perpendicular diameters. Antiovulatory activity was measured by administering the GnRH antagonists subcutaneously to rats at 1:00–2:00 P.M. on the day of proestrus. On the following morning the animals were sacrificed and the oviducts examined for the presence of ova.

Table 1. Amino acid sequences of two GnRH antagonists (ORF 21243 and 18260)

	1	2	3	4	5	6	7	8	9	10	
LHRH	*p*Glu	His	Trp	Ser	Tyr	Gly	Leu	Arg	Pro	Gly	NH_2
ORF 21243	Ac-D2Nal	4ClDPhe	D3Pal	Ser	Arg	DGlu (A.A.)	Leu	Arg	Pro	DAla	NH_2
ORF 18260	Ac-D2Nal	4FDPhe	DTrp	Ser	Tyr	DArg	Leu	Arg	Pro	Gly	NH_2

Table 2. A comparison of antiovulatory and anaphylactoid-like activities of ORF 21243 and 18260 in rats

Peptide	Antiovulatory activity rat ED_{50} µg/kg	Anaphylactoid activity rat ED (8.75 × 8.75 mm wheal) µg/wheal	Therapeutic index[b]
LHRH	NA	NA	–
ORF 21243	1.54[a] (1.16–2.06)	0.48[a] (0.20 –0.94)	0.312
ORF 18260	2.56 (1.85–3.41)	0.01 (0.0004–0.05)	0.004

[a] Significantly different than ORF 18260 ($p < 0.05$).
[b] Therapeutic index = anaphylactoid ED/antiovulatory ED.

Both ORF 18260 and ORF 21243 were potent inhibitors of ovulation with ED_{50} values of 2.56 and 1.54 μg/kg, respectively. ORF 21243 was 1.7 times more potent than ORF 18260. However, ORF 21243 was 48 times less potent than ORF 18260 in inducing a wheal response in the cutaneous anaphylactoid model. The doses required to cause a 8.75 × 8,75 mm wheal area in rats were 0.48 and 0.01 μg, respectively, for ORF 21243 and 18260. These studies suggest that the antiovulatory potency of a GnRH antagonist does not necessarily correlate with its ability to cause a cutaneous anaphylactoid-like response. These results suggest that it is possible to synthesize GnRH antagonists devoid of significant anaphylactoid activity. It appears that although some GnRH antagonists possess the potential for anaphylactoid-like activity, others do not. Thus GnRH antagonists, in general, offer potential for therapeutic use in all the clinical disorders for which GnRH agonists have been proposed as well as contraception.

GnRH Antagonist Suppression of Gonadotropins

GnRH antagonists are analogs of GnRH having a high affinity for the pituitary GnRH receptor but with no intrinsic biologic activity to stimulate follicle-stimulating hormone/luteinizing hormone (FSH/LH) secretion [9]. Persistent administration of GnRH antagonists suppress basal levels of gonadotropins creating a reversible "medical hypophysectomy" [10]. This suppression of the pituitary-ovarian axis is a dose-dependent phenomenon which can be demonstrated both in rodent and primate models.

In the following study the dose-dependent suppression of ovarian function in rats induced by chronic administration of GnRH antagonist (ORF 21243) is demonstrated by monitoring the alterations in vaginal cytology which change with the cyclic fluctuations in circulating hormonal levels. Rats were injected subcutaneously once daily with 20, 200, or 2000 μg/kg of ORF 21243 for 28 days. Cyclicity was completely suppressed with 2000 μg/kg, but only disrupted with 20 and 200 μg/kg. Periodic proestrus (P) which was observed with the two low doses was frequently followed by a prolonged period of estrus (E). When the mean number of days that proestrus was observed was calculated for each dose group, a dose-related effect on cyclicity was apparent. Bolus injections of 0, 20, 200, and 2000 μg/kg resulted in proestrus occurring 6.0, 3.6, 3.2, and 0 days, respectively, during the 28-day test period (Table 3).

Table 3. Effect of ORF 21243 on estrous cyclicity in the rat

Dose μg/kg per day	Number of days proestrus observed[a] mean ± SE bolus[b] ($n=5$)
0	6.0 ± 0
20	3.6 ± 0.4
200	3.2 ± 0.6
2000	0

[a] During the 28-day treatment period.
[b] Daily s.c. bolus injections.

It is interesting to note that although a single injection of 5 μg/kg of ORF 21243 is sufficient to inhibit ovulation on the day of proestrus (see Table 2), a dose of between 200 and 2000 μg/kg given chronically is needed to completely suppress ovarian function as indicated by the suppression of estrous cyclicity in rats. The significance of this point will be discussed below.

The dose-dependent suppression of ovarian function by GnRH antagonists is a direct result of these agents' ability to decrease pituitary secretion of FSH and LH, thus producing a hypogonadotropic state. This dose-dependent suppression of gonadotropin secretion by GnRH antagonists is observed following treatment of ovariectomized (8 weeks or more) female rhesus monkeys (*Macaca mulatta*). In this study ORF 21243 was administered intramuscularly, daily in a rising dose fashion: during the first 3 days, vehicle; days 4–6, 0.3 mg/kg per day of the GnRH antagonist; days 7–9, 1.0 mg/kg per day; days 10–12, 3.0 mg/kg per day; and days 13–15, vehicle alone (Fig. 1). Initial levels of plasma gonadotropins were in the ovariectomized range. After 3 days of vehicle treatment there were no meaningful changes in the tonic levels of gonadotropins. However, within 24 h after administration of 0.3 mg/kg of ORF 21243 there was a striking decrease in serum levels of FSH and LH. After 3 days of GnRH antagonist treatment at a dose of 0.3 mg/kg tonic FSH and LH serum concentrations decreased to near minimal detectable limits. After 3 days of treatment with 1 or 3 mg/kg per day of the GnRH antagonist, LH and FSH were suppressed below assay detection limits in all monkeys. Despite this prolonged suppression of tonic FSH and LH secretion by treatment with the GnRH antagonist the pituitary is, except during the 3.0 mg/kg per day

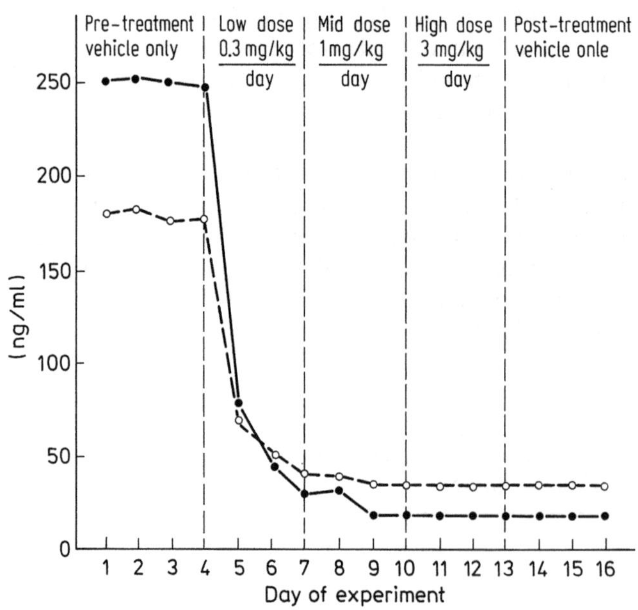

Fig. 1. Dose response of tonic FSH/LH to ORF 21243. The decrease of serum FSH (*closed circle*) and LH (*open circle*) throughout the study was significant ($p<0.02$ and $p<0.03$, respectively)

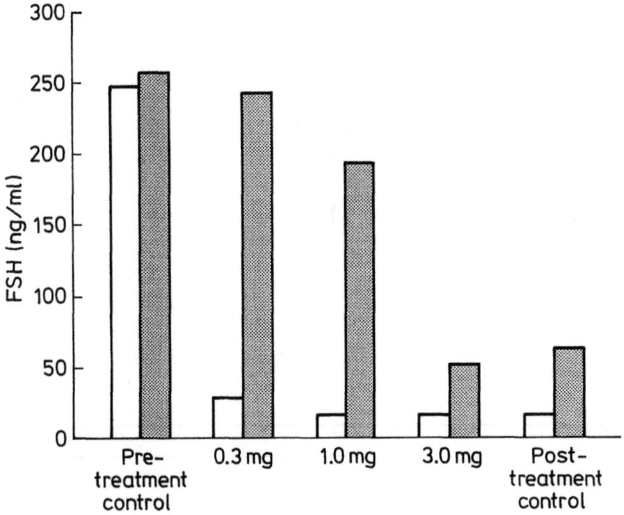

Fig. 2. Response of serum FSH to GnRH challenge test (100 μg i.v.); *open square*, 0 min; *closed square*, 30 min after GnRH bolus

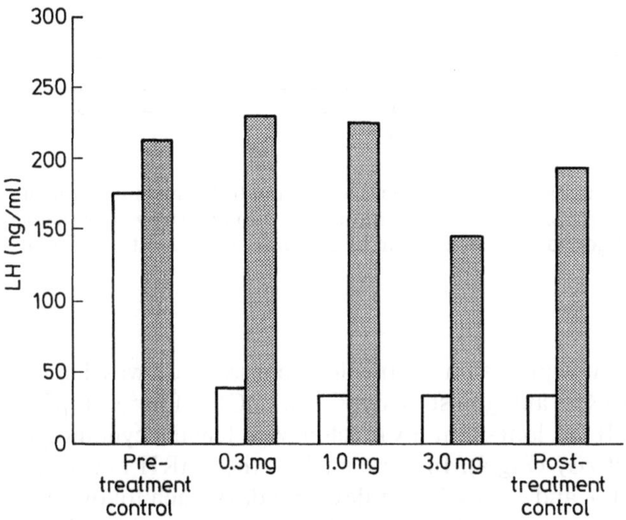

Fig. 3. Response of serum LH to GnRH challenge test (100 μg i.v.); *open square*, 0 min; *closed square*, 30 min after GnRH bolus

dose, equally responsive to a high dose of exogenous GnRH administered 1 h before the GnRH antagonist on days 4 (control), 7, 10, 13 (treatment), and 16 (recovery) (Figs. 2, 3). Importantly, the GnRH challenge test was performed 23 h after GnRH antagonist administration. Thus, the pituitary may have enough time to "recover" from the acute effects of the antagonist; antagonist occupation of the GnRH receptor is diminished and/or circulating GnRH antagonist levels are decreased.

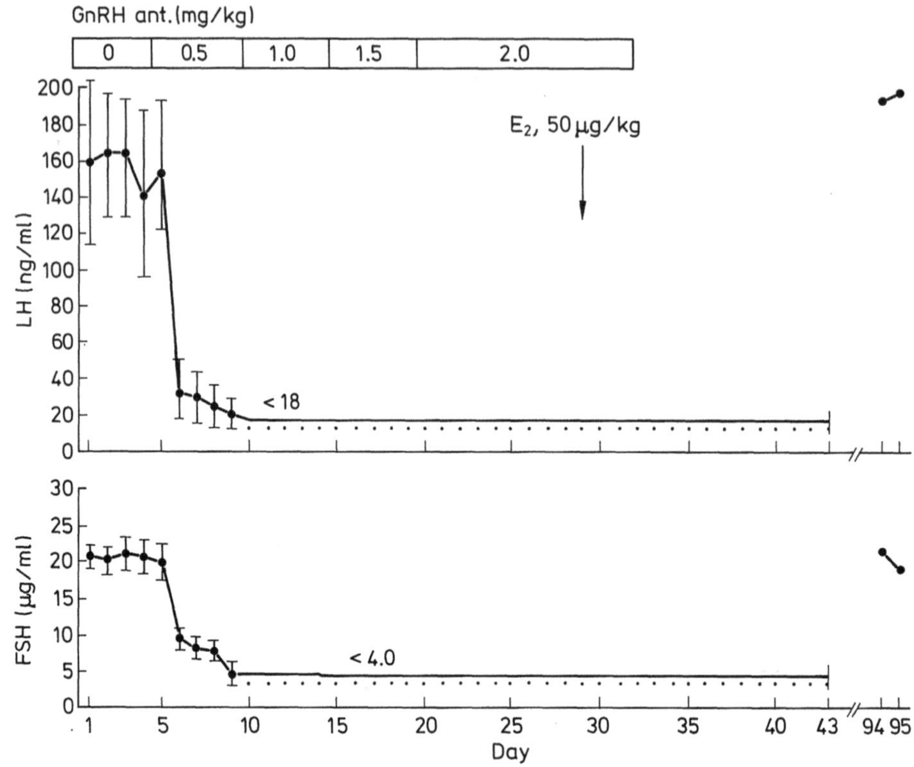

Fig. 4. GnRH antagonist suppresses FSH and LH levels in serum to below limits of assay detection. Long-term ovariectomized monkeys did not respond to an estrogen challenge test. Note the full recovery of gonadotropin secretion by 2 months after cessation of treatment. E_2, Estradiol

A similar dose-dependent suppression of gonadotropin secretion was demonstrated using another GnRH antagonist ([Ac-pC]Phe^1,pC1-D-Phe^2,D-Trp^3,D-Arg^6,D-Ala^{10}]-GnRH-HCl) in long-term ovariectomized female cynomolgus monkeys (*Macaca fascicularis*) (Fig. 4). In these studies, the GnRH antagonist was given at doses of 0.5, 1.0, and 1.5 mg/kg per day for 5 days, each followed by the treatment at a dose of 2.0 mg/kg per day for an additional 17 days. After 7 days of therapy, mean LH and FSH concentrations in serum were at or below the minimal detectable limits of the assays. These data indicate that within 24 h after a single dose of either GnRH antagonist a profound suppression of FSH and LH concentrations in peripheral serum occurs. It is interesting to note that although pituitary responsiveness to a large dose of GnRH is maintained despite prolonged GnRH antagonist treatment (see Fig. 2, 3), pituitary response to estrogen-positive feedback for LH/FSH release is abolished (Fig. 4). A single large dose of estradiol (50 µg/kg) had no effect on FSG or LH secretion. Reversibility of pituitary responsiveness was prompt; within 2 months after treatment endogenous gonadotropin elevations were restored to pretreatment, castrate levels.

GnRH Antagonist Suppression of Ovulation Without Estrogen Deficiency

There is considerable interest in the potential use of GnRH analogs for contraception. GnRH agonists effectively induce a hypoestrogenic state along with typical postmenopausal symptoms. Studies described previously in this paper demonstrate that GnRH antagonists (see Table 3) also inhibit ovulation. As noted earlier, however, it appeared to us that doses higher than antiovulatory doses of at least some GnRH antagonists are needed to totally suppress ovarian hormones. One possibility, then, is to find a dosage of GnRH antagonist which could inhibit ovulation without inducing hypoestrogenic side effects. While theoretically possible, however, this could be a significant task. However, in the following studies, we asked whether GnRH antagonists offer potential for female contraception with menopausal-like side effects when given using an intermittent (weekly) treatment regimen.

Monkeys previously having regular ovarian/menstrual cycles had no ovulation (32, or 32 treatment intervals) when the GnRH antagonist was administered once weekly [12]. The treatment consisted of a 4-week course of intermittent GnRH antagonist administered as a single dose (10 mg/kg; [Ac-pC]PHe^1,*p*Cl-D-Phe^2,D-Trp^3,D-Arg^6,D-Ala^{10}]-GnRH-HCl) beginning after spontaneous onset of menses and thereafter repeated at 7-day intervals. No ovulation sites were seen at laparoscopy. Moreover, the absence of ovulation was confirmed by the lack of serum progesterone (P_4) elevations; also, no LH surges were found. Most interestingly, there was no sustained suppression of estradiol-17β; that is, estradiol (E_2) concentrations remained near the level found in the early follicular phase on normal ovarian/menstrual cycles (Fig. 5).

After cessation of intermittent GnRH antagonist therapy, ovulation resumed promptly in six of eight monkeys. Results from a typical animal with ovulation inhibition and absence of LH surges during treatment, as well as resumption of an ovulatory ovarian cycle after treatment are shown in Fig. 6. After discontinuation of treatment with the GnRH antagonist, serum E_2 levels rose within 3 weeks and were followed by timely LH surges in six of eight monkeys. Presumed ovu-

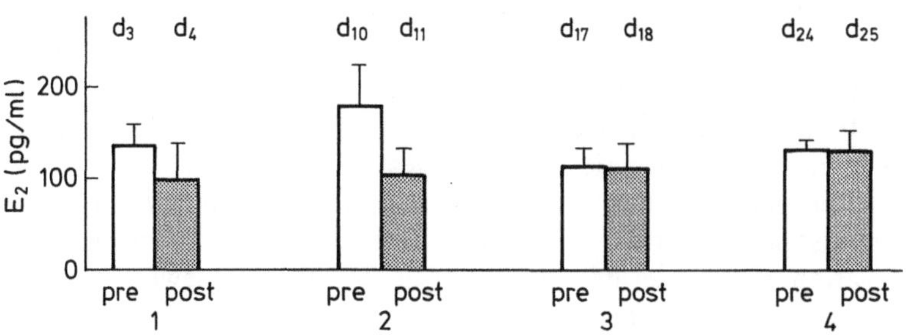

Fig. 5. Mean ± SE peripheral estradiol (E_2) levels immediately before (*solid bars*) and the day after (*hatched bars*) the four weekly treatments with GnRH antagonist in intact adult monkeys. There was no significant suppression of E_2 levels during these intermittent treatment intervals. d_3, day 3, etc

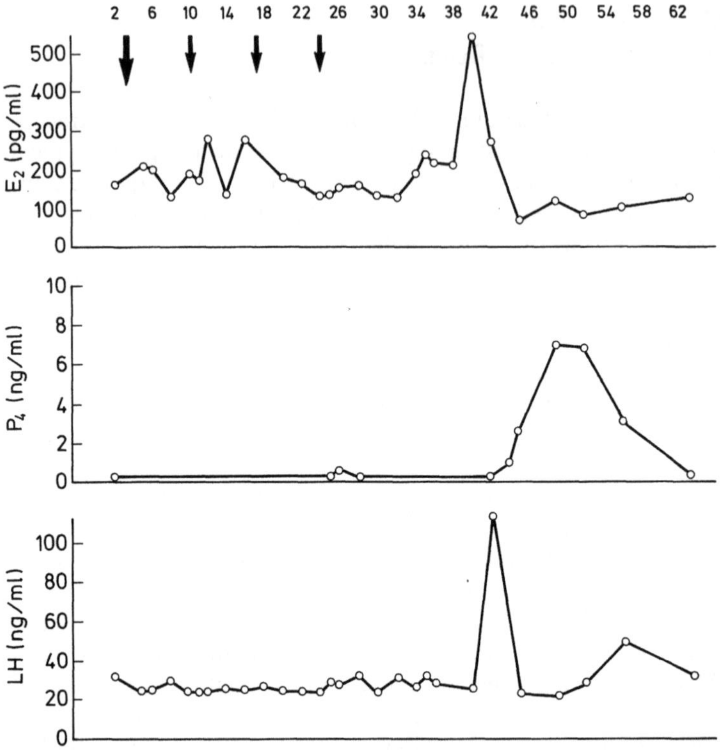

Fig. 6. Peripheral serum E_2, P_4 and LH levels in a monkey (six of eight) during and after weekly administration of GnRH antagonist (*arrows*). Note that within about 15 days after the last GnRH antagonist treatment, high serum E_2 levels and an LH surge occurred, followed by an increase in serum P_4. Day 1 was the spontaneous onset of menstruation (*top line*). Compared to the normal interval from menstruation to ovulation, the delay of apparent ovulation and next menses associated with GnRH antagonist treatment was highly significant ($p<0.01$)

lation was indicated by typical P_4 elevation in serum and an ensuing luteal phase of normal length. That some monkeys regained ovulatory status as soon as 8–10 days after the final dose of GnRH antagonist suggests that a weekly treatment interval may be near the upper limit for maintenance of ovulation inhibition at the dosage tested here. These observations correlate well with earlier experience in monkeys [15, 16] and women [17] undergoing surgical ablation of the putative dominant follicle, in whom destruction of the largest visible follicle delayed ovulation by causing reinitiation of a new follicular phase. Perhaps each-weekly dose of GnRH antagonist caused atresia of the newly selected dominant follicle. The intermittent elevation of E_2 in serum may reflect its secretion by newly recruited follicles in the next growing cohort [15].

In regard to the mechanism(s) by which the intermittent GnRH antagonist regimen prevented ovulation it appears that weekly GnRH antagonist treatment negates the estrogen-positive feedback for the LH surge. Figure 7 illustrates pituitary refractoriness to the E_2 benzoate challenge test given on cycle day 6 during

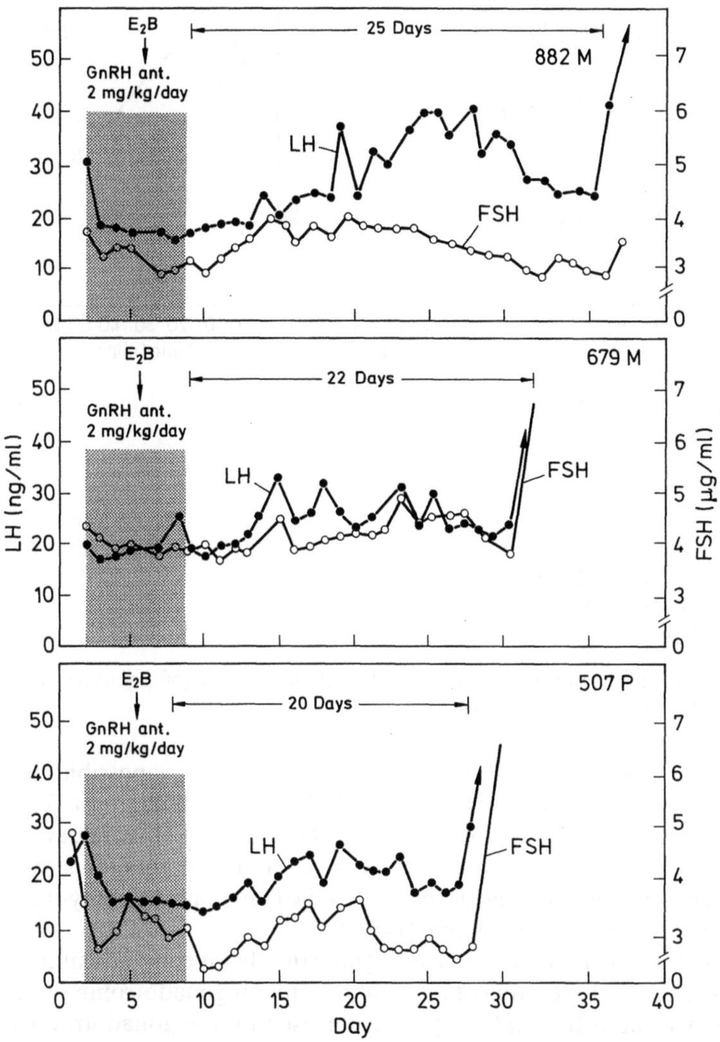

Fig. 7. E_2 benzoate (E_2B) challenge tests in monkeys receiving the GnRH antagonist (2 mg/kg per day, i.m.), from menstrual cycle days 2–9. Note the absence of gonadotropin surges, indicative of pituitary refractoriness to estrogen-positive feedback. Without the inhibitory effects of the GnRH antagonist, such exogenous estrogen treatment leads to preovulatory-like LH surge with 48 h (20–22)

a daily GnRH antagonist regimen from days 2 through 9 of the menstrual cycle. Notice the initial negative feedback effects of exogenous estrogen on LH and FSH secretion, the absence of familiar preovulatory-like LH surges and finally, the resumption of apparent ovulation about 3 weeks later. During the normal follicular phase, E_2 benzoate will induce midcycle-like LH surges within 48 h; the GnRH antagonist clearly negated this estrogen-positive feedback. In contrast, the response to GnRH was normal; GnRH administered as a 50-µg bolus dose on cycle day 6 during the daily GnRH antagonist regimen elicited unambiguous LH re-

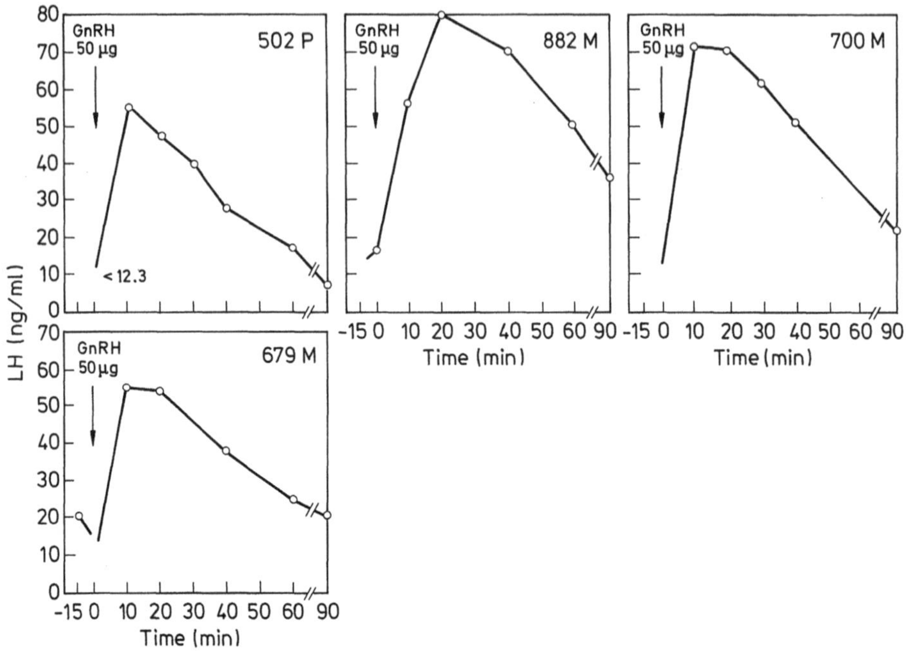

Fig. 8. Serum LH levels in four monkeys receiving a GnRH bolus dose (50 µg, i.v.) during concurrent administration on GnRH antagonist

sponses of seemingly normal magnitude and duration (Fig. 8). It is possible that the intravenous bolus doses of GnRH displaced the GnRH antagonist from gonadotropin receptors, so that the exogenous GnRH elicited LH secretory responses. An alternative interpretation is that the dose of GnRH antagonist was submaximal, since we previously achieved a "medical hypophysectomy-like" status with only 50% of the dose used here [14].

In conclusion, GnRH antagonists have significant therapeutic advantages over GnRH agonists in that they almost immediately inhibit gonadotropin secretion and ovulation without first inducing an acute rise in those gonadotropins. GnRH antagonists possessing anaphylactoid activity are clearly not acceptable, but studies presented here demonstrate that these two pharmacological properties are unrelated and that potent GnRH antagonists devoid of anaphylactoid activity can be synthesized.

GnRH analogs will be unacceptable as potential contraceptives to women, however, if a hypoestrogenic state and menopausal-like side effects accompany the contraceptive efficacy of these peptides. The studies described above suggest that it may be possible to avoid these undesirable side effects, but even so, the effects of long-term unopposed estrogenic stimulation and the potential risk of endometrial carcinoma may require periodic progestin supplementation to accommodate sloughing of proliferated endometrium. That we are making progress in our understanding of GnRH antagonists and their potential use as contraceptives is clear, but so too is the fact that development of these peptides as contraceptive agents will be a complex effort. Nevertheless, GnRH antagonists may offer potential as new contraceptives, especially for those for whom existing oral contraceptives are contraindicated.

Acknowledgements. The authors wish to thank Mrs. Peggy Westlake for her assistance in the preparation of this manuscript.

References

1. Matsuo H, Balea Y, Nair RM, Arimura A, Schally AV (1971) Structure of the porcine LH- and FSH-releasing hormone. I. The proposed amino acid sequence. Biochem Biophys Res Commun 43:1334
2. Burgus R, Butcher M, Amoss M, Ling N, Monahan MW, Rivier J, Fellows R, Blackwell R, Vale W, Guilleman R (1972) Primary structure of the ovine hypothalamic luteinizing hormone releasing factor (LRF). Proc Natl Acad Sci USA 69:278
3. Karten MJ, Rivier JE (1986) Gonadotropin-releasing hormone analog design, rationale and perspective. Endocr Rev 7(1):44
4. Rivier J, Rivier C, Perrin M, Porter J, Vale W (1984) LHRH analogs as antiovulatory agents. In: Vickery BH, Nestor JJ Jr, Hafez ESE (eds) LHRH and its analogs. MTP, Boston, p 11
5. Nekola MV, Coy DH (1984) LHRH antagonists in females. In: Vickery BH, Nestor JJ Jr, Hafez ESE (eds) LHRH and its analogs. MTP, Boston, p 125
6. Schmidt F, Sundaram K, Thau RB, Bardin CW (1984) [Ac-D-Nal(2)^1,4FD-Phe^2,D-Trp^3,D-Arg^6]-LHRH, a potent antagonist of LHRH, produces transient edema and behavioral changes in rats. Contraception 29:283
7. Phillips A, Hahn DW, Capetola RJ, McGuire JL (1986) The antiovulatory and anaphylactoid activities of two potent LHRH antagonists. Pharmacologist 28 Abs:#689
8. Hahn DW, McGuire JL, Vale WW, Rivier J (1985) Reproductive/endocrine and anaphylactoid properties of an LHRH antagonist, ORF 18260 [Ac-DNAL^1(2),4FDPhe^2,D-Trp^3,D-Arg^6]-GnRH. Life Sci 37:505
9. Schally AV, Arimura A, Coy DH (1980) Recent approaches to fertility control based on derivatives of LH-RH. Vitam Horm 38:257
10. Kenigsberg D, Littman BA, Hodgen GD (1984) Medical hypophysectomy: I. Dose-response using a gonadotropin-releasing hormone antagonist. Fertil Steril 42:112
11. Schriock ED, Monroe SE, Martin MC, Henzel MR, Jaffe RB (1985) Effect on corpus luteum function of luteal phase administration of a potent gonadotropin-releasing hormone analog (nafareline). Fertil Steril 43:844
12. Kenigsberg D, Hodgen GD (1986) Ovulation-inhibition by administration of weekly gonadotropin-releasing hormone antagonist. J Clin Endocrinol Metab 62:734
13. Werlin LB, Hodgen GD (1983) Gonadotropin-releasing hormone agonist suppresses ovulation, menses and endometriosis in monkeys: an individualized intermittent regimen. J Clin Endocrinol Metab 56:844
14. Kenigsberg D, Littman BA, Hodgen GD (1984) Medical hypophysectomy: I. Dose-response using a gonadotropin-releasing hormone antagonist. Fertil Steril 42:112
15. Goodman AL, Hodgen GD (1979) Between ovary interaction in the regulation of follicle's growth, corpus luteum function, and gonadotropin secretion in the primary ovarian cycle. I. Effects of follicle cautery and hemiovariectomy during the follicular phase in cynomolgus monkeys. Endocrinology 104:1304
16. diZerega GS, Nixon WE, Hodgen GD (1980) Intercycle serum FSH elevations: significance in recruitment and selection of the dominant follicle and assessment of corpus luteum normalcy. J Clin Endocrinol Metab 50:1046
17. Nilsson L, Wikland M, Hamberg L (1982) Recruitment of an ovulatory follicle in the human following follicle-ectomy and luteectomy. Fertil Steril 37:30

Desensitization of Pituitary Cells by Gonadotropin-Releasing Hormone in Vitro

K. Helm, L. Kiesel, T. Rabe, and B. Runnebaum

Department of Obstetrics and Gynecology, Division of Gynecological Endocrinology, Women's Hospital, University of Heidelberg, Voßstr. 9, 6900 Heidelberg, FRG

Introduction

Gonadotropin-releasing hormone (GnRH) stimulates the anterior pituitary gland to release luteinizing hormone (LH) and follicle-stimulating hormone (FSH). The decapeptide is secreted from the hypothalamus in a pulsatile manner in humans and animals. This secretory pattern results in a pulsatile release of gonadotropins in women (Kiesel et al. 1986 a). Continuous administration of high doses of GnRH or its potent analogues induces desensitization of the pituitary to physiological pulses of GnRH, thus leading to medical castration. This method of pituitary desensitization has already gained importance in the treatment of sex-hormone-dependent diseases, such as endometriosis, uterine leiomyoma, precocious puberty, prostrate and breast cancer, as well as in contraception (see review by Sandow 1986). The mechanism of this effect, however, has not yet been fully clarified.

Various authors have demonstrated changes of gonadotroph function following continuous administration of GnRH in vitro. Some reports have found a reduction of GnRH receptor numbers (Zilberstein et al. 1983); others have shown that mechanisms at the postreceptor level are also responsible for down-regulation of gonadotropin secretion (Badger et al. 1983; Smith and Vale 1981). The aim of this study was to characterize the time- and dose-dependent effects of GnRH on the desensitization of gonadotropin secretion using monolayer cell cultures from rat anterior pituitaries, taking an in vitro model to study GnRH use for contraception and hormone-dependent diseases.

Materials and Methods

Animals

Mixed-cyclic, female, Sprague-Dawley rats (250 g) were obtained from the Süddeutsche Tierfarm and housed, ten per cage, in a temperature-controlled room in which the lights were on between 0600 and 2200 h. All rats were fed Purina rat chow and water ad libitum.

Preparation of Pituitary Cells

For cell culture the rat anterior pituitary lobes were placed in a plastic tube containing medium 199 with 20 m*M* HEPES supplemented with 0.3% bovine serum

Female Contraception
Eds.: B. Runnebaum, T. Rabe, L. Kiesel

albumin (BSA, Sigma, Deisenhofen), 800 μML-glutamine (Seromed, Berlin), and 60 µg gentamycin/ml (Seromed, Berlin). The pituitaries were transferred into a glass petri dish and cut into six to eight pieces per gland in medium 199. The pieces were shaken for 15 min at 37 °C in medium 199 with 0.5% trypsin (Sigma, Deisenhofen) in a total volume of 1 ml per 10 pituitaries. For one further minute, 2 µg DNase (Sigma, Deisenhofen) was added to 10 pituitaries in medium 199. The supernatant was discarded, and medium 199 with 0.1% trypsin inhibitor (Sigma, Deisenhofen) was added to the pieces for 5 min at 37 °C to stop trypsinization completely. The supernatant was removed, and a 2 mM EDTA solution (Serva, Heidelberg) in Ca^{2+}-free Dulbecco's phosphate buffer saline (PBS, Seromed, Berlin) supplemented with 0.3% BSA was added for 5 min and incubated at 37 °C in the water bath. Finally, the pieces were shaken in 1 mM EDTA in solution 2 for 15 min after discarding the supernatant. The pieces were resuspended in Ca^{2+}-free PBS buffer. The supernatant containing the single cell suspension was transferred into a tube, and the remaining pieces were gently mixed in PBS buffer until no more fragments could be seen. Finally, the cells were filtered through nylon mesh and counted. The viability was determined by trypan blue staining. Cells were cultured in 24-well culture dishes with 1 ml medium per well at 37 °C in a humidified atmosphere of 5% CO_2 in air. Cells were allowed to recover from the preparation procedure for 1–2 days before GnRH challenge tests were started.

Preincubation of Pituitary Cells

Cells (3×10^5/culture dish) were preincubated in 1 ml of medium 199 "Earle" with 2.2 g/liter $NaHCO_3$ supplemented with heat-inactivated horse serum (HS, Seromed, Berlin) 800 μM L-glutamine, and 60 µg gentamycin/ml. The serum was heat inactivated at 56 °C for 30 min to prevent enzymes reacting with the cells.

GnRH Challenge Test in Vitro

Experiment A. Without washing the primary cultures, the cells were preincubated with 10^{-8} M GnRH (Peninsula Lab, San Carlos, CA) and stimulated up to 4 h with 10^{-8} M GnRH after washing twice to determine the kinetics of gonadotropin release after desensitization.

Experiment B. Without washing the primary cultures, the cells were preincubated with different concentrations of GnRH from 10^{-12} to 10^{-7} M for up to 24 h and stimulated with 10^{-8} M GnRH after washing twice to study the kinetics of the time- and dose-dependent preincubation period.

In both experiments medium 199 "Earle" with 10 mM HEPES and 1.1 g/liter $NaHCO_3$ was used for stimulation. Serum was replaced by 0.01% BSA. Following a 4-h GnRH challenge test, the supernatants were removed and frozen in order to be stored for radioimmunoassay.

RIA Determination of LH and FSH

LH and FSH release were determined by means of the RIA kits kindly supplied by the National Pituitary and Hormone Program, Baltimore, MD. Values are expressed as mean ng rat RP-2 LH/ml ± SD ($n=3$) or mean ng rat RP-11 FSH/ml ± SD ($n=3$). Radiolabeled LH (^{125}I-LH) and FSH (^{125}I-FSH) were provided by Dr. Sandow and Dr. von Rechenberg, Hoechst AG, Frankfurt.

Statistical Analyses

The significance of gonadotropin hormone suppression after GnRH desensitization was determined by regression analysis.

Results

Experiment A

Preincubation of rat anterior pituitary cells with 10^{-8} *M* GnRH reduced LH release induced by a 4-h GnRH challenge to 3.9-fold stimulation (7.4±0.8 ng/ml LH vs 1.9±0.3 ng/ml basal LH) as compared with controls (preincubation without GnRH) which showed a five-fold stimulation (14.5±1.3 ng/ml LH vs 2.9±1.4 mg/ml basal LH). After 2 h LH release was only 3.0±0.4 ng/ml LH in desensitized cells vs 7.1±1.6 ng/ml LH in the controls (Fig. 1 A). FSH release was diminished to three-fold (1.2±0.1 ng/ml FSH vs 0.4±0.1 ng/ml basal FSH) as compared with controls which showed a four-fold stimulation (1.6±0.1 ng/ml FSH vs 0.4±0.2 ng/ml basal FSH). After 2 h FSH release was only 0.6±0.1 ng/ml FSH vs 0.9±0.2 ng/ml FSH in the controls (Fig. 1 B). These experiments show that pretreatment with GnRH for 24 h results in a time-dependent reduction of LH and FSH release during a 4-h GnRH challenge test.

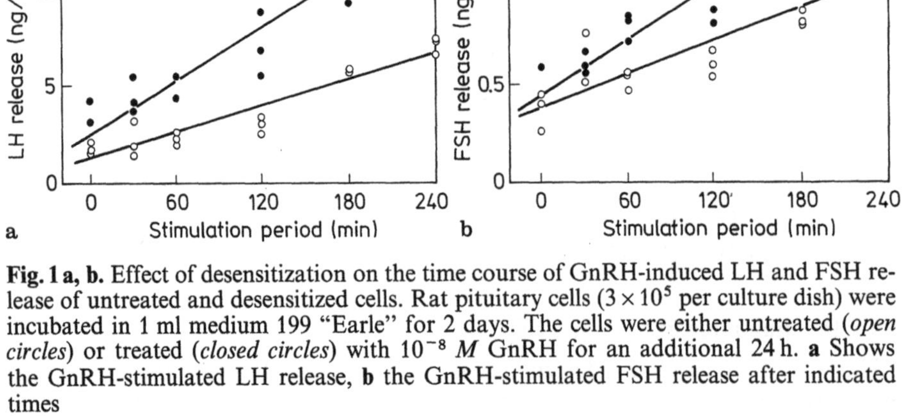

Fig. 1 a, b. Effect of desensitization on the time course of GnRH-induced LH and FSH release of untreated and desensitized cells. Rat pituitary cells (3×10^5 per culture dish) were incubated in 1 ml medium 199 "Earle" for 2 days. The cells were either untreated (*open circles*) or treated (*closed circles*) with 10^{-8} *M* GnRH for an additional 24 h. **a** Shows the GnRH-stimulated LH release, **b** the GnRH-stimulated FSH release after indicated times

Experiment B

The effect of the length of the preincubation period on gonadotropin secretion during a consecutive 4-h GnRH challenge test was examined. Down-regulation occurred after 3 h of 10^{-8} *M*, after 18 h of 10^{-9} *M* (LH release, not FSH release), and 24 h of 10^{-10} *M* preincubation with GnRH. LH release decreased from 27.7 ± 1.7 ng/ml (without GnRH pretreatment) to 21.3 ± 1.3 ng/ml after 3 h and to 9.9 ± 0.8 ng/ml after 24 h of 10^{-8} *M* GnRH challenge. FSH release decreased from 3.0 ± 0.1 ng/ml to about 2.5 ± 0.1 ng/ml after 3 h to 1.8 ± 0.1 ng/ml after 24 h of 10^{-8} *M* GnRH challenge. In Fig. 2, GnRH-stimulated LH release after preincubation periods of 1, 6, and 24 h with GnRH is shown (Fig. 2A, C, E). GnRH-stimulated FSH release occurs after preincubation periods of 0.5, 6, and 24 h (Fig. 2B, D, F) with GnRH. The results of GnRH-stimulated LH and FSH release after preincubation with 10^{-10} *M* and 10^{-8} *M* are shown in Fig. 3. These data demonstrate that the time course of GnRH-induced desensitization is dose-dependent.

Discussion

GnRH analogues are used for a variety of sex-hormone-dependent diseases and are under investigation for possible use in contraception. The gonadotropin release of rat pituitary cells can be down-regulated time- and dose-dependently by continuous GnRH exposure. Preincubation with the hypothalamic peptide at high doses results in a more rapid down-regulation, whereas preincubation at low doses requires a longer period of pretreatment. These results confirm our preliminary findings (Helm et al. 1987) and data published by other groups (Badger et al. 1983; Lui and Jackson 1984). Continuous administration of 1 n*M* GnRH in perfusion experiments decreased LH to basal values after 14 h (Smith et al. 1983). After this time the LH content in the cells was more than 55% of the original (Smith et al. 1983). Chronic exposure to saturating doses of GnRH caused pituitary refractoriness to further stimulation by GnRH, although the cells are capable of responding to other secretagogues (Smith and Vale 1981). It seems that the phenomenon of desensitization cannot be fully explained by receptor down-regulation. Coincidence of desensitization and receptor down-regulation in pituitary gonadotrophs stimulated by GnRH was reported (Zilberstein et al. 1983), but GnRH receptor down-regulation and the loss of responsiveness to GnRH were differently affected (Nett et al. 1981). GnRH receptor internalization and LH release can be uncoupled, but the loss of the GnRH receptor by internalization is not a sufficient explanation for GnRH-mediated desensitization of the gonadotroph (Gorospe and Conn 1987). A number of potential second messenger systems for the GnRH-induced gonadotropin secretion have been postulated (Kiesel et al. 1986b, c, 1987a, b; Kiesel and Catt 1987). A postreceptor mechanism has been reported to play a part in the process of desensitization of gonadotrophs (Baldwin et al. 1984; Hazum and Schvartz 1984). Ca^{2+} is necessary for pituitary responsiveness to GnRH stimulus (Bourne and Baldwin 1980; Conn et al. 1981; de Koning et al. 1982; Pickering and Fink 1979; Stern and Conn 1981), but it has been reported that GnRH-mediated desensitization of the pituitary

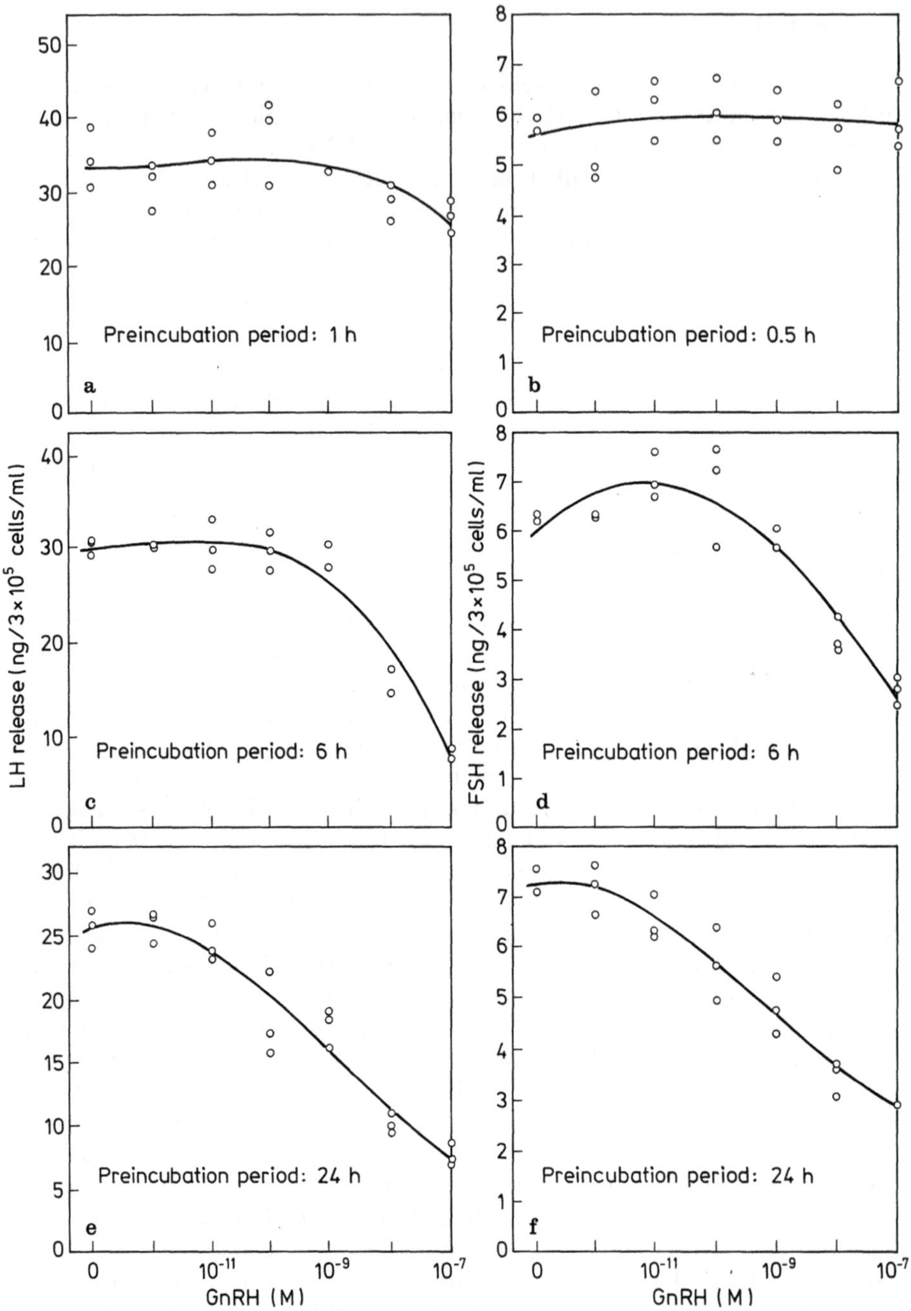

Fig. 2a–f. Effect of the length of the preincubation period with GnRH on subsequent GnRH-stimulated LH and FSH release. Rat pituitary cells (3×10^5 per culture dish) were incubated in 1 ml medium 199 "Earle" for 2 days. GnRH in the indicated concentrations was added to the monolayer cell cultures for 1 additional h (**a**), 0.5 h (**b**), 6 h (**c, d**) or 24 h (**e, f**). The 10^{-8} *M* GnRH-stimulated LH release is shown in **a, c, e**; the 10^{-8} *M* GnRH-stimulated FSH release is shown in **b, d, f**

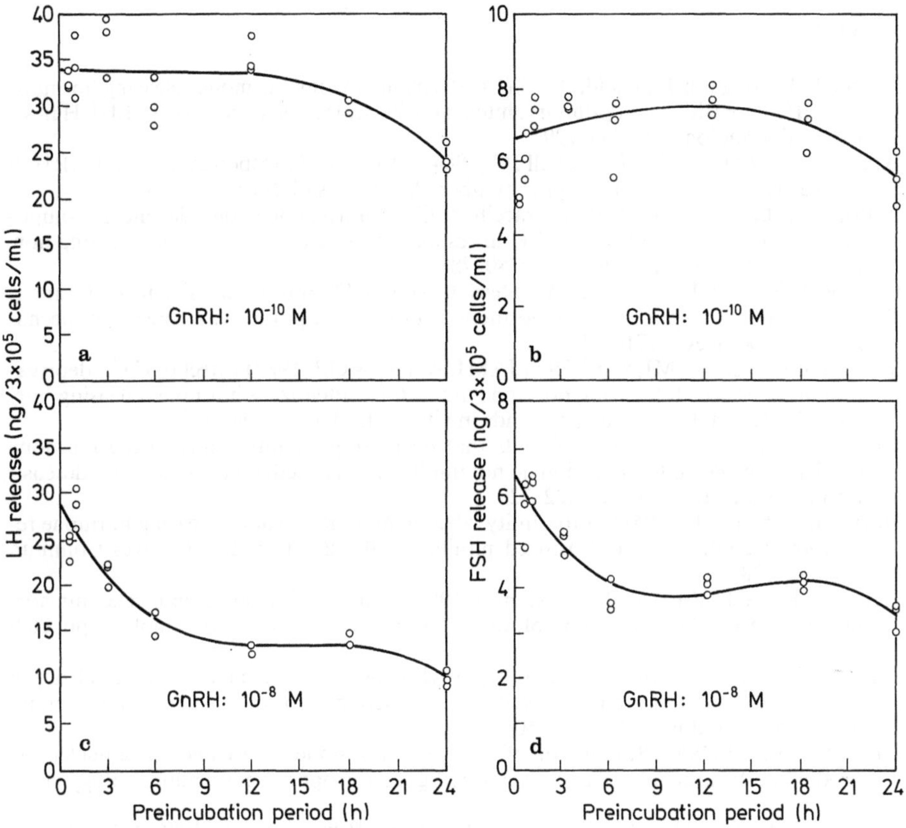

Fig. 3 a–d. Effect of preincubation with different concentrations of GnRH for different periods on subsequent 10^{-8} *M* GnRH-stimulated LH and FSH release. Rat pituitary cells (3×10^5 per culture dish) were incubated in 1 ml medium 199 "Earle" for 2–3 days. Then 10^{-10} *M* GnRH (**a, b**) or 10^{-8} *M* GnRH (**c, d**) was added to the monolayer cell cultures for different periods of time. Data show the subsequent GnRH-stimulated LH release (**a, c**) or FSH release (**b, d**)

gonadotroph is not Ca^{2+} dependent (Smith and Conn 1983). GnRH induces homologous desensitization only in the presence of Ca^{2+} ionophore, phorbol myristate acetate, or high potassium concentrations (Naor et al. 1982; Smith and Vale 1981; Yeo et al. 1981; Zilberstein et al. 1983). GnRH-mediated desensitization of cultured rat anterior pituitary cells can be uncoupled from LH release, because chelation of extracellular Ca^{2+} with ethylene glycol tetra-acetic acid blocked GnRH-stimulated LH release but did not prevent subsequent desensitization (Jinnah and Conn 1986). Taken together, it seems that receptor down-regulation as a postreceptor mechanism is also involved in the desensitization effect of pituitary gonadotrophs. Further studies will clarify the intracellular mechanism of the phenomenon.

Acknowledgements. This project was supported by the Deutsche Forschungsgemeinschaft/Bonn (Ki 283/2-1).

References

Badger TM, Loughlin JS, Naddaff PG (1983) The luteinizing hormone-releasing hormone (LHRH)-desensitized rat pituitary: luteinizing hormone responsiveness to LHRH in vitro. Endocrinology 112:793–799

Baldwin DM, Bourne GA, Marschall JC (1984) Pituitary LH responsiveness to GnRH in vitro as related to GnRH receptor number. Am J Physiol 247:E651–656

Bourne GA, Baldwin DM (1980) Extracellular Ca^{2+}-independent and -dependent components of the biphasic release of LH in response to luteinizing hormone releasing hormone in vitro. Endocrinology 107:780–788

Conn PM, Marian J, McMillian M, Stern J, Rogers D, Hamby M, Penna A, Grant E (1981) Gonadotropin releasing hormone action in the pituitary: a three-step mechanism. Endocr Rev 2:171–185

de Koning J, Tijssen AMI, van Dieten JAMJ, van Rees GP (1982) Effect of Ca^{2+} deprivation on release of luteinizing hormone induced by luteinizing hormone-releasing hormone from female rat pituitary glands in vitro. J Endocrinol 94:11–20

Gorospe WC, Conn PM (1987) Agents that decrease gonadotropin-releasing hormone (GnRH) receptor internalization do not inhibit GnRH-mediated gonadotrope desensitization. Endocrinology 120:222–229

Hazum E, Schvartz I (1984) Photoaffinity labeling of gonadotropin releasing hormone receptors in control and desensitized pituitary cells. Biochem Biophys Res Commun 125:532–538

Helm KJ, Kiesel L, Rabe T, Runnebaum B (1987) Kinetics of gonadotropin-releasing hormone induced desensitization of rat pituitary cells. Acta Endocrinol [Suppl 283] 114:184

Jinnah HA, Conn PM (1986) Gonadotropin-releasing hormone-mediated desensitization of cultured rat anterior pituitary cells can be uncoupled from luteinizing hormone release. Endocrinology 118:2599–2604

Kiesel L, Catt KJ (1987) Stimulation of luteinizing hormone release and cyclic nucleotide production by arachidonic acid in cultured gonadotrophs. Neuroendocrinology 46:1–9

Kiesel L, Rabe T, Schleef J, Schweizer M, Klinga K, Runnebaum B (1986a) Pulsatile secretory pattern of gonadotropins and steroids during the follicular and luteal phase of the menstrual cycle in women. In: Pulsatile GnRH 1985. Proceedings of the 3rd Ferring symposium on pulsatile GnRH, Noordwijk, 11–13 September 1985, Ferring, Haarlem, pp 43–49

Kiesel L, Bertges K, Rabe T, Runnebaum B (1986b) Gonadotropin releasing hormone enhances polyphosphoinositide hydrolysis in rat pituitary cells. Biochem Biophys Res Comm 134:861–867

Kiesel L, Przylipiak A, Rabe T, Runnebaum B (1986c) The role of novel arachidonic acid metabolites in GnRH action on gonadotropin release in vitro. Human Reprod 1:349–352

Kiesel L, Przylipiak A, Rabe T, Runnebaum B (1987a) Leukotrienes stimulated gonadotropin release in vitro. Gynecol Endocrinol 1:25–35

Kiesel L, Rabe T, Hauser G, Przylipiak A, Jadali F, Runnebaum B (1987b) Stimulation of luteinizing hormone release by melitin and phospholipase A_2 in rat pituitary cells. Mol Cell Endocrinol 51:1–6

Liu TC, Jackson GL (1984) Long-term superfusion of rat anterior pituitary cells: effects of repeated pulses of gonadotropin-releasing hormone at different doses, durations, and frequencies. Endocrinology 115:605–613

Naor Z, Katikineni M, Loumaye E, Vela AG, Dufau ML, Catt KJ (1982) Compartmentalization of luteinizing hormone pools: dynamics of gonadotropin releasing hormone action in superfused pituitary cells. Mol Cell Endocrinol 27:213–220

Nett TM, Crowder MD, Moss GE, Duello TM (1981) GnRH-receptor interaction. 5. Down-regulation of pituitary receptors for GnRH in ovariectomized ewes by infusion of homologous hormone. Biol Reprod 24:1145–1155

Nillius SJ, Gudmundsson J, Bergquist C (1985) A new superagonist of GnRH inhibition of ovulation in women. Contraception 31:119–122
Pickering AJ-MC, Fink G (1979) Priming effect of luteinizing hormone releasing factor in vitro: role of protein synthesis, contractile elements, Ca^{2+} and cyclic AMP. J Endocrinol 81:223–234
Sandow J (1983) Clinical applications of LHRH and its analogues. Clin Endocrinol 18:571–592
Sandow J (1986) Pharmacology of LHRH agonists. In: Furr, Vakeling (eds) Pharmacology and clinical uses of hormone secretion and action. Holt-Saunders, Eastbourne, pp 365–384
Smith WA, Conn PM (1983) GnRH-mediated desensitization of the pituitary gonadotrope is not calcium dependent. Endocrinology 112:408–410
Smith MA, Vale WW (1981) Desensitization to gonadotropin-releasing hormone observed in superfused pituitary cells on cytodex beads. Endocrinology 108:752–759
Smith MA, Perrin MH, Vale WW (1983) Desensitization of cultured pituitary cells to gonadotropin-releasing hormone: evidence for a post-receptor mechanism. Mol Cell Endocrinol 30:85–96
Stern JE, Conn PM (1981) Perifusion of rat pituitaries: requirements for optimal GnRH-stimulated LH release. Am J Physiol 240:E504–509
Yeo T, Grossman A, Belchetz P, Besser GM (1981) Response of luteinizing hormone from columns of dispersed rat pituitary cells to a highly potent analogue of luteinizing hormone-releasing hormone. J Endocrinol 91:33–41
Zilberstein M, Zakut H, Naor Z (1983) Coincidence of down-regulation and desensitization in pituitary gonadotrophs stimulated by gonadotropin-releasing hormone. Life Sci 32:663–669

Potency of Contraceptive Progestins to Inhibit Luteinizing Hormone Secretion in Vitro

L. Kiesel, T. Rabe, K. Helm, C. Maier, and B. Runnebaum

Department of Obstetrics and Gynecology, Division of Gynecological Endocrinology, Women's Hospital, University of Heidelberg, Voßstr. 9, 6900 Heidelberg, FRG

Introduction

Progestins are a major component of hormonal antifertility agents, and a large number of them are available for oral contraceptive (OC) use. Apart from the changes in dose the most recent developments in OC have arisen from newly synthesized progestational compounds.

It has been well established that sex steroids act through feedback mechanisms to modulate gonadotropin secretion. One main effect of OCs is their action at the hypothalamic and pituitary level. The physiologically present sex steroids in women such as estradiol-17β and progesterone have, for several years, been known to affect neuroendocrine function, but the exact regulatory mechanisms have not yet been fully understood.

Among the various other sites of antifertility action, contraceptive progestins alone can inhibit gonadotropin secretion via the hypothalamus and/or the pituitary. In order to be able to distinguish the effects on the pituitary from the action on the hypothalamus, an in vitro bioassay was established. In the present study a large number of progestational compounds are compared in their potency to inhibit gonadotropin-releasing hormone (GnRH)-induced luteinizing hormone (LH) release in a bioassay using altered rat anterior pituitary cells.

Methods

Rat Pituitary Cell Culture

Anterior pituitaries of female Sprague Dawley rats (250 g) were dispersed into a single cell suspension by trypsinization as described previously (Kiesel and Catt 1984). Cells (2×10^5 per culture dish) were incubated in 1 ml medium 199 "Earle" with 2.2 mg/ml $NaHCO_3$ (Seromed, Berlin) supplemented with 10% Serum Plus (KC Biological, Techomara, FRG), 800 μM L-glutamine (Seromed, Berlin), 100 units penicillin, and 100 mg streptomycin/ml (Seromed, Berlin). All steroids, which were dissolved in 0.1% dimethyl sulfoxide (DMSO, Serva, FRG), were added in the concentrations of 10^{-10}–10^{-5} M to each well. After 3 days in culture, the cells were washed twice and incubated in medium 199 "Earle" with 20 mM HEPES (Seromed, Berlin), supplemented with 0.85 mg/ml $NaHCO_3$, 800 μM L-glutamine, 100 units penicillin, 100 mg streptomycin/ml, and 0.25%

Female Contraception
Eds.: B. Runnebaum, T. Rabe, L. Kiesel

bovine albumin (Sigma, FRG). For stimulation of LH release, synthetic GnRH (Peninsula Laboratories, USA) was added to the medium in a final dilution of 10^{-7} *M*. After 4 h of incubation the supernatant was saved for radioimmunoassay of LH. Cultures with 0.1% dimethyl sulfoxide were used as controls, which were not different from controls without the solvent.

Studies on Incubation Conditions

In order to establish and optimize cell culture conditions for the study of contraceptive progestagens on LH secretion, various incubation conditions have been analyzed in vitro. Stimulation of pituitary cells was carried out as described above in various media such as medium 199 "Earle," medium 199 "Hank's," RPMI 1640, and McCoy's medium. In addition the effects of the steroid solvents DMSO and ethanol have been compared.

LH Secretion and Contraceptive Progestins

The effect of contraceptive progestins on LH was investigated under various conditions. To determine the time-dependence of steroid action, cells were preincubated with progestins for 0–72 h before being challenged with GnRH. The dose-dependent effect was studied using a 72 h incubation period, and steroid concen-

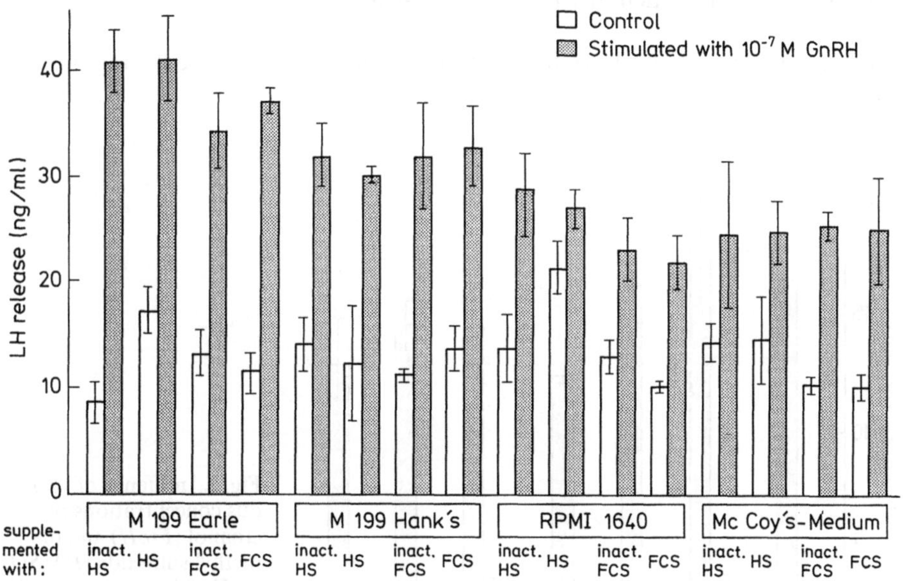

Fig. 1. Effect of various media on GnRH-stimulated LH secretion in primary rat pituitary cell cultures. Pituitary cells (2×10^5 cell/dish) were cultured for 2 days in medium supplemented with horse serum (HS) or fetal calf serum (FCS). Following two washes cells were stimulated by GnRH (10^{-7} *M*) for 4 h (*hatched column*) LH was determined in supernatants by RIA

trations were varied from 10^{-10}–10^{-5} *M*. To determine a shift in the sensitivity of the cells, GnRH progestins (10^{-5} *M*) were added to pituicytes for 72 h, and the cells were stimulated by GnRH (10^{-12}–10^{-6} *M*). Controls contained charcoal-extracted steroid-free media.

The following steroids were studied: progesterone, cyproterone, cyproterone acetate, chlormadinone acetate, ethynodiol diacetate, norgestimate, gestodene, norethinodrel, levonorgestrel, 3-keto-desogestrel, norethisterone, norethisterone acetate, norgestrel, lynestrenol, and desogestrel.

Results

Culture Conditions for the Study of Progestagens

The effect of different media on GnRH-stimulated LH release in rat anterior pituitary cell cultures in vitro is shown in Fig. 1. Secretory activity of pituicytes was highest in medium 199 using Serum Plus, which was chosen for further studies. Possible solvents for dissolving steroids in aqueous medium were tested to analyze their influence on pituitary cells in culture (Fig. 2). DMSO in a concentration not exceeding 0.1% did not alter GnRH-stimulated LH secretion and was used in the experiments with progestins.

Time Course of Inhibition by Progestins in Vitro

GnRH-stimulated LH release in rat pituitary cells was suppressed using progestational compounds.

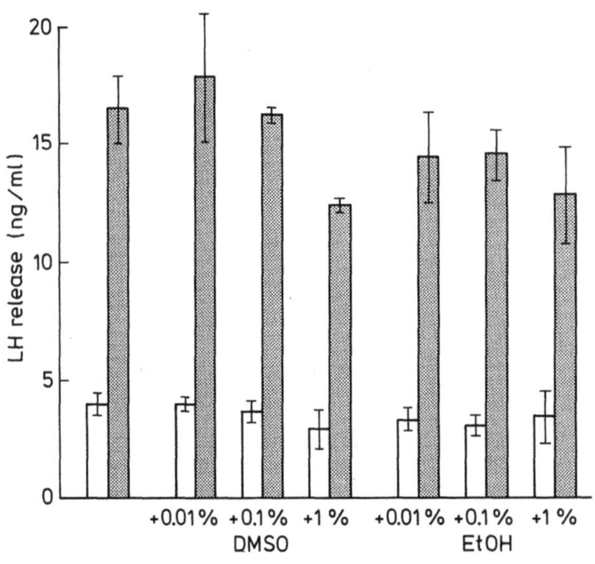

Fig. 2. Influence of various concentrations of ethanol (*EtoH*) and dimethyl sulfoxide (*DMSO*) on GnRH-stimulated LH release in pituitary cell cultures as described in Fig. 1

The time course of steroid effect is shown in Fig. 3. Some progestins administered for a short time (4 h) slightly enhanced gonadotropin release. With increasing preincubation time (23–72 h), the secretion of LH was progressively inhibited. Maximal inhibition was achieved at 72 h with 10^{-5} *M* progestin.

Dose-dependent Inhibition of Gonadotropin Release

Increasing progestin concentration caused a dose-dependent inhibition of 10^{-7} *M* GnRH-induced LH release, also in cells pretreated with steroids for 72 h (Fig. 4). Results were calculated as a percentage of the control. The difference between GnRH-stimulated and basal LH secretion was taken as 100%. All samples contained the solvent (0.1% DMSO) which had no significant effect on cell response during the time examined.

Various progestins (10^{-5} *M*) reduced the GnRH-induced LH secretion by different amounts (given as percent inhibition): lynestrenol (68%), 3-keto-desogestrel (53%), norgestrel (51%), norethisterone (55%), ethynodiol diacetate (53%), norgestimate (46%), gestodene (44%), chlormadinone acetate (43%), levonorgestrel (37%), norethisterone acetate (21%), desogestrel (15%), progesterone (15%), cyproterone acetate (9%), and cyproterone (0%).

Shift of GnRH-Response Curve of LH- and FSH-Release by Progestins

Progestins have been tested for their potency to shift the response curve of LH stimulated by GnRH (Fig. 5). Control was defined as the response of pituitary cells to GnRH (10^{-12}–10^{-6} *M*) without steroids. The effects of steroids on progestins were examined by preincubating cells with the steroids for 48 h using 10^{-5} *M* steroid concentrations. Progesterone had an inhibitory effect on LH release. Almost all contraceptive progestins tested caused a shift of the curve to the right and inhibited maximal cell response to GnRH. Cells pretreated with progestins have therefore become less sensitive to GnRH stimulation.

Half maximum stimulation (ED_{50}) of LH release by GnRH without steroid pretreatment was 3.2×10^{-10} *M* under the conditions examined. The ED_{50} value for GnRH response was increased by progestins (Table 1).

Discussion

In this study a comparison of progestagen effect on GnRH-stimulated LH release has been carried out in an in vitro bioassay system using primary cultures of rat anterior pituitaries. Since in vivo experiments do not allow the distinction between the hypothalamic and the pituitary sites of action, this model is useful for analyzing steroid modulations of gonadotrophs.

A number of other studies have taken advantage of this bioassay to investigate feedback mechanisms by naturally occurring steroids such as estradiol-17β (Apfelbaum 1983; Emons et al. 1986; Hsueh et al. 1979; Schally et al. 1973; Padmanabhan et al. 1978), progesterone (Apfelbaum 1982; Batra and Miller 1985; Ka-

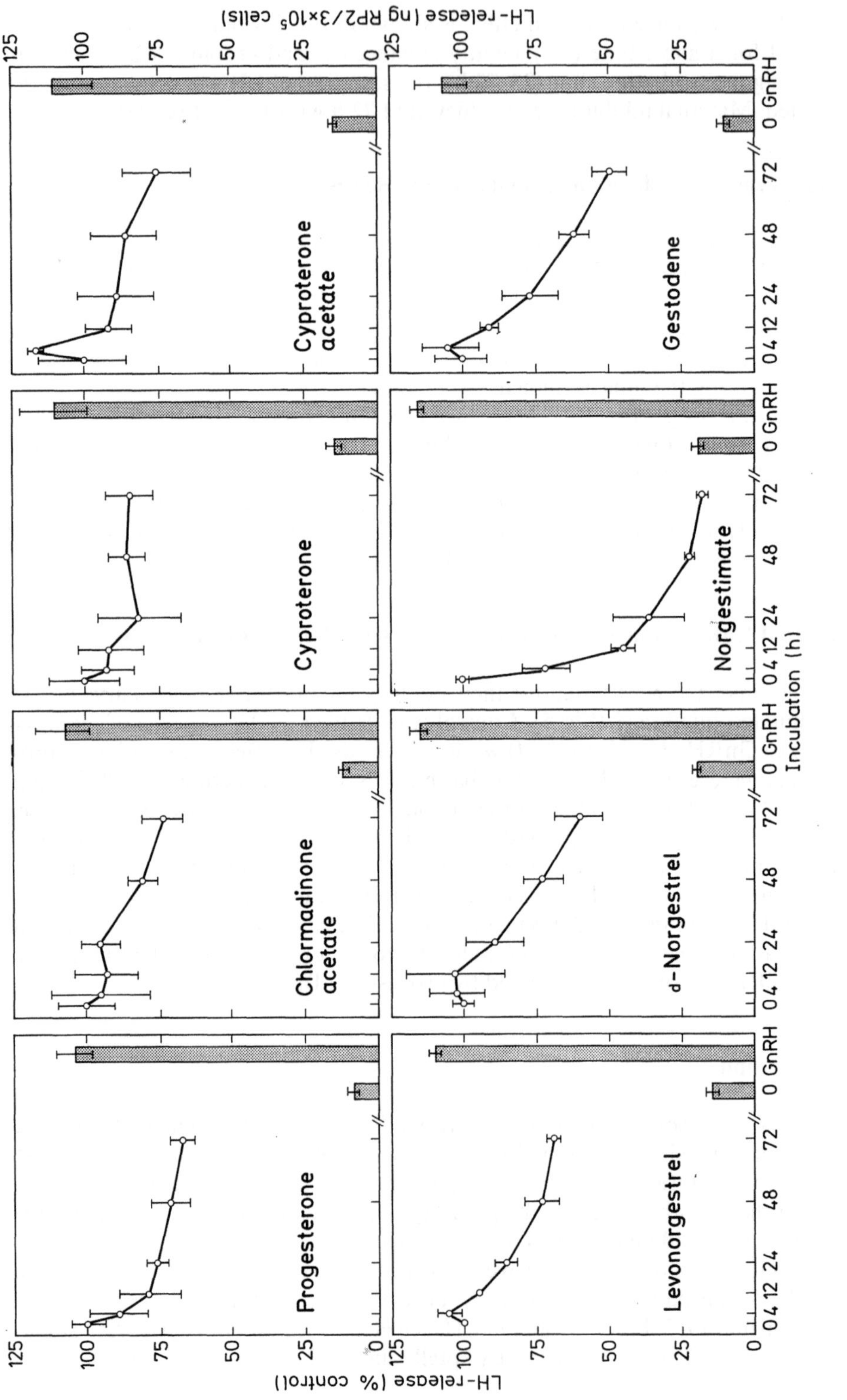
Progesterone
Chlormadinone acetate
Cyproterone
Cyproterone acetate
Levonorgestrel
d-Norgestrel
Norgestimate
Gestodene
LH-release (% control)
LH-release (ng RP2/3×10⁵ cells)
Incubation (h)
0 4 12 24 48 72
0 GnRH
0
25
50
75
100
125

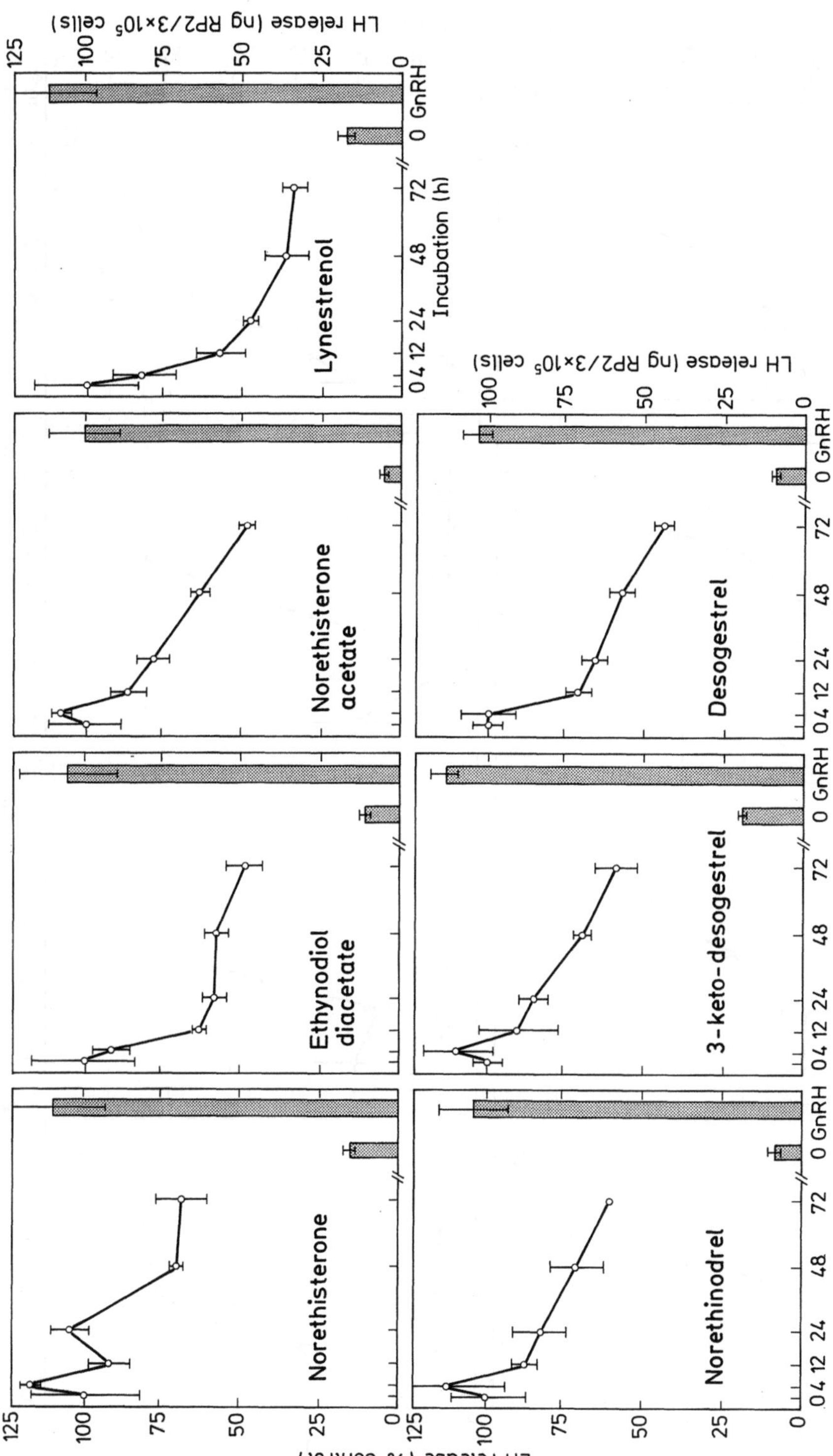

Fig. 3 Time-dependent effect of progestagen preincubation prior to GnRH challenge of pituitary cells

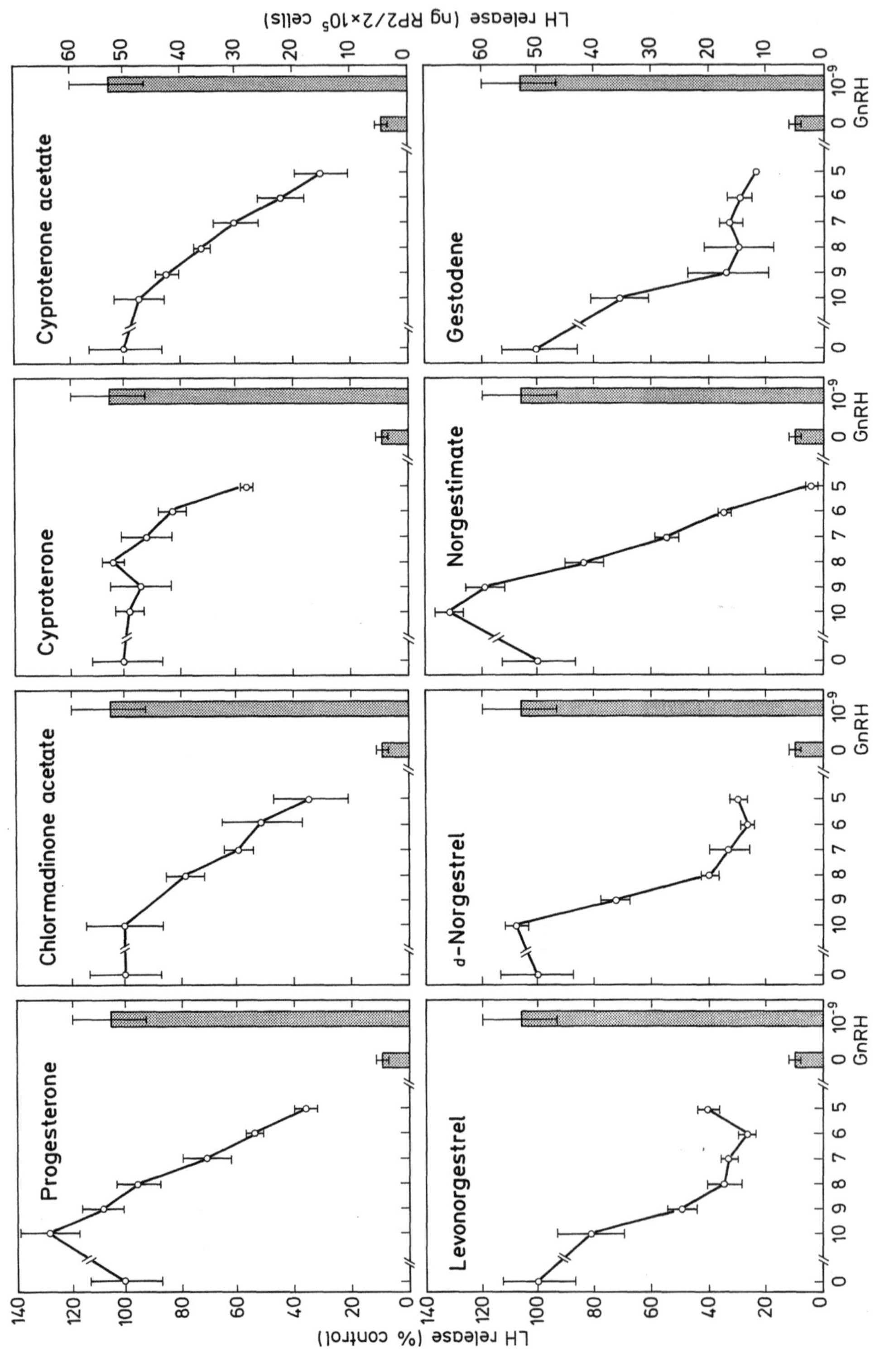
Progesterone
Chlormadinone acetate
Cyproterone
Cyproterone acetate
Levonorgestrel
d-Norgestrel
Norgestimate
Gestodene
LH release (% control)
LH release (ng RP2/2×10⁵ cells)
– Log steroid (M)
GnRH
0
10
9
8
7
6
5
10⁻⁹

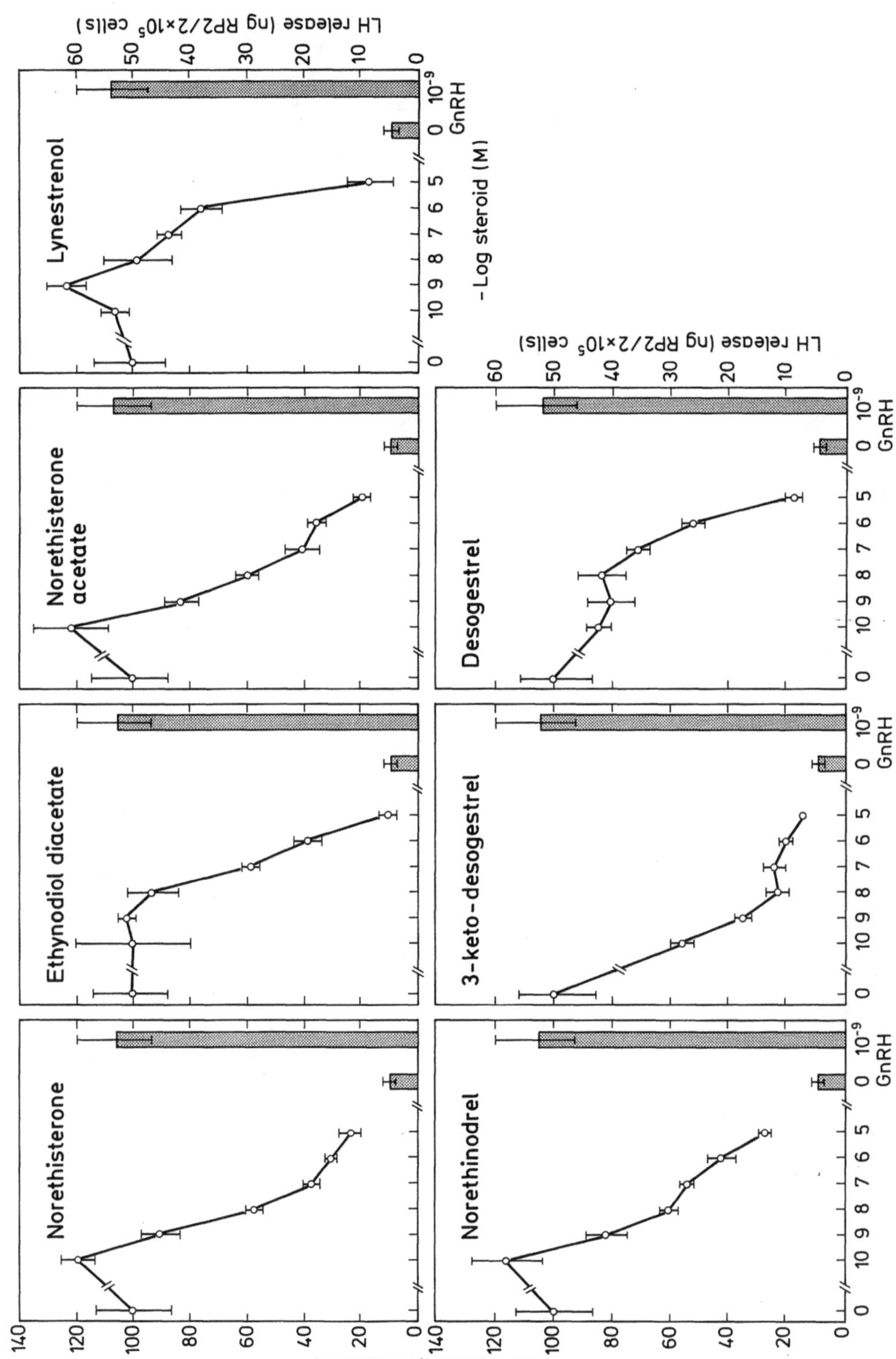

Fig. 4. Dose-dependent inhibition of GnRH-enhanced LH secretion by progestagens (10^{-10}–10^{-5} *M*) preincubated for 48 h

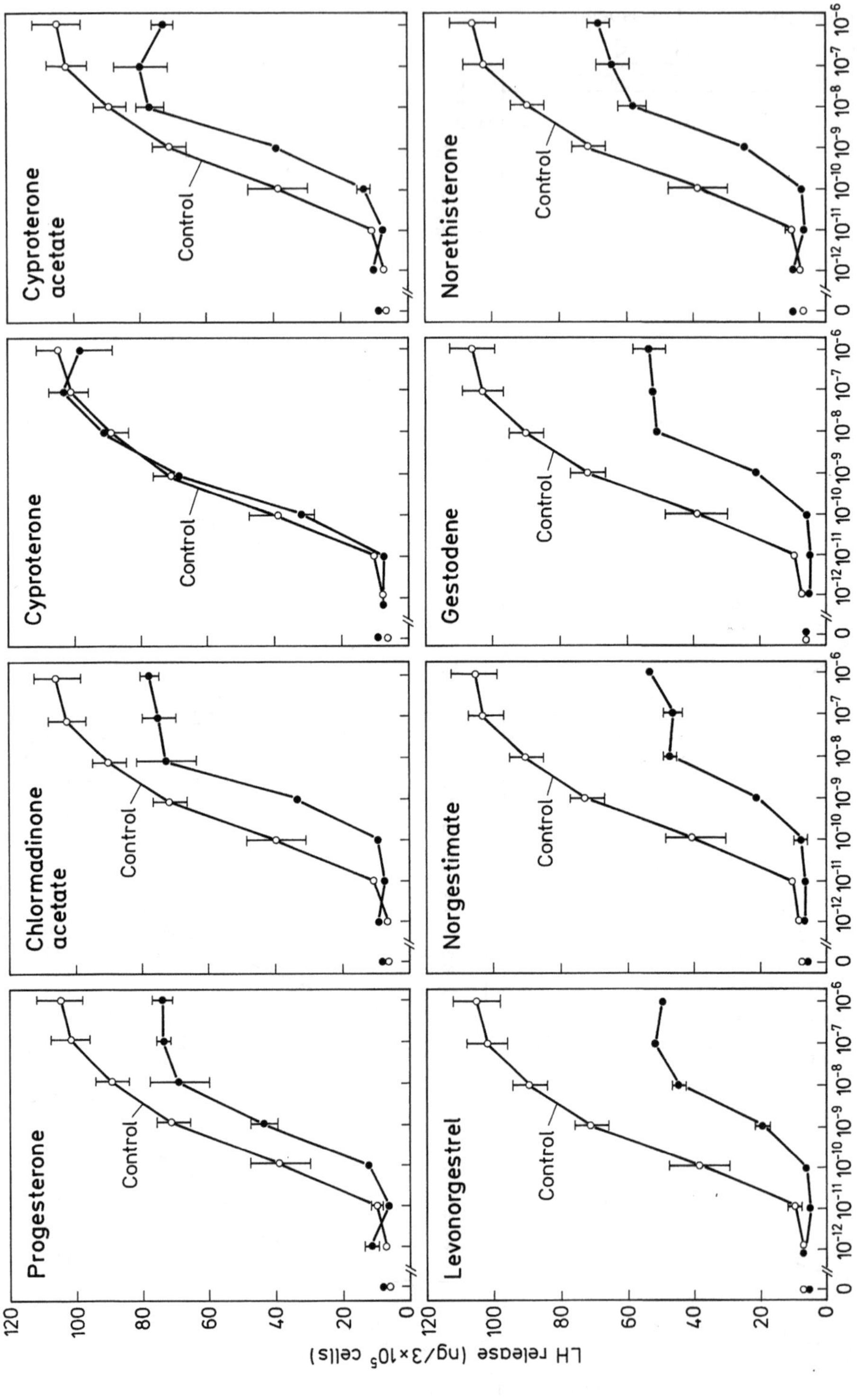
Progesterone
Chlormadinone acetate
Cyproterone
Cyproterone acetate
Levonorgestrel
Norgestimate
Gestodene
Norethisterone
Control
LH release (ng/3×10⁵ cells)
GnRH (M)
0
20
40
60
80
100
120
0 10⁻¹² 10⁻¹¹ 10⁻¹⁰ 10⁻⁹ 10⁻⁸ 10⁻⁷ 10⁻⁶

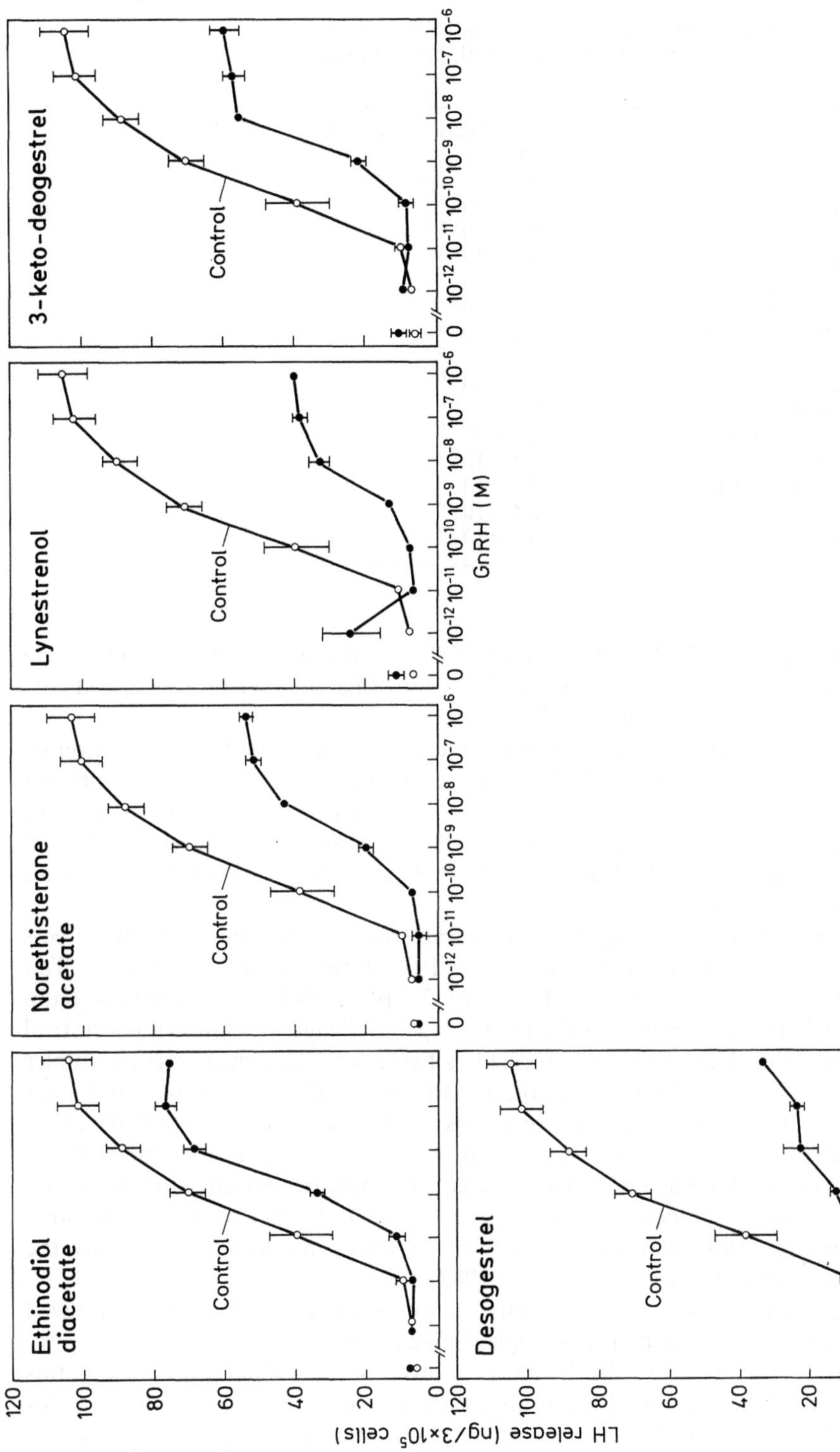

Fig. 5. Effect of progestins on the GnRH-stimulated LH secretion, altering the sensitivity of the gonadotrophs in vitro

Table 1. Half maximum concentration of GnRH for stimulation of LH secretion in cells pretreated with progestins in vitro

Steroid	LH release by GnRH (*M*)
Control	3.2×10^{-10}
Progesterone	$8\ \times10^{-10}$
Cyproterone	$4\ \times10^{-10}$
Cyproterone acetate	1.1×10^{-9}
Chlormadinone acetate	1.6×10^{-9}
Ethynodiol diacetate	1.6×10^{-9}
Norgestimate	1.6×10^{-9}
Gestodene	1.8×10^{-9}
Levonorgestrel	$2\ \times10^{-9}$
3-keto-Desogestrel	2.5×10^{-9}
Norethisterone	2.5×10^{-9}
Norethisterone acetate	2.5×10^{-9}
Lynestrenol	3.6×10^{-9}
Desogestrel	4.5×10^{-9}

washima et al. 1982; Kamel and Krey 1982), testosterone (Drouin and Labrie 1976; Labrie et al. 1977; Kao and Weisz 1975; Miller and Weites 1966), and corticosterone (Suter and Schwartz 1985).

The antifertility effects of OCs are numerous, including the modulation of the neuroendocrine function. So far it has remained unclear whether the inhibition of gonadotropin release occurs at the level of the hypothalamus (Kastin et al. 1972a; Kastin et al. 1972b; Vandenberg et al. 1974) or the pituitary (Robyn et al. 1974; Lemarchand-Beraud et al. 1974; Perez-Lopez et al. 1975; Krög et al. 1976; Mishell et al. 1977).

In vivo studies have attempted to characterize estrogen and progestin effects on the pituitary in humans (Mishell et al. 1977; Robyn et al. 1974; Dericks-Tan et al. 1976; Römmler 1982; Kuhl et al. 1982; Spona 1984) and in aminals (Kuhl et al. 1978; Bieslmayer et al. 1980a) following a challenge with GnRH. In one trial a double GnRH challenge was applied as two consecutive injections (Römmler 1982). The increase of serum LH and FSH following the first and second administrations was measured. Different doses of progestins were compared in Römmler's study and a dose-dependent inhibition of the pituitary function by progestins was demonstrated. The increase of gonadotropins after the second injection of GnRH indicated the capacity of the gonadotroph to secrete gonadotropins; progestagens seemed to antagonize the estrogen effect depending on the dose and type of progestin (Römmler 1982).

The progestins' site of contraceptive action at the cellular level is still not well defined, although their pharmacological effects have been widely studied (see review by Neumann 1978). At the receptor level, in the endometrium, progestins exhibit different affinities for the uterine progestagen receptor. In the gonadotroph, too, the intracellular action of steroids is still unclear. Progestins may affect GnRH stimulation of exocytosis at the receptor or postreceptor site. With steroids, changes in receptor numbers (Clayton and Catt 1981) as well as alterations of certain intracellular events (Kiesel et al. 1987a) have been observed in the pituitary. Other potential second messenger systems in gonadotrophs could be targets of these substances (Kiesel and Catt 1984; Kiesel et al. 1986a, b, 1987b; Emons et al. 1987; Kiesel and Catt 1987).

The present data show various synthetic progestins to be more potent than progesterone in reducing gonadotropic sensitivity to GnRH stimulation in enzymatically dispersed pituitary cells in vitro. Time course experiments analyzed the effect of the steroids preincubated with the cells for 0–72 h prior to the 4-h GnRH challenge.

Some progestagens potentiated gonadotropin release when present in the medium for only 4 h, while all of them caused an inhibition thereafter.

Using the same preincubation time progestagens showed a shift of the GnRH-induced LH curve in experiments with dose-dependent GnRH stimulation.

Data collected by others in pituitary in vitro bioassays show that the responsiveness of the pituicytes to GnRH can be decreased by progesterone and progestagens (Lagacé et al. 1980; Batra and Miller 1985; Bieslmayer et al. 1980b). The results of this paper confirm that progesterone acts directly on the gonadotroph function by inhibiting LH secretion. Furthermore, synthetic progestagens can also affect the pituitary and are more effective in blocking GnRH-enhanced gonadotropin release in cell culture. The potency of these progestational steroids can be compared by the inhibition of LH at the maximum steroid concentration used or by the shift of the GnRH-stimulated LH curve (ED_{50}). These in vitro findings demonstrate the usefulness of this system to investigate the relative potencies of steroids with regard to the inhibition of LH secretion. It has to be kept in mind, however, that this in vitro model can merely give results on one aspect of the antigonadotropic effect of progestagens, which in itself is only one partial characteristic of these compounds.

Acknowledgements. This project has been supported by grants from the Deutsche Forschungsgemeinschaft, Bonn (Ki 283/2-1).

References

Apfelbaum M (1983) Influence of gonadal steroids on the time-course of release and synthesis of luteinizing hormone, follicle-stimulating hormone and prolactin from rat pituitary glands in vitro. J Endocrinol 96:171–179

Batra SK, Miller WL (1985) Progesterone decreases the responsiveness of ovine pituitary cultures to luteinizing hormone-releasing hormone. Endocrinology 117:1436–1440

Bieslmayer C, Spona J, Schroeder R (1980a) Pituitary and hypothalamic action of progestagens in castrated female rats. Endocrinologica Experimentalis 14:17–25

Bieslmayer C, Spona J, Schroeder R (1980b) Modulation of LH-RH stimulated gonadotropin release by progestagens and 17β-estradiol in primary pituitary cell culture. Endocrinologica Experimentalis 14:171–182

Clayton R, Catt KJ (1981) Gonadotropin-releasing hormone receptors: characterization, physiological regulation, and relationship to reproductive function. Endocr Rev 2:186–209

Dericks-Tan JSE, Krög W, Aktories K, Taubert H-D (1976) Dose-dependent inhibition by oral contraceptives of the pituitary to release LH and FSH in response to stimulation with LH-RH. Contraception 14:171–181

Drouin J, Labrie F (1976) Selective effect of androgens on LH and FSH release in anterior pituitary cells in culture. Endocrinology 98:1528–1534
Emons G, Ortmann O, Fingscheidt U, Ball P, Knuppen R (1986) Short-term effects of oestradiol and 4-hydroxyoestradiol on gonadotrophin-releasing hormone induced luteinizing hormone secretion by rat pituitary cells in culture. Acta Endocrinol 111:312–320
Emons G, Frevert EU, Ortmann O, Kiesel L, Knuppen R (1987) Studies on the subcellular mechanisms mediating the negative estradiol effect of GnRH-induced LH-release. Acta Endocrinol (Copenh) 175:151
Hsueh AJW, Erickson GF, Yen SSC (1979) The sensitizing effect of estrogens and catechol estrogen on cultured primary cells to luteinizing hormone-releasing hormones: its antagonism by progestins. Endocrinology 104:807–813
Kamel F, Krey LC (1982) Gonadal steroid modulation of LHRH-stimulated LH secretion by pituitary cell cultures. Mol Cell Endocrinol 26:151–164
Kao IW, Weisz J (1975) Direct effect of testosterone and its 5alpha-reduced metabolites on pituitary LH- and FSH-release in vitro: change in pituitary responsiveness to hypothalamic extract. Endocrinology 96:253–260
Kastin AJ, Schally AV, Gual C, Arimura A (1972a) Release of LH and FSH after administration of synthetic LH-releasing hormone. J Clin Endocrinol Metab 34:753–756
Kastin AJ, Gual C, Schally AV (1972b) Clinical experience with hypothalamic releasing hormones. Part 2. Luteinizing hormone-releasing hormone and other hypophyseotropic releasing hormones. Recent Prog Horm Res 28:201–227
Kawashima M, Kamiyoshi M, Tanaka K, Hattori M, Wakabayashi K (1982) Effects of progesterone on pituitary cells of the hen (Gallus domesticus) during the ovulatory cycle for production and release of LH and FSH. Gen Comp Endocrinol 48:362–371
Kiesel L, Catt KJ (1984) Phosphatidic acid and calcium dependent actions of gonadotropin releasing hormone in pituitary gonadotrophs. Arch Biochem Biophys 231:202–210
Kiesel L, Catt KJ (1987) Stimulation of luteinizing hormone release and cyclic nucleotide production by arachidonic acid in cultured gonadotrophs. Neuroendocrinology 46:1–9
Kiesel L, Bertges K, Rabe T, Runnebaum B (1986a) Gonadotropin releasing hormone enhances polyphosphoinositide hydrolysis in rat pituitary cells. Biochem Biophys Res Commun 134:861–867
Kiesel L, Przylipiak A, Rabe T, Runnebaum B (1986b) The role of novel arachidonic acid metabolites in GnRH action on gonadotrophin release in vitro. Hum Reprod 1:349–352
Kiesel L, Helm K, Bertges K, Maier C, Rabe T, Runnebaum B (1987a) Contraceptive progestins and gonadotropin secretion in vitro. J Steroid Biochem (in press) 27(4–6):995–1002
Kiesel L, Przylipiak A, Rabe T, Runnebaum B (1987b) Leukotrienes stimulate gonadotropin release in vitro. Gynecol Endocrinology 1:25–35
Krög W, Aktories K, Dericks-Tan JSE, Taubert H-D (1976) Dose-dependent inhibition by oral contraceptives of the pituitary to release LH and FSH in response to stimulation with LH-RH. Contraception 14:171–181
Kuhl H, Sachs A, Rosniatowski C, Taubert H-D (1978) Time-dependent decrease of pituitary response to LH-RH after chronic treatment of intact female rats with ethinyloestradiol and norethindrone. Acta Endocrinol (Copenh) 89:240–250
Kuhl H, Dericks-Tan JSE, Taubert H-D (1982) Der Einfluß hormonaler Kontrazeptiva auf die hypothalamo-hypophysäre Achse. In: Hammerstein J (ed) Aspekte der hormonalen Kontrazeption. Excerpta Medica, Amsterdam, pp 28–36
Labrie F, Drouin J, De Léan A, Lagacé L, Ferland L, Beaulieu M (1977) Mechanism of action of LHRH and TRH in anterior pituitary gland and modulation of their activity by peripheral hormones. In: Porter J (ed) Peptide releasing hormone. Plenum Press, New York, p 157
Lagacé L, Massiocotte J, Labrie F (1980) Acute stimulatory effects of progesterone on luteinizing hormone and follicle stimulating hormone in rat anterior pituitary cells in culture. Endocrinology 106:684–689

Lemarchand-Beraud T, Rappoport G, Magrini G, Berthier C, Reymond M (1974) Influence of different physiological conditions on the gonadotropins and thyrotropin responses to LH-RH and TRH. Horm Metabol Res [Suppl] 5:170

Mishell DR Jr, Kletzky OA, Brenner PF, Subir R, Nicoloff J (1977) The effect of contraceptive steroids on hypothalamic-pituitary function. Am J Obstet Gynecol 128:60–73

Mittler JC, Meites J (1966) Effects of hypothalamic extract and androgen on pituitary FSH release in vitro. Endocrinology 78:500–504

Neumann F (1978) The physiological action of progesterone and the pharmacological effects of progestagens – a short review. Postgrad Med J [Suppl] 21:11–22

Padmanabhan V, Kesner JS, Convey EM (1978) Effects of estradiol on basal and luteinizing hormone releasing hormone (LHRH)-induced release of luteinizing hormone (LH) from bovine pituitary cells in culture. Biol Reprod 18:608–613

Perez Lopez FR, L'Hermite M, Robyn C (1975) Gonadotrophin hormone releasing test in women receiving hormonal contraception. Clin Endocrinol 4(5):477–485

Robyn C, Schöndorf H, Jürgensen O, Dericks-Tan JSE, Taubert H-D (1974) Oral contraception can decrease the pituitary capacity to release gonadotrophins in response to synthetic LH-RH. Arch Gynäkol 216:73–80

Römmler A (1982) Bestimmung der Östrogen- und Gestagenwirkungen oraler Kontrazeptiva auf die Hypophyse mit Hilfe des GnRH-Doppelstimulationstests mit gonadotropinfreisetzendem Hormon. In: Hammerstein J (ed) Aspekte der hormonalen Kontrazeption. Excerpta Medica, Amsterdam, pp 37–44

Spona J (1984) Androgenic action of progestins and possible synandrogenic properties of antiandrogens used in oral contraceptives. Gynaecol Obstet Invest 17:66–72

Suter DE, Schwartz NB (1985) Effects of glucocorticoids on secretion of Luteinizing Hormone and Follicle-Stimulating Hormone by female rat pituitary cells in vitro. Endocrinology 117:849–854

Schally AY, Redding TW, Arimura A (1973) Effect of sex steroids on pituitary responses to LH- and FSH-releasing hormone in vitro. Endocrinology 93:893–902

Vandenberg G, DeVane G, Yen SSC (1974) Effects of exogenous estrogen and progestin on pituitary responsiveness to synthetic luteinizing hormone-releasing factor. J Clin Invest 53:1750–1754

Implantables and Injectables

Long-Acting Injectable Steroidal Contraception Utilizing Norethindrone Microspheres

G. I. Zatuchni[1], L. R. Beck[2], and D. H. Lewis[3]

[1] General Obstetrics and Gynecology, Prentice Women's Hospital, Northwestern University, 333 East Superior Street, Chicago, Illinois 60611, USA
[2] New Product Development, Stolle Research and Development Corp, 2964 Sr. Rt. 42 S, Lebanon, Ohio 45036, USA
[3] New Product Development, Stolle Research and Development Corp. P.O. Box 5310, Decatur, Alabama 35601, USA

Introduction

Synthetic steroid hormones are generally accepted as a safe and efficacious means of fertility control. However, the formulations currently available fall short of ideal with regard to ease of administration and lack of side effects. There are questions regarding safety following long-term use of formulations containing estrogen, and efficacy may be compromised due to failure of user compliance.

To overcome these disadvantages, delivery systems are being developed to improve the benefit-to-risk ratio by providing continuous administration of low levels of contraceptive steroids for up to several years following a single administration.

The rationale, advantages, and disadvantages of long-acting, controlled-release, steroidal contraceptive systems have been previously reviewed [1, 5, 10, 12, 14]. The most advanced systems include depot steroid formulations, medicated intrauterine and intravaginal devices, and injectable small particulate systems.

This report provides an up-to-date summary of the research supported by the Program for Applied Research on Fertility Regulation (PARFR) to develop a long-acting, injectable, biodegradable, microsphere delivery system for the contraceptive steroid, norethisterone (NET).

To overcome some of the objections to the daily administration of steroid hormones, long-acting delivery systems have been developed, designed to provide a constant level of the steroid(s) in the blood that is maintained in the therapeutically effective dose range. As mentioned by Beck et al. [3–5, 7, 8] the ideal long-acting steroidal delivery system is one that provides steroid blood levels that remain within the therapeutic range, decreasing the likelihood of side effects; levels that are below the therapeutic level increase the risk of pregnancy.

The injectable controlled-release system meters the steroid into the blood at a controlled rate designed to maintain the blood level in the desired range, thereby achieving minimal intervention fertility control. Controlled release allows for reduction in the total amount of steroid administered over a prolonged period of time, and reduces the chance of human error by eliminating the need for repeated self-administration.

Female Contraception
Eds.: B. Runnebaum, T. Rabe, L. Kiesel

NET Microsphere Delivery System

The NET microsphere delivery system consists of microspheres composed of a biodegradable polymer and NET. Norethisterone was first synthesized in the Federal Republic of Germany, and clinical trials with norethisterone-enanthate as an injectable contraceptive began in 1957 [5]. The microspheres are prepared using a solvent evaporation process that has undergone substantial modification and improvement during the course of this program. Microspheres with diameters ranging from 10–240 μm have been used in studies of the rate and duration of NET release, injection efficiency, and biodegradation.

Initially, formulations capable of releasing NET at a near zero order rate were developed and tested in baboons. This prototype system was evaluated in clinical trials, and the results gave rise to an improved second generation formulation, which has been tested in multicenter clinical trials. Based on the results of these studies, further improvements in the delivery system have been made, and the final version is currently being evaluated in a phase II clinical study.

The microsphere formulation has been varied during the development phase of the research to optimize the NET release rates, biodegradation kinetics, and ease of administration. Details regarding the manufacture of the NET microspheres and the improvements made in the microencapsulation process have been published elsewhere [2, 9, 11] and will not be reviewed in this paper.

Prototype System

The polymer first evaluated as an excipient for making NET microspheres was DL-polylactic acid (PLA). PLA had previously been proven safe for human use in absorbable suture material, and long-term toxicity had been thoroughly evaluated. Early results showed that microspheres made from PLA using a solvent evaporation process had no adverse effects in rats, thus confirming the histocompatibility of the polymer and the fact that potentially irritating solvents and dispersing agents used in the manufacturing process had been removed.

Prior to animal testing, microspheres made of PLA containing NET were evaluated in vitro, in an attempt to define parameters that might be predictive of their performance in vivo. Scanning electron microscopy was used to monitor the spherical integrity and surface characteristics of the microspheres. The rate of NET release from each batch of microspheres was tested in vitro. These quality control procedures were repeated with each formulation and batch of the microspheres that was subjected to in vivo evaluation. Additionally, following the in vitro quality control analysis, each new formulation was tested in baboons to evaluate safety and pharmacokinetics.

Pharmacokinetics studies in baboons were used to demonstrate the dose response capabilities of the prototype system. Microspheres 10–240 μm in diameter containing 25% NET by weight were injected into baboons and serum estradiol (E_2), progesterone (P_4), and NET concentrations were determined by radioimmunoassay (RIA). The slopes of the NET release curves using different doses of the same batch were not significantly different from each other, and there was no difference in the duration of NET release. The differentiating feature among the different doses was the higher serum NET levels achieved with the higher doses. Two of the doses tested, 75 mg and 50 mg NET, were sufficient to inhibit ovarian cyclicity and ovulation in the baboons over a 6-month period. Parallel studies in rats demonstrated that release was occurring primarily by diffusion of the hormone from the microspheres. On the basis of these preclinical animal studies, this prototype formulation was judged safe for use in phase I clinical trials.

Phase I Clinical Trials

At three centers 63 women were treated with the prototype NET-PLA microsphere formulation. Poor injection efficiencies experienced by untrained practitioners with saline-suspended microspheres resulted in actual doses ranging from 7–95 mg of NET, expanding the dose-range of the study. Doses of microencapsulated NET ranging from 0.132–0.267 mg per kg body weight had no effect on ovarian function over the 6-month treatment period, whereas higher doses caused complete or partial suppression of ovarian function for varying periods after treatment [6, 13].

Menstrual abnormalities are the most common side effect of long-acting steroidal contraceptives. Although this sample size was too small to establish a meaningful correlation between the microsphere dose and the amount of menstrual bleeding, the higher doses caused a reduction in the quantity of blood lost in each episode and an increase in the interval between episodes in some subjects.

This preliminary trial reinforced the results of the animal pharmacodynamic and pharmacokinetic studies and demonstrated that higher doses would be necessary to achieve ovulation suppression in women for a 6-month period using this formulation.

It was concluded from these dose-response clinical studies that PLA microspheres are capable of delivering NET continuously for approximately 6 months and that the duration of ovarian suppression is dose dependent within a given microsphere formulation and size limit. The shape of the particular release curve within a given formulation is dependent upon microsphere size distribution and dose of NET contained in the microspheres.

Comparison of the serum NET profiles attained using different doses at three centers shows the influence of microspheres size on NET release rates. The size distribution of microsphere in the first study was 60–240 μm, whereas the size distribution used at the other two centers was 90–212 μm. Smaller microspheres provided more rapid release and higher initial serum NET levels, with a resulting steeper slope of the curve and shorter duration of action. A narrower size range results in flatter release curves coming nearer to zero order release. These curves, however, are characterized by a gradual decline in serum NET levels over the treatment period.

The early animal and human studies demonstrated the positive potential of the microsphere system; however, it was determined from biodegradation studies that up to 12 months were required for the PLA microspheres to biodegrade completely. Altering the molecular weight of the polymer and reducing the diameter of the microspheres did not significantly change the biodegradation interval.

There was concern that repeated injections of PLA microspheres at 6-month intervals might allow an undesirable build-up of PLA in the muscle tissues at the injection site. Additionally, small amounts of hormone associated with this residual polymer might be released at a later time. It was concluded that a PLA excipient that has a 12-month biodegradation time is not optimal for systems designed to provide steroid treatment for 6 months or less. Further research efforts were centered on developing a polymer formulation that provides better synchronization between duration of NET release and biodegradation of the polymer.

Second Generation NET Microsphere Formulation

To achieve faster biodegradation, polyglycolic acid (PGA) was incorporated into the polymer. It was found that when molar ratios of lactide:glycolide were decreased in stepwise fashion, the biodegradation time was reduced proportionately. NET microspheres made with the more rapidly biodegrading copolymers were evaluated in baboons to determine the pharmacokinetics of specific copolymer formulations. From these studies a copolymer with a lactide:glycolide molar ratio (85:15) that biodegrades in 6 months was selected.

Pharmacokinetic studies in baboons using NET microspheres made from the copolymer poly-lactide-co-glycolide (PLGA) resulted in release profiles uniquely characteristic of this formulation. The copolymer formulation produces a biphasic release curve. A diffusional release pattern characterized by decreasing NET levels with time, similar to those previously described for the PLA systems, occurs during the first 10 weeks postinjection. The duration of this diffusional release phase is variable, depending on formulation. A secondary rise in the serum NET level occurs later during the treatment period. This secondary phase corresponds to the period of rapid polymer biodegradation.

It was concluded from the pharmacokinetic studies in baboons that NET release from copolymer-fabricated microspheres occurs via both diffusion and bioerosion. We anticipated that this dual release mechanism could be exploited to develop formulations having more discrete release periods, uniform steroid levels, and less "tailing off" of NET release than occurs with the PLA formulation.

Clinical Trials with Improved NET Microspheres

Methods and Materials

The objectives of the phase I trial were to evaluate the safety of two microencapsulated NET dosage regimens (30 mg and 50 mg) and their effects on ovarian function. Each dosage was designed to provide a constant release of NET over a 90-day period. Each subject received a single NET injection given on day 3–6 of her menstrual cycle. The trial included 20 women, evaluated at a single clinic, who were randomly assigned to one of the two NET dosages. All women were evaluated weekly for 4 weeks prior to the NET injection, twice a week throughout the 90-day postinjection interval, and weekly until resumption of ovulation or resumption of normal menses. NET, progesterone, and estradiol levels were monitored for each woman during her participation in the trial. Serum progesterone levels of greater than 3 ng/ml were used to indicate ovulation. Throughout the study serial laboratory evaluations were performed to monitor serum liver enzymes, lipids, electrolytes, protein, and glucose. All women were 18–35 years of age, had regular menstrual cycles of 23–35 days in length, were generally healthy, and were not at risk of pregnancy. Women assigned to the 30 mg and 50 mg dosages were similar with respect to their age and parity distributions. Most women (80%) were 30–39 years of age and of parity 1–3 (80%).

The phase II study was designed to include a total of 120 women enroled at six clinics. At each clinic the study was conducted according to the same protocol. The object of the study was to evaluate the safety and contraceptive effectiveness of 65 mg and 100 mg microencapsulated NET regimens. Each subject was scheduled to receive four injections 90 days apart; the first one being given on day 3–6 of her menstrual cycle. Women were requested to return to the clinic for monthly follow-up evaluations throughout their participation in the study. After the last injection women were scheduled to be followed up until resumption of ovulation or the start of normal menses. The criteria for selection of subjects was the same as for the phase I study, except all women were at risk of pregnancy. Women did not use adjunctive contraceptive methods during the time they were "protected from pregnancy" by the NET microsphere injections. As in the phase I study, serial laboratory evaluations were performed to monitor serum liver enzymes, lipids, electrolytes, protein, and glucose. Serum NET levels were monitored for all subjects. Data were collected on serum progesterone and estradiol levels. At two centers, extensive endocrinologic studies were done. At each clinic women were randomly assigned to either the 65 mg or 100 mg NET dosages. Women assigned to the two dosages were similar with respect to their age and parity distributions. Overall, most women (72.3%) were under 30 years of age (mean age = 26.5 years) and were of parity 1–2 (60.6%). Of the group, 21% were nulliparous.

The data were analyzed using standard statistical techniques. Whenever statistical tests of significance were performed, only the associated significance levels (*P* values) are given in the text.

Results

Phase I Clinical Trials

During the 90-day period following NET injections five women (50%) who received the 30 mg dosage and two women (20%) who received the 50 mg dosage had serum progesterone levels suggestive of ovulation (> 3 ng/ml). Mean serum

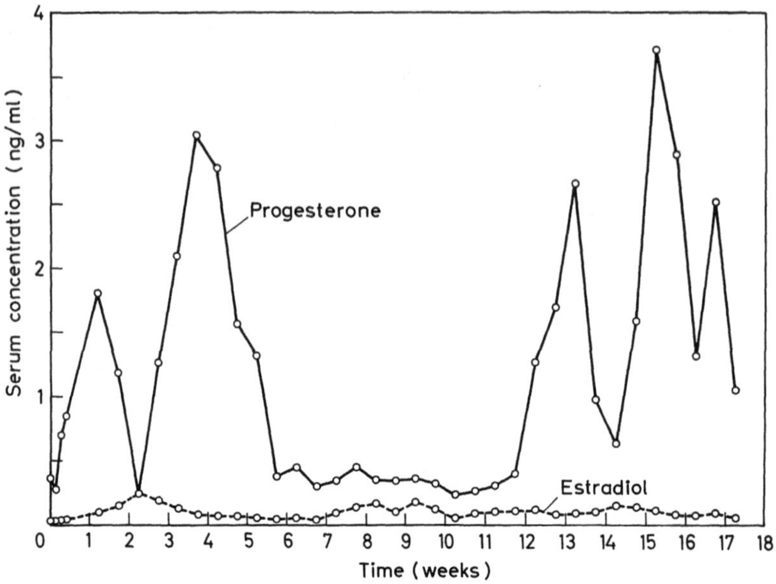

Fig. 1. Mean serum concentrations of progesterone and estradiol for women participating in the phase I 90-day NET microsphere study. NET dose of 30 mg ($n=10$)

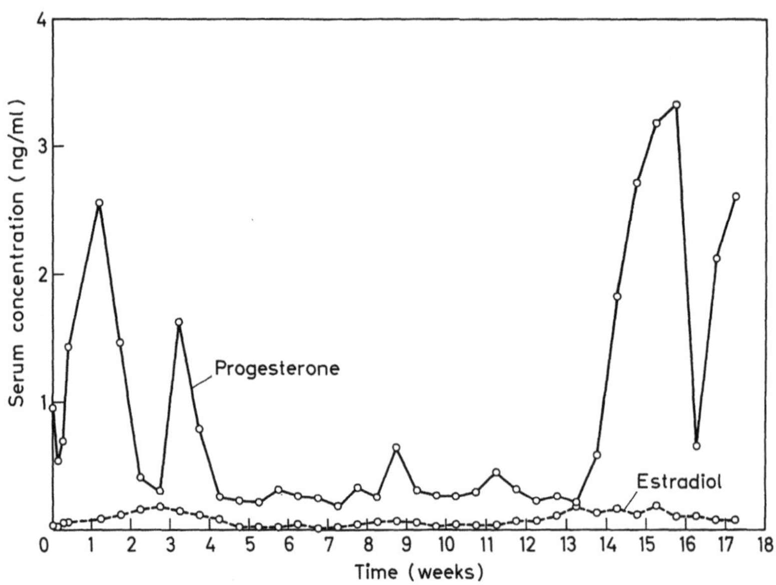

Fig. 2. Mean serum concentrations of progesterone and estradiol for women participating in the phase I 90-day NET microsphere study. NET dose of 50 mg ($n=10$)

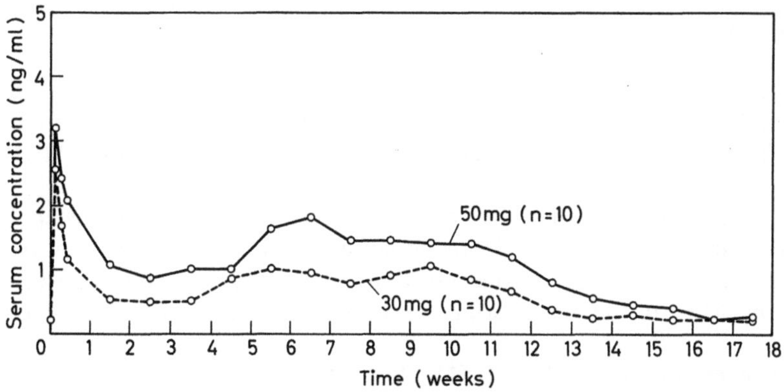

Fig. 3. Mean serum concentrations of NET for women participating in the phase I 90-day NET microsphere study

Table 1. Mean number of bleeding and/or spotting days for women assigned to the 30 mg or 50 mg NET dosages (phase I clinical trial)

	NET Dosage (mean and standard deviation)	
	30 mg (n=10)	50 mg (n=10)
Preinjection	6.9± 4.2	7.8±2.3
Postinjection:		
Days		
1– 30	5.7± 3.3	8.2±6.2
31– 60	12.3± 9.2	14.9±7.0
61– 90	16.6±11.9	10.7±8.7
91–120	4.6± 4.3	4.6±2.9

progesterone and estradiol levels for women assigned to the 30 and 50 mg dosages are shown in Figs. 1 and 2, respectively.

Mean serum NET values were consistently higher for the 50 mg as compared with the 30 mg dosage (Fig. 3). For both dosages there was an initial rise in NET levels shortly after the injection, a gradual decline in NET levels over about the next 3 weeks, followed by an increase in NET levels.

There were some out-of-range laboratory values for both groups of women. However, these values occurred at scattered, irregular times during the follow-up period and were not of clinical significance.

There were no significant side effects reported, except for an increase in the number of days of bleeding and/or spotting for women assigned to either dosage (Table 1). By 91–120 days after the injection the mean number of days of bleeding and/or spotting had returned to its preinjection level. By the end of the 23rd postinjection week all women had resumed normal menstruation.

Phase II Clinical Trial

To date (February 1987), 47 women have been assigned to each NET dosage. Of these women, 35 in the 65-mg group and 36 in the 100-mg group have received a second NET injection, and 19 women in both groups have received a third NET injection.

Figure 4 gives the mean serum NET concentrations for women administered 65 mg and 100 mg NET injections. There did not appear to be any consistent relationship between the serum NET concentration, NET dosage, and time between NET injections. Most of the mean serum concentrations were in the range of 1–3 ng/ml.

Of the women in the study, 11 (11.7%) withdrew for various reasons (Table 2). Four of the five withdrawals in the 65-mg group and three of the six withdrawals in the 100-mg group were for nonmedical reasons.

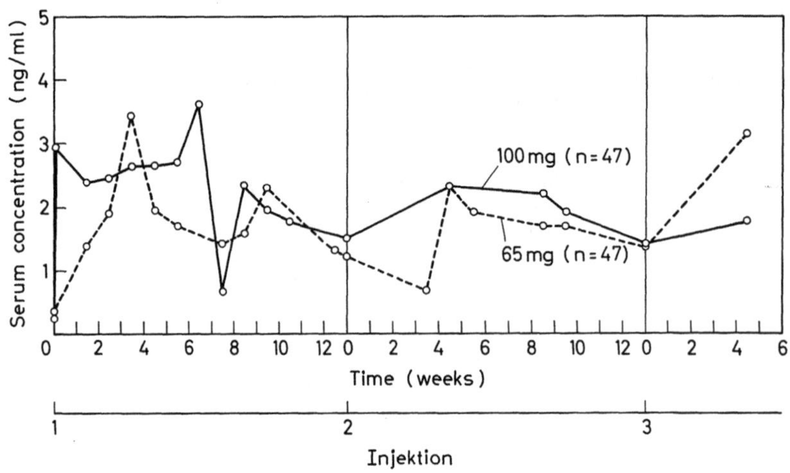

Fig. 4. Mean serum concentrations of NET for women participating in the phase II 90-day NET microsphere study

Table 2. Reasons for withdrawal from the phase II study

Withdrawal reason	NET dosage	
	Women on 65 mg ($n=47$)	Women on 100 mg ($n=47$)
Moved from clinic area	2	1
Planned pregnancy	1	
Did not return for follow-up	1	1
Failed to comply with protocol		1
Skin rash	1	
Migraine headaches		1
Headaches, insomnia		1
Amenorrhea		1

Table 3. Serious/unanticipated adverse reactions

Adverse reaction	NET dosage	
	Women on 65 mg (n=47)	Women on 100 mg (n=47)
Skin rash	2	1
Migraine headache	1	1
Decreased hemoglobin	1	

Table 4. Mean number of bleeding and/or spotting days for women assigned to the 65 mg or 100 mg NET dosages (phase II clinical trial)

	NET dosage			
	65 mg		100 mg	
	n	days	n	days
Preinjection	44	4.5±2.0[a]	42	4.4±2.3
Postinjection:				
Days				
1– 30	43	4.9±3.8	41	4.8±5.1
31– 60	38	7.1±7.2	35	7.4±8.9
61– 90	33	3.9±6.2	28	3.7±5.5
91–120	30	5.8±6.1	27	2.7±4.5
121–150	23	7.2±8.6	21	4.2±5.2
151–180	11	0.6±1.7	14	0.7±1.9

[a] Mean and standard deviation.
n, Number of subjects for whom bleeding/spotting data were available.

The investigators reported that four subjects in the 65 mg group and two subjects in the 100 mg group experienced serious or unanticipated reactions ($P>0.10$) (Table 3). Three of the six reactions were skin rashes; none of these subjects had a history of allergies. The data do not indicate any dose-related incidence of adverse reactions. Women were treated symptomatically, and all adverse reactions resolved spontaneously.

In general, out-of-range laboratory values were observed for some women at scattered, irregular times postinjection and in all cases were not of clinical significance. Changes in laboratory values were also not consistently observed in all study centers. There was no indication that one NET dose (either 65 mg or 100 mg) was associated ($P>0.10$) with a higher frequency of out-of-range laboratory values.

Table 4 gives the mean number of days of bleeding/spotting for consecutive 30-day periods following the first NET injection. The mean number of days of bleeding/spotting was significantly higher ($P>0.05$) for the women receiving the 65 mg dose. The principal menstrual complaint was dysmenorrhea, reported by 48.9% and 51.5% ($P>0.10$) of the women receiving the 65 mg and 100 mg NET dosages, respectively. Amenorrhea was reported by only one woman who received the 100 mg NET dose. No pregnancies were reported for women in either dosage group (65 mg, 236 woman months of observation; 100 mg, 24 woman months of observation).

Discussion

The results of the present study indicate that all microencapsulated NET dosages evaluated (30, 50, 65, and 100 mg) provide a safe method of contraception. The phase II study is still continuing and by the time of its completion (November 1987), sufficient data will have been obtained to determine the contraceptive effectiveness of the 65 mg and 100 mg dosages. The small phase I study of the 30 mg and 50 mg NET dosages indicates that neither may be an effective contraceptive since both were associated with relatively high rates of ovulation.

As expected, all NET dosages were associated with an increase in the monthly rates of bleeding and/or spotting. This is not unexpected since this has also been observed for women using progestogen-only contraceptives. In the phase II study, the data analyzed so far do not indicate any large differences in the monthly number of bleeding and/or spotting days for women using either the 65 mg or 100 mg NET dosages. Moreover, the phase II study did not indicate any dose-dependent side effects or adverse reactions.

The present evaluation shows that there are few significant differences between the 65 mg and 100 mg NET dosages. The mean NET serum levels provided by each dosage were similar and for the most part were in the range of 1–3 ng/ml. Higher serum levels were anticipated with the 100 mg dosage, but this was not always the case. There is no immediate explanation for this finding.

In an independent (two centers) endocrine evaluation of the 65 mg and 100 mg NET dosages that included 37 women, serum progesterone and estradiol levels indicative of ovulation were reported for two women (4.3%) given the 65 mg dose and none given the 100 mg dose. Since there are few differences between the two dosages with respect to the incidence of side effects and adverse reactions, the 100 mg dose is preferable to the 65 mg dose since it may be more effective as ovulation is more consistently inhibited. Before any choice of the two dosages can be made for evaluation in expanded phase III clinical trials, additional data must be collected and evaluated.

Conclusions

The injectable mircosphere contraceptive system offers a number of unique advantages over steroidal contraceptives such as daily pills and implants:

1. The microspheres can be administered by injection every 3 months.
2. The rate and duration of drug release in vivo can be predetermined by selection of the microsphere size and percentage loading of the steroid.
3. The microspheres biodegrade without causing any harmful effects at the injection site.

4. Steroid blood levels and the duration of effect can be programmed by selecting an appropriate distribution of microsphere sizes.
5. The system can be sterilized without affecting its performance.
6. Continuous progestational treatment utilizing the NET 90-day system inhibits ovulation effectively.
7. Once the system biodegrades (within 100 days) there are no carry-over effects on fertility.
8. Menstrual cycle irregularities are minor and well accepted.

Acknowledgements. The authors wish to thank the following investigators for their assistance in the clinical trials: David Archer, MD, Magee-Women's Hospital, University of Pittsburgh; Ramon Aznar, MD, Centro de Investigacion en Fertilidad, Mexico City; Jose P. Balmaceda, MD, The University of Texas Health Science Center at San Antonio; Giuseppe Benagiano, MD, The University of Rome; Horacio B. Croxatto, MD, Instituto Chileno de Medicina Reproductiva, Santiago; Charles E. Flowers Jr, MD, The University of Alabama at Birmingham; Jerome J, Hoffman, MD, Mount Sinai Medical Center, Miami; Andrew M. Kaunitz, MD, University Hospital of Jacksonville; Roberto Rivera, MD, Scientific Research Institute, Juarez University of Durango; Brij B. Saxena, PhD, The New York Hospital, Cornell Medical Center; Howard J. Tatum, MD, Emory University School of Medicine, Atlanta; Mokhtar Toppozada, MD, Shatby University Hospital, Alexandria, Egypt.

References

1. Beck LR, Pope VZ (1984) Controlled-release delivery system for hormones; a review of their properties and current therapeutic use. Drugs 27:528
2. Beck LR, Tice TR (1983) Poly (lactic acid) and poly (lactic acid-co-glycolic acid) contraceptive delivery system. In: Mishell DR Jr (ed) Long-acting steroid contraception, vol 2. Raven, New York, pp 175–199
3. Beck LR, Cowsar DR, Lewis DH, Cosgrove RJ Jr, Riddle CT, Lowry SL, Epperly T (1979) A new long-acting injectable microcapsule system for the administration of progesterone. Fertil Steril 31:545
4. Beck LR, Cowsar DR, Lewis DH, Gibson JW, Flowers CE Jr (1979) New long-acting injectable microcapsule contraceptive system. Am J Obstet Gynecol 135:419
5. Beck LR, Cowsar DR, Pope VZ (1980) Long-acting steroidal contraceptive systems. In: Zatuchni GI (ed) Research frontiers in fertility regulation, vol 1./1. PARFR/Northwestern University, Chicago
6. Beck LR, Ramos RA, Flowers CE Jr, Lopez GZ, Lewis DH, Cowsar DR (1981) Clinical evaluation of injectable biodegradable contraceptive system. Am J Obstet Gynecol 140:799
7. Beck LR, Flowers CE Jr, Pope VZ, Tice TR, Dunn RL, Gilley RM (1983) Poly (d,1-lactide-co-glycolide)/norethisterone microcapsules: clinical study. In: Zatuchni GI, Goldsmith A, Shelton JD, Sciarra JJ (eds) Long-acting contraceptive delivery systems. Harper and Row, Philadelphia, pp 407–417
8. Beck LR, Flowers CE Jr, Pope VZ, Tice TR (1983) Clinical evaluation of an improved injectable microcapsule contraceptive system. Am J Obstet Gynecol 147:815
9. Beck LR, Pope VZ, Flowers CE jr, Cowsar DR, Tice TR, Lewis DH, Dunn RL, Moore AB, Gilley RM (1983) Poly (d,1-lactide-co-glycolide) norethisterone microcapsules; an injectable biodegradable contraceptive. Biol Reprod 28:186

10. Goldzieher JW, Benagiano G (1982) Long-acting injectable steroid contraceptives. In: Mishell DR Jr (ed) Advances in fertility research, vol 1. Raven, New York, pp 75–115
11. Lewis DH, Tice TR (1983) Polymeric consideration in the design of microencapsulation of contraceptive steroids. In: Zatuchni GI, Goldsmith A, Shelton JD, Sciarra JJ (eds) Long-acting contraceptive system. Harper and Row, Philadelphia, pp 77–95
12. Mishell DR (ed) (1983) Long-acting steroid contraception. Raven, New York
13. Rivera R, Flores C, Aldaba S, Hernandez A (1984) Norethisterone microspheres 6-month system: clinical results. In: Zatuchni GI, Goldsmith A, Shelton JD, Sciarra JJ (eds) Long-acting contraceptive delivery systems. Harper and Row, Philadelphia, pp 418–424
14. Zatuchni GI, Goldsmith A, Shelton JD, Sciarra JJ (eds) (1984) Long-acting contraceptive systems. Harper and Row, Philadelphia

Monthly Injectable Contraception with Norethisterone Enanthate plus Estradiol Valerate

E. Kesserü[1] and R. Tozzini[2]

[1] First Gynecological Clinic, University of Buenos Aires, Argentina
[2] Gynecological Clinic, University of Rosario, Argentina

Introduction

Long-acting parenteral contraception was in its heyday from the late sixties through the mid-seventies [1]. At this time the method was based on estrogen-free depot-progestagens. The effect of a single dose lasted several months, providing high contraceptive efficacy, and was well accepted, especially amongst women of some developing countries [2, 3]. However, the main drawback consisted of poor cycle control, i.e., amenorrhea and/or intracyclic bleeding; this inconvenience accounted for the limitation of or even a decrease in the use of these preparations. The addition of an adequate estrogenic component and the monthly administration scheme were the obvious solutions. Thus, despite the fact that the first publication dates back to 1963 [4], the monthly injectables were somewhat neglected and became the focus of interest again only about 10 years ago. This may explain why, despite a large number of publications, the optimal drugs and doses for monthly injectables have still not been conclusively established [5, 6].

The present paper outlines a dose-seeking exercise. In a phase IIb clinical trial two doses of norethisterone enanthate (NET-EN) were compared, the estradiol valerate (EV) component being constant.

Material and Methods

Volunteers for the study were 194 healthy, fertile women recruited from two family planning services belonging to the University Gynecological Clinics of Buenos Aires and Rosario. The women were divided at random into two groups each being administered different doses of progestagen.

- Group HP (high progestagen): NET-EN (50 mg per ampoule) + EV (5 mg per ampoule
- Group LP (low progestagen): NET-EV (25 mg per ampoule) + EV (5 mg per ampoule)

The two compounds were administered over a 6-month period in a double-blind manner. The first injection was given on cycle day 4 ± 2; the following injections at intervals of 30 ± 3 days, irrespective of the stage of the menstrual cycle. Through monthly controls, the evolution of body weight, blood pressure, menstrual cycle patterns, and side effects was recorded. The number of women, the treatment period, and pretreatment characteristics are summarized in Table 1.

Female Contraception
Eds.: B. Runnebaum, T. Rabe, L. Kiesel

Table 1. Pretreatment characteristics of the women in the study (mean ± SD)

	HP	LP
Women (total)	90	104
Months (total)	480	507
Age (years)	28.21 ± 5.17	29.20 ± 4.94
Deliveries (*n*)	2.27 ± 1.53	2.52 ± 1.51
Abortions (*n*)	0.71 ± 0.96	0.86 ± 1.08
Cycle (days)	28.74 ± 5.17	29.48 ± 4.45
Bleeding (days)	4.28 ± 1.41	4.43 ± 1.58

HP, high progestagen group; LP, low progestagen group.

Results

First of all, three unwanted pregnancies occurred, one in the HP and two in the LP group. It should be pointed out that all three failures occurred in the 1st month, i.e., after the first and before the second injection.

Table 2 shows the variations of body weight. Although there was a trend of weight-gain, this was not statistically significant after 6 months. No differences between the two groups were observed.

The evolution of the duration of the cycles is shown in Fig. 1. The important finding was a marked shortening of the first treated cycle, in both HP and LP groups (comparison with control cycle, $P<0.0001$). However, after the second injection the cycle length returned almost to the pretreatment values. Through the third, fourth, fifth, and sixth cycles, the values remained unchanged, and even a trend towards an improvement by the narrowing of standard deviations was observed. Both groups did not differ in this parameter.

An increase in the duration of menstrual bleeding (Fig. 2) in the first treated cycle was observed in both groups ($P<0.05$). However, this increase reverted as from the 2nd month, although with a greater dispersion of individual values.

In Table 3 the incidence of side effects is shown. The occurrence of intracyclic bleeding (spotting or breakthrough bleeding) was more frequent in the LP group than in the HP group, enough so as to be of high statistical significance. Head-

Table 2. Body Weight variations (mean ± SD)

	HP	LP	*P*
Initial (kg)	58.74 ± 8.51	62.25 ± 10.78	<0.02
Final (6 months)	59.59 ± 9.34	62.46 ± 10.07	NS
Variation (kg)	+ 0.85	+ 0.21	NS
Variation ≧ 3 kg			
Increase (% cases)	22.4	22.1	NS
Decrease (% cases)	4.4	6.7	NS

HP, high progestagen group; LP, low progestagen group; NS, not significant.

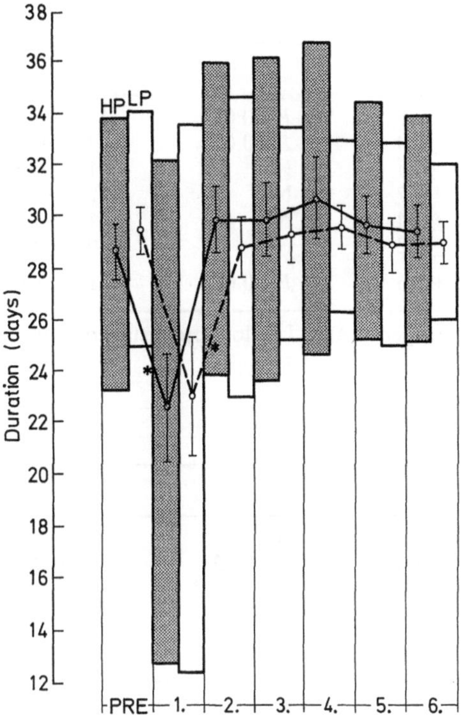

Fig. 1. Duration of the cycles. *HP*, high progestagen group (NET-EN 50 mg); *LP*, low progestagen group (NET-EN 25 mg). *Lines* represent mean ±2 SE and *bars* represent ±1 SD. *PRE*, Pretreatment control cycles; *ordinal numbers*, cycles under treatment; *, $P < 0.0001$

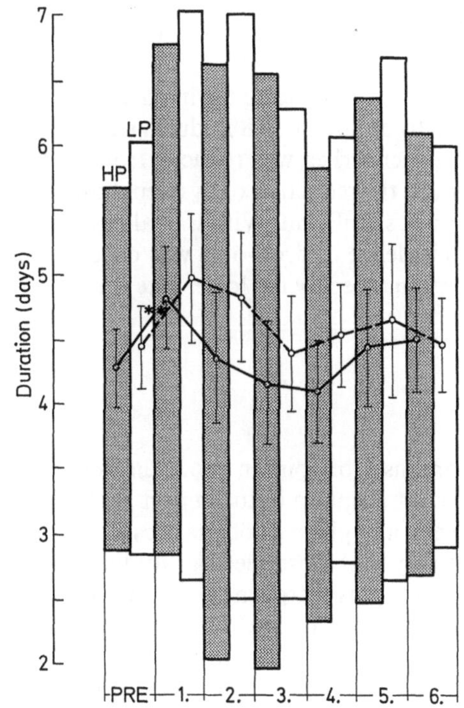

Fig. 2. Duration of menstrual bleeding. *HP*, high progestagen group (NET-EN 50 mg); *LP*, low progestagen group (NET-EN 25 mg). *Lines* represent mean ±2 SE and *bars* represent ±1 SD. *PRE*, Pretreatment control cycles; *ordinal numbers*, cycles under treatment; *, $P < 0.05$

Table 3. Side Effects (% cycles; mean ± SD)

	HP		LP
Spotting and BTB	6.3 ± 1.1	$P<0.01$	11.7 ± 1.4
Headaches	5.4 ± 1.0	$P \cong 0.05$	3.1 ± 0.7
Abdominal/pelvic/lumbar pain	1.5 ± 0.5	NS	1.8 ± 0.6
Nervous/dizziness	2.1 ± 0.7	NS	2.6 ± 0.7
Mastalgia	0.8 ± 0.4	NS	1.6 ± 0.5
Nausea/vomiting	0.2 ± 0.2	NS	0.4 ± 0.3
Total	16.3 ± 1.6	$P<0.05$	21.2 ± 1.8

BTB, breakthrough bleeding; HP, high progestagen group; LP, low progestagen group; NS, not significant.

Table 4. Withdrawals (% cases)

	HP		LP
Pregnancy	1.1 ± 1.1	NS	1.9 ± 1.3
Side effects	5.6 ± 2.4	$P<0.02$	16.4 ± 3.6
Personal reasons	5.6 ± 2.4	NS	6.7 ± 2.5
Lost to follow-up	6.7 ± 2.6	NS	7.7 ± 2.6
Total	19.0 ± 4.1	$P<0.05$	32.7 ± 4.6

HP, high progestagen group; LP, low progestagen group; NS, not significant.

aches were more common in the HP group without, however, being statistically significant.

The HP formulation had the beneficial effect of reducing the incidence of dysmenorrhea from 14.2% before treatment to as low as 1.8% during treatment ($P<0.01$). Likewise the incidence of hypermenorrhea was reduced from 10.8% to 2.6% ($P<0.05$). In the LP group, however, the reduction of dysmenorrhea and hypermenorrhea, although apparent, was not significant. Withdrawal figures are shown in Table 4. A significantly lower incidence of drop-outs was observed in the HP group, the difference largely being explained by the lower rate for side effects.

Discussion

The surprising fact that there is still no consensus of opinion about the best compounds and doses for monthly injectable contraception is due in part to the scarcity of information on their pharmacokinetic and pharmacodynamics [6, 7]. This increases the importance of drug-screening and dose-seeking studies [6, 8]. Through previous research, two progestagen plus estrogen combinations have proven useful: NET-EN plus EV and medroxyprogesterone acetate plus estradiol cipionate. The WHO is currently endeavoring through a multi-centric comparative exercise to match these two compounds (personal communication). The

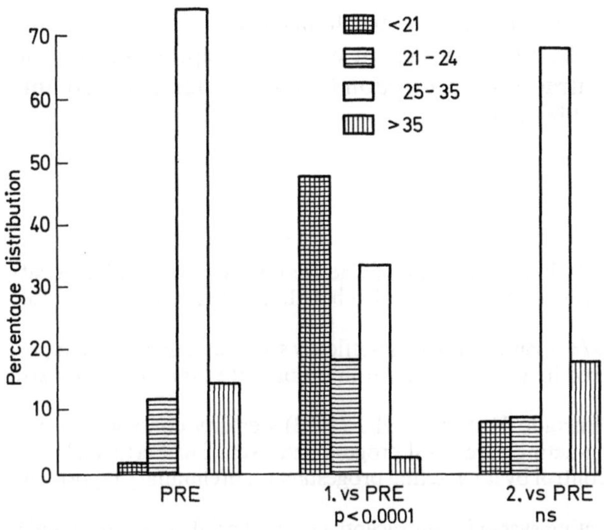

Fig. 3. Distribution of cycle length: percentage distribution observed in the *HP* (NET-EN 50 mg) group. *Bars* represent duration in days; *PRE*, pretreatment control cycle; *1st, 2nd*, treated cycles

NET-EN plus EV formulation they are using is identical to our HP-group dosage.

Our dose-seeking study confirms that the HP formulation (50 mg NET-EN + 5 mg EV) is superior to the LP (25 mg NET-EN + 5 mg EV) for the following reasons: fewer bleeding disturbances, better correction of dysmenorrhea and hypermenorrhea, and a lower withdrawal rate due to side effects. The differences on these points were statistically significant, the higher progestagen concentration being the probable explanation. On the other hand the HP and LP groups did not differ in any other parameter evaluated.

Because of its practical implications, a special comment should be made on the notable shortening of the first cycle under treatment in our study. This was not mentioned in the review publications [5, 6, 9] nor was it noted by the current WHO study, perhaps due to the screening design used (personal communication). The only reference to it was made by Saxena et al.'s Indian study [8]. With the same formulation as our HP, they obtained almost identical values for the cycle-length patterns. To explain this particular shortening of the first cycle, more pharmacodynamic studies are necessary [6, 7].

The frequency distribution of cycle lenth patterns (Fig. 3) shows that in the first cycle almost half the intervals are shorter than 21 days and only 32.5% of the cycles have a "normal" length of 25–35 days. In the second cycle the pretreatment patterns are resumed. One possible explanation is that, since the second injection is given 30 days after the first, the woman may have attained the middle of her second cycle, i.e., ovulation may have occurred, and no contraceptive protection is present.

In fact all three pregnancies in our study occurred within the 1st month of treatment, but in the second cycle. Of the four pregnancies in the WHO study, at least two may have responded to the same mechanism. In view of these findings, and to avoid changing the 30-day dosage, it would be helpful to advise the woman to use additional contraceptive protection (condom, vaginal foam) until she has been given the second injection.

References

1. Department of Medical and Public Affairs (1975) The George Washington University Medical Center: injectable progestogens – Official debate but use increases. Popul Rep [K] 1
2. Schwallie P, Assenzo JC (1973) Contraceptive use-efficacy study utilizing medroxyprogesterone acetate administered in an intramuscular injection once every 90 days. Fertil Steril 24:331–339
3. Kesserü E, Larrañaga A, Hurtado H, Scharff H-J (1973) Fertility control with norethisterone enanthate, a long-acting parenteral progestogen. Acta Eur Fertil 4:203–221
4. Siegel I (1963) Conception control by long-acting progestagens: preliminary report. Obstet Gynecol 21:666–668
5. Benagiano G (1977) Long-acting systemic contraceptives. in: Diczfalusy E (ed) Regulation of human fertility. Scriptor, Copenhagen, pp 323–360
6. Hall P, Fraser IS (1983) Monthly injectable contraceptives. In: Mishell DR Jr (ed) Long-acting steroid contraception. Raven, New York, pp 65–88
7. Aedo A-R, Landgren BM, Johannisson E, Diczfalusy E (1985) Pharmacokinetic and pharmacodynamic investigation with monthly injectable contraceptive preparations. Contraception 31:453–469
8. Saxena BN, Baweja R, Krishna U, Chaudhury SD, Bhattacharya SK, Philips FS, Manual M (1983) Monthly injectables: NET and estradiolvalerate/cypionate. In: Zatuchni GI, Goldsmith A, Shelton JD, Sciarra JJ (eds) Long-acting contraceptive delivery system. Harper and Row, Philadelphia, pp 537–542 (PAPFR series of fertility regulation)
9. Toppozada M (1977) The clinical use of monthly injectable contraceptive preparations. Obstet Gynecol Surv 32:335–347

Evaluation of the Norplant Subdermal Implant Contraceptive System – China

Gu Sujuan[1], Wang Suhua[1], Du Mingkun[2], Zhang Lingde[3], and Xu Meifang[4]

[1] Beijing Municipal Research Institute of Family Planning, Beijing, China
[2] Shanghai Medical University, Obstetrics and Gynecology Hospital, Shanghai, China
[3] Laoning Province Family Planning Research Institute, Shenyang, China
[4] Tianjin Medical College, Second Hospital, Tianjin, China

The Norplant system is a long-acting, low-dose, progestin-only contraceptive method for women. In 1984, a study was undertaken to determine how the Norplant implants are accepted by Chinese women.

This clinical trial in China was planned in two phases. Phase I commenced in October 1984 in four centers. By March–April 1985 1000 subjects for Norplant six capsules and 200 for Norplant two covered rods had been enrolled in the study. After a 1-year trial in four centers, phase II began in February 1986 in eight new centers in different provinces throughout the country. Implanting of 1200 Norplant six capsules was completed by May–June 1986. It is the methods and results of the 1-year trial in the four original centers which will be presented here.

Method

The Norplant subdermal implant system as approved by several countries consists of six silastic capsules containing a total of 216 mg of levonorgestrel. Norplant two covered rods, the more advanced model, consists of two rods, containing a total of 140 mg of levonorgestrel. The capsules and rods are placed under the skin through a small incision made with a No. 10 gauge trocar, and arranged in a fan shape. The effectiveness of the method is achieved by a steady release of the levonorgestrel into the blood. Removal of the implants is accompanied by the return of fertility.

Criteria for Accepting Subjects into the Study

Generally, requirements are that the women be of proven fertility, with no contraindication to the use of steroid contraceptive hormones, and willing to return for follow-up. Pregnant and breast-feeding women were excluded from the study.

Participants in Study. The total number of participants in the phase I study on Norplant six capsules was 1000 (250 per center), and for Norplant two rods there were 200 participants (50 per center).

The age distribution was not wide with more than 80% in the age group 25–34. There were few cases under 25. This reflects the fact that Chinese women marry later, and the requirement of our study that all women have at least one child. More than 90% of the women had only one child. Less than 1% had three or more children. The data reflect the fact that the participants are urban women living in the largest cities of China. It also indicates that many Chinese women prefer this long-acting, reversible method to sterilization.

Results

A single pregnancy was detected during the course of the study, but the age of the fetus, estimated at the time of abortion, strongly suggests that the pregnancy began at or prior to insertion of the implants. The pregnancy rate (including this case as a method failure) was 0.1 per 100 cases. Because there was no failure during use, there were no ectopic pregnancies.

Of all 1200 women in the four clinical centers, half or more had had some menstrual problems since the preceeding visit. Nevertheless, the withdrawal rate for menstrual problems was only around 10%. Among the 115 cases who withdrew in the first 12 months because of mentruals problems, complaints were primarily frequent, irregular, or prolonged bleeding, and spotting (94/115). To a lesser extent women withdrew because of amenorrhea (21/115). In the course of 1 year a significant reduction was recorded in the number of spotting days and duration of the longest bleeding and spotting episodes. Hemoglobin was measured in all women in the Shanghai clinic and remained essentially unchanged during the course of the year for women using either type of implants.

It is clear that the principal reasons for withdrawals were menstrual problems. These accounted for more than 70% of all withdrawals. Withdrawals for other medical reasons were at a net rate of 2% or less. The reasons were primarily of the kind previously reported in the literature.

The net termination rates per 100 participants at 1 year for Norplant six capsules and Norplant two rods were 12.4 and 9.1, respectively; the net continuation rates were 87.6 and 90.4, respectively.

There was no infection at the insertion site and no expulsion of the implants in the 1200 women recruited to the study.

Summary

One year of trials in China with both types of Norplant has demonstrated their high effectiveness and high continuation rate. The high continuation rate in this study undoubtedly reflects the intensive counselling about the menstrual and other side effects of the implant method. The continuation rate also indicates that the Norplant method is acceptable to Chinese women and to the medical and paramedical staff of the clinics.

Acknowledgments. We are grateful for the technical assistance and help given by The Population Council, Dr. John Gill, Irving Sivin, and David Leon.

Behavioral Methods of Contraception

The Sympto-thermal Method

J. J. Billings

St. Vincents Hospital 20 Milfay Avenue Melbourne 3101, Australia

This work in Melbourne, Australia, began in 1953 in response to the request for help in postponing pregnancy by couples who were seeking to achieve this by a natural technique. At that time the only natural method known was that of calendar Rhythm (Ogino-Knaus) which was soon demonstrated to lack the necessary reliability in some circumstances, or to impose inordinately long periods of abstinence. A review of the scientific literature resulted in attention being focussed upon the fact that the occurrence of fertility in a woman is accompanied by the secretion of a particular kind of mucus by the cervix of the uterus [1, 2]. From the 1930s this mucus was the subject of intensive laboratory study in both animals and humans. Remarkably little attention had been paid to the fact that the occurrence of this mucus secretion is often observed, as a vaginal discharge, by healthy, fertile women.

A number of people in different parts of the world were turning to the temperature method, based on the fact that the raised level of circulating progesterone following ovulation tends to elevate the body temperature. For more than 10 years therefore I taught a sympto-thermal method, similar to but not identical with, other sympto-thermal techniques which were being developed concurrently in other countries. Reference was included to other natural indicators of different phases of the cycle, including lower abdominal pain, bleeding, and breast tenderness. Our sympto-thermal method was different in that the primary emphasis was upon vulval observations of the cervical mucus pattern.

In 1962 James B. Brown took up an appointment in the Melbourne University Department of Obstetrics and Gynecology. He had previously been working with the Medical Research Council of the United Kingdom in Edinburgh were he had been assigned to the development of techniques for measuring oestrogen levels in blood and urine; Brown's method had already become known internationally. He willingly consented to submit my conclusions to laboratory evaluation, by measurement of the total oestrogens and progesterone (as pregnanediol) in 24-h specimens of urine. These were collected at first weekly and then daily throughout a menstrual cycle or a succession of cycles, sometimes for many months, in women who were breast-feeding or approaching menopause. It is impossible to exaggerate the debt of gratitude owed to the hundreds of women who have participated as volunteers in this collaborative clinical and laboratory research and continue to do so. Included in the study were young girls approaching menarche, women beyond menopause and women in all the different physiological stages of reproductive life and in the presence of many pathological disorders as well. Through

Female Contraception
Eds.: B. Runnebaum, T. Rabe, L. Kiesel

this, the teaching of mucus pattern observation, which was called the ovulation method, was refined and simplified.

In the 1970s I became aware of the studies of Erik Odeblad, Professor of Medical Biophysics at the University of Umea, Sweden. From the late 1950s he had been studying the physical properties of mucus taken from the cervix, using sophisticated modern techniques which had enabled him to identify different types of mucus in the cervix, varying in proportion in the different phases of the cycle. His observations offered independent confirmation of the conclusions reached from my clinical studies and laboratory analyses [3].

The various natural indicators of fertility and infertility were assessed with the following results.

1. Abdominal Pain

About 50% of women notice lower abdominal pain close to the time of ovulation. This is often described as an uncomfortable sensation in the lower abdomen extending towards the groin on either side. It may be brief, stabbing and confined to one side but even then cannot be reliably taken to mark the time of follicular rupture. In most cases the pain lasts for a day or so and is then probably an expression of the effect of the high level of oestrogens in the blood upon the uterine or tubal musculature. Hormonal monitoring has demonstrated a variable time relationship to ovulation, and most commonly the pain occurs in the few days before ovulation, less commonly shortly afterwards. Some women also notice that in the days just before ovulation, some degree of tenderness exists within the pelvis so that a momentary, deeply situated pain may be experienced immediately on sitting down on a firm seat; this tenderness may be an indication of distension of the follicle ahead of its rupture.

2. Intermenstrual Bleeding

It is common for a small amount of bleeding from the uterus to occur at about the time of ovulation and sometimes this may be more profuse, even sufficient to resemble the woman's menstrual flow. These studies have indicated that the bleeding is most often of a "break-through" character, occurring close to the time when there is a peak level of circulating oestrogen.

3. Sexual Inclination

It is only recently, particularly through knowledge of her cervical mucus pattern, that a woman has had any degree of certainty regarding the time of ovulation in her cycle. It was probably the existence of a sexual season in animals that gave rise to the idea that women experience sexual inclination maximally, or perhaps only, during times of fertility. However, this would mean that during the suppression of ovulation during breast-feeding for example, which may continue for 1–2 years, libido would be diminished or absent, which is not the case. Many women recognise that sexual responsiveness is under the control of the will and is prompted particularly by emotional influences, as well as by abstinence. Some women notice increased interest at the end of menstruation, around ovulation and premenstrually. It has been frequently observed that within a few months of adopting the use of a natural method of regulating fertility, sexual inclination is transferred to the infertile time in those women in whom it had previously been associated with times of fertility.

Self-Examination of the Cervix

As the level of oestrogen rises in the days before ovulation, the cervix tends to open, to become softer in consistency and to rise to a slightly higher position within the body [4]. None of these indications have proved sufficiently reliable to warrant close observation. Sometimes the tilt of the uterus forwards or backwards from the vertical position has been regarded as significant, but this is variable and is influenced by whether the bladder is full or empty.

There are many reasons why women should be advised against the use of the technique of self-examination of the cervix. Most women find its performance repugnant. Additionally, there is the possibility of damage to the cervix and of the introduction of different kinds of infection. Occasionally, the woman is disturbed because the examination produces an erotic stimulus.

The Basal Body Temperature

In an ovulatory cycle the body temperature is low during the menstrual period, sometimes tending to be even a little lower for several days before ovulation. Around the time of ovulation it rises, sometimes rapidly, sometimes gradually. Close to the next episode of menstruation or during menstruation the temperature returns to a lower level again. There is however no way of interpreting the temperature record which enables the time of ovulation to be determined accurately. Ovulation may occur as early as 5 or 6 days before or as late as 3 or 4 days after the time indicated by the temperature record, and sometimes the occurrence of ovulation is not reflected in the temperature record at all [5–10].

Exaggerated notions of the accuracy of the temperature record as an indicator of the time of ovulation have been responsible in the past for mistaken ideas of sperm survival time and also of ovum survival time. Another weakness of the temperature record with regard to natural family planning is that it can only define days of infertility following the occurrence of ovulation; no indication of the proximity or otherwise of ovulation is available in the pre-ovulatory phase. As far as infertility is concerned, the temperature record can provide evidence that the woman is ovulating but only in retrospect give much indication of the day in the cycle in which she had the greatest chance of conception.

The Cervical Mucus Pattern

The cervix of the uterus is closed by the presence of mucus during the reproductive cycle and during pregnancy, the mucus becoming dislodged to permit escape

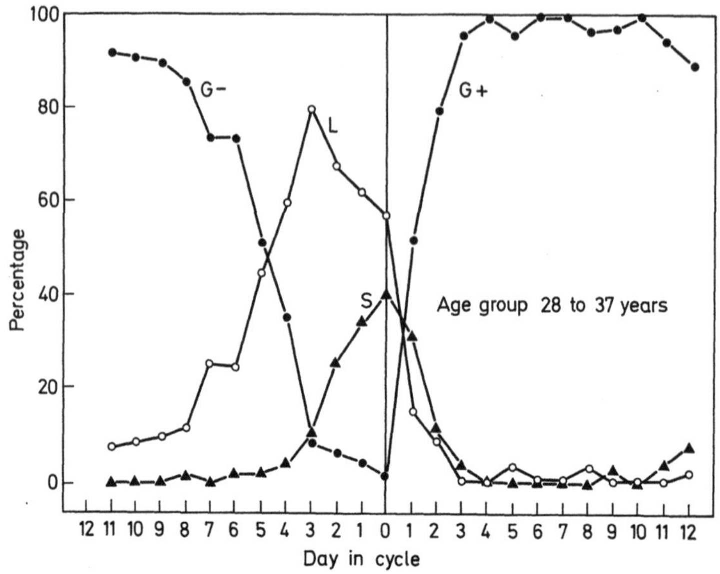

Fig. 1. Percentages of types of mucus (*L, S, G*) in the cervix at different times during a fertile cycle. There are slight physical differences between the pre-ovulatory (*G*−) and post-ovulatory (*G*+) G-mucus. This illustration was kindly supplied by Professor Erik Odeblad, Department of Medical Biophysics, University of Umea, Sweden

of the menstrual flow and delivery of the child. The cervix may also be described as being open during the fertile phase of the cycle because the mucus present in the canal at that time contains a number of channels to permit sperm migration.

At the end of menstruation the cervix is closed by a thick, sticky mucus which is impenetrable to the sperm cells and which by its physical and antibiotic properties provides protection of the reproductive tract and abdominal cavity against infection. Called G-mucus by Odeblad, this mucus forms when the circulating oestrogen level is low and also when the circulating progesterone level is high.

At the beginning of the fertile phase, when follicular development raises the circulating oestrogen level, the cervix produces two other kinds of mucus, called respectively L-mucus and S-mucus by Odeblad. The G-mucus progressively gives place to the L-mucus and then the S-mucus. The L-mucus which is formed in crypts along the whole length of the cervical canal, provides an architectural framework from which the strings of S-mucus are suspended. Odeblad has produced evidence that it is the L-mucus which is responsible for the phenomenon of sperm selection, a vital process which has been known to exist for many years although its basis was undetermined; this provides for the elimination of the defective sperm cells present in every ejaculate. The S-mucus provides channels which allow some sperm cells to pass into the cervical crypts and into the uterine cavity, so that some sperm cells may be found in the fallopian tubes within several minutes after coitus.

The L-mucus and S-mucus, especially the latter, have remarkable fluidity. As a result, their secretion causes the G-mucus to be dislodged from the cervix and the activity of the cervix to become apparent to the woman by observations made at the vulva. It has to be appreciated that these vulval observations are a matter of common experience to every healthy, fertile woman, recurring as they do and have done in every fertile cycle since she attained sexual maturity. Indeed, the phenomenon becomes apparent even as she approaches sexual maturity, intermittent days of mucus discharged from the vagina occurring perhaps for several months before menarche. It also needs to be appreciated that the most important observation the woman makes can be made even if she is blind; it is the sensation present at the vulva according to the presence or absence of mucus and the physical characteristics of any mucus which may be present which are significant. This observation she will make from time to time during the course of the day while in pursuit of her normal activities. At times she will also observe the visual appearance of the mucus, if it is there in a sufficient amount to be seen; it is not essential to touch the mucus with the fingers nor to use toilet tissue.

The woman may observe that close to ovulation the mucus is clear and stringy, tending to resemble raw egg-white but this is a description with which not all women can identify; when present, this spinnbarkeit phenomenon tends to be maximal a day or two before ovulation, as does the marked "ferning" of the mucus. The fern pattern is produced by the L-mucus and the marked threadability by a mixture of the L-mucus and S-mucus. In a number of women, especially those who have had difficulty in achieving pregnancy, the volume of mucus is smaller than usual, and its presence near ovulation may only be identified by its slippery, lubricative quality. The vulva has a soft swollen feeling at this time.

The woman identifies the last day on which the slippery, lubricative mucus is present as the day on which she is at the peak of her fertility and very close to the peak oestrogen level. Ovulation occurs on the day after the peak or on the peak day, rarely on a day on either side of those days; statistically, the peak day is 0.1 day before ovulation [11].

The Ovulation Method (Billings' Ovulation Method)

The development of the sympto-thermal method as a multiple indicator method arose from the recognised inaccuracy and at times inapplicability of the individual indicators used to attempt demarcation of the various phases of the menstrual cycle. Any newly reported indicator, especially if it is readily available, tends to be added, the eclectic approach sometimes signifying the insecurity experienced by the teacher and communicated to the pupil. As the temperature record is able to define post-ovulatory infertility with a good level of reliability, it came to be the dominant element and will remain so, until the exponents of the sympto-thermal method learn that *when the records of the cervical mucus pattern and the temperature are in contradiction, it is the temperature record which is giving incorrect information.* Until this is understood, the full potential of the cervical mucus observations will not be realised.

In Melbourne a different path was pursued. Careful observations of the cervical mucus pattern were quickly discovered to eliminate the weaknesses of the rhythm method, and temperature-taking was introduced only because it was not at first evident that by careful recording of observations of the cervical mucus, following competent instruction, every woman can recognise infertility and days of possible fertility. Indeed, she can define precisely all the phases of the reproductive cycle, menstrual bleeding, the days of pre-ovulatory infertility, the commencement of the fertile phase, the day of maximum fertility and the commencement of post-ovulatory infertility, and is able to predict confidently the time of her next menstruation. Because the woman is able to recognise pre-ovulatory infertility and the commencement of the fertile phase, the problem which had previously defied natural methods, that of reliable definition of days of pre-ovulatory infertility, was solved. In other words, the ovulation method (Billings' ovulation method) is a universal method, applicable in all the different circumstances which a woman may encounter during the reproductive era of her life. It has also become the primary means of management of the increasing problem of infertility.

During the 1960s the ovulation method was progressively refined and simplified, whilst it was at the same time subjected to scientific verification [12] and evaluation by field trials. The field trials have shown that when the couple follows these guidelines for the avoidance of pregnancy, the pregnancy rate is less than 1% [13–17].

An important practical and scientific concept in the pre-ovulatory phase is that of the basic infertile pattern of the cervical mucus. Before the rise in oestrogen which accompanies follicular development, the woman recognises dryness of the vulva or perhaps a slight discharge which remains the same day after day.

The couple is instructed to avoid coitus during the days of heavy menstrual bleeding as the bleeding may mask the presence of mucus warning of an early ovulation. It is advised that intercourse be confined to the evenings of days which have been recognised as infertile; the fluid consistency of the mucus which is formed during the fertile phase will cause it to leave the cervix and appear at the vulva when the woman is standing. The successive days are not used for coitus in order that the seminal fluid and vaginal transudates resulting from coitus do not mask the beginning of mucus secretion. The commencement of mucus secretion is the signal for the avoidance of all genital contact if pregnancy is to be avoided. In the ordinary cycle the woman observes the sequential changes in the physical characteristics of the mucus up to the peak; allowing time for ovulation to occur and 24 h for the survival of the ovum, she will know that from the beginning of the 4th day past peak she is infertile until the next cycle, so that safe intercourse is possible every day at any time of the day. In a long cycle and ahead of the return of fertility during breast-feeding, for example, there may be intermittent episodes of incomplete follicular development causing a day or a few days of mucus secretion; to be sure of avoiding pregnancy the couple must refrain from genital contact at this time, adding 3 days after the return of the infertile pattern to confirm that a basic low level of circulating oestrogen has returned. Ovulation will return later. Similar "mucus patches" occur in long cycles towards menopause, becoming less frequent as ovulation eventually ceases.

It is important for the couple to understand that all genital contact should be avoided during the fertile phase so that the changing mucus pattern can be closely followed and the peak identified. In other words, there are biological reasons for the exclusion of coitus interruptus and coitus with the use of barrier contraception at this time in order to avoid confusion and error. Additionally, it is a matter of common sense that pregnancy is avoided by the abstention from coitus during the fertile phase and by not using techniques which have a substantial pregnancy rate.

By the end of the 1960s it was realised that the best results in natural family planning were obtained by close attention to the cervical mucus pattern according to the principles and guidelines of the ovulation method and that the use of additional indicators were a source of confusion, discouragement and error. It then became evident that this most modern and most scientific of the natural methods was indeed universally applicaple. As a biological method which does not involve drugs, appliances or surgical procedures, it seemed likely to find a high level of acceptability and continued use amongst people of all cultures, and this has proved to be the case.

One colleague, Professor James Brown, has now produced an ovarian monitor to provide a quick, reliable method of measuring the level of oestrogen and progesterone conjugates in a timed specimen of urine. Oestrogene and oestriol glucuronide and pregnanediol glucuronide can be tied to bovine serum albumin; the carboxyl group links with the amino group. After this an anti-serum may be prepared in either rabbits or the sheep. It is possible to link the glucuronide to a lysozyme. If the anti-serum hooks on to this, the enzyme activity is destroyed, providing a test, as the measurement of the lysis of a micrococcus can be done by a photometer. It has been demonstrated that the method is highly accurate, inexpensive and gives a result within 5 min. It will have a wide application in the clinical practice of obstetrics and gynaecology and will greatly increase the use of the Billings' ovulation method, to which it is a natural companion. Brown's ovarian monitor is a monitor of the ovarian hormones, and *the cervical mucus pattern is the monitor of fertility.*

References

1. Smith WT (1855) The pathology and treatment of leucorrhoea. Churchill, London
2. Sims JM (1868) Illustration of the value of the microscope in the treatment of the sterile condition. Br Med J 2:465–466, 492–494
3. Odeblad E, et al. (1983) The biophysical properties of the cervical-vaginal secretions. Int Rev Nat Fam Plann (1):1–56
4. Keefe EF (1962) Self-observation of the cervix to distinguish days of possible fertility. Bull Sloane Hosp Columbia Presbyterian Med Cent 8:129
5. Buxton CL, Engle ET (1950) Time of ovulation; correlation between basal temperature, appearance of endometrium, and appearance of ovary. Am J Obstet Gynecol 60:539–551
6. Johansson EDB, Larsson-Cohn U, Gemzell C (1972) Monophasic basal body temperatures in ovulatory menstrual cycles. Am J Obstet Gynecol 113:933–937
7. Moghissi KS (1976) Accuracy of basal body temperature for ovulation detection. Fertil Steril 27:1415–1421
8. Lenton EA, Weston GA, Cooke ID (1977) Problems in using basal body temperature recordings in an infertility clinic. Br Med J 1:803–805
9. Hilgers TW, Bailey AJ (1980) Basal body temperature and estimated time of ovulation. Obstet Gynecol 55:333–338
10. Bauman JE (1981) Basal body temperature: unreliable method of ovulation detection. Fertil Steril 36:729–733

11. Billings EL, et al. (1972) Symptoms and hormonal changes accompanying ovulation. Lancet 1:282–284
12. Brown JB, et al. (1983) Correlations between the mucus symptoms and the hormonal markers of fertility throughout reproductive life. In: Billings JJ (ed) The ovulation method. Advocate, Melbourne
13. Weissman C, Foliaki L, Billings JJ, Billings EL (1972) A trial of the ovulation method of family planning in Tonga. Lancet 2:813–816
14. Klaus H, et al. (1979) Use of effectiveness and client satisfaction in six centres teaching the Billings ovulation method. Contraception 19:613–629
15. Billings EL (1980) Approaching the menopause. In: Billings E, Westmore A (eds) The Billings method. O'Donovan, Melbourne, pp 116–132
16. Stewart T (1978) Annual Report of The Happy Family Movement of Korea, September 1977–September 1978. Chun Cheon Diocese, Korea
17. World Health Organisation (1981) Task force on methods for the determination of the fertile period. A prospective multicentre trial of the ovulation method of natural family planning. II. The effectiveness phase. Fertil Steril 36:591–598

Temperature Computers

K. Loewit, H. G. Kraft, A. Ortlieb, and G. Wolfram

Institut für Medizinische Biologie und Genetik, Schöpfstraße 41,
6020 Innsbruck, Austria

Introduction

Behavioral methods of conception control or contraception have met with increasing interest [23] and constitute a growing – though still very small – segment of family planning methods. In recent surveys in Austria and the Federal Republic of Germany, 2.8% of females in fertile age reported the use of basal body temperature (BBT) [13], 3.9% the use of natural family planning (NFP), and 14% stated their intention to practise such methods in the future [6]. Contrary to previous calendar methods [8, 14] modern self-observation methods (SOM) like the symptothermal method (STM) [20] are safe and reliable [4, 7, 16–20].

However, they still suffer from two major handicaps: their generally bad reputation within the medical profession, dating from former unreliable attempts to calculate the fertile days of the cycle, and intrinsic methodological problems, especially regarding large scale practicability and acceptability, in particular concerning sexual abstinence. Therefore, to promote professional confidence in SOM, basic research into the theoretical foundations is still necessary to find a more knowledgeable and rational approach. With regard to their practicability, methodological improvements would be highly desirable. Thus, several devices have been designed using computer technology to facilitate the practicability of SOM in relieving women or couples of reading thermometers, drawing and interpreting graphs and charts, calculating fertile days, observing and correlating various symptoms of fertility, etc. Only some of these fertility indicators are temperature computers. Lately, two of them, "Anne" and "Rite Time" have been criticized for poor performance by Döring and Daucher [5]. "Baby comp," a promising temperature computer with a unique mathematical program, has recently been introduced [2] and is currently being tested. Other instruments measure tissue (e.g., vaginal) impedance, cervical mucus viscosity or salivary electrical resistance in order to detect or even to predict ovulation [1, 15, 22].

In an attempt to study further the physiological foundations of SOM, we have introduced a noninvasive method of hormonal ovulation detection by measuring luteinizing hormone (LH) in saliva [9] in order to accumulate a large body of data without putting an undue burden upon the volunteers. These studies showed that salivary LH was significantly correlated with serum-LH ($r=0.788$, $n=60$, $P<0.0001$) [10] and that it was also a suitable indicator of ovulation, as judged from simultaneous determination of serum LH and sonography of the maturing

Originally published in W. Eicher/G. Kockott (eds): Sexology, Springer 1988.

Female Contraception
Eds.: B. Runnebaum, T. Rabe, L. Kiesel

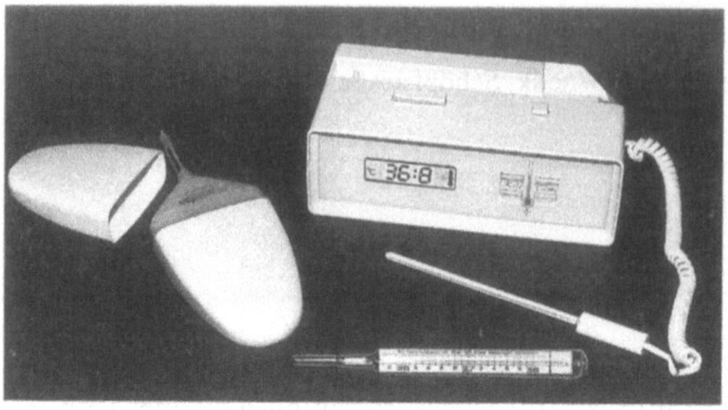

Fig. 1. The temperature computers "Rite Time" and "Bioself 110"

and rupturing follicle in 15 cycles. All salivary LH peaks were found ±1.5 days (60% ±0.5 days) around the time of ovulation [12].

Within the framework of these studies two temperature computers, "Rite Time" (RT) and "Bioself 110" (BS) could be tested for their performance and reliability (Fig. 1).

Participants, Methods and Devices

Participants

Of the 23 women (16 nulliparae and 7 parae) who volunteered for this study, with an average age of 27.0 ± 5.7 years, (range 22–42 years), each contributed between 1 and 17 (average 3) of the 84 cycles studied. The participants were either already experienced in SOM, mainly STM, or individually instructed and were highly motivated. Almost two-thirds were either engaged in or had completed an academic training. Thus, this group is not representative of the population in general. However, it reflects the predominance of women with higher education in the small segment practising SOM in Austria and the Federal Republic of Germany [6, 13] and is considered very suitable for basic research purposes.

In addition to recording and charting their BBT and cervical mucus patterns in the usual way, the volunteers also used one of the two temperature computers and kept records of the data displayed. Immediately after measuring temperature (i.e., before tooth-brushing, eating, drinking, etc.) they collected several milliliters of so-called early morning saliva, starting with the beginning of the mucus symptom, until the postovulatory higher level of BBT had been established. In this way usually between 10 and 15 samples of saliva were collected in small plastic tubes and stored frozen in a household refrigerator until delivery to the laboratory for LH determination.

Methods

Salivary LH has been determined radioimmunologically by modifying a commercially available LH Ria kit, as described in detail elsewhere [9, 10].

LH values exceeding $\bar{x}_{LH}+1$ SD have been tentatively regarded as LH peaks. The peak day was labeled day 0 and served as a reference point for ovulation detection. Cycle days were centered around day 0. According to well-established SOM rules (temperature method, STM [3, 4, 17, 20]), the postovulatory infertile period starts in the evening of the 3rd day of elevated BBT (BBT3). This was therefore used as a 2nd reference point for the reliability of the temperature computers under examination. No essential additional information came from correlations with cervical mucus patterns in general, although in individual cases they helped in detecting errors of the devices or in determining the first rise of BBT.

Devices

RT (Rite Time, England) is an electronic thermometer for oral measurement of BBT with a computer memory program for one cycle. It has a built-in time slot of 3 h during which measurements are registered in the device's memory; provided with daily BBT measurements, it is able to detect the postovulatory rise in BBT, having accounted for unphysiological temperature changes. Outside the time slot it may be used as a conventional thermometer. The time slot has to be set according to individual preference but is not to be changed during a particular cycle. At the beginning of each menstrual cycle (day 1 of the monthly period) the computer memory has to be set for day 1. From day 4 on, regular measurements of BBT are required, the temperature being displayed in degrees Celsius. The display window changes from blank (for the fertile time) to six bar lines at the beginning of the postovulatory infertile period. Thus RT only indicates infertility. The time of high fertility must be calculated from previous experience. The device can also be used as an ordinary clock or alarm clock. Experience with RT dates from a long-term case study with 17 of the 20 cycles studied being contributed by one 23-year-old nullipara over a period of 2.5 years. The average duration of the 20 cycles was 26.4 ± 1.9 (23–29) days.

BS (Bioself Distribution, Switzerland) is also an electronic temperature recording device for oral, rectal, or vaginal measurement of BBT. It is equipped with a microprocessor which calculates the fertile period of the cycle by subtracting 18 from the shortest and nine from the longest cycle recorded according to the calendar method [8, 14]. It detects the BBT shift by comparing each measurement with the eight previous ones according to the temperature method. Again, rises in temperature exceeding those typical for ovulation are rejected by the program. BS starts out from a hypothetical 28-day cycle and ajusts to the individual cycle pattern by storing the length of the last six menstrual cycles. It does not accept cycles longer than 39 or shorter than 19 days. A time slot of ± 2 h is set automatically at the time of the first temperature recording. Thereafter measurements are only accepted within this time slot, as indicated by a yellow light signal. The beginning of each cycle is recorded by pressing a special button. BBT is not shown; instead, light signals indicate the state of fertility. A constant red light denotes possible fertility (from day 5 to the beginning of flashing red and again thereafter until BBT3); a flashing red light indicates the most fertile period as calculated from the longest and shortest cycle; a constant green light is displayed during the infertile phase (from BBT3 for maximally 16 days), during the luteal phase, and again during the first 5 days of the following cycle. The memory of BS stores the temperature and light signals of the last 64 days, the length of the last six cycles and the remaining battery capacity. These data may be retrieved in graphic form by inserting the temperature probe of BS into a special printer. BS has been studied during 64 cycles in 22 women, the average cycle length being 28.3±3.2 (23–37) days.

Results and Discussion

Reliability in Comparison with the Salivary LH peak

As can be seen from Table 1, RT signaled infertility in 2 of 19 cycles at days +1 and +2, i.e., on probably or possibly fertile days. However, on day +1 cervical mucus of the fertile type was still present, the cervix was soft and open and thus the error of the device was obvious for someone experienced in SOM. On the other hand, on day +3, a certainly infertile day, infertility was signaled only in about one-quarter of the cycles in accordance with the manufacturer's contention that RT "is cautious and errs on the safe side". In 58% of all cycles the infertile

Table 1. First indication of infertility by two temperature computers related to the salivary LH peak (day 0)

Stage of cycle	(days)	Infertility signal			
		Rite time		Bioself 110	
		(*n*)	(%)	(*n*)	(%)
Before LH peak	3	–		1	1.6
	2	–		2	3.2
	1	–		–	
Simultaneously	0	–		1	1.6
After LH peak	1	1	5.3	–	
	2	1	5.3	1	1.6
	3	3	15.8	5	7.9
	4	3	15.8	9	14.3
	5	5	26.3	8	12.7
	6	2	10.5	2	3.2
	7	2	10.5	7	11.0
	8	–		3	4.8
	9	2	10.5	5	7.9
	10	–		1	1.6
	11	–		1	1.6
Never appeared		–		17	27.0
Appeared too early		2	10.6	5	8.0
Appeared after day +4		11	57.8	27	42.8[a]

[a] 58.5% of 46 cycles with green display (see Fig. 2)

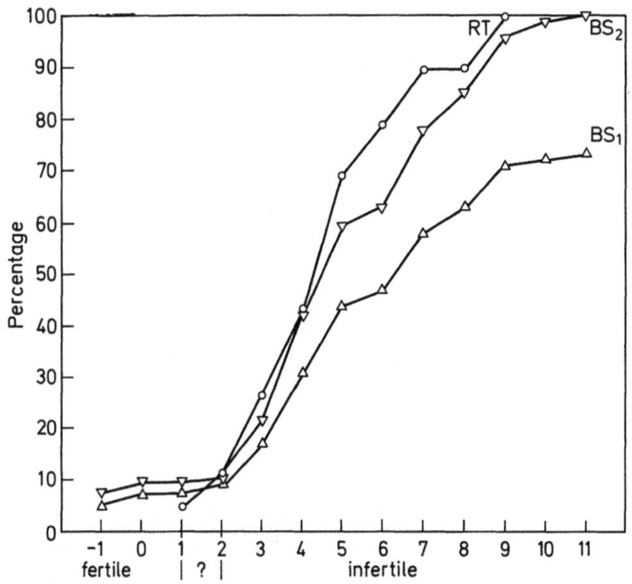

Fig. 2. Cumulative incidence of indication of infertility by two temperature computers in comparison with the salivary LH peak (day 0). *RT*, Rite Time, 19 cycles; *BS*, Bioself 110; BS_1, 63 cycles, no infertility indication in 17 cycles; BS_2, 46 cycles with infertility display

period was indicated after day +4, thus designating up to five infertile days as fertile. Figure 2 illustrates that even by day +5 fertility is still indicated in almost one-third of the cycles, the last signals changing to "infertile" as late as day +9.

Both in a study by Royston et al. [21], correlating RT data with ovarian ultrasonography in 14 cycles or with the serum LH peak in 13 cycles of six women, and in this study, the RT signal indicating infertility occurred after the salivary LH peak in all cases (mean $=4.9 \pm 2.1$ days; $n=19$). The corresponding values in Royston's study were 5.2 for the day of maximum follicular development and 4.3 for the day of the serum LH peak and had a range of 1–7 days. However, without hormonal control, a premature signal was suggested in only 2 of 73 cycles (3%).

The data for BS show that the green light appeared too early in 5 of 63 cycles. In all of these cases fertility was indicated by the appearance of the cervix or cervical mucus and the first green display occurred before the 14th day of the cycle. Thus, the error of the device was evident. Again, by day +3, infertility is signaled in only 16% of cases, the latest green display occurring on day +1. Thus, in 43% of all cases, the green light appears after day +4 and the BS estimate of the infertile period is somewhat more conservative even than that of RT. In this way, errors implying the danger of unwanted pregnancy are kept low (2.6% less than RT), but up to 7 infertile days are not recognized as such. However, in this study, due to the more sophisticated program of BS (which requires at least eight measurements before it can detect the BBT rise) and due to the fact that 34% of all cycles were first recordings for the device, the green light did not appear at all in 27% of the cycles. If only those cycles where the green light was present are compared, RT and BS closely parallel each other, as depicted in Fig. 2. In contrast to RT, BS indicates the most fertile time by flashing red signals. But even though BS adjusts to the individual cycle length after 6 months, it is no better than conventional observation of the cervix or cervical mucus in recognizing the optimal time for conception.

Reliability in Comparison with BBT3

In 15 of 20 RT cycles complete oral and rectal temperature records were available. In two-thirds of these cases (10/15), the first rise in BBT was recorded on the same day; in one-third it differed by ±1 day, RT showing the first rise in temperature twice 1 day before and three times 1 day after the respective rectal measurements. Thus, in this longitudinal study, the oral measurements were in better agreement with rectal BBT than in a recent report on 15 cycles of five women, which described opposite findings [5].

As shown in Table 2, on the day of BBT3 simultaneity was reduced to less than one-third (6/20) of the cases. In over two-thirds of the cases RT signaled infertility 1–4 days earlier (40%) or later (30%) than conventional BBT. In the study by Döring and Daucher [5] the variation was between 4 days earlier and 6 days later than BBT. The results of this longitudinal study, however, are in perfect agreement with data on 38 cycles of 20 women, showing that the RT signal occurred within 2 days of the user's own estimate in 82% of the cycles [21] which compared with 80% (16/20) in this study. Most of the BS measurements were taken rectally. Since, however, with BS the temperature is not displayed and also the printed graphs show only relative values, a direct comparison with con-

Table 2. Indication of infertility by two temperature computers related to the 3rd day of elevated basal body temperature (BBT3, day 0)

Stage of cycle	(days)	Infertility signal			
		Rite time		Bioself 110	
		(*n*)	(%)	(*n*)	(%)
Before BBT3[a]	4	1	5.0	–	
	3	–		–	
	2	5	10.0	2	5.0
	1	5	25.0	6	15.0
Simultaneously	0	6	30.0	13	32.5
After BBT3	1	2	10.0	8	20.0
	2	1	5.0	5	12.5
	3	2	10.0	3	7.5
	4	1	5.0	1	2.5
	5	–		1	2.5
	6	–		1	2.5
Appeared too early		8	40.0	8	20.0
Appeared late		6	30.0	19	47.5

[a] BBT was measured rectally with a mercury thermometer.

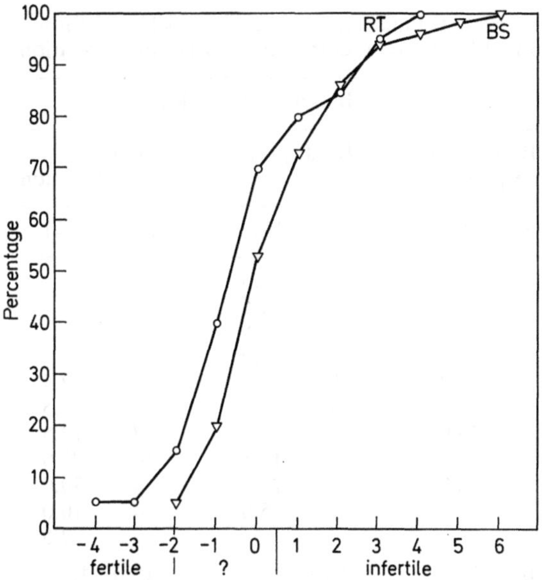

Fig. 3. Cumulative incidence of indication of infertility by two temperature computers versus the 3rd day of elevated basal body temperature (BBT3, day 0). *RT*, Rite time, 20 cycles; *BS*, Bioself 110, 40 cycles

ventionally taken BBT is not possible. Also, BS indicated infertility only in about one-third of the cases on the day of BBT3. However, as distinct from RT, the green light preceded BBT3 in only 20% of the cycles by 1 day (15%) or 2 days (5%). Thus, in comparison with the empirically well-established beginning of the infertile time after ovulation, BS seems to be the more reliable instrument.

These data conflict with the observation of only about 8%–11% of false infertility indications (Fig. 2) as compared with the LH peak. This discrepancy is explained by the time lag of BBT in regard to the LH peak. As we have seen BBT3 was delayed in 58% of 60 BS cycles or 52% of 194 cycles beyond day +4, thus occurring in these cases between 5 and even 10 days after the salivary LH peak [11]. Indeed, checking the relation with the LH peak in individual cycles where RT or BS infertility signals occurred before BBT3 reveals that only about one-quarter of cases fell on the possibly fertile days +1 and +2; the rest occurred between 3 and 7 days after the LH peak, although still before BBT3. This explains the high reliability of BBT3, which more often than not comes much too late. In addition, it underlines the need for a better marker of infertility. At the moment, however, BBT3 cannot be dispensed with. As shown in Table 2 and Fig. 3, the RT infertility display and the BS green light lag behind BBT3 in 30% and 48% of the cycles, respectively, BS reaching 100% of infertility display 2 days later than RT. Thus, the reliability of BS is again paid for by a shortening of the infertile period. This is once more borne out by the number of infertile days for each instrument as summarized in Table 3. While in the RT study the average number of postovulatory infertile days is practically the same whether indicated by RT or taken from BBT (as in the study by Royston et al. [21], even though absolute values differ), the period is almost 1 day shorter for BS than for BBT3. However, the standard deviation is larger for the instruments than for BBT3. Thus, the shortest periods of infertility, from 3 to 7 days per cycle, occur almost twice as often with the in-

Table 3. Postovulatory infertile days per cycle as indicated by Rite Time (RT) and Bioself 110 (BS) in comparison with conventional basal body temperature (BBT) interpretation

Infertile days per cycle	Rite time ($n=20$)				Bioself 110 ($n=40$)			
	RT display		BBT3 interpretation		BS display		BBT3 interpretation	
(n)	(n)	(%)	(n)	(%)	(n)	(%)	(n)	(%)
3	1	5.0	–		1	2.5	–	
4	1	5.0	1	5.0	1	2.5	–	
5	–		–		1	2.5	–	
6	2	10.0	2	10.0	2	5.0	–	
7	4	20.0	2	10.0	1	2.5	3	7.5
8	3	15.0	7	35.0	5	12.5	5	12.5
9	5	25.0	7	35.0	9	22.5	7	17.5
10	2	10.0	–		7	17.5	10	25.0
11	1	5.0	1	5.0	11	27.5	8	20.0
12	1	5.0	–		2	5.0	4	10.0
13	–		–		–		3	7.5
Average	7.9 ± 2.2		8.0 ± 1.5		$9.2 + 2.1$		10.0 ± 1.6	
Cycle length		26.4 ± 1.9				28.9 ± 3.1		

$\chi^2 = 6.6 < 15.51$ $(=\chi^2_{2;\,0.05})$ $\chi^2 = 10.92 < 18.31$ $(\chi^2_{2;\,0.05})$
$P > 0.05$

struments as with conventional BBT readings. These in turn comprise to a greater extent the longer infertility period of 8–12 days (75% vs 60% of the cycles) in the RT group and of 8–13 days (92% vs 85% of the cases) in the BS study. Finally, it should be noted that in principle both instruments were well accepted by their users. In the study by Royston et al. [21], 48% of the participants were willing to replace their usual methods with RT, although 55% stated being "not very confident" about the start of the infertile period as given by RT. In this study, most of the volunteers in the BS group would not rely solely on the instrument unless they could read the temperature themselves. This was the strongest criticism made. Instructing the user thoroughly is an indispensable prerequisite to high-use effectiveness, as is a basic understanding of SOM or cycle physiology in order to be able to detect possible errors of the device.

Thus, neither instrument can replace experience in SOM; such knowledge is neccessary if the instruments are to be used in a critical and safe way with confidence. Furthermore, neither the beginning of the fertile and infertile periods nor the optimal time for conception can be better recognized by using the temperature computers than from conventional SOM. In our limited experience (the results of BS may become better in longitudinal studies; those of RT may show greater variation in cross-sectional ones) the devices allow for an easier and more convenient way of practising SOM for already experienced or specially instructed women. They do not yet overcome the principal obstacles to large-scale use of SOM in the general population. Future instruments should be able to predict ovulation in good time and to detect its occurrence earlier than BBT in order to extend the pre- and postovulatory infertile periods, without jeopardizing the reliability and practicability of the devices. From past and present efforts it is obvious that this goal is still very difficult to reach.

Acknowledgements. The technical assistance of A. Friedl and S. Zennebe and the financial support granted to the first author by the Dr. Legerlotz Foundation are gratefully acknowledged.

References

1. Albrecht BH, Fernando RS, Regas J, Betz G (1985) A new method for predicting and confirming ovulation. Fertil Steril 44:200–205
2. Baby comp (1987) Dtsch Apotheker Z 127 (1/2)
3. Döring GK (1986) Die Temperaturmethode zur Empfängnisverhütung, 9th edn. Thieme, Stuttgart (1st edn 1954)
4. Döring GK (1986) Empfängnisverhütung, 10th edn. Thieme, Stuttgart
5. Döring GK, Daucher HK (1986) Bestimmung der unfruchtbaren Tage im Zyklus der Frau. Fortschr Med 104:941–942
6. Döring GK, Baur S, Frank P, Freundl G, Sottong G (1986) Ergebnisse einer repräsentativen Umfrage zum Familienplanungsverhalten in der Bundesrepublik Deutschland 1985. Geburtshilfe Frauenheilkd 46:892–897
7. Frank P, Raith E (1985) Natürliche Familienplanung. Springer, Berlin Heidelberg New York
8. Knaus H (1933) Die periodische Frucht- und Unfruchtbarkeit des Weibes. Zentralbl Gynakol 57:1393–1408
9. Kraft HG, Fischer-Korp C, Loewit KA (1984) A radioimmunological method for LH measurements in saliva. Contracept Delivery Syst 5:99
10. Loewit KK, Kraft HG, Ortlieb A (1985) Measurement of LH in saliva: a new approach to ovulation detection. In: Runnebaum B, Rabe T, Kiesel L (eds) Future aspects in contraception. MTP Press, Boston, pp 31–47
11. Loewit K, Ortlieb A, Kraft HG, Widhalm R, Wolfram G (1987) Wie erkennt man die „sicheren" Tage? Sexualmedizin 16:52–57
12. Loewit K, Huber J, Ortlieb A, Kraft HG, Widhalm R, Wolfram G (1987) Speichel-LH als Ovulationsindikator: Vergleich zwischen Speichel-LH, Serum-LH und Ultraschallbefund. Geburtshilfe Frauenheilkd 47:800–802
13. Münz R (1987) Empfängnisverhütung und Familienplanung. Prakt Arzt 41:11–30
14. Ogino K (1932) Über den Konzeptionstermin des Weibes und seine Anwendung in der Praxis. Zentralbl Gynakol 12:721–732
15. Rabe T, Kiesel L, Runnebaum B (1985) Future aspects in contraception: an overview. In: Runnebaum B, Rabe T, Kiesel L (eds) Future aspects in contraception, part I. MTP Press, Boston
16. Rice FJ, Lanctôt CA, Garcia-Devesa C (1981) Effectiveness of the sympto-thermal method of natural family planning: an international study. Int J Fertil 26:222–230
17. Rötzer J (1968) Erweiterte Basaltemperaturmessung und Empfängnisregelung. Arch Gynakol 206:195–214
18. Rötzer J (1978) The sympto-thermal method: ten years of change. Linacre Q 45:358–374
19. Rötzer J (1978) Sympto-thermal method and family planning. Acta Med Rom 16:339–348
20. Rötzer J (1986) Natürliche Geburtenregelung, 16th edn. Herder, Vienna
21. Royston JP, Humphrey SJE, Flynn AM, Marshall J, Zarzosa-Perez A (1984) An automatic electronic device (Rite Time) to detect the onset of the infertile period by basal body temperature measurements. Br J Obstet Gynaecol 91:565–573
22. Schenker JG, Mor-Yosef S (1985) Natural family planning. In: Runnebaum B, Rabe T, Kiesel L (eds) Future aspects in contraception. Part 2. MTP Press, Boston
23. WHO (1981) A prospective multicentre trial of the ovulation method of NFP. I. The teaching phase. Fertil Steril 36:152–158

Lactational Anovulation in Monkeys: Prolactin Secretion and Ovarian Function

R. F. Williams

The Jones Institute for Reproductive Medicine, Department of Obstetrics and Gynecology, Eastern Virginia Medical School, Norfolk, Virginia 23507, USA

In nonnursing women, pregnancy is followed by an interval of anovulation, which persists for an average of 2–3 months [1–3]. This puerperal infertility is extended if nursing occurs [1–5]. The interval of lactational anovulation and amenorrhea associated with nursing is highly variable, being dependent upon cultural practices in infant feeding and child rearing [2, 3, 5]. In Western cultures, lactational amenorrhea has been described as lasting less than a year [1, 3], while in developing countries 4-year interbirth intervals have been attributed to the inhibitory effects of breast-feeding [6]. These societal differences in postpartum infertility are specifically related to the frequency and duration of suckling [6, 8], and, in general, the cultural practices which reduce breast-feeding and thus the inhibition of the hypothalamic-pituitary-ovarian axis [4, 5]. Despite the importance of lactational anovulation in the control of population growth, the physiologic mechanisms sustaining lactational infertility are enigmatic.

Nonhuman primates have been utilized to investigate the mechanisms inducing and sustaining postpartum anovulation; the remainder of this paper will focus on those studied. Like women, old world primates (rhesus and cynomolgus monkeys, among others) exhibit postpartum anovulation in nonnursing and nursing mothers [9, 11]. The physiologic similarities in reproductive function (especially the menstrual cycle and postpartum interval) of women and these macaques warrants their use as research models for studies of the reproductive endocrinology of the postpartum interval [11]. These monkeys exhibit puerperal anovulation of 3 months' duration in nonnursing monkeys [9] and lactational anovulation of at least 5 months [11] and potentially of 1.5 years duration (personal observation, unpublished data). Like women, these postpartum monkeys exhibit: ovarian responsiveness to ovulatory doses of exogenous gonadotropin [9, 12, 14]; total inhibition during nursing of the surge mode of gonadotropin secretion induced by estrogen provocation, and early restoration of this process in nonnursing mothers [15, 18]; and recquired responsiveness to GnRH provocation coincident with the restoration of estrogen-positive feedback [19, 20].

Because of the putative inhibitory effect of prolactin on the function of the hypothalamic-pituitary-ovarian axis [21, 22] and the stimulatory effect of suckling on prolactin secretion [23, 26], patterns of prolactin secretion are characterized throughout the postpartum interval in nursing monkeys [27]. Frawley et al. [23] have described the prolactin secretory pattern associated with the initiation of a suckling bout. This study confirmed that in the rhesus and cynomolgus monkeys, unlike other species (including humans), maximum prolactin levels are not achieved until approximately 2 h after the initiation of suckling. Day and night

Female Contraception
Eds.: B. Runnebaum, T. Rabe, L. Kiesel

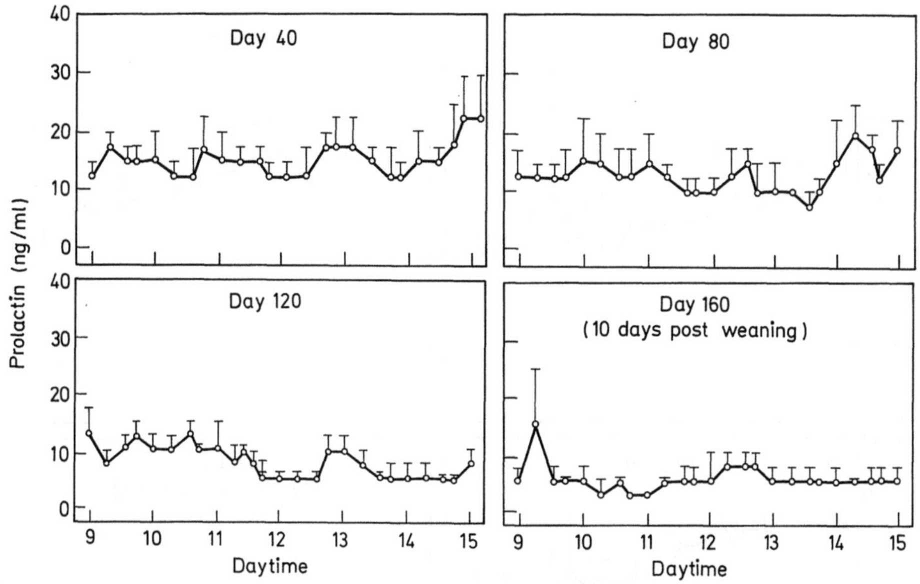

Fig. 1. Concentrations of maternal prolactin during the daytime (illumination, 0500–1700). Blood samples were collected via a cannula, protected by a vest and mobile tether. Mother-infant interactions were not disturbed by the protocol for these collections. Day 40, $n=5$; day 80, $n=5$; day 120, $n=3$; day 160, $n=4$. Data are presented as the mean ± SE ([27], used with permission)

prolactin levels were characterized throughout the postpartum interval in mothers housed with and temporarily without their infants.

In brief, five mother-infant pairs (rhesus and cynomolgus) were studied longitudinally at day 40, 80, and 120 postpartum and 10 days after weaning (day 160 postpartum). Blood samples were collected at 15-min intervals via a cannula from unanesthetized mother-infant pairs under the following conditions:

1. Undisturbed mother-infant pair (daytime, 0900–1500)
2. Undisturbed mother-infant pair (nighttime, 2100–0300)
3. Reunited mother-infant pair (daytime, 0900–1500; infant returned at 1100 following 5 or 17 h of separation)
4. Reunited mother-infant pair (nighttime, 2100–0300; infant returned at 2300 following 5 h of separation.

For monkeys at 160 days postpartum (10 days postweaning) only 1 and 2 were applied.

Figure 1 presents the mean (±SE) prolactin levels (PRL) associated with an undisturbed mother-infant relationship during daytime hours. Throughout the experiment mean daytime values were within normal limits (i.e., <25 ng/ml). By day 120, the PRL levels decreased significantly ($P<0.05$), with a further significant reduction after weaning ($P<0.05$).

Illustrated in Fig. 2 are the mean nighttime plasma PRL concentrations; the levels in each experimental segment were significantly different from one another ($P<0.05$). A dramatic reduction ($P<0.05$) in nighttime concentrations occurred

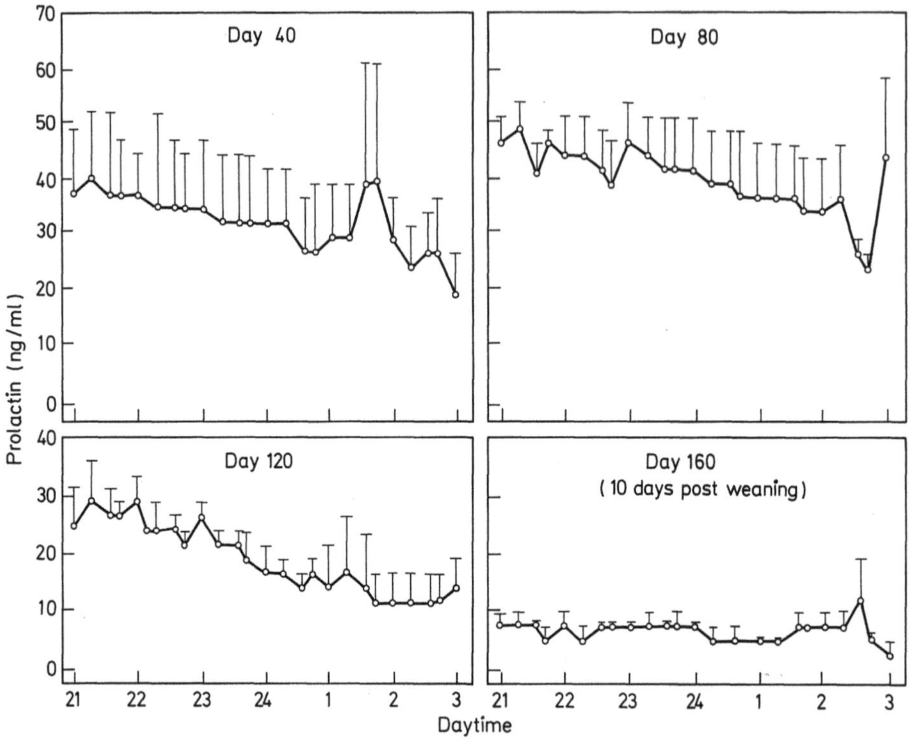

Fig. 2. Concentrations of maternal prolactin during the night (lights off, 1700–0500). Other conditions are outlined in Fig. 1. Day 40, $n=4$; day 80, $n=4$; day 120, $n=4$; day 160, $n=4$ ([27], used with permission)

after weaning. On days 40, 80, and 120, nighttime concentrations were two- to three-fold greater than daytime levels ($P<0.05$). In contrast, 10 days after weaning, there was no significant difference ($P>0.05$) between day- and nighttime values.

Such a nocturnal elevation of prolactin levels was not unexpected since both during ovulatory cycles [29] and in nonnursing postpartum mothers [20] there is a nocturnal elevation of prolactin levels. However, Fig. 3 demonstrates that the nighttime elevation is not solely the manifestation of the same neuroendocrine rhythm which regulates prolactin secretion in cycling females [28] and nonnursing postpartum monkeys [20]. In Fig. 3, peripheral plasma prolactin levels are compared for mothers with and temporarily without their infants during both day and night. There was no significant difference in daytime specimens whether the mother was with or without the infant. At night, if the infant was not with the mother, prolactin levels were not significantly different from daytime values. Only when the infant was with the mother were prolactin levels two- to three-fold greater than daytime levels. The increased secretion of prolactin at night (with the infant present) versus daytime levels (with the infant present) may be due to differences in mother-infant behavior.

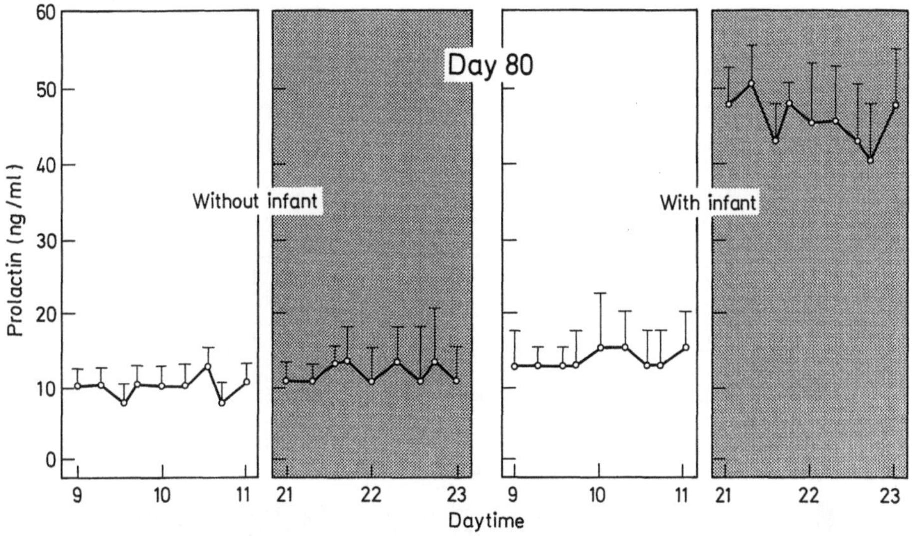

Fig. 3. Maternal prolactin concentrations during the day and night

On three occasions, observations were made via a television camera of mother-infant behavior throughout a 6-h interval during both day and night. During the daytime, the mother rarely held the infant. Typically, the infant roamed about the cage or played with the mother or food in the cage. Intervals of suckling were very brief (<1 min) and occurred infrequently (once every 2 h). In contrast, at night, the infant was held by the mother on her lap for the entire night. With the mother in this sitting position, the infant was constantly in contact with the mother's chest and was observed to hold a nipple in its mouth for intervals of 1 h or more. Frequently, though apparently sleeping (eyes closed), the infant actively suckled without disturbing the mother. Thus, the nocturnal elevation of PRL levels may be due to a disparity in nursing behavior between day and night.

If PRL is an agent via which the suckling stimulus sustains puerperal infertility, as has been suggested [21, 22], then one must question whether this nocturnal pattern of PRL secretion is of particular significance in the maintenance of lactational amenorrhea. From the current studies, the association of sustained lactational amenorrhea and the nocturnal elevation of PRL secretion does not answer this question. However, the importance of nighttime nursing is evident in several studies of women [6, 7, 30]. The common characteristic in two different groups of women with long-term lactational amenhorrhea was that the children slept with their mothers and had access to the mothers' breasts throughout the night, enabling suckling at will [6, 30]. Additionally, mothers in the Western culture who had the longest delay in the resumption of postpartum ovulation were those who breast-fed their infants at night [7].

That prolactin is the mediator of the suckling stimulus which sustains anovulation remains to be conclusively demonstrated in both women and nonhuman

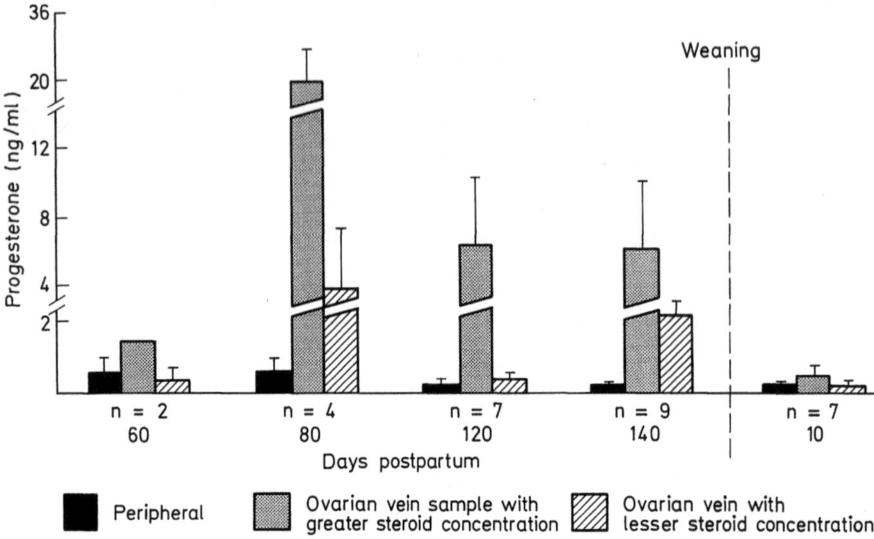

Fig. 4. Peripheral (femoral) (*black*) and ovarian (*shaded*) vein concentrations of progesterone in nursing monkeys before and after weaning (day 150). ([32], used with permission)

primates. In rhesus monkeys, one prolactin-mediated suckling effect is the sustained presence of the corpus luteum (CL) of pregnancy throughout the nursing interval. Weiss et al. [31] demonstrated histologically that the CL of pregnancy only partially involutes during the nursing interval. This CL remains until at least 86 days postpartum. They proposed that prolactin secretion induced by suckling may sustain this CL.

Throughout the nursing interval, an asymmetry exists in progesterone concentrations in ovarian venous effulent which reflects steroidogenesis by this partially involuted CL [32]. Figure 4 presents data on progesterone concentrations in peripheral sera and sera of both ovarian veins; mean progesterone concentrations in peripheral sera were near the limits of detection, but in ovarian venous effulent mean concentrations were as great as 20.7 ± 7.3 ng/ml; a 3- to 15-fold gradient existed in the concentrations between the two ovarian veins. This asymmetry persisted for the duration of nursing but was not evident 10 days after weaning (160 days postpartum). Subsequent studies have demonstrated that removal of the CL at delivery is associated with undetectable levels of progesterone in ovarian venous plasma, suggesting that the asymmetrical secretion of progesterone was attributable to the CL of pregnancy [32]. It is doubtful whether this progesterone secretion acts centrally in prolonging lactational anovulation since peripheral levels of progesterone did not exceed 0.6 ± 0.4 ng/ml (mean luteal phase peak is approximately 6.0 ng/ml). However, it is possible that the progesterone concentration within the ovary bearing the CL is great enough to affect folliculogenesis locally.

That this CL of the fertile cycle/pregnancy/lactation is sustained by prolactin has been demonstrated by the inhibition of prolactin secretion with bromocriptine [33]. In nursing monkeys, progesterone levels decline after delivery but remain elevated at 0.5–1.0 ng/ml during the 2nd and 3rd week postpartum. When postpartum prolactin secretion was inhibited with bromocriptine, progesterone concentrations fell to undetectable levels within the 1st postpartum week. Presumably, the inhibition of prolactin secretion by bromocriptine resulted in the further regression of the CL.

Whether this CL plays any role in the continuation of lactational anovulation remains entirely open to speculation. As stated earlier, the small concentration of peripheral progesterone probably does not play a central role in regulating gonadotropin secretion; however, the progesterone may act locally to inhibit folliculogenesis. More important is the possibility that through nonsteroidal compounds, this CL may centrally regulate gonadotropin secretion or act directly on both ovaries to suppress ovulation. It has been recently demonstrated that inhibin [34] and follicular regulator protein (FRP) [35] are secreted by the CL of the menstrual cycle. If the CL of pregnancy/lactation secretes inhibin, then suckling-induced prolactin secretion could act through the CL to suppress FSH and folliculogenesis, thus sustaining lactational anovulation. Alternatively, if the CL of pregnancy/lactation secretes FRP, as does the luteal phase CL, folliculogenesis could be inhibited directly at the ovarian level. It is proposed that FRP is an inhibitor of folliculogenesis, following its secretion from either the dominant follicle or the CL: It prevents the development of ovulatory follicles.

Despite this speculation, the hypopthesis remains that suckling primarily prolongs lactational anovulation by centrally inhibiting GnRH secretion and thus gonadotropin secretion, since in castrated nursing monkeys, gonadotropin concentrations remain suppressed relative to their levels in castrated nonnursing postpartum monkeys [36]. However, peptides secreted by the CL may act as a redundant or secondary mechanism in protecting against unwarranted folliculogenesis and/or ovulation.

In an unpublished study [37] nursing monkeys (120 days postpartum) were administered a regimen of pulsatile GnRH (6–9 μg every 90 min), which is known to induce folliculogenesis culminating in ovulation in monkeys with secondary amenorrhea. I hypothesized that diminished GnRH secretion, secondary to suckling, resulted in lactational anovulation; therefore, replacement therapy should stimulate folliculogenesis culminating in ovulation. Although it was demonstrated that the regimen was effective in inducing anovulation in monkeys with secondary amenorrhea within 3–5 weeks, it did not do so in nursing monkeys. In the course of 2 months, none of the six monkeys demonstrated endocrine patterns indicative of ovulation, nor was follicular maturation culminating in ovulation observed by laparoscopy. In three of the six nursing monkeys, a burgeoning CL developed during the GnRH treatment. Its emergence was not preceded by an ovulatory rise of LH and FSH, an antecedent estradiol rise, or an identifiable dominant follicle. After the initiation of GnRH therapy, peripheral progesterone levels were up to 4 ng/ml.

This burgeoning CL is probably a recrudescence of the CL of pregnancy/lactation. Prolactin secretion during lactation prevents total luteolysis of this CL; in turn, the rejuvenation of this CL may have been stimulated by LH secretion induced by the GnRH treatment. Additional experimentation is required to understand the physiology underlying the results of this experiment and the possible role of the CL of pregnancy/lactation in sustaining lactational anovulation.

In conclusion, from the studies of lactational anovulation reviewed here, there are two areas which need further investigation to determine whether they contribute to the mechanisms suppressing ovulation in the nursing monkey. Firstly, whether the infant-dependent nighttime increase of prolactin contributes to sustained anovulation in nursing mothers, and secondly, whether the corpus luteum of pregnancy/lactation inhibits, either centrally or locally, folliculogenesis culminating in ovulation during the nursing interval.

Acknowledgment. Appreciation is expressed to Ms. Dara Leary for excellent assistance in preparing the manuscript.

References

1. Cronin TJ (1968) Influence of lactation upon ovulation. Lancet 2:422
2. Robyn C, Meuris S (1982) Pituitary prolactin, lactational performance and puerperal infertility. Semin Perinatol 6:254
3. Howie PW, McNeilly AS, Houston MJ, Cook A, Boyle H (1982) Fertility after childbirth: post-partum ovulation and menstruation in bottle and breastfeeding mothers. Clin Endocrinol (Oxf) 17:323
4. McCann MF, Liskin LS, Piotrow PT, Rinehart W, Fox G (1981) Breastfeeding, fertility and family planning. Popul Rep [J] 9:525
5. Bonnar J (1982) Natural family planning including breastfeeding. In: Mishell DR Jr (ed) Advances in fertility research. Raven, New York, p 12
6. Konner M, Worthman C (1980) Nursing frequency, gonadal function and birth spacing among Kung hunter-gathers. Science 207:788
7. Howie PW, McNeilly AS, Houston MJ, Cook A, Boyle H (1982) Fertility after childbirth: infant feeding pattern, basal PRL level and post-partum ovulation. Clin Endocrinol (Oxf) 17:315
8. McNeilly AS, Glasier AF, Howie PW, Houston MJ, Cook A, Boyle H (1983) Fertility after childbirth: pregnancy associated with breastfeeding. Clin Endocrinol (Oxf) 18:167
9. Goodman AL, Hodgen GD (1978) Postpartum patterns of circulating FSH, LH, prolactin, estradiol and progesterone in nonsuckling cynomolgus monkeys. Steroids 31:731
10. Schallenberger E, Richards DW, Knobil E (1981) Role of prolactin in the lactational amenorrhea of the rhesus monkey (*Macaca mulata*). Biol Reprod 25:370
11. Williams RF, Hodgen GD (1983) Initiation of the primate ovarian cycle with emphasis on perimenarchial and postpartum events. In: Greep RO (ed) Reproductive physiology IV. University Park Press, Baltimore, p 1
12. Nakano R, Mori A, Kayashima F, Washio M, Tojo S (1975) Ovarian response to exogenously administered human gonadotropins during the postpartum period. Am J Obstet Gynecol 121:187
13. Adreassen B, Tyson JE (1976) Role of the hypothalamic-pituitary-ovarian axis in puerperal infertility. J Clin Endocrinol Metab 42:1114
14. Maneckjee R, Moudgal RN, Banavar SR (1977) Ovarian responsiveness to exogenous gonadotropins during lactation in the rat and monkey. Fertil Steril 28:986
15. Williams RF, Johnson DK, Hodgen GD (1979) Resumption of estrogen induced gonadotropin surges in postpartum monkeys. J Clin Endocrinol Metab 49:422
16. Plant TM, Schallenberger E, Hess DL, McCormack JT, Dufy-Barbe L, Knobil E (1980) Influence of suckling on gonadotropin secretion in the female rhesus monkey (*Macaca mulatta*). Biol Reprod 23:760

17. Baird DT, McNeilly AS, Sawers S, Sharpe M (1979) Failure of estrogen-induced discharge of luteinizing hormone in lactating women. J Clin Endocrinol Metab 49:500
18. Canales ES, Fonseca ME, Mason M, Zarate A (1981) Feedback effect of estradiol on follicle-stimulating hormone and prolactin secretion during the puerperium. Int J Gynaecol Obstet 19:79
19. Canales ES, Zarate A, Garrido J, Leon C, Soria J, Schally A (1974) Study on the recovery of pituitary FSH function during puerperium using synthetic LRH. J Clin Endocrinol Metab 38:1140
20. diZerega GS, Williams RF, Hodgen GD (1981) Pregnancy induced anovulation in the primate ovarian cycle. In: Schwartz NB, Hunzicker-Dunn M (eds) Dynamics of ovarian function. Raven, New York, p 147
21. Maneckjee R, Srinath BR, Moudgal NR (1976) Prolactin suppresses release of luteinizing hormone during lactation in the monkey. Nature 262:507
22. McNeilly AS, Glasier A, Johassen J, Howie PW (1982) Evidence for direct inhibition of ovarian function by prolactin. J Reprod Fertil 65:559
23. Frawley LS, Mulchahey JJ, Neil JD (1983) Nursing induces a biphasic release of prolactin in rhesus monkeys. Endocrinology 112:558
24. Tyson JR, Carter JN, Andreassen B, Huth J, Smith B (1978) Nursing-mediated prolactin and luteinizing hormone secretion during puerperal lactation. Fertil Steril 30:154
25. Aono T, Shioji T, Shoda T, Kurachi K (1977) The initiation of human lactation and prolactin response to suckling. J Clin Endocrinol Metab 44:1101
26. Howie PW, McNeilly AS, McArdle T, Smart L, Houston M (1980) The relationship between suckling-induced prolactin response and lactogenesis. J Clin Endocrinol Metab 50:670
27. Aso T, Williams RF (1985) Lactational amenorrhea in monkeys: effects of suckling on prolactin secretion. Endocrinology 117:1727
28. Quadri SK, Spies HG (1976) Cyclic and diurnal patterns of serum prolactin in the rhesus monkey. Biol Reprod 14:495
29. Williams RF, Hodgen GD (1980) Reinitiation of the diurnal rhythm of prolactin secretion in postpartum rhesus monkeys. Biol Reprod 23:276
30. Duchen MR, McNeilly AS (1980) Hyperprolactinemia and long-term lactational amenorrhea. Clin Endocrinol (Oxf) 12:621
31. Weiss G, Dierschke DJ, Karsch FJ, Hotchkiss J, Butler WR, Knobil E (1973) The influence of lactation on luteal function in the rhesus monkey. Endocrinology 93:954
32. Williams RF, Hodgen GD (1983) Mechanism of lactational anovulation in primates: Nursing increases ovarian steroidogenesis. In: Greenwald GS, Terranova PF (eds) Factors regulating ovarian function. Raven, New York, p 17
33. Richardson DW, Goldsmith LT, Pohl CR, Schallenberger E, Knobil E (1985) The role of prolactin in the regulation of the primate corpus luteum. J Clin Endocrinol Metab 60:501
34. Baird DT, Messinis IE, Templeton AA, McNeilly AJ, Tosnis CG (1987) Inhibin levels in gonadotropin-treatment cycles (Abstr PS-018). 5th World Congress on In Vitro Fertilization and Embryo Transfer, April 5–10, Norfolk, Virginia
35. di Zerega GS, Katt EL, Yanagaharia D, Mishell D, Holst P, Tonetta S, Rodgers K, et al. (1987) Characterization of follicle regulatory protein in urine during the menstrual cycle (Abstr 3685). 34th Annual Meeting of the Society of Gynecologic Investigation, March 18–21, Atlanta
36. Weiss G, Butler WR, Dierschke DJ, Knobil E (1976) Influence of suckling on gonadotropin secretion in the postpartum rhesus monkey. Proc Soc Exp Biol Med 153:330
37. Williams RF, Aso T (1984) (Abstract 181). 7th International Congress of Endocrinology, Quebec City, Canada

Barriers and Sterilization

New Approaches in Vaginal Contraception

I. Gerhard

Division of Gynecological Endocrinology, University of Heidelberg, Voßstraße 9, 6900 Heidelberg, FRG

The use of barrier methods increased dramatically between 1973 and 1982 in North America as well as in Europe (Pratt et al. 1984; Döring and Schicketanz 1986). In 1982 one-third of married women using contraception to delay pregnancy were using condoms or diaphragms, compared with only 16% in 1973. Of sexually active never-married women aged 15–19 years who were using contraception, 28% were using condoms (22%) or diaphragms (6%) (Pratt et al. 1984).

The acceptability of barrier methods may be more strongly influenced by the perceived disadvantages of other methods than by the advantages of the method selected, for instance, possible linkage of hormonal contraceptives to heart disease and cancer or the increased risk of pelvic inflammatory disease, pain, and bleeding in IUD users. The availability of safe, legal abortion probably increases the willingness of some women in developed countries to use methods such as spermicides that show higher failure rates but at present no risk of systemic effects or other health hazards. The increasing popularity of vaginal contraceptives in the past 3 years may be due to the estimated protective effect against sexually transmitted diseases (STD) and acquired immune deficiency syndrome (AIDS).

Compounds

The following vaginal contraceptives are available: chemical barriers (creams, jellies, suppositories, foams), physical barriers (cervical cap, diaphragm, sponge), combined chemical-physical barriers, and vaginal delivery systems for spermicides and female sex hormones.

There are several active ingredients used in spermicides (Table 1). Enzyme inhibitors disrupt the enzymes necessary for intermediary metabolism of spermatozoa. Many of these are toxic so only a few are used commercially. The sulfhydral-binding substances suspend sperm motility by oxidizing, by forming mercaptides, or by alkylating essential substrates or enzymes of the spermatozoa. The surface-active agents include the most popular spermicidal compounds in use today, such as nonoxynol-9 (N9). These disrupt the outer lipoprotein surface layer of spermatozoa, thus altering cell permeability and allowing intracellular components, proteins and enzymes, to escape. On an equal weight basis octoxynol is half as active as nonoxynol, and benzalkonium chloride is 4–10 times more active. In addition to being spermicidal, benzalkonium chloride coagulates cervical mucus so that it becomes impermeable to spermatozoa, which might be another added barrier mechanism (Mendez et al. 1986). The combination of low concentrations

Female Contraception
Eds.: B. Runnebaum, T. Rabe, L. Kiesel

Table 1. Active ingredients in spermicides

Enzyme inhibitors	Trisodium salt of sulfuric acid ester of a polysaccharide (Agen 53)
Surface-active agents	Nonoxynol-9 (Lady, Agen 53 N, Ortho cream, Patentex oval) Octoxynol-9 Menfegol (Menfegol tablets) Benzalkonium chloride (Benzaltex) Dioctyl sodium sulfosuccinate + nonoxynol-9 (Contraceptivum E)
Electrolytes	
Acids	Boric acid Tartaric acid Lactic acid

of N9 with dioctyl sodium sulfosuccinate (DONS) results in a faster sperm-immobilizing effect and fewer side effects. Electrolytes such as sodium chloride disrupt spermatic metabolism. Acids are used in conjunction with other active ingredients to lower the pH of the compound.

Vehicles

The vehicles used to carry spermicidal agents are creams, suppositories, and jellies. A waiting time of 10–15 min is necessary to ensure maximal dispersion of the spermicide. Contraceptive foams in pressurized containers, commonly called aerosols, disperse well in the vagina and require no wait between application and coitus (in contrast to foaming tablets). After placement, spermicidal capacity rapidly decreases, so renewed application is recommended before subsequent coital activity. Excessive lubrication, smell, taste, and messiness associated with the use of spermicides are additional disadvantages. The advantages are that no physician must be contacted, they are always available, and they lack systemic side effects.

Chemical-Physical Barriers

The diaphragm is the most widely used female barrier method. It acts as a mechanical barrier to the entrance of sperm into the cervical os and as a receptacle for spermicidal creams held adjacent to the cervix. It must be fitted by a physician, and the woman must be trained to use it correctly. Although Leitch (1986) showed that Orthocreme had good spermicidal activity 12 h after insertion, it is recommended that the diaphragm be refilled after 4 h and repeatedly in case of multiple coital episodes.

Cervical caps are not commonly used, mostly because self-insertion is too difficult for many women. Firmer cervical caps could be left in place between menses, but cap dislodgement and pregnancies were too frequent, although the spermicide Orthocreme used in cervical caps was still active 5 days after insertion (Leitch 1986). If the cap is directly placed over an active infection of the cervix,

Table 2. Contraceptive sponges

Type	Vehicle	Size (cm)	Spermicide
Collagen sponge	Collagen fibrous protein (bovine skin)	6.0–7.0 wide 2.0–2.5 thick	–
Today sponge	Polyurethane	6.0 wide 1.5–2.5 thick	1 g nonoxynol-9
Intravaginal insert	Polyester	3.5 wide 4.5 thick	Nonoxynol-9
Benzaltex sponge	Polyvinyl alcohol	4.0 wide 2.0 thick	0.06 g benzalkonium chloride

it could increase the chances of trapping pathogenic organisms at the cervical os and encouraging their ascent into the uterus and fallopian tubes. Vaginal injury due to a sharp-edged rim may occur.

Sponges (Table 2) act as a physical and a mechanical barrier by their ability to release the agent and absorb semen. Cylindrical collagen sponges made from the fibrous protein collagen isolated from bovine skin were first developed. However, viable spermatozoa in the cervical mucus were found in 25% of the tests with these nonmedicated sponges, as compared to 6% with sponges containing N9 (Chvapil et al. 1985). Therefore clinical trials with various medicated sponges for single use were initiated. The Today sponge used in North America and Europe contains 1 g N9. After 2 h of wear almost 50% of N9 was lost from the sponge. In sexually inactive women only about 20% of the original amount of N9 was left in the sponge worn for 24 and 48 h. Intercourse significantly increased the release of N9 from sponges (Chvapil et al. 1985; Lemberg 1984; Vorhauer et al. 1984). The Benzaltex sponge developed in France is made of polyvinyl alcohol and contains benzalkonium chloride. The vehicle is more resistant to rupture than polyurethane. It is easy to insert but sometimes difficult to remove, as it gives the impression of vaginal mucosa.

Sponges should not be retained in the vagina for more than 30 h because of malodor developing in the presence of ejaculate (soon after insertion the initial pH is neutralized by vaginal secretions, and polyamines such as spermine and spermidine are metabolized to propylamine and butylamine by aminooxidases) (Chvapil et al. 1985). Some women experience dryness of the vagina, others uncontrollable loss of fluid (dripping) which may be a hypersensitivity phenomenon analogous to contact dermatitis. The recovered vaginal and/or cervical fluid amounted to 20 ml over a 24-h period (Chvapil et al. 1985).

The sponge offers users several advantages over other vaginal contraceptive methods. It is easy to use and is not messy. It does not need to be fitted. It is available in a single size and can be purchased without prescription. After insertion it provides immediate and continuous protection against pregnancy for at least 24 h, regardless of the frequency of intercourse. It permits a greater degree of sexual spontaneity in that it may be inserted up to 24 h before intercourse (Edelman et al. 1984).

Chvapil et al. (1985) compared several sizes of sponges and came to the following conclusions: The sponge must be larger than 6 cm in diameter in order to serve as a mechanical barrier that will not be dislodged during physical activity. In multiparous women one of 7–8 cm is necessary, which may become difficult to insert. It must be at least 2.5 cm thick, otherwise it often folds in the vagina. Application with an inserter results in more reproducible and appropriate placement of the sponge. Retention in the vagina should not exceed 24 h. Only 6 h after the last coitus the sponge may be removed.

Safety

Although spermicides are generally considered to be a safe method of contraception, several recent reports have raised questions about their use around the time of conception. As surfactants cause irreversible membrane alteractions, resulting in immediate devitalization of spermatozoa, and are partly resorbed from the vagina, these membrane changes might also occur in other cells.

Of N9, 85% is recovered in the urine and feces (Chvapil et al. 1985). The detergent was detected in the milk of lactating rats and the serum of their pups within 2 h after the intravaginal dose (Chvapil et al. 1980a–c). Fibroblasts in tissue culture were found to be more sensitive than spermatozoa to the effect of N9 (Chvapil et al. 1980a–c). Evidence of hepatotoxicity and nephrotoxicity in rats and rabbits was given when high doses of N9 were administered in the peritoneal cavity or the vagina (Chvapil et al. 1985). In pregnant rats 44% of intravaginally administered N9 was absorbed from the vagina; over 6 h 17% was recovered in urine and feces. After 6 h, concentrations in the uterus and placenta were similar to that in maternal plasma, whereas mean concentrations in amniotic fluid and in the fetus were approximately one-third that of maternal plasma (Buttar 1982).

When octoxynol-9, at 6 times the clinical doses, was administered intravaginally to pregnant rats during organogenesis, no differences in treated and control groups were found as to maternal and fetal toxicity, malformations or developmental variations (Saad et al. 1984). Comparable experiments were performed with benzalkonium chloride in pregnant rats and rabbits. Vaginal application of doses 6–360 times the clinical dose could not be measured in the uterus and did not produce any toxic or teratogenic side effects. In the serum of women who had used the benzalkonium sponge over 24 h benzalkonium chloride could not be detected with most sensitive HPLC methods (below 50 ng/ml serum).

In the beginning of the 1980s cohort and case-control studies implicated an increased risk of malformations, Down's syndrome, abortion, or low birth weight in offspring of spermicide users compared to nonusers (Jick et al. 1981, 1982; Janerich et al. 1980; Rothman 1982). The absence of a single, well-defined syndrome among infants whose mothers used spermicides raised doubt about a causal connection. In addition, the precise time of exposure had not been established in most of these studies and the active substances were not explained further. Several of these spermicides contained borates, which have been associated with fetal skeletal abnormalities in animals. Some of the observed positive connections may be related to this compound.

Table 3. Malformation rate in spermicide users: 34660 prenatal questionnaires evaluated during 1974–1977 (Mills et al. 1985)

Group	Number of patients	Malformation rate
Spermicide before LMP	3146	0.132
Spermicide after LMP	2282	0.128
Others before LMP	13148	0.126
Others after LMP	2831	0.127

LMP, last menstrual period.

Table 4. Adjusted odds ratios comparing spermicide use in trisomic cases and controls (Strobino et al. 1986)

Maternal age	Sample sizes (n) in matched samples		Ratios duration of use	
(years)	Trisomies	Controls	≦1 year	>1 year
≦ 24	67	1009	1.0	0.8
25–29	72	488	0.7	0.9
30–34	77	470	1.2	2.6
≧ 35	93	272	0.8	2.6

Mills et al. (1985) documented contraceptive exposure in 34660 women at the first prenatal visit during 1974–1977 (Table 3). Of these 3146 had used spermicides before the last menstrual period and 2282 after the last menstrual period. No increased risk of malformation, abortion, etc. could be detected in either of these groups compared to nonspermicide users. Spermicide groups were subdivided as to different substances and different dosages without an indication of positive associations with fetal toxicity. Thus, findings of previous studies which could not detect teratogenic effects of vaginal spermicides were confirmed (Shapiro et al. 1982; Abrutyn et al. 1982).

Strobino et al. (1986) successfully karyotyped 1556 out of 6339 spontaneous abortions during 1974–1982 (Table 4). The mothers were interviewed with respect to spermicide exposure. Controls were 2766 pregnant women with healthy offspring. There was no association between spermicide use and the various types of chromosomally abnormal abortion except for trisomic abortions. At a ratio of 1.9 spermicide use for more than 1 year at any time prior to conception was significantly more common in the cases aborting trisomic conceptions than in the control group. This association was confined to women over 30 years of age and to long-term use. The authors assume that factors causing trisomy may act upon the ovum at any time between the onset of meiosis I in the embryonic ovum through the completion of meiosis I at ovulation and the completion of meiosis II at fertilization.

Adverse Effects of Spermicides

When the vagina of rabbits or rats is exposed to increasing doses of N9 over 5 days, inflammatory changes of the epithelium are induced. Changes in the continuity of the epithelial lining, edema of the submucosal layer, and cell infiltrations were proportional to the amount of N9. Increased DNA and collagen was demonstrated. The increased cell membrane permeability produced by binding of the monomeric detergent molecules to lipids of the membrane activated the cellular inflammatory response in the tissues. These changes may explain the irritation produced by spermicidal formulations containing this surfactant reported by some women or their sexual partners (Chvapil et al. 1980a–c).

Foaming solid spermicides generate heat when dissolving, which both partners are likely to sense. While this heat-releasing effect apparently disturbs some users (without rejecting the method because of this), the sensation of heat is pleasurable for others, so that in some countries advertisements now cite the sensation of warmth as an added benefit.

Benefits of Spermicides

Prevention of sexually transmitted diseases (STD) is one of the outstanding benefits of spermicides. Spermicides have been shown in vitro to inhibit the growth of *Neisseria gonorrhoeae, Treponema, Mycoplasma*, and *Chlamydia trachomatis* (Singh et al. 1972; Bolch and Warren 1973). In clinical studies the risk of gonorrhea was 2–10 times lower in spermicide users than in non-users (Keith et al. 1976).

In vitro N9 and benzalkonium chloride inactivated HTLV III (Hicks et al. 1985; Chermann 1987) at concentrations used in contraceptive compounds. Laboratory studies suggest that most spermicides have antiparasitic and antifungal effects. Strains of herpes simplex virus exposed to various dilutions of surface-active agents were shown to be inactivated after only 10 s (Asculaii et al. 1978; Singh et al. 1976). Electron-microscopic evaluation showed that the chemicals act as solvents of the lipid membrane, so that the virus loses its infectivity.

A large study of Kelaghan et al. (1982) showed that women using spermicides alone had a 30% lower risk of hospitalization for first-episode pelvic inflammatory disease compared with women not using contraceptives. Although in vitro the antimicrobial and antiviral effects were proved for solutions of nonoxynol, benzalkonium chloride, povidone, and the trisodium salt of a sulphuric acid ester of a polysaccharide (Thurner et al. 1983), the in vivo effects vary greatly due to different chemical compositions of the spermicides and variations in the concentrations needed for irreversible damage of the microorganism, so that STD can be significantly reduced, but not totally prevented.

Evidence that the rate of cervical cancer might be associated with different methods of contraception began to accumulate in the 1960s. In studies comparing patients with cervical cancer and controls a more frequent use of barrier methods among noncancer groups was reported (Boyd and Doll 1964; Vessey et al. 1976). However, up to the present no differentiation has been possible between mechanical and spermicidal barriers. As the role of papillomavirus in the development of cervical dysplasia and carcinoma appears to be established, the antiviral potencies of spermicides may be responsible for this antineoplastic effect (Syrjanen et al. 1984).

Adverse Effects of Chemical-Physical Barriers

In diaphragm users allergic reactions to the rubber are sometimes observed. Sponge users may show a hypersensitivity phenomenon (Chvapil et al. 1985). As the anterior rim of the diaphragm may produce a mechanical irritation of the urethra and thus facilitate the entry of microorganisms into the lower urinary tract, urinary infections and urethral stricture are reported with a frequency of 1.7 per 1000 women-years (Vessey et al. 1976). Fihn et al. 1985 conducted a case-control study on 199 women and a retrospective cohort investigation on 374 women to assess the relationship between diaphragm use and urinary tract infection (UTI). The estimated risks of UTI were very similar in both studies with ratios of 2.0 and 2.5 for diaphragm users compared to women on oral contraceptives. It could be demonstrated that peak urinary flow rates were significantly reduced when the diaphragms were in place (Gillespie 1984). In most of the UTI patients *Escherichia coli* was cultured. This is consistent with the finding that in diaphragm users, concomitant with a rise in vaginal pH, the normal vaginal flora is replaced by aerobic gram-negative bacilli which are frequently recovered in the vaginal introitus as a reservoir for ascending infection (Watt et al. 1981; Percival-Smith et al. 1983; Peddie et al. 1984; Thurner et al. 1983; Chow et al. 1986). Hemorrhoids, too, are observed in 2.1 per 1000 women-years; the risk increases if the diaphragm does not fit exactly (Vessey et al. 1976).

The most severe side effect reported was toxic shock syndrome (TSS). This is an acute febrile exanthematous illness associated with toxin-producing staphylococci. The use of highly absorbent tampons as well as barrier devices retained in the vagina over a prolonged time influence the pH and the microbial colonization and may lead to mucosal alterations. Although some women harbor large numbers of staphylococci in the lower genital tract, these rarely become symptomatic. Which conditions are involved in the production and absorbance of toxins to produce clinical illness is still questioned, as the incidence of TSS is as low as 10 cases per 100000 menstruating women per year using tampons (Davis et al. 1980) and ten cases per 100000 women per year using sponges and diaphragms, respectively (Reingold 1986). Some predisposing factors could be identified, such as the continuous retention of diaphragms or tampons, and this resulted in the recommendation to remove the diaphragm after 24 h. Fragmentation of the sponge and retention was sometimes observed. As N9 at any concentration was noninhibitory to two strains of *Staphylococcus aureus* and a strain of β-hemolytic streptococcus, the replenishment of the spermicide after some hours did not prevent TSS (Baehler et al. 1983; Chvapil et al. 1985).

In vivo no measurable growth of *S. aureus* was observed at $pH < 4.2$ in women using nonoxynol sponges (Chvapil et al. 1985). However, within less than 6 h the slightly alkaline vaginal secretion with high buffering capacity neutralized the pH of the sponge. The attempt to increase the buffering capacity of the citrate buffer above a strength of 0.2 mol/l resulted in irritation of the vagina (itching). Contrary to nonoxynol, benzalkonium chloride produced a strong inhibitory effect on *S. aureus* in vitro.

During menstruation and during the postpartum period, vaginal barriers should not be used. Women with vaginal lesions or a history of recent vaginitis are predisposed to acute TSS because the disruption of the normal indigenous microflora alters the resistance to pathogenic microorganisms. An approximate doubling of the incidence rate of TSS is observed for women reporting a history of vaginitis in the previous year (Lanes et al. 1986).

Benefits of Chemical-Physical Barriers

Of course, all the benefits outlined above for spermicides are found for diaphragms, too. However, the protection against STD is even more pronounced. Austin et al. (1984) reported a 20% reduction in the risk of gonorrhea with spermicides alone. When spermicides were used with either condoms or diaphragms, the risk was reduced to 60%. Besides the lessened likelihood of diaphragm users having gonorrhea, they showed a significantly lower risk of hospitalization for pelvic inflammatory disease compared with women using no contraceptives (Kelaghan et al. 1982). As cervical cancer behaves epidemiologically like a STD (Kessler 1976; Rosemann et al. 1984), the relative risk of severe cervical dysplasia and neoplasia for diaphragm users drops to 0.2 compared with users of other contraceptives (Wright et al. 1978; Harris et al. 1980).

As the only serious side effect of sponge use is the risk of death due to nonmenstrual TSS, Reingold (1986) estimated a relative risk of 1.5, taking into account baseline incidence, case-fatality rate, and failure rate. Sponge nonuse results in exposure to other risks of potentially greater magnitude, for instance, those related to pregnancy (8.3) or to use of hormone contraceptive pills (0.1–5.2).

Effectiveness

The main objections to barrier methods is their high failure rate. Vaughan et al. 1977 reported the following contraceptive failure rates among married women in the United States in 1970–1973: about 2% of pill users, 4% of IUD users, 8% of diaphragm users, 10% of condom users, and 15% of spermicide users became pregnant within the first 12 months of use (Table 5). Effectiveness rates expressed in a Pearl Index assume equal probability of failure in every month of exposure: if the observation period is short, the failure rate will appear misleadingly high; if the period is long, the success of long-term use will be overrepresented. Life tables can avoid this distortion, calculating failure rates of specific intervals after contraceptive use begins, normally after 12 months, as in this study and the following tables.

Although in this report women using barrier methods had the highest failure rate, pregnancy rates as low as 1–7 per 100 women-years were shown in small

Table 5. Contraceptive failure rate among married women in the United States 1970–1973 (Vaughan et al. 1977)

Method	Failure rate[a] (%)
Pill	2
IUD	4
Diaphragm	8
Condom	10
Spermicide	15

[a] Number of women with pregnancies within the first 12 months of use.

clinical studies run by private physicians. On the one hand, this may reflect the individual characteristics of these women (e.g., education, motivation); on the other, however, lower failure rates may also reflect greater care and effort on the part of the provider to ensure that women understand how to insert and use spermicides.

For this reason three types of contraceptive failures must be considered: (a) physiological failure, in which the product did not protect against pregnancy even though it was correctly used; (b) provider failure, in which the contraceptor failed to use the product correctly because the provider did not supply accurate guidance; and (c) psychological failure, in which the contraceptor failed to use the product or used it uncorrectly despite adequate instructions.

Regarding physiological failure, first, the potencies of the spermicidal agents commonly used (N9, octoxynol, benzalkonium chloride) are well documented, and dose-effectiveness curves are available. Differences in total dosage influence effectiveness especially in women with large amounts of vaginal fluids. The content of the base material also influences effectiveness, as some bases themselves can immobilize spermatozoa. The ability of the vehicle to spread rapidly and evenly over the cervical os and to hold spermicides in place as long as possible differs markedly between compounds. Foams and creams are dispersed best, suppositories need body heat to melt, and foaming tablets need moisture to produce foam. Solid preparations may require more than 10 min between insertion and intercourse to ensure melting or foaming action. Diaphragms, cervical caps, and sponges hold the spermicide in place over a longer period so that effectiveness is increased. Benzalkonium chloride is not yet commercially availably in the Federal Republic of Germany, but it appears to have promising effectiveness in various vehicles. The Pearl Index for cream, suppositories, and sponges has been measured at around 2.0 in different countries where these preparations were used by more than 4000 women. Mendez et al. (1986) reported a life table pregnancy rate after 1 year of suppository use of 3.7; 52% of these failures could be traced to error or failure to use.

Provider failure is that due to inadequate instructions in contraceptive packages or insufficient guidance and support from family planning personnel. Reports on effectiveness are controversial: in clinical studies usually low failure rates

Table 6. Factors influencing the effectiveness of diaphragms: calculated from 19101 cycles in 778 women (mean Pearl Index 4.34) (Döring and Schicketanz 1986)

Factors		Number of cycles	Pearl index
Age (years)	18–29	13167	4.74
	30–50	5934	3.43
Previous deliveries	Yes	3475	5.86
	No	15626	3.99
Desire for later pregnancy	Yes	8048	5.22
	Unclear	7073	4.22
	No	3285	2.92
Previous information	Bad	1678	7.14
	Medium	2924	5.74
	Good	14069	3.75
Duration of use	<1 year	5349	6.28
	1–2.5 years	9115	4.61
	>2.5 years	4637	1.55

are given, as for instance less than one pregnancy per 100 women-years in studies concerning Patentex oval. However, reports on women seeking abortion and estimates of the proportion of all users suggest failure rates between 4 and 10 per 100 women-years. These differences possibly reflect the difference between the majority of spermicide users who buy these products over the counter and the small sample of women who receive extensive medical care.

Psychological failures, however, account for most of the discrepancy between pregnancy rates calculated on the basis of the spermicidal potency of a compound and actual failures. Some characteristics of spermicide users producing high effectiveness could be found: high motivation, good education, positive communication between the partners, and long experience.

Döring and Schicketanz (1986) evaluated the various factors influencing the effectiveness of diaphragms in 778 women (Table 6). Lower failure rates were reported in women over 30 without previous deliveries, no desire for later pregnancy, good previous information, and longer duration of use. In recent years method failures account for only about one-third or fewer of all failures. It is possible to achieve 95% protection or more by using proven spermicides regularly and correctly. However, in actual practice failure rates are about 3 times higher, representing only 85% protection, because many users are not as careful as they need to be.

Only few studies have been conducted in recent years in which various barrier methods were prospectively tested in a well-defined population (Table 7). In the United States Edelman et al. (1984) compared the effectiveness of the Today sponge and the diaphragm, both loaded with N9. The pregnancy rate was significantly higher in the sponge users. Related to this study, McIntyre and Higgins (1986) proved that for nulliparous women the sponge was as effective as the diaphragm (pregnancy rate 13.9 versus 12.8). However, parous women using the sponge were twice as likely to become pregnant (28.3 versus 13.4). Although the

Table 7. Pregnancy and continuation rates in prospective studies

Method	Number of patients	Pregnancies Parous	(%)	Nulli-parous	1-year contin-uation rate (%)	Source
Today sponge	723	28.3	17	13.9	54.1	Edelman et al.
diaphragm and N9	721	13.4[a]	12.5[a]	12.8	57.3	(1984) (USA)
Today sponge	245	35.5		21.9		Bounds and Guille-
diaphragm and N9	246	14.1[a]		8.0[a]		baud (1984) (UK, Canada)
Today sponge	184		10.4		72.9	Borko et al. (1985)
neo sampoon	187		12.8[a]		71.6	(Yugoslavia)
Today sponge	554		11.2		56.3	Edelman (1986)
neo sampoon	553		12.3		67.8	(Yugoslavia, Taiwan, Bangladesh)
Today sponge	86		4.7		58	Jeker amd Mall-
benzaltex sponge	71		11.3		58	Haefeli (1986) (Switzerland)

[a] Statistically significant in the overall 12-month cumulative life table pregnancy rate.

continuation rate was not significantly different between sponge and diaphragm users, the event rates leading to discontinuation from the study differed significantly ($p < 0.05$), with a higher rate of accidental pregnancies, allergic-type reactions, and discomfort in the sponge users. Personal reasons accounted for 19% dropping these methods. Sponge users had more problems with the correct placement and removal of the sponge, which sometimes tore. They were less confident in the method. On the other hand, diaphragm users more frequently reported too much trouble to use, objections of the partner and the desire for an alternative method.

The comparison of the Today sponge with the diaphragm in a study in the United Kingdom and Canada gave significantly higher pregnancy rates even in nulliparous women (Bounds and Guillebaud 1984).

In Yugoslavia, Taiwan, and Bangladesh the Today sponge was compared to Neo Sampoon, a Japanese foaming tablet containing menfegol, a surface-active agent. The report of Borko et al. (1985) on Yugoslavia gave a significantly higher pregnancy rate for Neo Sampoon users, with a good continuation rate of over 70% in both groups. At the conclusion of the trial 41% of users asked to be provided with a barrier contraceptive method for additional months. The recent publication of Edelman (1986) with a greater number of women did not state significant differences between these methods, but the discontinuation rate was higher in sponge users. In Switzerland Jeker and Mall-Haefeli (1986) conducted a study with the Today and the Benzaltex sponge. Although the number of patients was limited, the pregnancy rate was higher in the Benzaltex group but comparable to the world-wide Today results. They observed that 50% of failures happened in

Table 8. Recommendations for barrier methods

Indications	Contra-indications
1. Women having infrequent intercourse 2. Reliable Women 3. Birth spacing 4. Intolerance of hormonal contraception 5. Temporary interruption of hormonal contraception 6. If a pill was missed during hormonal contraception 7. High risk of sexually transmitted deseases 8. Previous pelvic inflammatory disease	1. All methods: Sensitivity to the spermicide Pregnancy (absolute contraindication) Women who dislike touching their genitals 2. Diaphragm, sponge: Sensitivity to rubber or synthetic material Descensus uteri Vaginal infection Anamnestic toxic shock syndrome Postpartum, postabortum 3. Sponge: Retroflected uterus

women with a retroflected uterus. While over 60% of their patients were satisfied with the sponge barrier methods, 42% wished to discontinue after 1 year.

As cervical caps lack popularity, no prospective studies have included this method. In view of theoretical considerations and according to a clinical trial performed by Koch (1982a, b) in 413 women who were perfectly selected and trained, the cap can be as effective as the diaphragm.

Recommendations

Based on the results of practicability, safety, and effectiveness the following recommendations for the use of barrier methods can be made (Table 8). Barrier methods are particularly convenient for women who have intercourse infrequently (because these are only used at coitus) and for intelligent and reliable women. They are better suited for women who are spacing births than for women who may not become pregnant. They are well acceptable for women objecting to pills for medical reasons. They are effective means for prevention against STD and pelvic inflammatory disease in risk groups.

Barrier methods cannot be recommended for women in whom an absolute contraindication for conception exists, because of the 10% failure rate. Women who dislike touching their genitals would probably also dislike using spermicides. Women who dislike sexual activity are more likely to dislike the consistent, active participation in contraception that vaginal methods require. Sensitivity to the spermicide, the rubber, or the synthetic material of the sponge may rule out using these methods. Dislocation of diaphragm, cap, and sponge is possible in descensus uteri. In addition, the mechanical protection of the cervical os by the sponge is not complete in women with a retroflected uterus. Because of the increased risk fo TSS, diaphragm, cap and sponge should not be used in women with vaginal infection, anamnestic TSS, and during postpartum and postabortion periods as long as the lochial secretion persists.

Along these lines, barrier methods should have their place beside other methods, as they fill the special needs of certain women and provide contraception for some who otherwise would do without. At present, mechanical barriers (diaphragm, cap, sponge, condom) combined with spermicides yield the best effectiveness and safety.

Prospective Research

Prospective research is currently under way to identify spermicides and vehicles which are longer acting, more effective, more acceptable and more specific (Table 9). There are enzyme inhibitors which work on a different principle than spermicides, for instance, the synthetic substance *p*-nitrophenyl, *p*-guanidinobenzoate which inhibits acrosin activity necessary for impregnation (Zaneveld et al. 1985). Its therapeutic index is 100–1000 times higher than that of N9. Many guanidinobenzoates caused significant reductions in fertilization at dose levels that had no spermicidal effects (Kaminski et al. 1985). Tetradecyl sodium sulfate is also an inhibitor of sperm acrosin and hyaluronidase activity (Burck and Zimmermann 1984; Joyce et al. 1979). The antiinflammatory agents phenylbutazone and oxyphenbutazone are inhibitors of hyaluronidase and cyclooxygenase. In relatively low, nonspermicidal doses they prevent fertilization (Joyce and Zaneveld 1985).

RS 37367, a 1-substituted imidazole, caused immediate spermatostasis by generalized stripping of the outer acrosomal membrane. This compound was 50-fold more active than N9 in immobilizing spermatozoa in vitro and in vivo. Extensive washing of the spermatozoa was not able to reverse this effect, in contrast to spermatozoa transiently exposed to N9 (Zaneveld et al. 1984; Vickery et al. 1983).

Another compound, ORF 13904, was tested in vitro and in vivo. It lacks spermicidal properties, yet possesses potent vaginal contraceptive activity by agglutinating the spermatozoa, altering sperm-mucus interaction, and inhibiting acrosin activity (Foldesy et al. 1986; Homm et al. 1985).

Gossypol is a substance isolated from cottonseed oil (Tso and Lee 1982; Ratsula et al. 1983). It inhibits spermatozoal motility by uncoupling the respiratory chain and oxidative phosphorylation. Allitridum, an active principle of garlic, was shown to have spermicidal effects equal to or more than that of gossypol (Qwian et al. 1986). It produced no vaginal irritation reaction or other side effects. It had no bacteriostatic action on the lactic acid bacilli.

Table 9. Novel vaginal contraceptive compounds

1. *p*-Nitrophenyl, *p*-guanidino benzoate (synthetic substance): inhibition of acrosin activity
2. Tetradecyl sodium sulfate: inhibitor of acrosin and hyaluronidase activity
3. Phenylbutazone, oxyphenbutazone
4. RS 37367 (1-substituted imidazole)
5. ORF 13904 (long-chain, sulfonated polystyrene polymer)
   (a) Agglutination of spermatozoa
   (b) Inhibition of acrosin activity
6. Gossypol (isolated from cottonseed oil): inhibition of spermatozoal motility
7. Allitridum
8. Propanolol: inhibition of sperm motility

Table 10. Life table rates for accidental pregnancy at 1-year of use in selected studies (Gao et al. 1986)

Method	Rate
Oral contraceptives	
30 mg levonorgestrel only	9.5
150 mg levonorgestrel, 30 mg ethinylestradiol	3.5
Vaginal ring	
20 mg levonorgestrel per day	3.3
levonorgestrel, ethinylestradiol	1.8
IUD	
Progesterone-releasing	2.4

Propanolol is a potent inhibitor of sperm motility in vitro and in vivo. Daily administration during the cycle resulted in five pregnancies in 198 women, a life table pregnancy rate of 3.4 per 100 women (Zipper et al. 1983). It appeared that sperm motility was inhibited whether intercourse occurred shortly after insertion of the tablet or was delayed up to 10 h. As propanolol is extensively absorbed from the vagina, some systemic actions preventing implantation are possible.

Research on the mechanic vaginal barrier is directed towards disposable, single-sized diaphragms that gradually release N9 over a 24-h period. Custom-fitted cervical caps made of flexible plastic that stay in place through surface tension resulting from contact with a thin film of mucus are currently being studied. Semipermeable material should allow the release of cervical secretion and menstrual blood and at the same time prevent the ascension of spermatozoa. Contraception sponges are to be produced in different sizes, shapes, synthetic materials, and spermicides. Vaginal rings left in place for several days or weeks, which release the spermicide or sperm-immobilizing agent at a constant rate, are under trial.

Vaginal delivery systems have recently been used for female contraceptive hormones. From the vagina the systemic bioavailability is greater than from the gastrointestinal tract. Drugs inserted into the vagina show a smaller first-pass effect than when taken by mouth, since blood from the vagina enters the systemic circulation directly without passing through the liver.

Silastic polysiloxane rings contain a core with either a gestagen alone (Gao et al. 1986; Landgren et al. 1986) or an estrogen-gestagen mixture (Ahren et al. 1983). The gestagen-loaded rings are used successively for 90 days, while the combined estrogen-gestagen rings are inserted at the 7th day and removed after 3 weeks in order to allow menstrual bleeding. Life table rates for accidental pregnancies show that the failure rate is equal to that of comparable oral contraceptives or even lower (Table 10). Vaginal delivery systems remain in place at all times during the period between menses, so that the act of contraception is independent of coitus. They free the user from a daily commitment to contraception. They can be inserted by the user, unlike an intrauterine device. The main advantages of these methods are the steady plasma levels of the hormones and the lacking enterohepatic circulation. Because of this, influences on the renin system, sex hormone-binding globulin, and the lipoprotein pattern may be quite different from those observed in oral hormone users, resulting in higher safety for women usually at risk with oral contraceptives. The main adverse effects are vaginal discharge, reported in 10%–20% of patients, and 40%–60% of the patients experienced expulsion at least once. Of these expulsions, 80% occurred during urination or defecation (Gao et al. 1986). Several women complained of interference with coitus.

In order to overcome these objections to the use of vaginal rings, but with a view to the preservation of the advantages of the vaginal route, daily vaginal administration of normal oral contraceptives containing a progestagen in combination with an estrogen were evaluated. Although the plasma levels were lower than after oral administration at any day in a 21-day treatment cycle, patients did not ovulate. The vaginal pills were completely absorbed after 1–2 h (Coutinho et al. 1984; Souka et al. 1986). They did not even interfere with vaginal treatment for yeast or bacterial infections.

Based on these results, vaginal administration of spermicides, sperm-immobilizing agents, or hormones may become an effective alternative form of contraception.

References

Abrutyn D, McKenzie B, Nadaskay N (1982) Teratology study of intravaginally administered nonoxynol-9-containing contraceptive cream in rats. Fertil Steril 37:113–117

Ahren T, Victor A, Lithell H, Vessby B, Jackanicz TM, Johansson ED (1983) Ovarian function, bleeding control and serum lipoproteins in women using contraceptive vaginal rings releasing five different progestins. Contraception 28:315–327

Asculaii SS, Weiss MT, Rancourt MW, Kupferberg AB (1978) Inactivation of herpes simplex viruses by nonionic surfactants. Antimicrob Agents Chemother 13:686–690

Austin H, Louv WC, Alexander WJ (1984) A case-control study of spermicides and gonorrhea. JAMA 251:2822–2824

Baehler E, Dillon W, Dryia D, Neter E (1983) The effects of prolonged retention of diaphragms on colonization by Staphylococcus aureus of the lower genital tract. Fertil Steril 39:162–166

Bolch OH Jr, Warren JC (1973) In vitro effects of Emko on Neisseria gonorrhoeae and Trichomonas vaginalis. Am J Obstet Gynecol 115:1145–1148

Borko E, McIntyre S, Feldblum P (1985) A comparative clinical trial of the contraceptive sponge and Neo Sampoon tablets. Obstet Gynecol 65:511–515

Bounds W, Guillebaud J (1984) Randomized comparison of the use-effectiveness and patient acceptability of the Collatex (Today) contraceptive sponge and diaphragm. Br J Fam Plann 10:69

Boyd JT, Doll R (1964) Aetiology of carcinoma of the cervix. Br J Cancer 18:419–434

Burck P, Zimmermann R (1984) An intravaginal contraceptive device for the delivery of an acrosin and hyaluronidase inhibitor. Fertil Steril 41:314–318

Buttar HS (1982) Transvaginal absorption and disposition of nonoxynol-9 in gravid rats. Toxicol Lett 13:211–216

Chermann IC (1987) Gutachten bezüglich der Untersuchung einer den Aids-Virus hemmenden Wirkung des Spermizides Benzaltex. Institut Pasteur, Paris

Chow AW, Percival-Smith R, Bartlett KH, Goldring AM, Morrison BJ (1986) Vaginal colonization with E. coli in healthy women. Determination of relative risks by quantitative culture and multivariate statistical analysis. Am J Obstet Gynecol 154:120–126

Chvapil M, Droegemueller W, Owen J, Eskelson C, Betts K (1980 a) Studies on nonoxynol-9. I. The effects on the vaginas of rabbits and rats. Fertil Steril 33:445–450

Chvapil M, Eskelson C, Stiffel V, Owen J, Droegemueller W (1980b) Studies on non-9. II. Intravaginal absorption, distribution, metabolism and excretion in rats and rabbits. Contraception 22:325–339
Chvapil M, Ulreich J, O'Dea K, Betts K, Droegemueller W (1980c) Studies on non-9. III. Effect on fibroblast and spermatozoa. Fertil Steril 33:521–525
Chvapil M, Droegemueller W, Heine MW, MacGregor JC, Potters D (1985) Collagen sponge as a vaginal contraceptive barrier: critical summary of 7 years of research experience. Am J Obstet Gynecol 151:325–329
Coutinho E, da Silva A, Carreira C, Rodrigues V, Goncalves M (1984) Conception control by vaginal administration of pills containing ethinylestradiol and dinorgestrel. Fertil Steril 42:478–481
Davis JP, Chesney PJ, Wand PJ, La Venture M (1980) The investigation and laboratory team: toxic shock syndrome. N Engl J Med 303:1429–1435
Döring GK, Schicketanz R (1986) Über die Zuverlässigkeit des Scheidendiaphragma als kontrazeptive Methode. Geburtshilfe Frauenheilkd 46:33–36
Edelman D, McIntyre S, Harper J (1984) A comparative trial of the Today contraceptive sponge and diaphragm. Am J Obstet Gynecol 150:869–876
Edelman (1986) Collaborative Study
Fihn S, Latham R, Roberts P, Running K, Stamm WE (1985) Association between diaphragm use and urinary tract infection. JAMA 254:240–245
Foldesy R, Homm R, Levinson S, Hahn D, Running K, Stamm W (1986) Multiple actions of a novel contraceptive compound ORF 13904. Fertil Steril 45:550–554
Gao J, Sun HZ, Song GY, Ma LY (1986) Clinical investigation of a low-dose levonorgestrel-releasing vaginal ring. Fertil Steril 46:626–630
Gillespie L (1984) The diaphragm: an accomplice in recurrent urinary tract infections. Urology 24:25–30
Harris RWC, Brinton LA, Cowdell RH, et al. (1980) Characteristics of women with dysplasia or carcinoma in situ of the cervix uteri. Br J Cancer 42:359–369
Hicks D, Martin L, Getchell J, Heath J, Francis D, McDongal J, Curran J, Voeller B (1985) Inactivation of HTLV III/LAV-infected cultures of normal human lymphocytes by nonoxynol-9 in vitro. Lancet 2:1422–1423
Homm R, Foldesy R, Hahn D (1985) ORF 13904 – a new long-acting vaginal contraceptive. Contraception 32:267–274
Janerich DT, Piper JM, Glebatis DM (1980) Oral contraceptives and birth defects. Am J Epidemiol 112:73–79
Jeker P, Mall-Heafeli M (1986) Vaginale Kontrazeption mit Today- und Benzaltex-Tampons. Ther Umsch 43:411–416
Jick H, Walker AM, Rothman KJ, Hunter KR, Holmes LB, Watkins RN, d'Ewart DC, Danford A, Madsen S (1981) Vaginal spermicides and congenital disorders. JAMA 245:1329–1332
Jick H, Shiota K, Shepard T, Hunter JR, Stergachis A, Madsen S, Porter JB (1982) Vaginal spermicides and miscarriage seen primarily in the emergency room. Teratogenesis Carcinog Mutagen 2:205–210
Joyce C, Freud M, Peterson RN (1979) Contraceptive effects of intravaginal application of acrosin and hyaluronidase inhibitors in rabbits. Contraception 19:95
Joyce K, Zaneveld L (1985) Vaginal contraceptive activity of hyaluronidase and cyclooxygenase (prostaglandin synthetase) inhibitors in the rabbit. Fertil Steril 44:426–428
Kaminski J, Nuzzo N, Bauer L, Waller D, Zaneveld L (1985) Vaginal contraceptive activity of aryl-4-guanidinobenzoates. Contraception 32:183–189
Keith L, Berger GS, Moss W (1976) Cervical gonorrhea in women using different methods of contraception. J Am Vener Dis Assoc 3:17–19
Kelaghan J, Rubin GL, Ory HW, Layde PM (1982) Barrier-method contraceptives and pelvic inflammatory disease. JAMA 248:184–187
Kessler II (1976) Human cervical cancer as a veneral disease. Cancer Res 36:783–791
Koch J (1982a) The preventif contraceptive, cervical cap: acceptability aspects and their implications for future cap design. Contraception 25:161–173
Koch J (1982b) The preventif contraceptive cervical cap: a contemporary study of its clinical safety and effectiveness. Contraception 25:135–159

Landgren BM, Aedo AR, Cekan SZ, Diczfalusy E (1986) Pharmacokinetic studies with a vaginal delivery system releasing levonorgestrel at a near zero order rate for one year. Contraception 33:473–485
Lanes SF, Poole C, Dreyer N, Lanza LL (1986) Toxic shock syndrome, contraceptive methods and vaginitis. Am J Obstet Gynecol 154:989–991
Leitch WS (1986) Longevity of Ortho Creme and Gynol II in the contraceptive diaphragm. Contraception 34:381–393
Lemberg E (1984) The vaginal contraceptive sponge (Today). A new nonprescription barrier contraceptive. Nurse Pract 9:24–25
McIntyre SL, Higgins JE (1986) Parity and use-effectiveness with the contraceptive sponge. Am J Obstet Gynecol 155:196–801
Mendez F, Castro A, Ortega A (1986) Use effectiveness of a spermicidal suppository containing benzalkonium chloride. Contraception 34:353–362
Mills J, Reed G, Nugent R, Harley E, Berendes H (1985) Are there adverse effects of periconceptional spermicide use? Fertil Steril 33:442–446
Peddie BA, Bishop V, Bailey RR, McGill H (1984) Relationship between contraceptive method and vaginal flora. Aust NZ J Obstet Gynecol 24:217–218
Percival-Smith R, Bartlett KH, Chow A (1983) Vaginal colonization of Eschericha coli and its relation to contraceptive methods. Contraception 27:497–504
Pratt WF, Mosher WD, Bachrach CA, Horn MC (1984) Understanding U.S. fertility: findings from the National Survey of Family Growth, cycle III. Popul Bull 39:20–24
Quian YX, Shen PJ, Xu RY, Lin GM, Yang HQ, Lu YS, Sun P, Zhang RW, Qi LM, Lu QH (1986) Spermicidal effect in vitro by the active principle of garlic. Contraception 34:295–302
Ratsula K, Haukkamaa M, Wichmann K, Luukainen T (1983) Vaginal contraception with gossypol: a clinical study. Contraception 27:571–576
Reingold A (1986) Toxic shock syndrome and the contraceptive sponge (Today). JAMA 255:242–243
Rosemann DS, Ansell JS, Chapman WH (1984) Sexually transmitted diseases and carcinogenesis. Urol Clin North Am 11:27–43
Rothman K (1982) Spermicide use and down syndrome. Am J Public Health 72:399–401
Saad D, Kirsch R, Kaplan L, Rodwell D (1984) Teratology of intravaginally administered contraceptive jelly containing octoxynol-9 in rats. Teratology 30:25–30
Shapiro S, Slone D, Heinonen OP, Kaufmann DW, Rosenberg L, Mitchell AA, Helmrich SP (1982) Birth defects and vaginal spermicides. JAMA 247:2381–2384
Singh B, Cutler JC, Utidjian HMD (1972) Studies on the development of a vaginal preparation providing both prophylaxis against veneral disease and other genital infections and contraception. Br J Vener Dis 48:57–64
Singh B, Postic B, Cutler JC (1976) Viricidal effect of certain chemical contraceptives on type 2 herpes virus. Am J Obstet Gynecol 126:422–425
Souka AR, el Sokkary H, Kamel M, Hassan M (1986) The effect of vaginal administration of low-dose oral contraceptive tablets on human ovulation. Contraception 33:365–371
Strobino B, Kline J, Lai A, Stein Z, Susser M, Warburton D (1986) Vaginal spermicides and spontaneous abortion of known karyotype. Am J Epidemiol 123:431–442
Syrjanen K, Vayrynen M, Castren O (1984) Sexual behaviour of women with human papilloma-virus (HPV) lesions of the uterine cervix. Br J Vener Dis 60:243–248
Thurner J, Poitscheck C, Kopp W (1983) Der Einfluß von Spermiciden auf die physiologische und pathologische Genitalflora. Wien Med Wochenschr 10:265–268
Tso W-W, Lee C-S (1982) Gossypol uncouppling of respiratory chain and oxidative phosphorylation in ejaculated boar spermatozoa. Contraception 25:649–655
Vaughan B, Trussel J, Menken J, Jones EF (1977) Contraceptive failure among married women in the United States 1970–1973. Fam Plann Perspect 9:251
Vessey MP, Doll R, Peto R, Johnson B, Wiggins P (1976) A long-term follow-up study of women using different methods of contraception – an interim report. J Biosoc Sci 8:373–427

Vickery BH, Goodpasture JC, Bergstrom K, Walker KAM, Overstreet JW, Katz DF (1983) Assessment of a new spermicidal agent against ejaculated dog and human spermatozoa in vitro. Fertil Steril 40:231–236

Vorhauer B, Edelman D, North B, Soderstrom R (1984) A review of the safety and effectiveness of the Today-vaginal contraceptive sponge. Siegfried, Zofingen

Watt B, Goldacre MJ, Loudon N (1981) Prevalence of bacteria in the vagina of normal young women. Br J Obstet Gynaecol 88:588–595

Wright NH, Vessey MP, Kenward B, McPherson K, Doll R (1978) Neoplasia and dysplasia of the cervix uteri and contraception: a positive protective effect of the diaphragm. Br J Cancer 38:273–279

Zaneveld LJD, Bruns J, Goodpasture J, Vickery B (1984) Evaluation of the in vitro efficacy of a new vaginal contraceptive agent in stumptailed macaques. Fertil Steril 31:455–459

Zaneveld LJD, Kaminski JM, Waller D, Anderson RA, Bauer L (1985) Chemistry, contraceptive activity and toxicology of aryl-guanidinobenzoates: inhibitors of sperm acrosin. In: Runnebaum B, Rabe T, Kiesel L (eds) Future aspects in contraception. MTP Press, Boston, pp 23–29

Zipper J, Wheeler RG, Potts DM, Rivera M (1983) Propranolol as a novel, effective spermicide: preliminary findings. Br Med J 287:1245–1246

New Techniques of Female Sterilisation

G. M. Filshie

Department of Obstetrics and Gynaecology, University Hospital,
Queen's Medical Centre, Nottingham NG 7 2 UH, U.K.

Female sterilisation continues to be a highly effective method of female contraception. Every effort is being made to simplify present methods and to explore new methods which could be even simpler and safer. New developments focus around both non-surgical and surgical techniques. Most of these methods are still in an experimental stage.

Non-surgical Techniques

Tissue Toxins. Non-surgical techniques include the installation of tissue toxins into the uterus and also into the lumen of the fallopian tubes. These tissue toxins attempt to ablate the endometrium and endosalpinx, the end result of which is to produce blocked fallopian tubes and to inactivate the endometrium. Such tissue toxins, so far tried, include formaldehyde, phenol, tetracycline and phenolmucilage. Of these tissue toxins quinacrine has been extensively investigated and has been instilled into the uterine cavity as a solution, as a solid attached to the upper part of an intrauterine contraceptive device or as pellets instilled through the cervix. The latter seems to be the most practical. On the first application 75% of patients may expect to be rendered sterile. Repeated applications at monthly intervals are therefore necessary. After three applications approximately 98% of fallopian tubes may be blocked. A hysterosalpingogram is necessary to confirm the success of the procedure. Repeated visits to the hospital, repeated hysterosalpingogram and re-application of the tissue toxins have made the procedure less popular. Phenolmucilage also needs repeated application. Further testing of these tissue toxins will be necessary to establish a more acceptable delivery system.

Tissue Adhesives. Methylcyanoacrylate (MCA), a tissue glue, has been used to ablate the lumen of fallopian tubes. A carefully designed applicator which administers a metered amount of MCA (0.6 ml) is available under the name of Femcept. After two applications nearly 98% of tubes become blocked. A post-operative hysterosalpingogram or Rubin test is necessary to confirm the successful blockage of the fallopian tubes. Both tissue adhesives and tissue toxins sverely damage the lining of salpinx and endometrium. Reversibility is therefore impossible after such a procedure. The method is therefore unsuitable for young patients and patients of low parity.

Female Contraception
Eds.: B. Runnebaum, T. Rabe, L. Kiesel

Hysteroscopic Techniques

Cornual Cautery. The interstitial part of the fallopian tube may be cauterised by electro-coagulation or cold-coagulation (cryocautery). Although these methods are relatively easy to perform, they both have a significant failure rate, which renders them so far unacceptable. There are also an unusually large number of complications with electrical cautery, as bowel burns have been noted, as have ectopic pregnancies.

Tubal Plug Devices. There has been an assortment of tubal plug devices including ceramic plugs, silicone rubber plugs, titanium/silicone rubber plugs, stainless steel plugs and more recently a hydrogenic plug (P-Block) from Sweden. These are inserted hysteroscopically through the ostea so that it can set and form an intratubal device is very appealing, but, once again, the results of this method have not come up to expectations, particularly when considering the potential reversibility of these methods.

New Surgical Techniques: The Filshie Clip

In the mid-1970s laparoscopic tubal diathermy – usually unipolar cautery – achieved much publicity, and this method became widely accepted. As more and more women were sterilised, more and more complications were noted. The more serious complications, namely bowel burns resulting in faecalant peritonitis, and some deaths promoted a relook at the method. A rationalisation to bipolar techniques took place which reduced but did not eliminate these serious complications of bowel burns. A further safety precaution was to introduce endo-coagulation: a method of using electrical cautery having a maximum temperature of 120°–130 °C.

In an attempt to eliminate complications of cautery altogether, mechanical methods of sterilisation were developed. The Yoon ring was developed, as was the Hulka clip, following on from the Weck clip. These two methods became established. The high initial failure rate and difficulties encounted using instrumentation led to the introduction of a new method of tubal occlusion using a clip made from titanium and silicone rubber: the Filshie clip.

Original research on this was started in 1974 using prototypes in pigs. A year later smaller prototypes were used in humans. The principle was to line a malleable metal (e.g., an enlarged Weck clip) with silicone rubber. When it is placed over the fallopian tube both the rubber and the silicone are compressed. As the tube undergoes a vascular necrosis, it shrinks, the dead space being taken up by the compressed rubber. During the experimental period many prototypes were tested until the final model emerged. It was tested in 1980 and became generally available in 1981. The final model is 4 mm wide, 3.5 mm broad and 14 mm long. It has a hinge at one end and may be opened and partially closed many times before final application.

The clip may be applied by mini-laparotomy, by laparoscopy or at the time of caesarean section. There are a number of applicators available depending on the circumstances. A "mini gun" is available for mini-laparotomies or for application of the clip at caesarean section. A double puncture applicator is available for use with any type of diagnostic laparoscope. There are three different types of applicators for use with single puncture operating laparoscopes. There is an 8 mm diameter applicator for an 8 mm channel operating laparoscope, a 7.4 mm diameter applicator for the Storz Universal operating laparoscope and a 5 mm diameter applicator for any operating laparoscope with a 6 mm operating channel. This last applicator must be assembled within the laparoscope prior to use. The clip can be applied using local or general anaesthetic techniques.

The instrumentation is relatively easy to use, and where the clip is applied correctly, there is a low failure rate. However, some studies have shown a high failure rate, and others have shown a very low failure rate.

Because the Filshie clip has an apparently low method failure rate with a variable operator failure rate, careful teaching programmes can be recommended and implemented. The clip should be placed 1–2 cm from the cornu on the isthmic portion of the fallopian tube. The clip should be inspected to check that it is totally occluding the tube. If there is any doubt as to the placement of the clip on the tube, a second clip should be applied. Should the rare event be encountered that the tube is too large for the clip, another method of tubal occlusion should be adopted.

In a personal series conducted by the author on 269 patients no failures were encountered; these patients were operated on under local anaesthesia. An interim report from Family Health International, who are conducting a multi-centre comparative study in 15 countries and 33 centres, so far has results on 1858 patients who had the operation performed as an interval procedure with follow-up over 8819 months. So far two failures have been reported, making a cumulative life table pregnancy rate at 1 year of 0.1 and a Pearl rate of 0.27. Of 503 patients clipped post-partum, there have been three pregnancies, giving a cumulative life table pregnancy rate at 1 year of 0.9 and a Pearl rate of 0.82. Of the three failures two were noted to be operator-related failures. Major complications so far reported have not been significant. Minor problems encountered include the closing of the clip prior to application and dropping the clip into the peritoneum. Placing a second clip on the tube is also noted in 5%–7% of cases. Abdominal discomfort following the operation was noted but was not regarded as an important problem.

A number of reversals of the procedure have been performed, and approximately 80% of patients have become pregnant after the operation. This method appears to be satisfactory in virtually all cases of sterilisation but is particularly suitable for young patients with low parity.

Recent Experience with the Cervical Cap in the United States

R. Chalker

Ballantine Books, Publicity Department, 201 East 50th Street, New York, N.Y. 10022, USA

The cervical cap is a barrier method of birth control similar to the diaphragm, but far superior in several respects: it can be left in place for several days, or even a week at a time, does not require the repeated application of spermicide and cannot be felt by the woman once it is in place. Because the cap is more compact, less messy and easier to use, women have reported an increase in both libido and frequency of sexual activity.

An Historical Note

The invention of the cervical cap has traditionally been attributed to German gynecologist Friedrich A. Wilde, but this supposition remains controversial. In 1838 Wilde [1] described the method for making plaster casts of the cervix and custom-fit cervical caps but does not specifically name himself as inventor. No other contemporary account has come to light. In the 1840s or 1860s an American cap also appears to have been invented by E. B. Foote, an activist physician, but documentation of this invention is apparently lost. Foote [2] reports that his application to a patent was denied – on the grounds that the device could be used for obscene purposes. Consequently, he claims, his device was widely counterfeited; poor copies were made and the public lost interest in it.

Emma Goldman [3] and later Margaret Sanger [4] brought other cervical caps to the United States as they sought to make contraception a public issue. English activist Marie Stopes found the cervical cap to be superior to the diaphragm and had one especially designed for use in her clinic. As much as anything it was Sanger's personal preference for the diaphragm, perhaps acquired on a visit to the Netherlands, where the diaphragm appears to have been universally provided, which did the cap in the United States. Sanger promoted the domestic manufacture of the diaphragm, leaving practitioners who wished to provide caps dependent upon foreign supply. However, Sanger never repudiated the cap and apparently felt that it had a definite place in the birth control armamentarium [5]. By the early 1960s, when the contraceptive pill and the IUD appeared on the scene, cervical cap use had all but died out. Hans Lehfeldt, a New York gynecologist who fitted caps in Germany in the 1920s and 1930s, may have been the only physician in the United States who was still providing cervical caps.

Today, there are only five cervical caps manufactured commercially. Lamberts of London produces three types of caps: the Prentif cavity rim, the most widely used cervical cap and the only one considered for approval by the United

Female Contraception
Eds.: B. Runnebaum, T. Rabe, L. Kiesel

States Food and Drug Administration (FDA); the Dumas, which looks like a diaphragm but has no spring rim and stays in place by suction; and the Vimule, a bell-shaped cap. Two hard plastic caps are manufactured in the Federal Republic of Germany: the KaWe, made by Kirchner and Wilhelm of Stuttgart, and the Contracon, made by Schweitzer of Berlin.

The Cervical Cap Renaissance

In response to the deepening birth control crisis, interest in the cervical cap appears to have sprung up spontaneously in several different quarters. Feminist author Barbara Seaman [6] concluded a chapter in *Women and the Crisis in Sex Hormones*, saying, "If the diaphragm is the Queen of birth control, then the cervical cap is the Anastasia, or lost Princess." Irene Snair, a nurse practitioner in New Hampshire and James Koch, a Boston gynecologist, were the first practitioners in the United States to provide caps in 1977. Because of the work of the New Hampshire Feminist Health Center interest soon spread to other practitioners and to a nationwide network of feminist clinics.

In 1980 the FDA regulated the cap and mandated a $2-million study [7] comparing the cervical cap to the diaphragm. During the 5-year study period nearly 100 practitioners provided the cap to clients under Investigational Device Exemptions (IDEs). The results of these studies and the commonalities and diversity of their experience is reviewed thoroughly in *The Complete Cervical Cap Guide* [5].

Before the cervical cap was regulated an estimated 10000 women received cervical caps (estimate by the New Hampshire Feminist Health Center), and during the 6-year study period more than 30000 caps were dispensed by IDE holders. Although there were few exclusionary requirements imposed by the cap investigators, most of the women who sought cervical caps were 25- to 35-year-old, white, middle-class "refugees" from the pill and IUD or women who disliked the diaphragm.

Results of Cervical Cap Studies in the United States

A survey of cervical cap investigators reveals the following trends in cap use: (a) Women overwhelmingly preferred the cap to the diaphragm. (b) The time of continuous wear ranged from 8 h to 1 week, but the average length of wear was 12–48 h. (c) A high percentage of women in almost all studies used spermicide consistently, although a few women in most studies said they used it inconsistently or not at all; half the women in one study [8] did not use spermicide.

Cap Fitting

Cervical cap pioneers in the United States quickly realized that there is far more to a cap fitting than to the standard diaphragm visit. There are considerably more variables in a cap's fit, and judgements tend to be far more subjective than those required in fitting a diaphragm. A woman must be motivated to use the cap and must be highly involved in her fitting session. Both fitting and training, which can be done separately or simultaneously, require more time and attention from the practitioner.

Cervical cap investigators in the United States are overwhelmingly in agreement that the cap visit should offer a woman an opportunity to see her cervix with the aid of a light and a mirror and speculum and to locate it manually. This direct visualization appears to be essential to proper placement of the cap on the cervix.

In the United States there is considerable variation in criteria for cap fitting. Some providers fit 95% of women who ask for caps, while others fit as few as 30% –50%; most, however, fit 80%–85%. By far the most frequently fitted size is the Prentif 22-mm cap; a minority of practitioners, however, fit primarily the 28-mm cap. Those who fit primarily the 22-mm size seldom fit the 31-mm cap, the largest size, while those who tend to fit a high proportion of 28-mm caps also fit some 31-mm caps.

There seems to be a general consensus among experienced cap practitioners that an ideally fit Prentif cavity rim cervical cap should entirely cover the cervix, with its rim tucked snugly and evenly into the fornix; this provides good suction and cannot easily be dislodged. Eliot, who directed a multicenter cap study in the Midwest of the United States, has suggested that in addition to a secure fit new cap users need to be given confidence that the cap will work for them. Eliot [9] found, in fact, that confidence in the cap was the single strongest predictor in cap acceptance and continuation.

The most frequently cited contraindications to cap use have been the following: (a) history of toxic shock syndrome (TSS), (b) in utero exposure to diethylstilbestrol, (c) current or history of pelvic inflammatory disease (PID), (d) unresolved abnormal Pap smear, (e) poor fit, and (f) discomfort in touching genitals.

Effectiveness

In the FDA-mandated study [7] the cervical cap was found to be as effective as the diaphragm. Twelve-month cumulative pregnancy rates by the life table method were 11.7 for the cap, compared to 12.6 for the diaphragm (user failures). The cap had 6.4 method failures compared to 4.6 for the diaphragm. Combined failure rates were 17.4 for the cap and 16.7 for the diaphragm. Almost all other cervical cap investigators have reported failure rates within this range.

Problems

Cervical cap users report a few problems which are, for the most part, similar to those encountered with the diaphragm. A small percentage of women in each study experienced initial difficulties with insertion and removal (more with removal than with insertion), but less than 5% discontinued the cap for this reason. Positive support and encouragement from practitioners is the surest cure for this problem.

Although odor either with or without infection has been reported by diaphragm users, this problem appears to be far more prevalent among cap users. Bernstein identified a number of anaerobic bacteria that may grow inside caps left in place for longer periods of time and noted, along with several other practitioners, an "odor threshold" at about 3 days of continuous cap wear. Cultures may be taken to identify the specific types of pathogens present, but the simplest solution to odor problems is shorter periods of cap wear. Women who have frequent intercourse may have two or three caps and rotate their use. Many women have successfully cleaned them, using a number of natural substances, such as lemon juice, or household products such as bleach or alcohol.

A few women experience dislodgement during intercourse and some also find that the cap may come off during strenuous activity or during a strong bowel movement. Many practitioners require a woman to return for a refit session if more than one or two unexplained dislodgements occur. Several investigators have noted that dislodgements occur most often in the early months of use, but a well-fitted cap should not become dislodged during intercourse or otherwise.

A small percentage of women and their partners have reported experiencing discomfort during sex while the cervical cap is in place. A few women find that the rim of the Prentif cap is pushed against the vaginal walls during vigorous sex and may be uncomfortable or actually hurts. Between 5% and 15% of male partners say that they can feel the cap in place, but generally this is simply an "awareness that the cap is there." A few men, however, find that the cap interferes with the enjoyment of sex or causes pain. Some couples have solved their problem by experimenting with sexual positions or switching to different type of cap such as the Dumas or the Vimule.

Impact on Sexuality

Very early in the cervical cap renaissance in the United States Koch [10] reported an increase in both libido and frequency of sexual activity among the women in his study. In fact, this phenomenon was a recurrent theme among cap users. Many cap users reported that use of the cap enhances sexual spontaneity, and because it is less intrusive, promotes greater relaxation and enjoyment of sex.

Unlike the diaphragm, the cervical cap does not cover the roof of the vagina and therefore leaves the urethral sponge uncovered. This spongey structure surrounds and protects the urethra, fills with blood and becomes erect during sexual response, and perhaps acts as a back-up in preventing the flow of urine. This structure, identified and named by the Federation of Feminist Women's Health Centers [11] has also been identified as the locus of the "G spot" [12].

The Cervical Cap and AIDS

At this time it is not known how AIDS is transmitted vaginally. No studies have been done on the major types of vaginal secretions – with the exception of menstrual blood – to see whether differences exist. Menstrual blood is a known carrier of the AIDS virus. In this case, a cervical cap worn during intercourse could protect a woman's partner from exposure. Because of the remote risk of TSS the cap should be removed promptly after 6–8 h. When using the cap, the virus-bearing blood would mix with nonoxynol-9 in the cap dome. The diaphragm offers similar protection, but more because of the nonoxynol in the dome rather than because it provides a physical barrier.

The condom is the best known protection against AIDS during intercourse, but the rate of breakage has been estimated to be as high as 20%. In general, a back-up to condoms is desirable whenever possible, and both the cervical cap and the diaphragm may offer some protection to men from exposure to menstrual blood.

The issue as to whether or not AIDS virus-bearing semen is absorbed through the vaginal walls is difficult to resolve and is likely to remain controversial for a long time. If it is readily absorbed, the condom represents a woman's best protection against AIDS during intercourse. If it is not, both the cervical cap and the diaphragm offer some protection: men may be protected from infected menstrual blood and virus-bearing sperm may be prevented from entering a woman's body through the cervical canal.

Is the Cervical Cap the Wave of the Future?

In spite of dramatic breakthroughs in contraceptive technology, we are in the midst of a profound and enduring birth control crisis. Women and their partners are resorting to surgical sterilization in record numbers and many pill and IUD users discontinue each year because of unwanted physical effects and fears about infertility. The pill, which has been the method of choice among family planning providers and population control advocates, may no longer be appropriate for certain groups at risk of AIDS. In these cases barriers may be the only appropriate option. Pills, IUDs, and sterilization appear to offer no protection against the sperm- and blood-borne AIDS virus.

In the United States, at least, the legal climate – with prohibitively high malpractice premiums and astronomical liability awards – have effectively stifled contraceptive research. Furthermore, the FDA has designated all new contraceptive devices as well as old devices with "new" uses as "significant risk" devices, placing all new candidates – including the cervical cap – in the category with heart pacemakers, joint replacements, and other implantable devices. The significant risk cited by the FDA Advisory Committee, which met in November 1977, is *pregnancy*.

Given the current legal and regulatory climate, women, their partners, and practitioners may well be forced to take a hard look at existing low-risk birth control alternatives.

Approval of the Prentif cavity rim cervical cap by the FDA is bound to attract a good deal of media attention and may have the effect of stimulating cervical cap research. Already some work is underway. Koch has patented two new cap models and plans to begin human trials shortly. The Contracap, a custom-fit device which has been under development in Chicago for the past 12 years, may soon begin trials in the People's Republic of China. And Lamberts, the manufacturer of the Prentif, Dumas, and Vimule caps, may decide to promote its products more vigorously.

The cap designs currently produced by Lamberts are at least 30 or 40 years old and do not vary greatly from much earlier models. Certainly modern research, which can send people to the moon and can almost literally make angels dance on the head of a pin, can design a device that will be unobtrusive, as easy to insert and remove as contact lenses, will fit almost all women, and, above all, be highly effective.

References

1. Wilde FA (1838) Das weibliche Gebärunvermögen. Berlin
2. Foote EB (1875) A step backward. Murray Hill, New York
3. Goldman E (Undated) Why the poor should not have many children (pamphlet)
4. Sanger M (1914) Family limitation, 5th edn. Privately printed
5. Chalker R (1987) The complete cervical cap guide. Harper and Row, New York
6. Seaman B, Seaman G (1987) Women and the crisis in sex hormones. Bantam, New York
7. Bernstein GS, et al. (1987) Final report: use-effectiveness study of cervical caps. July 1, 1981 to Mar. 31, 1986 (contract no NO1-hd-1-2804). Contraceptive Development Branch, Center for Population Research, National Institute of Child Health and Human Development, National Institutes of Health, Bethesda
8. Stein L (1986) Third Annual Progress Report to U.S. Food and Drug Administration. Alternative Health Center, Seattle
9. Eliot J, Anderson L, Bernstein S (1985) Progress, report on a study of the cervical cap. J Reprod Med 30(10)
10. Koch JP (1982) Prèntif contraceptive cervical cap: a contemporary study of its clinical safety and effectiveness. Contraception 25(2)
11. The Federation of Feminist Women's Health Centers (1981) A new view of a woman's body. Simon and Schuster, New York
12. Ladas AK, Wipple B, Perry JD (1982) The G spot. Holt, Rinehart and Winston, New York

Aryl 4-Guanidinobenzoates: Potential Vaginal Contraceptives*

L. J. D. Zaneveld[1], J. M. Kaminski[2], D. P. Waller[2], J. Quigg[2], R. A. Anderson[2], S. R. Mack[2], and L. Bauer[2]

[1] Department of Obstetrics and Gynecology and Department of Biochemistry, Rush University, Rush-Presbyterian-St. Luke's Medical Center, Chicago, Illinois, USA
[2] Department of Pharmacodynamics and Department of Medicinal Chemistry, College of Pharmacy, University of Illinois at Chicago, Chicago, Illinois, USA

Introduction

A significant amount of evidence supports the use of sperm enzyme inhibitors as contraceptive agents [1, 2]. Of particular interest are inhibitors of the acrosomal enzyme acrosin. Numerous animal investigations have shown that acrosin is essential for fertilization [2]. The same appears to be true for the human. Infertile men are known to possess 2–3 times lower acrosin levels than asymptomatic men [3, 4]. Procedures known to reduce the fertilizing capacity of spermatozoa, such as sperm banking (cryopreservation), also reduce sperm acrosin levels, even in cases where sperm motility is retained [5, 6]. Finally, sperm acrosomal abnormalities are known to be associated with male infertility [7]. Thus, inhibition of sperm acrosin should lead to infertility. Indeed, a large number of animal studies have shown that acrosin inhibitors prevent fertilization whether they are administered vaginally, into the uterus, or intraperitoneally [1, 2]. Several different types of acrosin inhibitors have been evaluated for their vaginal contraceptive use [1, 2, 8–12], but the aryl 4-guanidinobenzoates are the most potent inhibitors of acrosin, and several may have clinical application. The following summarizes the data obtained with these aryl 4-guanidinobenzoates by our laboratories [2, 13–33, and unpublished results].

Synthesis and Biochemical Properties

Twenty-seven aryl 4-guanidinobenzoates have been synthesized, including nine that possess phenols currently marketed for human use. Such marketed phenols include, among others, acetaminophen (AGB), ethylparaben (EGB), and methylsalicylate (MSGB). Guanidinobenzoic acid is also relatively nontoxic. Thus, it was felt that the combination of guanidinobenzoic acid and a marketed phenol should lead to a relatively nontoxic and clinically acceptable agent. This, indeed, appears to be the case (see further). The results summarized in this chapter primarily describe the studies done with the guanidinobenzoic-acid derivatives containing the marketed phenols.

The nine synthesized aryl 4-guanidinobenzoates containing marketed phenols and a tenth, the methylumbelliferone (MUGB) derivative, which was purchased, were found to be potent inhibitors of human acrosin with I_{50} values ranging from

* This research was supported by PARFR-338 (AID) and by NIH HD 19555.

Female Contraception
Eds.: B. Runnebaum, T. Rabe, L. Kiesel

3×10^{-7} to 7×10^{-10} M. The compounds form pseudoirreversible complexes with human acrosin. The K_{app} of selected aryl guanidinobenzoates ranges from 10^{-8} to 10^{-9} M and the k_2 (acylation constant) is about 10^{-2} s. The acrosin-aryl 4-guanidinobenzoate complex dissociates only after extensive dialysis at pH 3.0 over a 2-day period with frequent changes of dialysate (each time 1000-fold the volume of the dialyzed material). Therefore, no dissociation of acrosin and inhibitor will occur during the period that the sperm are in the vagina (approximately 6 h). Once the sperm enter the cervical mucus and the uterus, the pH of the surrounding medium changes to about 7, which prevents dissociation. These data imply that acrosin will remain tightly bound to inhibitor while the sperm are in the female genital tract, even if the sperm remain stored for 4 days or longer in the cervical mucus or uterus. The contraceptive studies in animal models support this.

Treatment of whole human semen with selected aryl 4-guanidinobenzoates, the guanidinobenzoate derivatives containing AGB, EGB, MSGB, and MUGB, for less than 2 min inhibited sperm acrosin in a dose-dependent manner. The ED_{50} values of the agents ranged from 5×10^{-5} to 6×10^{-7} M. Thus, the aryl 4-guanidinobenzoates react extremely quickly with human spermatozoa at very low concentrations even when added to the ejaculate. This is essential, because at midcycle spermatozoa may rapidly enter cervical mucus.

In order to determine how tightly the aryl 4-guanidinobenzoates bind to human spermatozoa, whole human semen was treated with AGB, MSGB, EGB, or MUGB (at the concentrations described above) for maximally 2 min and immediately washed by centrifugation over Ficoll. Free aryl guanidinobenzoate will not pass through the Ficoll. The acrosin on the spermatozoa remained inhibited, showing that the aryl 4-guanidinobenzoates cannot be washed away from the spermatozoa. This is important because the spermatozoa are in essence washed when they enter cervical mucus because seminal plasma does not enter the mucus.

Recent studies further indicate that AGB inhibits not only acrosin but also the activation of proacrosin to acrosin. Proacrosin is the inactive form of acrosin that is present on spermatozoa.

Antifertility/Contraceptive Properties

Selected aryl 4-guanidinobenzoates were tested for their ability to prevent in vitro fertilization using: (a) mouse gametes, and (b) the human sperm-zona free hamster oocyte penetration assay ("humster test"). At very low inhibitor concentrations (10^{-4}–10^{-6} M) penetration was prevented in the humster test. At even lower concentrations fertilization was inhibited in the mouse in vitro fertilization system (the I_{50} was approximately 10^{-8} M). The antifertility activity of the inhibitors was shown to parallel their acrosin inhibitory activity. The lower amounts required for antifertility activity in the mouse system is not surprising since the mouse eggs possessed a zona pellucida, whereas this layer was removed from the hamster egg. The latter test primarily indicates the ability of human spermatozoa to undergo capacitation, the acrosome reaction, and to fuse with investment-free (denuded) oocytes. Acrosin may be particularly important for the penetration of spermatozoa through the zona pellucida of the egg, although this enzyme is also involved in the acrosome reaction. Thus, it can be expected that even lower concentrations of the inhibitor than those observed for the humster test will inhibit fertilization of zona-intact human eggs by human spermatozoa.

In order to verify that aryl 4-guanidinobenzoates can prevent the acrosome reaction, the effect of an aryl 4-guanidinobenzoate (the nitrophenyl derivative) on the guinea pig acrosome reaction was studied. The guinea pig was used because the acrosome reaction is readily visible in this species. At 10^{-5} M complete inhibition of the acrosome reaction occurred.

Nonoxynol-9 immobilized all human spermatozoa at 257 μg/ml in the Sander-Cramer assay (30-s incubation). No antimotility effect was observed at nonoxynol-9 concentrations below 5.1 μg/ml. For MUGB, EGB, and AGB complete immobilization and no immobilization were obtained, respectively, at 213 and 71 μg/ml, 228 and 30 μg/ml, 1460 and 146 μg/ml. These results show that the aryl guanidinobenzoates also have antimotility properties. However, the primary mechanism of contraception will remain their acrosin inhibitory activity.

Comparative rabbit vaginal contraceptives studies were performed with all nine derivatives containing marketed phenols, as well as with nonoxynol-9. Low concentrations (100 μg/ml) of the aryl 4-guanidinobenzoates were used which did not effect sperm motility. Two milliliters (200 μg/rabbit) were applied. Seven of the nine aryl guanidinobenzoates greatly depressed fertility (the percent fertilization with these agents varied from 0.5% to 33%, as compared with 85% to 90% in the controls). The most potent inhibitors, AGB, EGB, and MSGB, depressed fertility to 6%, 0.5% and 7%, respectively. By contrast, much higher concentrations of nonoxynol-9 (2000 μg and 20000 μg per rabbit) were required to depress fertility to 25% and 17%, respectively. Thus, even at these high doses of nonoxynol-9 the decrease in fertilization did not reach that of the much lower doses of these three aryl 4-guanidinobenzoates. The results with nonoxynol-9 confirm previous data which showed its relatively poor in vivo efficacy [34–38]. Higher concentrations of the aryl 4-guanidinobenzoates should reduce fertility to zero, but such concentrations were not employed since it would not have been possible to differentiate between the acrosin-inhibitory activity of the compounds and their antimotility effect. These results suggest that certain aryl 4-guanidinobenzoates are at least 100 times more potent as vaginal contraceptives than nonoxynol-9.

Vaginal contraceptive experiments in the primate with 4′-nitrophenyl 4-guanidinobenzoate (NPGB) also indicate that low doses of aryl 4-guanidinobenzoate are contraceptive. These studies show that NPGB, even at 100 times lower concentrations than the nonoxynol-9 content in Delfen Vaginal Cream (Ortho), has the same or slightly higher contraceptive potency than Delfen Vaginal Cream.

Toxicity Studies

Acute toxicity (LD_{50}) studies were performed in mice with all the aryl 4-guanidinobenzoates containing marketed phenols and nonoxynol-9. The agents were injected intraperitoneally. Nonoxynol-9 (LD_{50} = 180 mg/kg under the same conditions) was more toxic than any of the aryl guanidinobenzoates. Several aryl guanidinobenzoates, including MSGB, possess LD_{50} values of about 1000 mg/kg with some (including MUGB) having an $LD_{50} > 2000$ mg/kg.

Based on the above contraceptive and acute toxicity studies, four aryl guanidinobenzoates were selected for further study: the guanidinobenzoic acid derivatives of AGB, MSGB, EGB, and MUGB.

The acute toxicity studies were repeated with two of these compounds in mice and rats. The results were similar in both species, with respective LD_{50} values of 829 and 1000 mg/kg for AGB and of 261 and 250 mg/kg for EGB. Based on the acute toxicity evaluations and the rabbit vaginal contraceptive studies it can be calculated that the therapeutic index (toxic dose/contraceptive dose) for these selected aryl guanidinobenzoates is at least 125–500 times higher than the therapeutic index of nonoxynol-9.

The Ames test was performed with all four aryl guanidinobenzoates (MUGB, MSGB, EGB, and AGB), and none showed mutagenicity. A mixture of nonoxynol-9 and one of the aryl guanidinobenzoates was also tested and shown to be nonmutagenic.

Preliminary subchronic vaginal toxicity studies were performed with all four aryl 4-guanidinobenzoates and nonoxynol-9 by applying them for 50 days to the vagina of rats at 100 mg/rat (the highest amount that could be used due to the small vagina of the rat and viscosity of the suspension). None of the animals died in any of the treatment groups. None of the compounds caused a significant increase in organ or tissue pathology, including that of the vagina, as compared to the controls.

These studies were subsequently repeated with AGB under GLP conditions (United States Food and Drug Administration). AGB was applied to rats for 30 days either alone or mixed with nonoxynol-9. Histopathological studies concluded that neither AGB alone or mixed with nonoxynol-9 resulted in any significant changes in any of the organs examined, including the vagina.

Vaginal irritation studies were performed under GLP conditions using the rabbit as animal model. Dose levels were employed that were about 20 times higher than those that are expected to be used (or are being used in case of nonoxynol-9) in the human. The compounds were applied daily for 10 days. During the first series of tests MUGB, AGB, MSGB, and EGB were compared to nonoxynol-9. AGB did not cause any vaginal irritation, i.e., no differences from the control (vehicle-treated) animals were observed. The other aryl 4-guanidinobenzoates did cause some vaginal irritation but none were as severe as nonoxynol-9. EGB was the only inhibitor which approached the irritation observed after nonoxynol-9 administration. Since AGB was the least irritating to the vagina, it was selected for further study. During the second series of tests the observations with AGB were confirmed, and it was further shown that the mixture of nonoxynol-9 and AGB was no more irritating to the vagina than nonoxynol-9 alone.

Development of a Vaginal Delivery System

Saxena at VLI incorporated AGB into the Today sponges. The AGB was pulverized to a very small particle size, mixed with the other components of the Today sponge to get uniform distribution, and the sponges were constructed by the usual VLI process. Nonoxynol-9 was either also incorporated or was omitted. The highest amount of AGB that could be incorporated and uniformly distributed in the sponge was 350 mg.

In vitro testing of the AGB released from the sponge showed that the chemical and biochemical properties of AGB were not altered by the sponge construction. HPLC analysis of the released AGB indicated that it was not hydrolyzed into its subunits. Also, the enzyme-inhibitory and spermicidal properties of AGB were not altered.

To measure the release rate and to roughly mimic "infinite sink" conditions in order to simulate the fact that AGB is probably rapidly removed from the vagina, the sponges were placed in a beaker containing 900 ml of formic acid buffer at pH 4.0 (the approximate pH of the vaginal fluid). The buffer was replaced after 12, 24, 36, 48 h and once daily thereafter for 7 days. The amount of AGB released at each time point was determined by analyzing a sample by HPLC. The amount of AGB released over a 1-day period from the sponge containing 350 mg AGB was 75 mg if the sponge did not contain nonoxynol-9 and 120 mg if the sponge did contain nonoxynol-9. Thereafter, the release rate decreased but significant amounts of AGB were still released after 1 week of incubation.

Stability studies with AGB were performed at pH 4.0, 6.0, and 8.0. At the approximate vaginal pH (pH 4.0) AGB was stable over a 3-month period. It was slightly less stable at pH 6.0 and somewhat more unstable at pH 8.0. Thus, it can be expected that AGB will not destabilize while the sponge is in the vagina.

Summary

Aryl 4-guanidinobenzoates that contain an already marketed phenol have been synthesized and were shown to be potent inhibitors of the sperm enzyme acrosin. These agents also prevent the conversion of proacrosin to acrosin. When mixed with human ejaculates, the aryl 4-guanidinobenzoates rapidly bind to spermatozoa, inhibit acrosin, and cannot be removed from the sperm by washing. These compounds inhibit the in vitro fertilizing capacity of mouse spermatozoa, the guinea pig acrosome reaction, and the penetration of human spermatozoa into zona-free hamster oocytes. Rabbit vaginal contraceptive studies indicate that at least three of the compounds, the AGB, EGB, and MSGB derivatives, are orders of magnitude more potent than nonoxynol-9. These three aryl 4-guanidinobenzoates are also less toxic than nonoxynol-9 and are less irritating to the vagina, particularly AGB. A vaginal delivery system for AGB was developed utilizing the Today sponge. Clinical trials with AGB are planned.

Acknowledgements. The investigators appreciate the manuscript preparation of Ms. Barbara Hartrampf.

References

1. Zaneveld LJD (1976) Sperm enzyme inhibitors as antifertility agents. In: Hafez ESE (ed) Human semen and fertility regulation in men. Mosby, St Louis, p 570
2. Zaneveld LJD (1982) Sperm enzyme inhibitors for vaginal and other contraception. In: Zatuchni GI (ed) Research frontiers in fertility regulation. (PARFR, vol 2/2)
3. Goodpasture JC, Zavos PM, Cohen MR, Zaneveld LJD (1982) Relationship of human sperm acrosin and proacrosin to semen parameters. I. Comparisons between symptomatic men of infertile couples and asymptomatic men, and between different split ejaculates. J Androl 3:151
4. Mohsenian M, Syner FN, Moghissi KS (1982) A study of sperm acrosin in patients with unexplained infertility. Fertil Steril 37:223
5. Goodpasture JC, Zavos PM, Cohen MR, Zaneveld LJD (1981) The acrosin system of human spermatozoa. Effects of various conditions of semen storage. J Reprod Fertil 63:397
6. Jeyendran JS, van der Ven HH, Kennedy W, Perez-Pelaez M, Zaneveld LJD (1984) Comparison of glycerol and a zwitter ion buffer as cryoprotective media for human spermatozoa: motility, hamster oocyte penetration and acrosin/proacrosin levels. J Androl 5:1
7. Jeyendran RS, van der Ven HH, Kennedy WP, Heath E, Perez-Pelaez M, Sobrero AJ, Zaneveld LJD (1985) Acrosomeless sperm: a cause of primary male infertility. Andrologia 17:31
8. Drew JH, Loeffler LJ, Hall IH (1981) Antifertility activity of N-protected glycine activated esters. J Pharm Sci 70:60
9. Hall IH, Drew JH, Sajadi Z, Loeffler LJ (1979) Antifertility and antiproteolytic activity of activated N-carbobenzoxy amino acid ester. J Pharm Sci 68:696
10. Burck PJ, Zimmerman RE (1980) The inhibition of acrosin by sterol-sulphates. J Reprod Fertil 58:121
11. Burck PJ, Thakkar AL, Zimmerman RE (1982) Antifertility action of sterol sulphate in the rabbit. J Reprod Fertil 66:109
12. Zimmerman RE, Nevin RS, Allen DJ, Jones CD, Goetel ME, Burck PJ (1983) Antifertility effects of tetradecyl sodium sulphate in rabbits. J Reprod Fertil 68:257
13. Zaneveld LJD, Beyler SA, Kim DS, Bhattacharyya AK (1979) Acrosin inhibitors as vaginal contraceptives in the primate, and their acute toxicity. Biol Reprod 20:1045
14. Kaminski JM, Bauer L, Zaneveld LJD, Bhattacharyya AK, Nuzzo N, van der Ven HH (1981) Synthesis and evaluation of enzyme inhibitors with contraceptive potency. 19th Annual Meeting of Medicinal Chemistry, Iowa City
15. Van der Ven HH, Bhattacharyya AK, Kaminski J, Binor H, Bauer L, Zaneveld LJD (1981) Inhibition of human sperm capacitation by proteinase inhibitors and a high molecular weight factor from human seminal plasma. Biol Reprod [Suppl 1] 24:38a
16. Kaminski JM, Zaneveld LJD, Bauer L (1982) Aryl 4-guanidinobenzoates as inhibitors of human acrosin. National American Chemical Societies Meeting, Kansas City
17. Beyler SA, Zaneveld LJD (1982) Antifertility activity of systemically administered proteinase (acrosin) inhibitors. Contraception 26:137
18. Kaminski J, Diao X-H (1984) Kinetics of interaction of aryl 4-guanidinobenzoates with human acrosin. Biol Reprod [Suppl 1] 30:137
19. Zaneveld LJD (1985) Sperm enzymes and fertilization: development of acrosin inhibitors as vaginal contraceptives. In: Zatuchni GI (ed) Fertility regulation. Harper and Row, Philadelphia, p 1c (Gynecology and obstetrics, vol 6, sect A)
20. Van der Ven HH, Kaminski J, Bauer L, Zaneveld LJD (1985) Inhibition of human sperm penetration into zona-free hamster oocyts by proteinase inhibitors. Fertil Steril 43:609
21. Kaminski JM, Nuzzo NA, Bauer L, Waller DP, Zaneveld LJD (1985) Vaginal contraceptive activity of aryl 4-guanidinobenzoates (acrosin inhibitors) in rabbits. Contraception 31:183

22. Zaneveld LJD, Kaminski JM, Waller DP, Anderson RA, Bauer L (1985) Chemistry, contraceptive activity and toxicology or aryl guanidinobenzoates: inhibitors of sperm acrosin. In: Runnebaum B, Rabe T, Kiesel L (eds) Future aspects in contraception. MTP Press, Lancaster
23. Kaminski J, Reid DS, Kennedy W, Jeyendran RS, Zaneveld LJD (1985) Effect of aryl 4-guanidinobenzoates on the acrosin activity of whole human spermatozoa. Biol Reprod [Suppl 1] 32:102
24. Burns JW, Kaminski J, Miller IF, Zaneveld LJD (1985) Development of a contraceptive intrauterine releasing device. 38th Annual Conference on Engineering in Medicine and Biology, Chicago
25. Kennedy WP, Reid DS, Kaminski JM, Jeyendran RS, Zaneveld LJD (1985) Development and evaluation of a clinical assay for determination of the acrosin activity of human spermatozoa. 41st Annual Meeting of the American Fertility Society, Chicago
26. Zaneveld LJD, Kaminski JM (1985) Aryl 4-guanidinobenzoates (acrosin inhibitors) for vaginal contraception. 3rd National Congress, Indonesia Society of Andrology, Jakarta
27. Zaneveld LJD, Kaminski J, Waller D, Bauer L (1986) Capacitation and fertilization; Acrosin inhibitors (aryl 4-guanidinobenzoates) as vaginal contraceptives. In: Zatuchni GI, Goldsmith A, Spieler JM, Sciarra JJ (eds) Male contraception: advances and future prospects. Harper and Row, Hagerstown, p 209
28. Nuzzo NA, Anderson RA, Phillips JF, Zaneveld LJD (1986) Role of acrosin in guinea pig sperm capacitation and the acrosome reaction. J Androl 7:22P
29. Kaminski JM, Bauer L, Zaneveld LJD (1986) The development of aryl 4-guanidinobenzoates (acrosin inhibitors) for clinical use as vaginal contraceptive agents. 4th Annual Meeting of the Society for Advancement of Contraception, Chicago
30. Kaminski JM, Bauer L, Mack SR, Anderson RA, Waller DP, Zaneveld LJD (1986) Synthesis, inhibition of human acrosin and trypsin, and acute toxicity of aryl 4-guanidinobenzoates. J Med Chem 29:514
31. Quigg JM, Kaminski J, Waller DP, Zaneveld LJD (1986) Development of a vaginal sponge delivery system for an aryl 4-guanidinobenzoate with and without nonoxynol-9. 4th Annual Meeting of the Society for Advancement of Contraception, Chicago
32. Kaminski JM, Smith D, Reid DS, Kennedy W, Jeyendran RS, Zaneveld LJD (1987) Effect of aryl 4-guanidinobenzoates on the acrosin activity of human spermatozoa. Biol Reprod, (in press)
33. Kaminski JM, Mack SR, Zaneveld LJD (1987) Interaction of aryl 4-guanidinobenzoate (AGB) with human proacrosin. 20th Annual Meeting of the Society for the Study of Reproduction. Urbana
34. Zaneveld LJD, Bhattacharyya AK, Kim DS, Schumacher GFB, Beluhan Z (1977) Primate model for the evaluation of vaginal contraceptives. Am J Obstet Gynecol 129:368
35. Chang MC (1960) Effect of commercial contraceptive jellies placed into the rabbit vagina before mating. Fertil Steril 11:109
36. Homm RE, Doscher GE, Hummel EJ, Greenslade FC (1976) Relative antifertility activity of three vaginal contraceptive products in the rabbit: relationship to in vitro data. Contraception 13:479
37. Newell SD, Polakoski KL, Williams WL (1972) Inhibition of fertilization by proteinase inhibitors. 7th International Congress on Animal Reproduction and Artificial Insemination, Munich
38. Zaneveld LJD, Polakoski KL, Robertson RT, Williams WL (1971) Trypsin inhibitors and fertilization. In: Fritz H, Tschesche H (eds) Proceedings of the first international research conference on proteinase inhibitors. de Gruyter, New York, p 236

New IUD Technology

Intrauterine Devices: Efficacy and Side Effects

T. Rabe, B. Ellwanger, K. Grunwald, L. Kiesel, and B. Runnebaum

Department of Obstetrics and Gynecology, Division of Gynecological Endocrinology, Women's Hospital, University of Heidelberg, Voßstr. 9, 6900 Heidelberg, FRG

Introduction

Despite early methods described in Egypt in 2000 B.C. for contraception in camels, the first known human application of intrauterine contraceptives in terms of vaginal and uterine pins occurred 100 years ago. In Germany the development of intrauterine devices originated with a device developed by Richter in 1909 consisting of a natural silk ring (Fig. 1). Later Gräfenberg (1926) introduced a metal ring consisting of a mixture of brass, bronze, and copper. The development of new IUDs stopped abruptly when multiple pelvic inflammatory diseases and deaths lead to prohibition of this method for contraception. In 1959 intrauterine devices had a renaissance when the original metal ring of the Japanese Ota was replaced by one made out of plastic and the device used by 20000 Japanese women. In 1962 the Gräfenberg ring was admitted to the United States market. The second generation of IUDs are the inert plastic Margulis devices and Dalkon Shield. Since 1970, third-generation copper-containing IUDs have been available, and during recent years progesterone-releasing devices have also become available.

The main hazards for IUD users are disturbances of the menstrual cycle (breakthrough bleeding and spottings), lower abdominal pain, pelvic inflammatory disease, expulsions of the IUD and lower contraceptive safety in comparison to oral hormonal contraceptives. Pelvic infections caused by the Dalkon Shield and insufficient package information led to the withdrawal from the market in the United States of all intrauterine devices except the progesterone-releasing Progestasert.

Intrauterine devices available in the Federal Republic of Germany (except TCu-220C) are shown in Fig. 2; the major characteristics of these IUDs are summarized in Table 1. Before approval of IUDs in the Federal Republic of Germany by the Federal Health Agency (Bundesgesundheitsamt, BGA) in Berlin (West) the regulations of the new drug law (AMG 1976) must be met; for this, evidence of the efficacy, the quality, and harmlessness of the drug must be given. For the period of IUD use (e.g., 3 or 5 years) efficacy must be demonstrated for at least 500–1000 women per year. The following clinical parameters must be considered: expulsion rate, pregnancy rate, bleeding rate, and side effects.

Female Contraception
Eds.: B. Runnebaum, T. Rabe, L. Kiesel

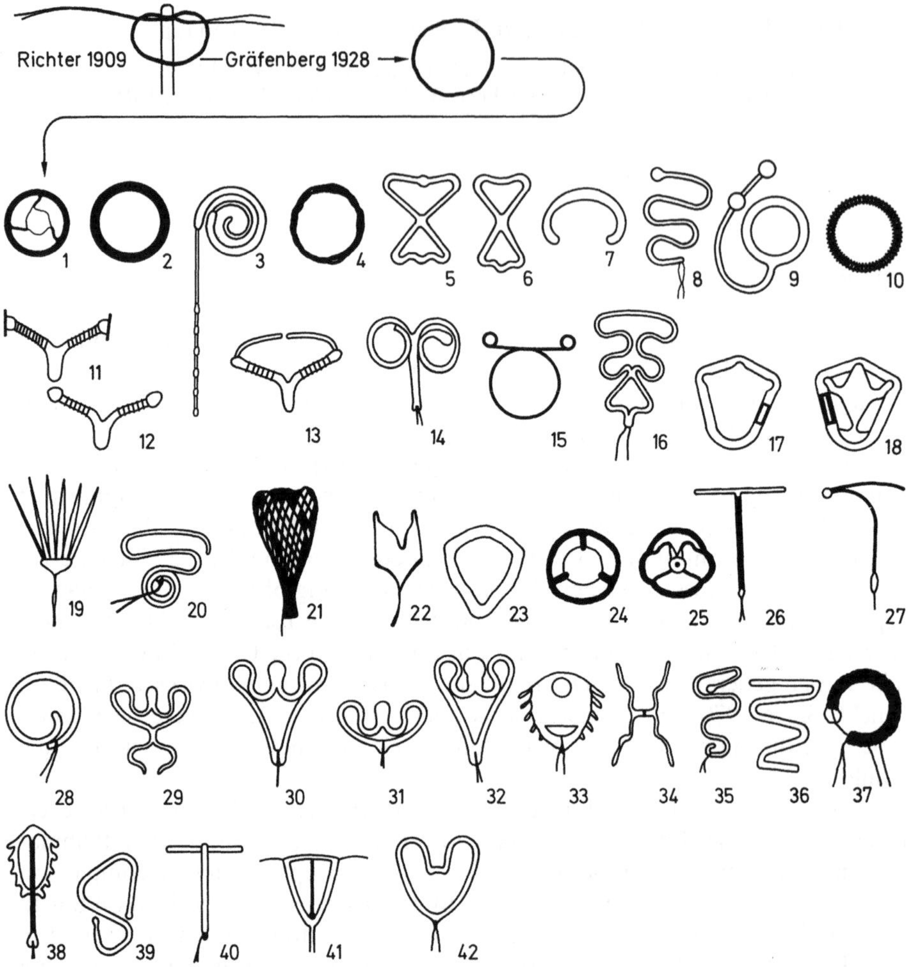

Fig. 1. Intrauterine devices
1 Ota ring (A. Ishihama 1959)
2 Steel ring (H.H. Hall and M.L. Stone 1962)
3 Margulies IUD (L.C. Margulies 1964)
4 Silk ring (K. Fuchs, S. Grünstein, and A. Peretz 1964)
5 Birnberg bow (C. Birnberg and M.S. Burnhill 1964)
6 Birnberg bow (C. Birnberg and M.S. Burnhill 1964)
7 Birnberg bow (C. Birnberg and M.S. Burnhill 1964)
8 Lippes loop (J. Lippes 1965)
9 Comet (J. Schwartz and F.C. Reyner 1966)
10 Intraband (H.H. Hall 1966)
11 Wing IUD (A. Naim and H.M. Hasson 1966)
12 Wing IUD (A. Naim and H.M. Hasson 1966)
13 Wing IUD (A. Naim and H.M. Hasson 1966)
14 Saf-T-coil (R.C. Seymour 1967)
15 Silent protector (H.M. Knoch 1967)
16 Dana Super (J. Sracek 1967)
17 Antigon (M. Osler and P.E. Lebech 1968)
18 Winged Antigon (M. Osler and P.E. Lebech 1972)
19 Solish-Majzlin-Feather (G.I. Solish and G. Majzlin 1968)
20 Coiled loop (S.F. Rifai 1969)
21 Corolle (J. Cohen 1969)
22 M (E. Silbermann, M.L. Stone, and E.B. Connell 1969)
23 Incon (E.B. Leerich, L.L. Doyle, and D.L. Barcley 1969)

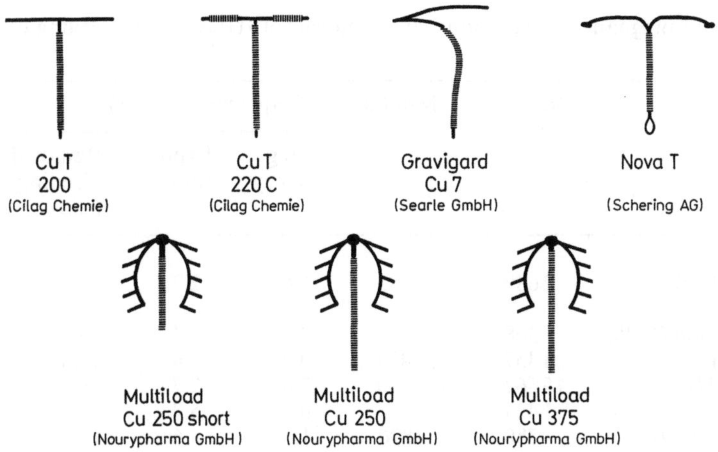

Fig. 2. Intrauterine devices analyzed in this paper

Table 1. Intrauterine devices

FRG brandname	Width (mm)	Length (mm)	Copper weight (mg)	Copper surface (mm^2)	Material	Producer
Gyne T	32	36	100	208	Polyethylene +22% $BaSO_4$	Cilag
Gravigard Kupfer 7	28	36	89	200	Polypropylene	Searl
Minigravigard	22	28		200	Polypropylene	Searl
Kupfer T 200	31	35	115–120	200	Polyethylene	Schering
Kupfer T 375						
Nova-T	30	34	107–141	208+13	Polyethylene	Schering
Multiload Cu 250	18	35		250	Polyethylene	Nourypharma
Short	18	25		250	Polyethylene	
Multiload Cu 375	13	30		375	Polyethylene	

←

24 Japanaise ring (C.L. Armstrong and P.S. Anderson 1969)
25 Yusei ring (Y. Hata, Y. Ishihama, N. Kudo, Y. Nakamura, Z. Miyai, T. Makino, and T. Kagabu 1969)
26 Copper-T (T-Cu 200) (J.A. Zipper, H.J. Tatum, L. Pastena, M. Medel, and M. Rivera 1969)
27 Copper-7 (J.A. Zipper, H.J. Tatum, L. Pastena, M. Medel, and M. Rivera 1969)
28 Open ring (S. Rozin and A. Adoni 1970)
29 OM-GA GBBI (S. Espagno 1970)
30 OM-GA 1 (S. Espagno 1970)
31 OM-GA 2C (S. Espagno 1970)
32 OM-GA 0 (S. Espagno 1970)
33 Dalkon shield (H.J. Davis 1970)
34 Petal or LEM (W.K. Rashbaum and R.C. Wallach 1971)
35 Organon A (F. Subeck, R. Belsky, R. Lardner, W.J. Shack, and P.Y. Tam 1971)
36 Organon B (F. Subeck, R. Belsky, R. Lardner, W.J. Shack, and P.Y. Tam 1971)
37 Spiral loop (N.N.)
38 Multiload (Cu 250) (van Os 1972)
39 Soonawala (H.P. Sonnawala 1972)
40 Biograviplan*
41 Butterfly (H. Massouras 1972)
42 Cairo heart (N.N.)

Table 2. Frequency of pregnancies, expulsions, and removals of IUDs due to bleeding or pain

Author/year	Insertions	Months	Frequency (%/year)[a]		
			Pregnancy	Expulsion	Removal bleeding/ pain
TCu-200					
Timonen and Luukkainen (1974)	2689	29143	1.6	2.2	7.1
Nygren and Johansson (1975)	368		2.7	2.4	6.8
Tejuja et al. (1975)	4357	37429	0.9	7.4	10.8
Jain and Sivin (1977)	15662	121300	2.6	7.7	8.6
Snowden (1977)	1429		0.4	5.7	7.6
Luukkainen et al. (1979)	780	7896	1.8	4.6	11.9
Thiery et al. (1980a, b)	730	7467	1.0	2.7	1.4
Luukkainen et al. (1981)	974	608	1.9	4.2	11.4
Nielsen et al. (1983)	947	26683	2.1	4.6	12.2
Luukkainen et al. (1983)	650	9245	2.2	4.8	13.9
Tatum (1984)	9641	68000	2.6	8.1	9.0
Van der Pas et al. (1983)	230	2451	3.3	4.1	4.9
Zipper (1984)	846	8782	2.1	3.6	1.9
Thiery et al. (1985)	134		3.6	5.3	5.9
Total or mean	39410		2.2	6.8	8.8
TCu-220C					
Goh et al. (1983)	401	4288	0.8	3.0	5.2
Tatum (1984)	86	9439	1.2	3.7	2.7
Van der Pas et al. (1983)	230	2566	1.0	4.0	3.7
Shih et al. (1984)	887	9588	0.3	1.6	3.3
Total or mean	1604		0.6	2.4	3.8
TCu-380Ag					
Shih et al. (1984)	892	9720	0.1	4.3	6.8
Cole et al. (1985)	737	6984	0.3	3.3	3.6
TCu-380A					
Tatum (1984)	3536	57000	1.1	8.5	26.7
Cu-7					
Gibor et al. (1972)	8065	83676	1.4	5.9	8.9
Tejuja et al. (1975)	854	5177	2.4	6.4	10.9
Jain and Sivin (1977)	1831	12289	2.8	15.5	10.0
Snowden (1977)	8098		2.1	11.7	9.4
Jepe et al. (1979)	1439		2.0	5.1	2.7
Goh et al. (1983)	398	3942	3.9	5.7	4.2
Goh et al. (1983)		2095	4.4	6.1	4.5
Zipper (1984)	514	5448	3.7	4.4	2.1
Zipper (1984)	554	5754	2.2	4.8	1.7
Hasson (1985)	239	5364	2.3	2.5	10.6
Total or mean	21992		2.0	8.7	8.4
MLCu-375					
Van Os et al. (1984)	746	7625	0.1	2.1	2.6
Van Os et al. (1984)		5234	0.0	0.5	4.1
Timonen et al. (1982)	324	3380	0.4	9.2	9.9
Thiery et al. (1983)		9536		0.5	

Table 2 (continued)

Author/year	Insertions	Months	Frequency (%/year)[a]		
			Pregnancy	Expulsion	Removal bleeding/pain
Thiery et al. (1983)	455	5234	0.0	0.5	4.1
Van der Pas et al. (1983)	1650	21762	0.4	1.8	5.9
Van der Pas et al. (1983)	456	5245	0.2	0.5	4.1
Van der Pas et al. (1983)	100	1110	0.0	3.1	2.1
Tauber and Nohlen (1985)	281	2756	0.0	2.1	8.8
Thiery et al. (1985)		84411		2.4	
Thiery et al. (1985)		1200	0.4	2.4	5.1
Thiery et al. (1985)	134		0.0	4.7	4.9
Cole (1985)	740		0.8	4.1	3.8
Thiery, unpublished	1979	26423	0.4	2.4	5.1
Total or mean	6865		0.3	2.5	5.1
MLCu-250 (Standard)					
Thiery et al. (1980a)	3729	50380	0.45	2.0	3.6
Thiery et al. (1980b)	664	6805	0.5	1.2	2.3
Van Os (1980)	2782	29669	0.5	2.2	3.7
Van Os (1980)		4907	2.3	0.8	5.7
Thiery et al. (1982)	4412	56213	0.4	1.9	3.4
Thiery et al. (1982)	556	7663	1.3	6.6	6.0
Goh et al. (1983)	400	7808	1.5	2.3	4.3
Goh et al. (1983)	455	4907	2.3	0.8	5.7
Van der Pas et al. (1983)	877	9440	1.2	1.3	5.7
Van der Pas et al. (1983)	456	4970	2.2	0.7	5.6
Van der Pas et al. (1983)	100	1131	0.0	4.1	1.0
Thiery et al. (1985)	136		1.8	3.1	2.4
Total or mean	14567		0.7	2.1	3.8
MLCu-250 (Short)					
Van Os (1984)	813	10132	0.6	3.0	4.9
MLCu-250 (Mini)					
Van Os (1984)	444	4373	0.8	3.6	8.5
Nova T					
Luukkainen et al. (1979)	741	7402	0.7	4.2	10.5
Altmann et al. (1981)	45	527		4.4	
Luukkainen et al. (1981)	907	8790	0.7	5.8	12.3
Timonen et al. (1982)	346	3615	2.0	6.7	9.3
Luukkainen et al. (1983)	918	76260	0.7	5.5	10.8
Nielsen et al. (1984)	918	24947	0.8	5.8	11.9
Tauber and Nohlen (1985)	262	2506	0.8	2.3	8.8
Total or mean	4092		0.8	5.3	11.1
Progestasert					
Alza Corp. (1976)					
Nulliparae	1231	10109	2.5	7.5	12.1
Parae	4264	35739	1.9	3.1	9.7
Mall-Haefeli et al. (1984)					
Nulliparae	1393	11423	2.4	7.9	12.1
Parae	4463	39813	1.8	3.1	9.3

Table 2 (continued)

Author/year	Insertions	Months	Frequency (%/year)[a]		
			Pregnancy	Expulsion	Removal bleeding/pain
Totals and means					
Nulliparae	2624		2.5	7.7	12.1
Parae	8727		1.9	3.1	9.5
Lippes Loop D					
Tietze and Lewit (1970)	3489	31032	3.2	19.1	11.0
Andolesk et al. (1972)	851		2.0	2.8	
Snowden (1977)	4067		1.2	7.4	12.3
Hasson et al. (1985)	122	3301	0.0	5.7	18.2
IFRP (1979)	1417		2.7	14.0	10.0
IFRP (1979)	2502		2.9	11.1	10.0
Snowden (1977)	2082		1.4	5.2	10.1
Tietze and Lewit (1970)	7553	72046	2.7	12.7	11.7
WHO (1979)	894	9725	2.0	8.3	8.2
Total or mean	22126		2.4	11.7	11.1
Lippes Loop C					
Andolesk et al. (1972)	851		2.8	9.8	

[a] Column means respresent means weighted by respective number of insertions.

Methods

In this review cumulative published data obtained from life table analysis of various clinical trials with various IUDs are analyzed with respect to the different types of IUDs. For each study the number of events is calculated, based on the percentage of events reported. The absolute number of events of all studies concerned with the same IUD is summed and the mean cumulative rate is calculated; additionally, the range (lowest and highest incidence) of the event is reported.

Studies will be reviewed here which compare the major side effects of several IUDs, such as pregnancy and expulsion. In addition, the reasons for withdrawals are summarized, e.g. bleeding, pain or wish to become pregnant. The frequency rate of undesired pregnancies, expulsions, and withdrawals because of bleeding and pain after 1 year of IUD use, excerpted from major studies and compiled for each type of IUD are shown in Table 2; studies are listed here in order of the year of publication of the respective study. From these data the weighted mean event rate was taken: frequencies (percent) of the events, multiplied by the number of insertions, added across all studies and divided by the total number of insertions. The advantage of using weighted means lies in the fact that studies with a larger number of cases exert a stronger influence on the evaluation of the respective IUD.

Contraceptive Safety

Mode of Action. Contraceptive safety of IUDs depends on various factors. The size of the IUD plays an important role; contraceptive efficacy can be improved by enlargement of the IUD, although simultaneously the rate of complications increases (i.e., more irregular bleedings and expulsions). Contraceptive safety can be improved by using medicated IUDs, such as those of copper, which do not affect the rate of bleedings and expulsions. Consequently, modern copper IUDs can be designed to be smaller because they have large copper surfaces which provide a high contraceptive safety and a low complication rate. For contraceptive efficacy it is furthermore important that contraceptive action cover even the area of the insertion of the fallopian tubes either mechanically or by drug release (e.g., copper). If the surface of a copper-loaded pessary is encrusted, pregnancy rate increases to that of a nonmedicated IUD.

Pregnancy in IUD Users. A pregnancy may be due to a method failure or to a dislocation of the IUD. In most cases patients became pregnant after an unobserved IUD expulsion. In some cases, however, a pregnancy may occur despite the correct placement of the IUD. If the IUD is dislocated from the uterine cavity into the cervical canal a pregnancy can develop in the fundus uteri without interference. The risk of a spontanous abortion in these cases is particularly high (with an IUD in situ, 50%), although the risk of malformations of the child is not significantly increased. Septic abortions may occur in pregnant patients with an IUD in situ. Therefore the IUD should be removed and a bacteriological screening done. After an IUD removal without complications a termination of the pregnancy is not indicated.

Extrauterine Pregnancies. The rate of extrauterine pregnancies increases significantly with the use of IUDs; consequently, in women with a history of extrauterine pregnancies an IUD should not be used. The mean rate of extrauterine pregnancies for Nova T and TCu-200 was approximately 1.5% (Nielsen et al. 1983).

Pearl Index and Life Table Analysis. The Pearl index for IUDs ranges between 0.5 and 5.0 and is higher than that for oral contraceptives (0.05–0.9). The mean pregnancy rate after the 1st year of use in the studies analyzed in this paper ranged between 0.3% and 2.4%, depending on the type of IUD.

Pregnancy Rates with various IUDs

The cumulative pregnancy rate after 1 year of use is summarized in Fig. 3. In the following the pregnancy rates of the various IUDs are discussed. (Figures in parentheses represent the annual pregnancy rates of the respective year.)

Lippes Loop D. The cumulative pregnancy rate of the Lippes Loop in the 1st year was found to be 2.0%; 4.5% (+2.5%) after the 2nd year; and 5.8% (+1.3%) after the 3rd year (Andolesk 1972). The pregnancy rate in the first 3 years according to this study, ranged from 1.3% to 2.5%. The mean cumulative pregnancy

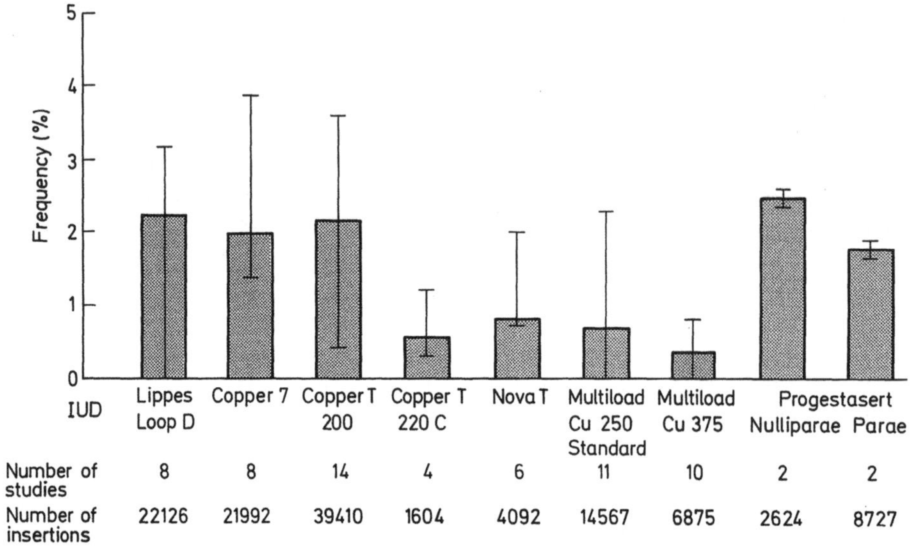

Fig. 3. Pregnancy rate after 1 year of IUD use. Cumulative life table events in patients using intrauterine devices as described in various studies (mean cumulative rate ± range)

rate over all studies after 1 year for the nonmedicated Lippes Loop D (2.4%) is similar to that of copper IUDs as well as that of the progesterone-releasing Progestasert (2.5% for nulliparae and 1.9% for parae).

Nova T. In a comparison trial of TCu-200 and Nova T, Luukkainen et al. (1983) found for Nova T the following cumulative pregnancy rates during the first 5 years: 1st year, 0.8%; 2nd year, 1.8% (+1.0%); 3rd year, 2.7% (+0.9%); 4th and 5th years, 2.9% (+0.2%) and 3.4% (+0.5%), respectively (Luukkainen et al. 1983). Except for the MLCu devices the Nova T had the lowest annual pregnancy rates during the observed 5 years, being lower than 1%. The mean cumulative rate after 1 year of use for all studies was 0.8%.

TCu-200. Under the use of TCu-200 a pregnancy rate of 2.1% was found in the 1st year; 2nd year, 4.8% (+2.7%); 3rd year, 6.5% (+1.7%), 4th year, 7.1% (+0.6%); and 5th year, 8.7% (+1.6%) (Luukkainen et al. 1983). TCu-200 had high pregnancy rates in the first 2 years (2.1%, 2.7%), but the rate decreased in the following years (below 2%). The mean cumulative pregnancy rate over all studies for TCu-200 users in the 1st year was 2.2%.

Cu-7. In a long-term study by Zipper (1984) the cumulative pregnancy rates of Cu-7 IUD users over 5 years were: 3.2% after the 1st year; 4.6% (+1.4%) after the 2nd year; 6.4% (+1.8%) after the 3rd year; 6.7% (+0.3%) after the 4th year; and 9.0% (+2.3%) after the 5th year. With a relatively high rate in the 1st year (3.2%) this fell in the following years to levels between 0.3% and 2.3%. After 1 year of use, over all studies, a mean cumulative rate of 2.0% was found.

TCu-220C. In the 1st year of use the pregnancy rate was found to be 1.2%; 2.8% (+1.6%) after the 2nd year; 4.9% (+2.1%) after the 3rd year; 4.9% (+0.0%) after the 4th year; and 5.2% (+0.3%) after the 5th year (Tatum 1984). The pregnancy rate for Cu T 220 C over 5 years ranged constantly between 0% and 2%. After 1 year of use, over all studies, the mean cumulative pregnancy rate was 0.6%.

MLCu-250. In a 4-year trial with MLCu-250 cumulative pregnancy rates were 0.4% in the 1st year; 1.0% (+0.6%) in the 2nd year; 1.2% (+0.2%) in the 3rd year; and 1.2% (+0.0%) in the 4th year (Thiery et al. 1982). Van der Pas et al. (1983) observed in a study with 100 women over a period of 3 years no pregnancies at all. In another 3-year study with 456 women Van der Pas et al. (1983) reported cumulative annual pregnancy rates of 2.2%, 3.1% (+0.9%) and 3.8% (+0.7%) and 3.8% (+0.7%). Over all studies, the annual pregnancy rate was below 1%, and the mean cumulative pregnancy rate for theMLCu-250 after 1 year was 0.7%.

MLCu-375. In a comparison trial Van der Pas et al. (1983) found pregnancy rates of 0.2% in the 1st year; 0.8% (+0.6%) in the 2nd year; and 1.5% (+0.7%) in the 3rd year of IUD use. In a study with 1979 women the cumulative pregnancy rate went from 0.4% in the 1st year to 2.9% in the 5th year (Thiery et al. 1985, unpublished). MLCu-375 had a low pregnancy rate similar to that of MLCu-250 and reported to be 0.6%–0.7%. The overall mean cumulative pregnancy rate was 0.3% after 1 year.

Progestasert (1 Year Progesterone Dosage). After the 1st year the pregnancy rate under progesterone-containing IUDs was 2.4% in nulliparae and 1.8% in parae. After the 1st year the progestasert was replaced by a new one. In the second year 1.7% of the nulliparae and 1.7% of the parae became pregnant (Mall-Haefeli and Spornitz 1984). Over all studies the cumulative rate for nulliparae after 1 year was 2.5%, for parae 1.9%.

Summary. Copper IUDs give the best results when the uterine bleeding pattern is taken into account. The pregnancy rate depends directly on the copper surface area and secondarily on the size of the IUD. Thus, the lowest pregnancy rate was found for the MLCu-375 (0.3%), which had the largest copper surface area (375 mm^2) followed by the IUD with the second largest copper surface area (MLCu-250; surface 250 mm^2) with a pregnancy rate of 0.7%. Contraceptive safety was correlated with the copper surface for other IUDs: TCu-220C (0.6%), the Nova T (0.8%), the Cu-7 (2.0%), and the TCu-200 (2.2%), in order of ascending pregnancy rate and descending copper surface area. The high pregnancy rate of the Cu-7 and TCu-200 may be due to the small copper surface and its sharp edged design, whereas the pessaries with rounded edges (Nova T) adapt better to the uterine cavity and thus lead to lower pregnancy and expulsion rates.

The highest pregnancy rate was found for unmedicated pessaries, i.e., the Lippes Loop with a pregnancy rate of 2.4%; in order to provide a sufficient contraceptive safety it must have a larger size, which in turn is responsible for the higher complication rate. The cumulative pregnancy rate of 2.5% for nulliparae and 1.9% for parae in Progestasert users is in the range of IUDs with smaller copper surface areas. Over an observation period of 5 years the highest pregnancy rates have been observed in users of the Lippes Loop (1.3%–2.0%) and the Progestasert (1.7% and 2.4%, nulliparae; 1.8% and 1.7%, parae); the TCu-200 had a high rate of pregnancies in the first 2 years (2.1, 2.7) but fell below 2% in the following years. Similarly, the Cu-7 had a high rate in the 1st year (3.2%), with a marked decrease thereafter (below 2%). Low pregnancy rates were found for Nova T, MLCu-250, and MLCu-375 (below 1%).

Side Effects

Patient selection (e.g., no multiple sexual partners, no previous pelvic inflammatory disease), insertion, and the type, size, and medication of IUDs play important roles in contraceptive efficacy and side effects. Pregnancy rate decreases and frequency of complications increases with the size of the IUD. Side effects of all IUDs depend on their acting as a foreign body and, for medicated IUDs, also on their release of several substances.

When inserting an IUD, cervical lesions, bleedings, perforations, pain, and vasovagal reactions such as bradycardia, vomiting and syncopes may occur.

During IUD use the main side effects are bleeding and disturbances of the menstrual cycle (e.g., intermenstrual bleeding, prolonged, enhanced or painful bleeding). In addition, some women complain of other side effects such as crampus-like or diffuse pain in the lower pelvic region. Bleedings occur if the type of IUD does not fit the size of uterus, in cases of improper insertion, or when the body shows a strong reaction to the IUD by contractions of the uterus. Menstrual disorders and pain are the most frequent indications for IUD removal.

Further severe complications are pelvic infections. These are hazardous because they can result in tubal occlusion and subsequent sterility. The incidence of salpingitis depends on several factors, such as hygiene, previous infections, parity (multiparae become sick much more rarely than nulliparae), duration of IUD use, and the number of sexual partners.

Extrauterine pregnancies are more frequent in patients using progesterone-releasing pessaries.

Removal Due to Bleeding or Pain

The cumulative removal rate after 1 year of IUD use due to bleeding or pain is summarized in Fig. 4. In the following, the bleeding rates of the various IUDs are discussed.

Multiloads. The cumulative bleeding rate of MLCu-250 was 5.0% after the 1st year; 7.4% (+2.4%) after the 2nd year; 7.9% (+0.5%) after the 3rd year; and 8.1% (+0.2%) after the 4th year (Thiery et al. 1982). Cumulative removal rates

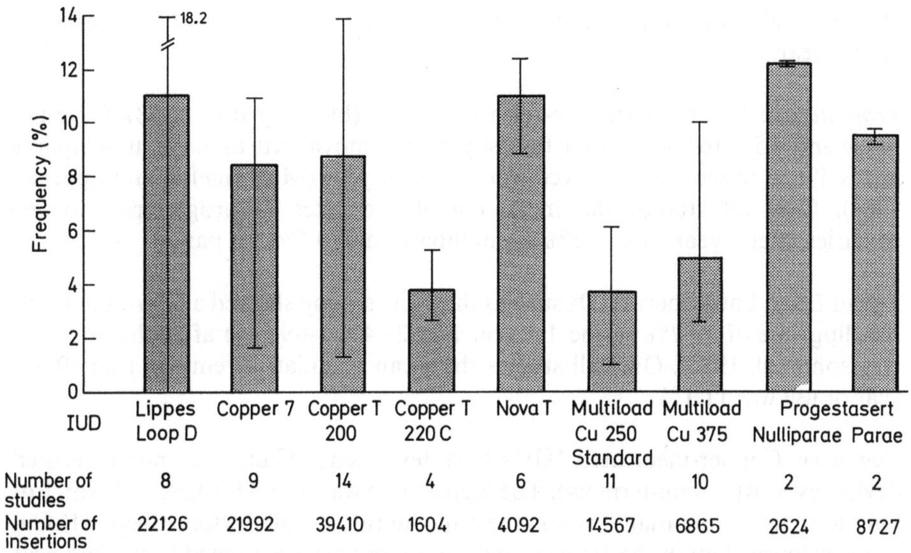

Fig. 4. IUD removal rate after 1 year of use due to pain and/or bleedings. Cumulative life table events in patients using intrauterine devices as described in various studies (mean cumulative rate ± range)

for MLCu-375 were 5.1%, 9.6% (+4.5%), 12.9% (+3.3%) and 17.4% (+4.5%) in 4 years; after 5 years in 20.8% (+3.4%) of the women removal of the IUD was required because of bleeding (Thiery et al. 1985). With the MLCu-375 there was a high removal rate, ranging between 5.1% and 3.3% over 5 years. Though the MLCu-375 had a lower bleeding rate than MLCu-250 in the 1st year, the bleeding rates in the following years remained constantly high, whereas the rates for MLCu-250 after the 2nd year decreased. Over all studies, the mean cumulative rate after 1 year of use was 3.8% for MLCu-250 and 5.1% for MLCu-375.

Cu-7. For Cu-7 the cumulative removal rate due to bleeding was reported at 4.5% after the 1st year and 6.9% (+2.4%) after the 2nd year (Goh et al. 1983). Over all studies, the mean cumulative rate after 1 year of use was 8.4%.

TCu-200. During the first 2 years the cumulative removal rate was found to be 5.4% and 8.0% (+2.6%), respectively, and 12.6% (+4.6%) in the 3rd year (Van der Pas et al. 1983). Over all studies the mean cumulative rate was 8.8% after 1 year of use.

Nova T. During the first 2 years the cumulative removal rate for Nova T remained constant at 8.8% (+0.0%) (Tauber and Nohlen 1985). Over all studies the mean cumulative rate after 1 year was 11.1%.

TCu-220C. The cumulative removal rates for TCu-220C because of bleeding were 5.9% and 6.5% (+0.6%) during the first 2 years of use (Goh et al. 1983).

Over all studies the mean cumulative removal rate because of bleeding was 3.8% after 1 year.

Progestasert. For progesterone-releasing IUDs (bleeding rate 12.1% for nulliparae and 9.5% for parae after the 1st year) a removal rate of 3.8% in nulliparae and 3.4% in parae was observed after the 2nd year (Mall-Haefeli and Spornitz 1984). Over all studies the mean cumulative rates of progesterone-loaded pessaries after 1 year was 12.1% for nulliparae and 9.5% for parae.

Lippes Loop. Large inert IUDs such as the Lippes Loop showed a high cumulative bleeding rate of 18.2% in the 1st year and 27.4% (+9.2%) after the 2nd year (Hasson et al. 1985). Over all studies the mean cumulative removal rate after 1 year of use was 11.1%.

Summary. Copper-medicated IUDs have fewer side effects than nonmedicated devices even after long-term use. The highest rate was found for Lippes Loop. For long-term use (more than 2 years) the removal rate for all devices except MLCu-375 was lower than in the 1st year and for copper devices ranged in the 2nd year between 0% and 2.6%. Good results are found for the Nova T, which in the 2nd year caused no more bleedings. The highest removal rates were found for the MLCu-375, with removal rates above 3.3% (3.3%–5.1%).

Copper IUDs show after 1 year of use the lowest impact on the menstrual bleeding pattern and have the lowest removal rate. This is due to the fact that copper-loaded IUDs are of smaller size and therefore act less as an foreign body. At the same time, the copper content did not cause an increase in bleeding frequency with the Cu-7, the TCu-220, the TCu-200, and, in the 1st year of use, MLCu-375. When long-term use is considered, a steady decrease of the annual removal rate can be found in all copper-medicated devices, although less marked in the users of MLCu-375. After 1 year of use the cumulative rate of bleeding disturbances with the MLCu-375 in comparison to MLCu-250 differed by only 1.2% (from 3.8% to 5.0%), whereas the copper surface had been increased by 175 mm^2.

Being the largest of all copper-containing IUDs (width 300 mm, length 34 mm), the Nova T showed the highest removal rate (11.1%). The high rate of bleedings is caused by the side arms of the Nova T, which come up to the interstitial part of tube and therefore have a lower expulsion and pregnancy rate.

The cumulative removal rate after 1 year of Gravigard Copper 7 use was found to be 8.4%. With the TCu-200 a cumulative removal rate of 8.8% was reported. The TCu-220C had a cumulative removal rate of 3.8%. In comparison with the copper-loaded devices, the nonmedicated and rather large Lippes Loop D had a high removal rate of 11.1%.

Expulsion

The cumulative expulsion rate after 1 year of use of different IUDs is summarized in Fig. 5. Based on a study by Lippes (1984), who did not observe any expulsions

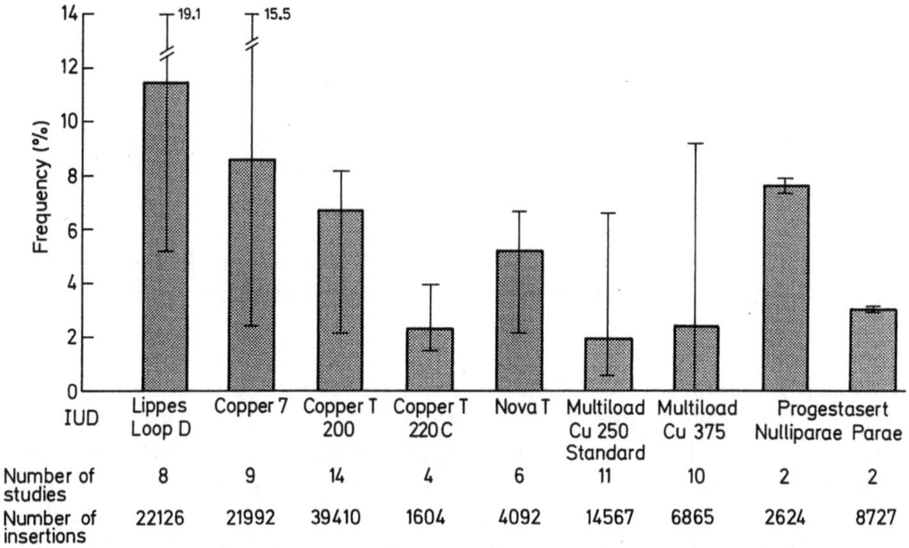

Fig. 5. Expulsion rate after 1 year of IUD use. Cumulative life table events in patients using intrauterine devices as described in various studies (mean cumulative rate ± range)

between the 4th and 10th year, in general the expulsion rate decreases during the time of use.

TCu-220C. The cumulative expulsion rate for TCu-220C was 3.7% in the 1st year; 4.7% (+1.0%) in the 2nd year; 5.5% (+0.8%) in the 3rd year; and 6.3% (+0.8%) in the 4th year of IUD use (Tatum 1984). Over all studies, the mean cumulative expulsion rate after 1 year was 2.4%.

MLCu-250. In the 1st year cumulative expulsion rate of MLCu-250 was 2.0%; in the 2nd year 2.6% (+0.6%); in the 3rd 3.0% (+0.4%); and in the 4th year 3.9% (+0.9%) (Thiery et al. 1980a, b). Over all studies, after 1 year of use a mean cumulative expulsion rate of 2.1% was found.

MLCu-375. Annually cumulative expulsion rates from the 1st year to the 4th year of use for the MLCu-375 were as follows: 3.5%, 4.2% (+0.7%), 4.9% (+0.7%), and 5.6% (+0.7%) (Thiery et al. 1985). Over all studies, the mean cumulative expulsion rate after 1 year of use for MLCu-375 was 2.5%.

Lippes Loop. Expulsion occurred in 2.8%, 3.9% (+1.1%), and 4.4% (+0.5%) of users from the 1st to the 3rd year (Andolesk 1972). Over all studies the Lippes Loop had a cumulative expulsion rate of 11.7% after 1 year.

Nova T. The cumulative expulsion rates for Nova T observed over a period of 4 years were as follows: 5.5%, 6.9% (+1.4%), 8.1% (+1.2%), 8.7% (+0.6%). Over all studies the mean cumulative expulsion rate for Nova T was 5.3% after 1 year of use.

TCu-200. The annual cumulative expulsion rate remained at 4.1% for the first 3 years (+0.0%) (Van der Pas et al. 1983). Over all studies the mean cumulative rate after 1 year was 6.8%.

Cu-7. The expulsion rate for Cu-7 increased during the first 2 years from 6.1% to 7.5% (+1.4%) (Goh et al. 1983). Over all studies the mean cumulative expulsion rate after 1 year of use was 8.7%.

Progestasert. The cumulative expulsion rates of progesterone-loaded pessaries are in the range of those of the larger copper-loaded pessaries (7.7% for nulliparae and 3.1% for parae after 1 year of use).

Summary. In the 1st year of IUD use there is a correlation between the size of the IUD and the expulsion rate. The expulsion rate of those IUDs with a width of between 28 mm and 31.8 mm (Lippes Loop, Progestasert, TCu-200, Nova T, Cu-7) ranged between 5.3% and 8.7%, whereas the remaining three IUDs (MLCu-375, MLCu-250 and TCu-220C), which had widths below 18 mm, were expelled in less than 3% of the cases in the 1st year. Among the IUDs with a similar size the IUDs with rounded edges (MLCu-250, MLCu-375, Nova T, TCu-220C) have the lowest expulsion rates. This is due to the fact that the round design of these IUDs adapts better to the cavum uteri.

After 1 year of use the MLCu-250 (expulsion rate 2.1%), the MLCu-375 (expulsion rate 2.5%), and the TCu-220C (expulsion rate 2.4%) had lower cumulative expulsion rates than the Nova T, which was almost twice the size (5.3%). The expulsion rates for larger copper pessaries such as Gravigard Copper 7 and TCu-200 are 8.7% and 6.8%. The highest expulsion rate (mean 12.6%) was in users of the nonmedicated IUDs (Lippes Loop). In a study fo Tietze and Lewit (1970) the expulsion rate was 19.1%. This high expulsion rate can be explained by the size of these IUDs. In order to reach a Pearl index comparable with other pessaries this IUD must be markedly larger and consequently will be more easily expelled than other pessaries.

During long-term use we no longer find any difference between the various kinds of IUDs. The annual expulsion rates stabilized at below 1% for TCu-220C, MLCu-250, MLCu-375, and TCu-200. The remaining Nova T, Progestasert and Lippes Loop still reached a value below 1.5% of expulsions per year. It seems that if the device is not expelled in the 1st year it will only be expelled in very few cases during the following years.

Acceptance of IUDs in Parae and Nulliparae

Studies with various IUDs have shown that acceptance is better in parae than in nulliparae. This can be proven both by the incidence of bleeding and pain and by the expulsion rate.

TCu-200. The expulsion rates in nulliparae and parae are 12.9% and 5.2%, respectively. As to the bleeding rate we find a similar situation, with 30.4% in nulliparae compared to 21.9% in parae. The Pearl index of TCu-200 was 1.5 (parae) and 3.6 (nulliparae) (Luukkainen et al. 1983).

Nova T. The Pearl index of Nova T was 0.6 in parae compared with 0.9 in nulliparae (Luukkainen et al. 1983).

MLCu-250. Kaiser et al. (1983) found no significant difference in acceptance rate of MLCu-250 between parae and nulliparae. The expulsion rate for parae (0.7%) was lower than for nulliparae (2.3%), but there were higher rates of bleeding and pain in parae (2.3%) than in nulliparae (2.0%). Fewer pregnancies occurred in nulliparae (0.0%) than in parae (0.7%). In a study comparing women over 30 years of age to those under 30, where parity was assumed, a lower expulsion rate in older (1.2%) than in the younger women (3.5%) was found. In younger women IUDs had to be removed because of bleeding more frequently (5.7%) than in older women (4.4%) (Thiery et al. 1985).

MLCu-375. No data about MLCu-375 IUDs regarding acceptance rates in parae and nulliparae are yet available.

Progestasert. Progesterone-releasing IUDs give much better results in women who have given birth to children. These women had an expulsion rate of only 3.1% (nulliparae, 7.9%), a bleeding rate of 9.3% (nulliparae, 12.1%) and a pregnancy rate of 1.8% (nulliparae, 2.4%) (Mall-Haefeli and Spornitz 1984).

Summary. With Nova T the bleeding rate in women with more than three children was 27.6% compared to 32.9% in women without children. The expulsion rate of Nova T was 8.8% in parae in comparison to 11.7% in nulliparae (Luukkainen et al. 1983).

In conclusion, independent of the IUD used, acceptance is better in parae than in nulliparae. This can be proven both by the incidence of bleeding and pain and by the expulsion rate.

Conclusions

Modern IUDs can be classified into a group of inert nonmedicated IUDs (Lippes Loop) and a group of medicated IUDs. Medicated IUDs release either copper (MLCu-250/375, Nova T, TCu-200, TCu-220C, Cu-7) or steroids (progesterone, Progestasert). If oral contraceptives cannot be used for certain reasons, the IUD is a suitable alternative method for contraception. The Pearl index of IUDs ranges between 0.5 and 5.0 and is thus higher than that of oral hormonal contraceptives. The main side effects of IUDs are expulsions (2.1–11.7%), removal for bleeding and pain (3.8–11.1%), and unwanted pregnancies (0.5–2.5%). Complications caused by medicated IUDs depend on its design, its size, and its copper surface. Low expulsion and bleeding rates are achieved by using small devices with rounded edges (Nova T), which act less as a foreign body. Enlargement of the copper surface seems to increase contraceptive safety, whereas the rate of side effects such as bleeding and expulsions increases only slightly. The lowest pregnancy rates were found for MLCu-375 (0.3%), TCu-200C (0.6%), MLCu-250 (0.7%), and Nova T (0.8%). The lowest removal rates due to bleeding and pain were found for MLCu-250 (3.8%), TCu-220C (3.8%), and MLCu-375 (5.1%), whereas the lowest expulsion rates were observed for MLCu-250 (2.1%), TCu-220C (2.4%), MLCu-375 (2.5%), and Nova T (5.3%). The devices with the highest complication rates were Progestasert, TCu-200, Cu-7, and Lippes Loop. New studies show that the main risk factor for the incidence of pelvic infections is not the age of the patient but the number of sexual partners. For young females (16–35 years of age) without previous pelvic inflammatory disease and one sexual partner intrauterine devices are the second-choice method for contraception after oral hormonal contraceptives.

References

Andolsek L (1972) Experience with immediate post-abortum insertions of the IUD. Excerpta Med Int Congr Ser 255:62–67

Altmann G, Feichtinger W, Havelec L, Beck A (1981) Die klinische Wirksamkeit der kupferhaltigen Intrauterinpessare Nova T und Kupfer-T-200 Ag im randomisierten Vergleich. Wien Klin Wochenschr 17:556–558

Alza Corporation (1977) The progestasert. Intrauterine progesterone contraceptive system release 65 µg/day progesterone for one year. Alza Product Information, Palo Alto

Cole PL, Malcolm Potts D, Aranda C, Behlilovic B, Etman ES, Moreno J, Randic L (1985) An evaluation of the TCU 380 Ag and the Multiload Cu 375. Fertility and Sterility 43:214–217

Gibor Y, Zipper J, Stewart WC (1973) The association between the amount of copper on copper carrying IUDs and their contraceptive efficacy. J Reprod Med 11:209

Goh TH, Sinnathuray TA, Sivanesaratnam V, Sen DK, Lim LS, Ratnam SS, Karim SMM, McCarthy T, Hutapea H, Hanafiah MJ, Simandjuntak P (1983) A randomized comparative evaluation of the Copper 7, Multiload Copper 250 and T Copper-220C IUD's. Contraception 27:75–84

Hasson HM (1985) Clinical experience with intrauterine devices in a private practice. Advances in Contraception 1:51–61

IFRP (1979) IUP's – Update on safety, effectiveness and research. In: Intrauterine devices. John Hopkins University, Baltimore (Population Information Program, series B, no 3, Population report 1979)

Jain AK, Sivin I (1977) Life-table analysis of IUD's: problems and recommendations. Stud Fam Plann 8/2:25

Luukkainen T, Nielsen NC, Nygren KG, Pyörälä T, Allonen H (1979) Combined and national experience of postmenstrual IUD insertions of Nova-T and Copper-T in a randomized study. Contraception 19:11–19

Luukkainen T, Nielsen NC, Nygren KG, Pyörälä T, Kosonen A (1981) Randomisierter Wirkungsvergleich von zwei kupferabgebenden Intrauterinpessaren (Nova-T und Kupfer-T 200) in Dänemark, Finnland und Schweden. Extracta gynaecologica 5:187–198

Luukkainen T, Allonen H, Nielsen NC, Nygren KG, Pyörälä T (1983) Five years' experience of intrauterine contraception with the Nova-T and the Copper-T-200. Am J Obstet Gynecol 147:885–892

Mall-Haefeli M, Spornitz UM (1984) Das Progestasertsystem. In: Beller FK, Schweppe KW, Wagner H (eds) Intrauterinpessare – Entwicklung, Wirkungsweise, Anwendung, Nebenwirkung. pp 279–293 (Edition medizin, Weinheim)

Nielsen NC, Pyörälä T, Allonen H, Nygren KG, Luukkainen T (1983) Nova T und Kupfer T 200: Eine Vergleichsuntersuchung über vier Jahre zwischen zwei IUP. Extracta gynaecologica 7:243–254

Nygren KG, Johansson EDB (1975) Post-abortion insertion of the intrauterine copper-T (T Cu 200). In: Hefnawi F, Segal SJ (eds) Analysis of intrauterine contraception. Elsevier/North Holland, Amsterdam, p 115
Shih S, Li-juan Q, Xuan L (1984) Comparative clinical experience with 3 IUDs, TCu 380 Ag, TCu 220 C and Mahua Ring in Tianjin. Contraception 29:228–238
Snowden R (1977) The statistical analysis of menstrual bleeding patterns. J Biosoc Sci 9:107–120
Tatum HJ (1984) Erfahrungen mit Kupfer-T-Intrauterinpessaren. In: Beller FK, Schweppe KW, Wagner H (eds) Intrauterinpessare – Entwicklung, Wirkungsweise, Anwendung, Nebenwirkung. pp 245–250 (Edition Medizin vol 8)
Tauber PF, Nohlen M (1985) IUP-Modelle im Vergleich. Sexualmedizin 7:400–401
Tejuja S, Saxena NC, Malhotra U, Choudhury SD (1975) Experience with the copper T in India. In: Hefnawi F, Segal S (eds) Analysis of intrauterine contraception. Elsevier/North Holland, Amsterdam, p 165
Thiery M, Van der Pas H, Van Os W (1980a) The effective intrauterine life span of the ML Cu 250. Br J Fam Plann 6:85–86
Thiery M, Van der Pas H, Delbeke L, Van Kets H (1980b) Comparative performance of two Copper-Wired IUDs (ML Cu 250 and T Cu 200). Immediate postpartum and interval insertion. Contracept Deliv Syst 1:27–35
Thiery M, Van Kets H, Van der Pas H, Van Os W, Dombrowicz N (1982) The ML Cu 250; clinical experience in Belgium and the Netherlands. Br J Obstet Gynecol [Suppl] 4:51–53
Thiery M, Van der Pas H, Van Os W (1983) Clinical evaluations of IUDs: performance of multiload IUD model with different copper loads. Contracept Deliv Syst 4:227–230
Thiery M (1985) personal communication
Thiery M, Van der Pas H, Van Kets H (1985) The ML Cu 375 intrauterine contraceptive device. Contraception 1:37–44
Tietze C, Lewit S (1970) Evaluation of intrauterine devices: ninth progress report of the cooperative statistical program. Stud Fam Plann 55:1–40
Timonen H, Luukkainen T (1974) The use-effectiveness of the copper T-200 in a simulated field trial. Contraception 9:1
Timonen H, Nylander P, Kivijarvi A, Hirvonen E, Kajanoja P, Kajvola S, Kotilainen A, Savia E, Saure A, Lonnblad R, Terava M, Venhola M, Mannikko H, Kaar K, Vierola H (1982) Comparative performance of three copper IUD's (ML Cu-375, Fincoid, Nova T) after one year's follow-up in randomized multicenter trial. Contracept Deliv Syst 3:226
Van der Pas H, Thiery H, Van Os W (1983) Ergebnisse mit Multiload Cu 375. In: Bonnar J, Thompson W, Harrison RF (eds) Research in family planning.
Van Os WAA (1984) Erfahrungen mit vier verschiedenen Modellen des Multiload-IUP. In: Beller FK, Schweppe KW, Wagner H (1984) Intrauterinpessare – Entwicklung, Wirkungsweise, Anwendung, Nebenwirkung. pp 256–267 (Edition Medizin vol 8)
WHO (1979) IUP's – update an safety, effectiveness and research. In: Intrauterine devices. John Hopkins University, Baltimore (Population Information Program, series B, no 3, Population report 1979
Zipper J (1984) Four years experience with the Cu 7-200 devices. Endouterine copper in fertility control. Contraception 13:7–16. In: Beller FK, Schweppe KW, Wagner H (eds) Intrauterinpessare – Entwicklung, Wirkungsweise, Anwendung, Nebenwirkung. pp 252–253 (Edition Medizin, vol 8)

Hazards of IUDs and Their Prevention

M. Thiery

Department of Obstetrics, University Hospital, Gent, Belgium

Introduction

The IUD has an important place in family planning, and if proof of its acceptability is still needed, one must merely note that this method of contraception continues to be disproportionately popular among female American gynecologists (Zbella et al. 1986). Since its revival in the early 1960s as a modern contraceptive method the IUD has contributed greatly to the health of women. Today it remains one of the few options open to those who want a reliable method of reversible birth control. Three decades of IUD research have produced "better" IUDs and have taught physicians how such devices can be used more safely. The future of intrauterine contraception cannot be predicted, but I remain confident that other countries will respond more responsibly to the external pressures of the kind which drove American pharmaceutical companies to withdraw their devices from the market (Forrest 1986).

All methods of contraception have advantages and disadvantages, and the IUD is no exception. Because the disadvantages of IUD use are specific, IUDs must be considered complementary to oral contraceptives for reversible birth control. Some of the disadvantages of IUD use have been designated as hazards by the scientific committee of this Congress. Besides sounding frightening, the term "hazards" is too vague. For this discussion, "hazards" will be applied to cover all "somatic" problems, ranging from trivial side effects connected with insertion or retrieval to more serious complications which may even endanger the life of the IUD wearer.

Before reviewing IUD-related problems and their prevention we should note one particular advantage of the IUD that has greatly increased the accessibility and acceptability of the method: IUDs can be inserted at almost any time; indeed, the clinical performance of an IUD is hardly affected by the time in the menstrual cycle at which it is inserted (Thiery 1985 b). Furthermore, results of IUD insertion, whether postcoitally (Gottardi et al. 1986) or during first-trimester interruption, are comparable to those for interval insertion (Thiery 1985 b). Admittedly, expulsion rates are higher when insertion occurs during late abortion or within 10 min after expulsion of the placenta, but such timing does not increase the hazards of perforation and infection or increase the pregnancy rate in patients with proper follow-up (Thiery et al. 1985 b; Thiery 1985 b). To our dismay, all attempts to reduce the ease of expulsion of the IUD – the sole drawback of immediate postplacental insertion – have so far failed, and neither specially designed IUDs (Petal IUD) nor adapted models (sutured IUDs, Thiery et al. 1983; Nova T

Female Contraception
Eds.: B. Runnebaum, T. Rabe, L. Kiesel

PP, Van Kets et al. 1986) have improved retention rates conspicuously. But research goes on, and we are anxiously awaiting the results of a pilot study on a new anchoring system for IUDs, which will be discussed in due course (Wildemeersch et al. 1986). One word of caution must be added here: IUD insertion should probably be discouraged in lactating women on grounds of the current suspicion that the procedure is accompanied by a higher risk of uterine perforation (Chi and Kelly 1984). Recently published preliminary results concerning IUD insertion during cesarean section were similar to those obtained with immediate postplacental insertion (Van Kets et al. 1985; Chi et al. 1986 b).

Problems with IUDs may be related to the insertion or the retrieval of the device or may be coincident with wearing of the IUD. The problems related to each of these three phases are examined here.

Insertion-Related Problems

The main complications of interval insertion of the IUD are pain, syncope, bleeding, and perforation.

Pain. The *pain* caused by insertion of a sound or introduction of the loaded inserter tube is caused primarily by dilatation of the isthmic region of the uterus. After long-term use of oral contraceptives – especially sequential preparations – the uterine os may be thight, and in an occasional patient touching of the fundal area with such instruments will elicit unbearable pain. Severe pain at interval insertion can to some extent be anticipated because it is known to occur more frequently in women of higher education, low parity, and with a longer open interval between the end of pregnancy and IUD insertion (Chi et al. 1986 a). Insertion-related pain can be prevented by local anesthesia (e.g., intracervical block and uterine lavage), but paracervical block (PCB) analgesia is more effective, and the use of dental equipment adds to the acceptability of this procedure (Thiery 1985 a).

Uterine pain which persists after the first 24–48 h is usually that of cramps and may recur before menstruation. Spastic dysmenorrhea is probably attributable to enhanced prostaglandin (PG) synthesis, which explains the beneficial effect of administration of PG synthesis inhibitors. With time, uterine cramps tend to decrease and gradually disappear as the myometrium adapts to the IUD. However, uterine pain which persists or increases may accompany impending or partial expulsion, and IUD wearers should be encouraged to examine themselves, at least after each menstrual period. If pain persists beyond the 1st week after insertion, the physician must perform an examination to rule out pelvic infection.

Syncope. Sudden loss of consciousness or a sudden feeling of faintness is caused by dilatation of the cervical canal inducing a vasovagal reflex. The risk of syncope is probably greater in anxious and tense women. Although some women may benefit from having the procedure explained in advance and being told that the insertion may cause some pain, these precautions may increase anxiety in other women. It should be kept in mind that analgesia is supremely effective for the prevention of syncope at IUD insertion.

Bleeding. The occurrence of bleeding during and after insertion is the result of cervical dilatation or laceration of the portio by a vulsellum (Thiery 1984). Complications during and after insertion can be avoided by dilating the cervical canal with urethral bougies before insertion of the device and using an Allis forceps instead of a tenaculum, respectively. Pain, syncope, and/or mild cervical laceration were found not to affect subsequent IUD performance (Chi et al. 1986c).

Uterine Perforation. Whether at the fundal or the isthmic level and whether partial or complete, perforation of the uterus is a potentially dangerous complication. Reportedly, perforation is a rare event (1 in 2000–4000 insertions). The incidence varies according to the IUD model and the insertion technique (push-out or retraction) but, most of all, with the experience accumulated by and the care taken by the operator.

Preventive measures consist of pelvic examination with empty bladder and straightening of the uterine axis by steady traction on the vulsellum. If the sound or the loaded inserter meets the slightest resistance, the cervical canal must be dilated, preferably under PCB. The norgestrel Nova-T IUD (NG-Nova-T) is particularly difficult to insert because of the disproportion between the diameter of the inserter tube and that of the IUD. Difficult insertion of the IUD often leads to failure and enhances the risk of perforation and expulsion due to faulty placement.

Complications Related to IUD Retrieval

An IUD is easily removed by pulling on the marker strings with a pair of forceps. Extraction may be more difficult long after the menopause, and it has been shown that the maximum pull needed to retrieve current IUD models varies so widely that some IUD models (e.g., those of the Multiload family) can tax the skill of even the most experienced operator (Thiery 1986). To prevent the marker strings from raveling or breaking we use curved arterial forceps after dilatation of the cervical canal under PCB whenever IUD removal proves difficult.

Lost IUD tails call for invasive extraction procedures after exclusion of complete expulsion and incipient pregnancy. We have tested most IUD retrievers proposed in recent years, but found none of them particularly helpful for the extraction of IUDs with missing strings (Thiery 1986).

Complications Related to IUD Wearing

Bleeding. The menstrual pattern of the IUD wearer is so characteristic that current IUD use can usually be inferred from a glance at the woman's menstrual calendar. Compared with the pre-IUD pattern, the bleeding phase is longer and the number of pads or tampons is higher. In addition, pre- and postmenstrual spotting or bleeding is almost universal. Net average blood loss is lower for copper IUDs than for inert models (Table 1) because, although the copper itself causes some extra bleeding (Tatum and Connell 1985), the smaller platform of

Table 1. Average menstrual blood loss per cycle in four groups

Groups	Loss (ml/cycle)
No IUD	30–40
Nonmedicated IUDs	60–75
Copper IUDs	40–50
NG-Nova-T	<30

From Tatum and Connell (1985).

copper devices reduces blood loss significantly. Intermenstrual bleeding or spotting is frequent and tends to increase with long-term use of both nonmedicated and copper-bearing IUDs, probably due to the deposition of calcium which roughens the surface of the platform and traumatizes the endometrium (Tatum and Connell 1985).

There are two types of abnormal IUD-related bleeding which often occur in combination: excessive menstrual bleeding (menorrhagia) and intermenstrual bleeding (metrorrhagia) or spotting. Spotting is embarrassing to the woman and may be culturally unacceptable. Menorrhagia depresses body iron stores significantly, and this makes it a major health hazard, especially in those parts of the world where iron stores are already endemically depleted (Thiery et al. 1986).

Clinical trials have indicated that although patient acceptance of abnormal bleeding is difficult to forecast, bleeding problems are the main reason for the discontinuation of IUD use. Prevention is difficult, however, mainly because the etiopathology of abnormal bleeding is insufficiently understood. Metrorrhagia is probably related to an endometrial trauma caused by the IUD frame (Sheppard and Bonnar 1980), but the increased incidence of spotting associated with progestin-only IUDs suggests that hormonally mediated endometrial changes may also play a role. This led to the hypothesis that the reduction of frame size and the addition of a tissue-regenerating agent (e.g., an estrogen) could solve the problems of acyclic bleeding (Gibson et al. 1985). For the control of menstrual hemostasis – an even more complex phenomenon, involving platelet aggregation, fibrin formation, and prostanoid release (Chrstiaens et al. 1982) – estrogens might be helpful and accelerate reepithelialization of the uterine cavity.

To test this hypothesis we carried out a double-blind randomized trial to compare the bleeding pattern in women wearing a plain MLCu-250 IUD with that in a group with a MLCu-250 dip-coated with estradiol and releasing 1–3 μg hormone per day. Unlike the encouraging results obtained with intrauterine estriol systems in the baboon (Dmowski et al. 1980), our clinical trial showed no difference between estrogen-medicated IUDs and controls as to intensity or duration of bleeding (Kleinhout et al. 1987). It is not clear whether this line of research is worth pursuing, and it seems probable that few investigators will be found who, because of the possible hazards of unopposed stimulation of the endometrium, would be prepared to test estrogen-only devices. On these grounds, IUDs releasing both an estrogen and a progestin seem more acceptable, because such devices might retain the favorable qualities of the progestin-only devices without the bleeding problem.

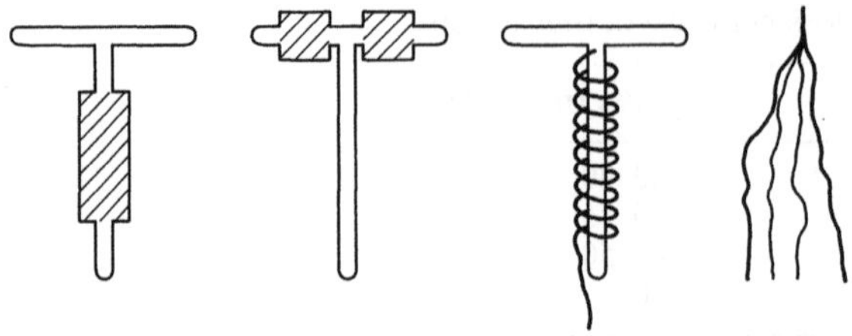

Fig. 1. Types of IUDs. From *left* to *right*: one- and two-compartment IUDs for release of progesterone and estrogen; fiber-wrapped T IUD for steroid release; and device composed of estrogen- and progestogen-releasing fibers lying loose in the uterine cavity and permanently attached to the uterine fundus

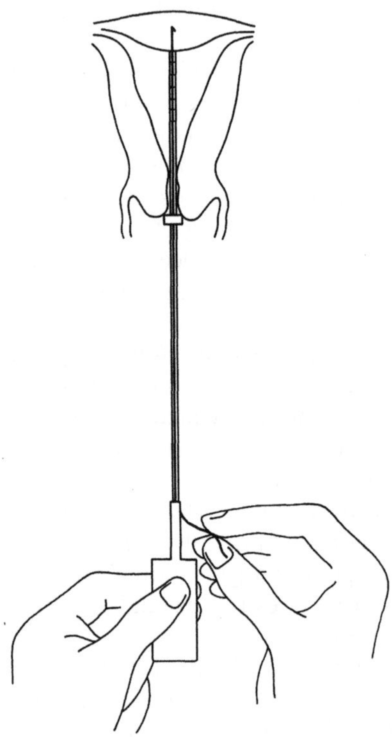

Fig. 2. The Cu-Fix IUD inserted at interval

Theoretically, the two steroids could be released from a reservoir, as in the Progestasert System and the NG-Nova-T (Fig. 1), but because these hormones diffuse through polymer membranes at different rates, two-compartment systems would be needed. Such systems are difficult and costly to produce. A much simpler solution is to use fibrous delivery systems wrapped around a given IUD platform (Gibson et al. 1985). Both monolithic and sheathed fibers, made of various plastic materials and loaded with progesterone or estradiol which they deliver at a steady rate, can be produced easily. Because the rate of drug release is es-

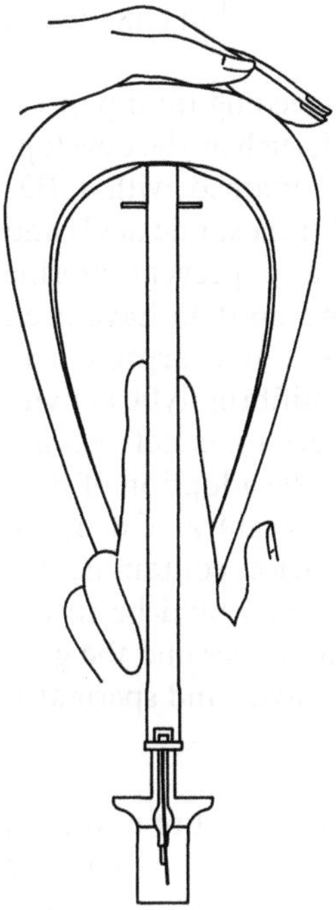

Fig. 3. Immediate postplacental insertion of T IUD using the Wildemeersch principle for attachment of the device to the uterine fundus

sentially dependent on fiber length, relative rates of steroid delivery can be adjusted by altering the length of the fibers. This novel approach to IUD technology could be extended further by using estrogen- and progestin-releasing fibers lying loose in the uterine cavity instead of fiber-wrapped IUDs (Fig. 1). By doing away with the bulk of the IUD frame such devices would automatically solve the problems of IUD-associated bleeding and pain.

The expulsion of frameless devices must of course be prevented. This could be accomplished by affixing the thread- or ring-type IUD to the uterus permanently. Bauer (1984) proposed a variety of anchoring systems analogous to those currently used to attach pacemaker electrodes to the myocardium, but neither the screw-type nor the barbed attachment have been tested clinically. Wildemeersch (1985) proposed a much simpler solution to the problem, and we are currently testing his Cu-Fix implant which, according to a pilot study, may significantly reduce bleeding and pain in women fitted with this high-load copper model. The Cu-Fix-360, which is still bench-made, consists of copper sleeves threaded on a length of surgical nylon suture material (Fig. 2). The sleeves are prevented from sliding off the nylon material by two smaller sleeves crushed onto the thread at both of its ends. The proximal end of the thread is provided with a knot which at insertion is pushed into the fundal myometrium with a needle inserter for permanent fixation of the device. As already mentioned, we are currently testing the same principle for attaching a TCu-380A IUD, introduced immediately after expulsion of the placenta (Fig. 3). For this trial, however, we have replaced the nylon by chromic catgut, which we hope will prevent expulsion of the device during the period of uterine involution. This system seems to be effective, but conclusive, hard data are not yet available (Wildemeersch et al. 1986).

Although a means to prevent abnormal IUD-induced bleeding (and pain) is in view, other research avenues are currently being explored, such as the development of IUDs releasing styptic drugs. However, results obtained with IUDs coated with antifibrinolytic agents (e.g., aminocaproic and tranexamic acid) and PG synthesis inhibitors (indomethacin) – which might also prevent uterine cramping – are not convincing (Srivastava et al. 1984), and no data have been published concerning a reservoir-type T model releasing isoaminocarproic acid (Levrier 1983). Because aminocaproic acid has only weak antifibrinolytic activity and is highly diffusible, much larger reservoirs would be needed for effective long-lasting release of this drug. This gave rise to two proposals: the adoption of flexible carriers, provided with a cavity designed to receive the concentrated drug solution (Shaw 1981) and the use of solid flexible polymeric matrices containing dispersed antifibrinolytics (Yolles 1982). An alternative solution would be to use more potent antifibrinolytic drugs, such as the aromatic diamidines and the guanidines, which besides styptic effects were found to have ovotoxic and spermatotoxic potencies (Shaw 1981).

Pain. Discontinuation of IUD use is not frequently due to pain: out of a total of 76 ML devices extracted because of bleeding and/or pain, only 13 were removed for pain only (Thiery, unpublished). Menstrual cramping tends to recur in older IUD users, especially those with a history of spastic dysmenorrhea.

Since uterine pain may be caused by disproportion between the IUD and the uterine cavity, especially in nulligravidae, use of short or mini-IUD models may help. The expectations concerning the Cu-Fix with respect to decreasing pain have already been discussed; and dysmenorrhea often vanishes after insertion of a NG-Nova-T. As already mentioned, sustained low-abdominal pain calls for the ruling out of expulsion, infection, and ectopic pregnancy.

Expulsion. Partial or complete expulsion of the IUD leaves the woman unprotected. Expulsion is frequently associated with menstrual bleeding and accompanied by cramping. It occurs more frequently in the nulligravid and nulliparous patient. Although the risk of expulsion differs somewhat according the type of IUD used, nonretainability is due mainly to faulty placement of the device.

The following measures have a preventive effect:

History: Do not insist on continued IUD use in patients known to have expelled a device (Van der Pas 1985). If an informed patient insists, choose an IUD model with a low expulsion rate, e.g., a Multiload (Thiery 1985c) or an Ombrelle-380 (Van der Pas et al. 1987).

Technique: Make every effort to achieve high fundal placement at insertion of the IUD. As already mentioned, the chances of correct placement are increased by pelvic examination, sounding of the uterus, and the use of a vulsellum (Van der Pas et al. 1980).

Device: Use an IUD model with good retainability and adequate size. The use of uterine metrology has been reported to decrease the risk of expulsion, and Kurz has repeatedly underlined the advantages of tailoring the TCu-200 to the size of the individual's uterus (Thiery 1986).

Teach the woman (or her partner) how to diagnose impending IUD expulsion and insist on periodic (self-) examination after each period and when abnormal bleeding/pain occurs. An increase in the length of the IUD tail felt in the vagina suggests expulsion, and feeling the presence of the tip of the IUD at the cervical os is diagnostic.

Future developments: We have already commented on an experimental IUD model (the Cu-Fix) attached to the fundal myometrium.

IUD Replacement. A drawback of the use of medicated IUDs is the need for periodic replacement. Attempts to extend the effective life span of Cu IUDs have resulted in the manufacture of devices with a silver-cored copper filament and multisleeved copper IUDs (TCu-220C, TCu-380A) (Thiery et al., 1985).

Late Perforation. We are not inclined to believe in the occurrence of delayed perforation (Tatum and Connell 1985), i.e., the hazard of erosion of the fundal myometrium by the sharp points of a wrongly placed device. Even in cases with somersaulted Multiload devices we have never observed delayed partial or complete expulsion of the device, nor has the perforation suggesting hysterographic appearance of the T-Cu-200 been proven to be associated with erosion of the uterine wall. Only for the original Cu-7 has genuine delayed perforation been documented, but here the sharp end of the stem was found to have penetrated the cervix.

For those who believe in the existence of delayed migration the most likely pathogenesis seems to be partial perforation by the device at the time of insertion with subsequent migration resulting from intermittent uterine contractions. If this hypothesis is correct, prevention of delayed perforation would demand fundal placement of an atraumatic IUD model (e.g., ring-type IUDs) or a three-point model with blunted arms and stem.

Intrauterine Pregnancy. The occurrence of intrauterine pregnancy in association with an IUD is uncommon and is usually due to partial expulsion. Hence, prevention of gestation coincides with prevention of expulsion and enhancement of the antifertility effect of IUDs. The TCu-380A and MLCu-380 are probably the most effective models now available.

Intrauterine pregnancy is associated with an enhanced risk of miscarriage, preterm birth, and – most important of all – spontaneous intrauterine sepsis, usually developing during the second trimester of gestation. Sepsis, although rare, is a life-threatening complication that can only be prevented by early extraction of the IUD. If the marker strings cannot be reached easily, hysterographic IUD removal tends to increase the chances of continuing pregnancy (Van der Pas 1987). IUDs provided with multifilament marker strings (Dalkon Shield) are currently thought to increase the hazard of uterine sepsis (Tatum et al. 1975). Women with a history of intrauterine pregnancy associated with an IUD should be advised to use other methods of contraception, because the chance of recurrence is substantial.

Extrauterine Pregnancy. An IUD protects against an intrauterine pregnancy but not against ectopic gestation, hence the rule of thumb: "Whenever suspicion arises about possibilities of pregnancy in an IUD wearer, *think ectopic* which is a life-threatening complication" (Tatum and Connell 1985). There is no way to prevent ectopic pregnancy in IUD wearers. It may be said, however, that progesterone-releasing IUDs (Progestasert System) probably represent a greater hazard for extrauterine pregnancy (Sivin 1985), whereas the reverse has been claimed for the NG-Nova-T (Haukkamaa et al. 1985).

Infection. Concern has frequently been expressed that women using an IUD might be at an increased risk of acquiring pelvic inflammatory disease (PID) leading to tubal sterility. Most case-controlled studies show that IUD users have a higher risk of developing PID than women using other contraceptive methods, but the results of case-controlled studies are not in agreement with those of cohort studies which, considered collectively, show that PID rates of IUD wearers are similar to those in the general population in the absence of abortion, childbirth, and surgery (Edelman and Porter 1986). Whatever the truth, it was the publication of two epidemiologic studies indicating an association between tubal infertility and the use of IUDs (Daling et al. 1985; Cramer et al. 1985) which gave the final blow to the IUD in the United States in 1986. What we should not forget (Mishell 1985) is that the risk enhancement was very small for copper IUD users and insignificant for multiparae with only one sexual partner.

In his excellent appraisal of the risk of IUD-related genital infections, Defoort (1985) discussed the currently available preventive measures for IUD-related PID: identify those women who should not receive an IUD, take sensible and consistent precautions, and use proper techniques for insertion. Although the IUD itself does not play a prominent role in the genesis of PID, both copper-bearing and gestagen-delivering IUDs (NG-Nova-T) are considered safer in this respect because of the bacteriostatic properties of the copper and the modification of physicochemical properties of the cervical mucus, respectively. As already mentioned, the opposite holds for the Dalkon Shield; but the lack of safety of this device is unique and must be ascribed to defective construction (Tatum et al. 1975).

A substantial proportion of pelvic infections originate at insertion (Defoort 1985), and because it is inevitable that the device will carry microorganisms present in the vagina and cervix to the uterus, it would be logical to develop IUDs medicated with an antiseptic compound capable of neutralizing the most important agents causing pelvic infection or to use antibiotics to prevent the development of infections. Sparks is currently conducting a microbiologic study in Birmingham (United Kingdom) to assess the prophylactic value of an ML IUD dip-coated with chlorhexedrine (personal communication 1986). Other microbicidal compounds and more sophisticated delivery systems have been proposed recently, but these must await clinical testing (Gallop and Korb 1985; Yolles 1982; Costerton 1985).

Why some IUD wearers develop PID long after device insertion is still not clear (Defoort 1985). One of the factors under suspicion is the presence of the transcervical appendage, which might serve as a "ladder" for bacteria to ascend from the vagina into the uterus (Tatum 1983). In this connection there are impressive results of a study in which a multiple-biopsy approach was used to assess

Table 2. Mortality associated with pregnancy and childbirth, legal abortion, oral contraceptives (by smoking status), and IUDs, by age

Age	Pregnancy and childbirth[a]	Legal abortion[b]	Oral contraceptives		IUDs[c]
			Nonsmokers	Smokers	
15–19	10.4	1.0	0.6	2.1	0.8
20–24	9.5	1.4	1.1	4.2	0.8
25–29	12.1	1.8	1.6	6.1	1.0
30–34	22.8	1.8	3.0	11.8	1.0
35–39	43.7	2.7	9.1	31.3	1.4
40–44	68.2	2.7	17.7	60.9	1.4

[a] Per 100000 live births (excluding abortion).
[b] Per 100000 first-trimester abortions.
[c] Per 100000 users per year.
From Tietze and Lewit (1980).

the effect of various types of tailed and tailless IUDs on the bacterial status of the uterus. All uteri containing tailless models were found to be sterile, but the majority of those with a tailed device showed bacteria (Sparks et al. 1981). The species of bacteria found do not represent the survival of organisms introduced at insertion, because they were not present in the uteri with tailless IUDs. Thus, the tail was clearly implicated in the introduction of bacteria into the uterine cavity. This led to the suggestion that use be restricted to stringless IUDs. So far, however, clinical trials comparing devices with and without strings have not proven the validity of this assumption, probably because the series were too small, and it is hoped that the ongoing FHI-sponsored multicenter random trial will yield unequivocal evidence (Wheeler et al. 1985).

Because removal of the strings from the IUD would complicate device localization and retrieval, the use of medicated appendages has also been suggested. Laufe (personal communication 1986) is currently working on the development of coated monofilament strings that release povidone-iodine for over a period of three months. For protracted prevention of infection, Levrier (1983) patented flexible copper-silver strings, whereas Fox et al. (1986) proposed the use of strings made of synthetic polymeric materials rendered infection-resistant by the incorporation of antimicrobial agents, such as nalidixic acid derivatives. The already described fibrous delivery systems for progesterone release produced by Gibson et al. (1985) could also be good candidates, because such filaments would modify the rheologic characteristics of the cervical mucus and thus render it inpenetrable for both spermatozoa and bacteria for up to 3 years.

Mortality. The level of mortality associated with IUD use is of the order of 12 per 1000000 women using the method for 1 year (Pepperell 1986). Thus, the risk of death from IUD use is significantly lower than the mortality associated with pregnancy/childbirth and the use of oral contraceptives except by women under 30 who do not smoke (Tietze and Lewit 1980) (Table 2). Most IUD-related deaths have been due to septic abortion and ectopics. Since 13 of the 17 women who died of septic abortion between 1972 and 1974 had used a Dalkon Shield, mortality from septic abortion has probably declined since that time (Cates 1976). Ectopic pregnancies probably contribute fewer than 0.2 deaths per 100000 women per year to the method-related mortality of IUD users (Tietze and Lewit 1980). In view of all this, prevention of IUD-related mortality means mainly the prevention, early diagnosis, and correct management of pregnancy associated with an IUD.

Conclusions

Safety, effectiveness, and acceptability of intrauterine contraception overlap considerably. The mainstay of safe IUD use continues to be the combination of correct selection of candidates and expert IUD insertion, and both the contraceptor and the physician must be made aware of symptoms that may herald serious complications related to IUD use.

References

Bauer HA (1984) Intrauterinpessar. European Patent Office No.0.100.924 Al
Cates W (1976) The intrauterine device and deaths from spontaneous abortion. N Engl J Med 295:1155–1165
Chi I-C, Kelly E (1984) Is lactation a risk factor of IUD- and sterilization-related uterine perforation? Int J Gynaecol Obstet 22:315–317
Chi I-C, Gallich LF, Tauber PF, Wilkens LR, Waszak CS, Siemens AJ, Lippes J (1986a) Severe pain at interval IUD insertion. Contraception 34:483–495
Chi I-C, Gao JI, Siemens AJ, Waszak CS (1986b) IUD insertion at cesarean section. Adv Contracept 2:145–153
Chi I-C, Waszak CS, Wilkens LR (1986c) Do insertion-related problems affect subsequent IUD performance? Contraception 34:497–503
Christiaens GC, Sixma JJ, Haspels AA (1982) Hemostasis in menstrual endometrium. Obstet Gynecol Surv 37:281–303
Costerton JW (1985) Microbicidal and antimicrobial biomedical devices. European Patent Office No. 0.147.970 Al
Cramer DW, Schiff I, Schoenbaum SC, Gibson M, Belisle S, Albrecht B, Stillman RJ, Berger MJ, Wilson E, Stadel BV, Seibel M (1985) Tubal infertility and the IUD. N Engl J Med 312:941–947
Daling JR, Weiss NS, Metch BJ, Chow WH, Soderstrom RM, Moore DE, Spadoni LR, Stadel BV (1985) Primary tubal infertility in relation to the use of an IUD. N Engl J Med 312:937–941
Defoort P (1985) An appraisal of the risk of IUD-related genital infections. In: Zatuchni GI et al. (eds) Intrauterine contraception. Harper and Row, Philadelphia, pp 390–397
Dmowski WP, Kapetanakis E, Scommegna A (1980) Contraceptive effect of intrauterine estriol delivery systems in rabbits and baboons. Contracept Deliv Syst 1:11–16
Edelman DA, Porter CW (1986) Pelvic inflammatory disease and the IUD. Adv Contracept 2:313–325
Forrest JD (1986) The end of IUD marketing in the United States: what does it mean to American women? Fam Plann Perspect 18:52–56
Fox CL, Modak S, Reemtsma K (1986) Infection-resistant materials. US Patent No. 4.563.485
Gallop PM, Korb DR (1985) Polymeric compositions and hydrogels formed therefrom. US Patent No. 4.543.371

Gibson JW, Dunn RL, Perkins BH, Scommegna A (1985) Development of a fibrous IUD delivery system for estradiol/progesterone. In: Zatuchni GI et al. (eds) Intrauterine contraception. Harper and Row, Philadelphia, pp 215–227
Gottardi G, Spreafico A, de Orchi L (1986) The postcoital IUD as an effective continuing contraceptive method. Contraception 34:549–558
Haukkamaa M, Allonen H, Heikkilä M, Luukkainen T, Lähteenmäki P, Nilsson CG, Toivonen J (1985) Long-term clinical experience with levonorgestrel-releasing IUD. In: Zatuchni GI et al. (eds) Intrauterine contraception. Harper and Row, Philadelphia, pp 232–237
Kleinhout J, Thiery M, Van der Pas H, Van Os WAA, De Nooyer CC, Clements J (1987) Extradiol-medicated IUDs. Adv Contracept (in press)
Levrier H (1983) Système endo-utérin contraceptif. Institut Propriété Industrielle, Paris. Patent No 83.003.02
Mishell DR (1985) Current status of IUDs. N Engl J Med 321:984–985
Pepperell RJ (1986) Beneficial and adverse side-effects of hormonal contraception. Med J Aust 144:169–170
Shaw ST (1981) European Patent Office No. 0.024.779 Al
Sheppard BL, Bonnar J (1980) The response of endometrial blood vessels to intrauterine contraceptive devices. Br J Obstet Gynaecol 87:143–154
Sivin I (1985) IUD-associated ectopic pregnancies. In: Zatuchni GI et al. (eds) Intrauterine contraception. Harper and Row, Philadelphia, pp 340–353
Sparks RA, Purrier BGA, Watt PJ, Elstein M (1981) Bacteriological colonisation of uterine cavity. Br Med J [Clin Res] 282:1189–1191
Srivastava K, Srivastava UK, Dasgupta PK (1984) Inhibition of fibrinolytic activity by KR2. A medicated device. SAC 2nd Ann Meet, Jakarta, Abstr No 81
Tatum HJ (1983) Milestones in IUD development. Fertil Steril 39:141–143
Tatum HJ, Connell EB (1985) Managing patients with intrauterine devices. Creative Informatics, Durant, pp 74–75
Tatum HJ, Schmidt FH, Phillip D, McCarty M, O'Leary WM (1975) The Dalkon Shield controversy. JAMA 235:704–705
Thiery M (1984) Use of a tenaculum. Br J Fam Plann 9:135–136
Thiery M (1985a) Pain relief at insertion and removal of an IUD: a simplified technique for paracervical block. Adv Contracept 1:167–170
Thiery M (1985b) Timing of IUD insertion. In: Zatuchni GI et al. (eds) Intrauterine contraception. Harper and Row, Philadelphia, pp 369–374
Thiery M (1985c) Multiload devices. In: Zatuchni GI et al. (eds) Intrauterine contraception. Harper and Row, Philadelphia, pp 87–94
Thiery M (1986) Intrauterine contraception: new developments. Tempo Medical 61:51–60
Thiery M, Laufe L, Parewijck W, Van der Pas H, Van Kets H, Derom R, Defoort P (1983) Immediate postplacental IUD insertion: a randomized trial of sutured and non-sutured models. Contraception 28:299–313
Thiery M, Van Kets H, Van der Pas H (1985) Immediate postplacental IUD insertion: the expulsion problem. Contraception 31:331–349
Thiery M, Martens G, Van der Eecken A (1986) Iron stores in users of oral and intrauterine contraception. IRCS Med Science 14:725 (1p.)
Tietze C, Lewit S (1980) Mortality associated with reversible methods of fertility regulation. In: Keith LG et al. (eds) The safety of fertility control. Springer, Berlin Heidelberg New York, pp 42–48
Van der Pas H (1985) Are current reporting methods of clinical IUD experience up to date? In: Zatuchni GI et al. (eds) Intrauterine contraception. Harper and Row, Philadelphia, pp 115–121
Van der Pas H (1987) Hysteroscopy retrieval of IUD in first trimester of pregnancy. Acta Obstet Gynecol Scand (in press)
Van der Pas H, Thiery M, Delbeke L, Van Kets H, Haspels A (1980) Six years' experience with the TCu220C IUD. Contracept Deliv Syst 1:1–10

Van der Pas H, Thiery M, Van Kets H, Parewijck W (1987) The Ombrelle-380 IUD: a pilot study. Adv Contracept (in press)
Van Kets H, Thiery M, Van der Pas H (1985) IUD insertion during cesarean section. Adv Contracept 1:337–340
Van Kets H, Thiery M, Van der Pas H (1986) Immediate postplacental insertion: Nova T and Nova T-PP. Adv Contracept 2:227–228
Wheeler RG, Cole LP, Galvez RS (1985). IUDs with or without strings. In: Zatuchni GI et al. (eds) Intrauterine contraception. Harper and Row, Philadelphia, pp 420–426
Wildemeersch D (1985) Dispositif anticonceptionnel intra-utérin nouveau et perfectionné et son dispositif d'insertion et de fixation á la matrice. Ministère Affaires Economiques, Bruxelles. Patent No. 901.652 (A 61F)
Wildemeersch D, Defoort P, Thiery M, Tatum H (1986) A new insertion-fixation instrument and technique for immediate postplacental insertion of IUDs. Fertil Steril [Suppl]: Abstr 235 (Ann Meet, Toronto, Sept 27–Oct 2)
Yolles S (1982) US Patent No. 4.344.431
Zbella EA, Vermesh M, Gleicher N (1986) Contraceptive practice of female physicians. Contraception 33:423–436

The Endometrium and the IUD

D. Serfaty[1] and H. Yaneva[2]

[1] Hôpital Saint-Louis, Centre de Régulation des Naissances, Paris, France
[2] Hôpital Necker, Paris, France

Mechanism of Action of IUDS

In mammals, the primary effect of intrauterine foreign bodies is to prevent pregnancy. How? The mechanisms of action are as yet uncertain and vary depending on the type of device [1]. In the case of inert and copper IUDs, the endometrium is the site of the essential contraceptive effect. This is an antiimplantation effect that is secondary to the changes in the endometrium and its functioning [2]. The IUD first causes *injury* to the endometrium, the extent of which depends on the shape and, especially, the size of the IUD. When in contact with the IUD, the mucosa becomes flattened, crushed, atrophic, and eroded. The second important change is a nonspecific *inflammatory response* (that of an endometrium reacting to a foreign body). This response consists of a focal inflammatory infiltrate containing polymorphonuclear cells, lymphocytes, plasma cells, macrophages, and, infrequently, giant cells. The inflammatory reaction is especially marked where the endometrium is in contact with the IUD. The IUD also causes *vascular changes*: altered permeability and diffuse microthrombosis of the capillaries in the endometrial stroma in contact with the IUD. These vascular changes, together with the presence of inflammatory cells, induce the release of numerous substances such as histamine, prostaglandins (PGE_2 and $PGE_{2\alpha}$) – the levels of which are increased in the uterus with an IUD (which explains some cases of uterine pain) – and plasminogen activators, especially a proteolytic enzyme responsible for enhancing the fibrinolytic activity of the endometrium (this may be the cause of certain cases of uterine bleeding and may damage the blastocyst and/or prevent its implantation).

The stroma in contact with the IUD is often the site of premature predecidualization, thought to be related to local trauma by the device [1]. In the presence of an IUD the endometrium may sometimes be the site of disturbance of maturation (usually a delay of several days in maturation) which render it unsuitable for implantation. This dysmaturation is thought to be due to the inflammatory response and to vascular changes rather than to a systemic effect of the IUD on ovarian function. The anti-implantation effect resulting from these often interwoven actions of the IUD on the endometrium is demonstrated by the absence in the blood of IUD users of β-HCG (human chorionic gonadotropin), which is the indicator of trophoblastic implantation.

Other mechanisms of action include the following: (a) the effect of copper on cervical mucus (rendering it hostile to movement of spermatozoa), on spermatozoa, and perhaps the blastocyst (toxic effect), and on endometrial steroid recep-

Female Contraception
Eds.: B. Runnebaum, T. Rabe, L. Kiesel

tors (in particular, progesterone receptors with which they may compete); (b) the increased contractility of the myometrium (role of prostaglandins) which may favor expulsion of the blastocyst; and (c) alteration of fallopian tube motility, which may adversely effect transportation of the gametes and blastocyst, and of the epithelium of the fallopian tube, which sometimes shows evidence of inflammation.

As regards progesterone IUDs, local injury to and inflammatory response of the endometrium are similar to those seen with other IUDs but do show a number of characteristic features. (a) The progesterone released in situ (and which does not affect the hypothalamus-pituitary-ovarian axis) exerts a continuous antiestrogen effect which enhances the contraceptive effect of the device. (b) Vascular changes consist primarily of extensive dilatation of the capillaries of the endometrial stroma in contact with the IUD (shown in the research by Sheppard using the electron microscope [2]). (c) Above all, the endometrium is usually thinned and is the site of an extensive decidual reaction where in contact with the IUD. (d) The progesterone diffused by these IUDs has a slight and inconstant action on cervical mucus.

With levonorgestrel IUDs injury to the endometrium and the resulting inflammatory response are comparable to those seen with other IUDs. Furthermore, the appearance of the endometrium is similar to that seen with progesterone IUDs, but there is extensive and highly uniform atrophy of the endometrium, and the stroma is the site of extensive decidualization. In addition, the levonorgestrel diffused by the IUD acts strongly on the cervical mucus (which becomes hostile to the ascent of spermatozoa). And, finally, levonorgestrel has systemic effects, although these rarely occur and only slightly affect ovarian function.

Normal Cytologic and Histologic Features with IUDs. The vaginal smear is not modified by the presence of an IUD. In contrast, 80% of cervical smears contain numerous inflammatory cells, and cellular atypia is found in 5% of cervical smears (usually discrete squamous abnormalities). Endometrial smears have a special appearance which is poorly known by cytologists, who tend to classify them as doubtful. They contain aggregates of polymorphonuclear cells, a few macrophages, a few lymphocytes, and occasional monocytes. There are numerous endometrial cells, often in large patches as they become readily detached. They have a decidual appearance when the smear contains a fragment taken near the IUD.

The endometrium is of uneven thickness. At the site of IUD insertion it is thin, but elsewhere it may be moderately hyperplastic with a lumpy surface. Around the IUD the glands are unevenly distributed; they have a polymorphic appearance, and secretion is irregular. The stroma around the IUD is heterogenous; it shows decidual-like patches, small hemorrhagic patches, patches of fibrosis and sometimes of edema. It always contains a few polymorphonuclear and mononuclear cells, but these are dispersed and do not form an abscess. Blood supply around the IUD is unevenly distributed. The blood vessels are of unequal size and often have thickened walls. The endometrium at a distance from the IUD is normal.

Relationship between Endometrial Changes and Adverse Effects

Uterine Bleeding

Bleeding is more or less unavoidable and is related to the mechanism of action of IUDs. Whether isolated or associated with pelvic pain, uterine bleeding is, however, the single most frequent cause of discontinuation of intrauterine contraception. Indeed, pain and bleeding are the cause of IUD removal in 7%–15% of cases after 1 year.

Certain types of bleeding indicate a complication; these are (a) infection, e.g., endometritis (see below) and pelvic inflammatory disease; and (b) pregnancy, including possible ectopic pregnancy, which must be suspected in women with IUDs who present abnormal bleeding, however slight, with or without pelvic pain and/or delayed menstruation. When both of these diagnoses are ruled out, the following should be suspected: (a) concurrent genital disease unrelated to the IUD (especially endometrial and cervical cancer); and (b) IUD not appropriate for the uterine cavity (IUD too large, of inappropriate shape, or incorrectly inserted).

Other types of bleeding are an increased or prolonged menstruation and mild metrorrhagia. The latter usually occurs during the first few months following insertion of the IUD and may be, for instance, pre- or postmenstrual metrorrhagia, bleeding during ovulation, irregular metrorrhagia, or postcoital bleeding.

All IUDs, with the exception of progesterone and progestin (levonorgestrel) IUDs, increase menstrual blood loss, and most prolong menstruation. With inert and copper IUDs blood loss is increased by 50%–100% with respect to preinsertion blood loss. This seems to be especially related to an increase in fibrinolytic activity of the endometrium. Several authors, including Christiaens et al. and Audebert also insist on other alterations of hemostasis (prostaglandin and histamine release, alteration of platelet function) and on IUD-induced vascular changes (vascular compression, capillary rupture). Furthermore, Audebert has suggested the possibility of a hormonal imbalance towards luteal insufficiency.

There is also a mechanical explanation: like the remainder of the endometrium, it is the fate of the endometrium around the IUD to desquamate. But in this case, regrowth is much slower because of the presence of a foreign body which fosters endometrial injury, resulting in microhemorrhage.

All the aforementioned changes thus favor endometrial bleeding. This affects patients to varying degrees and tends to decrease after several weeks or months. Prophylaxis of this abnormal blood loss is not always possible. Nevertheless, the following points are to be observed: (a) The appropriate IUD should be chosen and correctly inserted. (b) An inert or copper IUD should not be inserted in women who usually present menorrhagia, who have prolonged menstruation or a disturbance of hemostasis, or who are anemic. (c) All IUDs are contraindicated in women with unexplained bleeding.

Treatment of such blood loss is necessary even if it only occasions discomfort. Treatment may include the following: (a) hemostatics, uterotonics, fibrinolysis inhibitors, vascular protectors, progestins (if there is luteal insufficiency); (b) antiprostaglandins, which have a beneficial effect on menstrual blood loss (Roy et al. 1981), [quoted in 3] bearing in mind that anti-inflammatory agents may affect the contraceptive effectiveness of IUDs [4–6]; (c) in women with prolonged menstruation, estrogens may theoretically be used to hasten endometrial regrowth – to our knowledge, however, this type of treatment has never been attempted for this indication.

In any case, the consequences of such blood loss should not be overlooked. Indeed, in 10% of cases anemia was evidenced (by a hemoglobin level below 12 g/dl) after 1 year of nonhormonal IUD use in Finnish women. These findings are not found by all authors. According to the aforementioned study, the incidence of anemia does not correlate with the amount of blood lost in women with IUDs. According to Guillebaud et al. in 45% of women who have had an IUD for 1 year the serum ferritin level (16 μg/l) is in the range of iron deficiency (versus 19% before IUD use); this occurs even more frequently if menstrual blood loss is more than 80 ml. These authors suggest serum ferritin determination, which is a more sensitive predictor of iron deficiency in women with IUDs than hematocrit or serum iron. In any case, either iron should be prescribed to anemic women with IUDs, or the IUD should be removed if possible and replaced by a progesterone or levonorgestrel IUD. The latter types of IUDs are, in effect, the only IUDs that may be inserted in anemic women. In women who are at risk of iron-deficiency anemia (i.e., whose serum iron level or ferritin level before IUD insertion was near the lower normal limit) it is prudent to determine hemoglobin (or better yet, ferritin) every 6–12 months.

Uterine Bleeding with Progesterone IUDs. Endometrial fibrinolytic activity is not altered by the progesterone IUD. This has been demonstrated experimentally on the uterus bicornis in female rabbits by Liedholm and Sjöberg [16].

Furthermore, menstrual blood flow is significantly decreased (by approximately 40%) with respect to preinsertion blood flow. This action is thought to be due to endometrial involution and local vascular development. A number of studies have demonstrated this action, which has a clinically beneficial effect on blood loss.

This decrease in menstrual blood flow is an essential therapeutic aspect of this type of IUD, which, again, is to be preferred in anemic or menorrhagic women. This decrease is also thought to be the cause of a decrease in the risk of uteroadnexal infections with Progestasert. This has been emphasized in particular by Söderstrom and Luukkainen. In contrast, Progestasert may be associated with a slight increase in duration of menstruation. This is generally well-accepted by patients who have been properly informed. In a French multicenter study [7], prolonged menstruation with Progestasert led to discontinuation of this type of contraception in 4 of 221 women. Progestasert may also be associated with spotting or metrorrhagia, especially frequent in the first 3 months following insertion of the IUD.

Abnormal blood loss during the first 3 months following insertion is the most frequent cause of IUD removal (21 of 221 insertions after 18 months of usage), but the incidence decreases with time (9.6% at 3 months, 5.4% at 12 months, 2.5% at 18 months). Uterine bleeding in women with progesterone IUDs is thought to be histologically related to marked vascular congestion and, especially, to marked dilatation of the capillaries of the endometrium close to the device; these are venules that may burst and result in spotting and/or prolonged menstruation.

Uterine Bleeding with Levonorgestrel IUDs. Nilsson et al. [22] have reported a decrease in menstrual flow (compared to preinsertion level) in 90% of women after 1 year with the levonorgestrel IUD. Duration of menstruation was also significantly decreased. These facts, together with the action on cervical mucus of the levonorgestrel diffused by this device, probably explain the "anti-infectious" effect of this type of IUD (uteroadnexal infections are very infrequent in women with these IUDs).

The beneficial effect of the levonorgestrel IUD on blood loss and duration of menstruation (as well as its remarkable effectiveness) are related to the extensive and very uniform atrophy of the endometrium; levonorgestrel has a more potent atrophying and antiestrogenic action than does progesterone. However, 3–6 months are necessary before a decrease in blood loos, sometimes quite marked, becomes apparent. Indeed, during the first 3 months this device, on the contrary, results in more days with menometrorrhagia and/or spotting than do copper IUDs. Patients should be thoroughly informed. Furthermore, an increase in duration of menstrual cycles with levonorgestrel IUDs has been shown in almost 50% of users.

To our knowledge, this is the only IUD associated with a change in duration of the menstrual cycle. Our experience suggests that the increase in duration of menstrual cycle is common (80%?) in women with nonhormonal IUDs; this lengthening may be due to the longer follicular phase. More importantly, after 1 year of use 11% of women present amenorrhea. This is a nonhormonal amenorrhea of "endometrial" origin, which is rapidly reversible (in approximately 1 month) after removal of the IUD. The physician should also inform patients of this before suggesting this IUD.

Lastly, in women with levonorgestrel IUDs the stroma of the endometrium shows an increase in lipid and carbohydrate content (metabolic effect of levonorgestrel on the endometrium). However, this IUD does not affect plasma lipids or lipoproteins; it also does not affect blood pressure or weight.

Pelvic Pain

An increase in prostaglandin synthesis (especially $PGF_{2\alpha}$) by endometrial tissue with respect to the preinsertion level has been reported by several authors (Hillier et al. 1976) [quoted in 10] both in animals and in women.

This increase in synthesis and diffusion of prostaglandins results in hypercontractility of the myometrium, which may play a role in the mechanism of action of IUDs and also be the cause of pelvic pain: dysmenorrhea and/or pelvic pain unrelated to menstruation. In women presenting this type of pain complications – in particular, uteroadnexal infection – should first be ruled out.

Dysmenorrhea is more frequent and usually more severe in patients with IUDs, except in those who have a progesterone or levonorgestrel IUD, the beneficial effects of which have been well demonstrated in the literature. Other types of pelvic pain are due to an inappropriate IUD (too large, or its shape does not correspond to that of the uterine cavity) or an incorrectly inserted IUD.

Women with IUDs who complain of dysmenorrhea should be treated with nonsteroidal anti-inflammatory agents (such as mefenamic acid, ibuprofen, or naproxen) during the painful phase of menstruation. Hormonal IUDs should be preferred in women who are known to suffer from dysmenorrhea.

Other types of pelvic pain have become less common with the availability of smaller IUDs (made possible by adding copper) and better IUDs (flexible plastics, models that are less traumatic for the endometrium). If simple medical management, excluding anti-inflammatory agents (analgesics, antispasmodic agents, muscle relaxants, etc.), does not result in rapid pain relief, the IUD must be removed and the patient placed under observation.

Disorders of the Endometrium with an IUD

Endometritis

Definition. According to Hendrickson [1], endometritis can be defined as an abnormal infiltration of the endometrium by inflammatory cells. The diagnosis of endometritis in women with IUDs is particularly difficult, especially for the inexperienced physician, because (a) the normal endometrium, even without an IUD, contains a variety of inflammatory cells that have no pathological significance (more importantly, during menstruation the endometrium shows acute inflammation and necrosis); and (b) because a certain degree of endometritis is "normal" in women with IUDs (see below) and appears to be essential to the contraceptive effect of these devices.

Normally, the endometrial cavity is sterile, which indicates that the endocervix serves as an effective barrier against ascent of bacteria. In women with IUDs the normal cervical barrier is disrupted by the presence of the IUD string, allowing entry of cervical mucus into the endometrial cavity. The cervical mucus may be contaminated by microorganisms, in particular by germs responsible for sexually transmitted diseases. Insertion of the IUD favors this route of contamination. This serves to emphasize the absolute necessity of treating any vaginal discharge; especially, of checking that the cervical mucus is normal before inserting the IUD; of thoroughly cleansing the cervix and vagina before inserting the IUD; and of using the no-touch method which avoids any contact between the device and the walls of the vagina during insertion.

Moyer and Mischell have often found bacterial contamination of the uterine cavity similar to that of the cervical mucus during the first 48 h following insertion of the Lippes Loop IUD. In most cases, bacterial infection of the endometrial cavity disappears several days after insertion of the IUD.

Lastly, the "normal" inflammatory state of the endometrium due to the presence of the foreign body (the IUD) undoubtedly favors this superinfection of the endometrium; the inflammatory response is, as we have seen, an essential part of the mechanism of action of IUDs.

Incidence. According to Jessen et al. acute or chronic endometritis of varying severity occurs in 10.1% of women with IUDs. In our experience more or less significant endometritis probably exists in approximately 20% of women with IUDs.

Classification. There are two forms of endometritis, acute and chronic. Acute endometritis is histologically defined by: (a) massive inflammatory infiltration of the stroma and glands, with the presence of inflammatory cells in the lumen of the glands; (b) more or less extensive focal necrosis; (c) hemorrhagic zones; and, especially, (d) formation of *microabscesses* – which suffice to establish the diagnosis of acute endometritis. The presence of microorganisms is considered pathological only if associated with acute endometritis.

Bacteriologically, any microorganism may be responsible. This may be a sexually transmitted microorganism, in particular *Chlamydia* or *Gonococcus* (some authors insist on the high incidence of *Gonococcus* associated with copper IUDs). However, this may also be of endogenous bacteria. Pathological diagnosis is sometimes difficult, and all degrees may be seen.

One should be particularly careful before establishing a diagnosis of acute endometritis when the endometrium is in the late secretory phase or during menstruation. Indeed, in the latter two circumstances, all the criteria of acute inflammation may be present: (a) exudative reaction (consisting primarily of neutrophils and serum protein such as fibrin); (b) hyperemia, edema, interstitial hemorrhage; (c) tissue necrosis; and (d) regeneration.

Cytologically, in acute endometritis there is usually an abundance of polymorphonuclear cells and necrotic endometrial cells. Giant cells may occasionally be found.

The differential histological diagnosis of nonspecific acute endometritis which may arise is that of tuberculous endometritis, which is histologically evidenced by the presence of follicles containing giant cells and epithelioid cells. The other type of specific endometritis, syphilitic endometritis, is no longer found.

Chronic endometritis is diagnosed much more frequently than acute endometritis in women with IUDs, probably because acute endometritis can rapidly become chronic if this has been left untreated, or if treatment has been ineffective. In this case, the endometrium has the characteristics of that in women with IUDs but with the following additional characteristics: (a) there are organized foci of round cells (lymphocytes, macrophages, and more rarely, plasma cells, etc.), and (b) there is discrete fibrosis. Lesions are usually localized to the endometrium in contact with the IUD.

As with a recent pregnancy, salpingitis, pelvioperitonitis (more often chronic than acute), endouterine necrotic tissue, and mechanical obstacles to evacuation of menstrual blood, the presence of an IUD represents one of the circumstances in which chronic endometritis can be seen; acute endometritis, however, may also be present in these circumstances.

In women with IUDs, chronic endometritis, diagnosed on the pathological examination, is usually clinically silent and therefore should not be systematically treated. But concurrent chronic salpingitis must be suspected whenever chronic endometritis has been correctly diagnosed on the presence of mononuclear cell infiltrates (lymphocytes, monocytes, plasma cells). Indeed, according to Cadena et al. [quoted in 1], inflammation of the fallopian tubes is present in 25% of cases of chronic endometritis. Management (anti-infectious treatment, removal of the IUD, or nontreatment) should be tailored to the individual case.

In practice, one should keep in mind that (a) all IUD users may pathologically present any degree of endometritis from chronic to acute; and (b) a certain degree of endometritis appears to be required for IUDs to be effective.

Clinical Aspects. The diagnosis of endometritis in women with IUDs should be considered when the patient presents [27] vaginal discharge (especially when foul), mild but repeated metrorrhagia, and/or pelvic pain without fever. These symptoms are important particularly when they occur several months after insertion of an IUD. On physical examination there are two positive signs: turbid mucus, sometimes purulent or containing blood, and pain on palpation and mobilization of the uterus. There are also two negative signs: no palpable adnexal mass through the vaginal fornices and normal blood count and sedimentation rate.

A resolution of symptoms may result from a short and intensive antibiotic therapy[1], initiated immediately after obtaining a complete blood count, sedimentation rate, and culture of the endometrium (by endometrial aspiration if there is no clinical sign of mucopurulent cervicitis) and of mucus and discharge (with testing for aerobes, anaerobes, and chlamydia). Systematic treatment of the sexual partner should be undertaken if the cultures show a sexually transmitted microorganism.

The IUD should be removed (a) systematically in the young nullipara who nevertheless has an IUD (in our opinion, this type of contraception is contraindicated in these women) and in women at high risk of infection, especially if they are young and wish to have children; and, more commonly, (b) if symptoms persist despite correct antibiotic treatment. The IUD along with endometrial fragments obtained at the same time should be cultured on appropriate media for aerobes, anaerobes, and chlamydia.

In our opinion, an essential procedure is to perform a pathological examination of the endometrial fragments obtained with the IUD. This procedure will make it possible to confirm the diagnosis of endometritis, to identify the type (more or less acute or chronic), and to rule out any other endometrial disease which may be associated with endometritis.

Course. In the absence of appropriate treatment, endometritis may be complicated by: (a) salpingitis, followed by pelvioperitonitis, with all the possible consequences on subsequent fertility; (b) abscess of the cul-de-sac; and (c) ovarian abscess.

Exogenous microorganisms may follow several routes [9] including: (a) from vagina to cervix to endometrium (endometritis) to fallopian tubes (salpingitis) to peritoneum (pelvioperitonitis); or (b) vagina to cervix to endometrium to myome-

[1] J. Henry-Suchet advises a combination of Augmentin (amoxicillin plus clavulanic acid), Vibramycine (doxycyclin) and Naxogyn (nimorazole) while awaiting the results of bacterial examination.

trium to lymphatics and metastasis to a fallopian tube or ovary. The latter route would explain unilateral adnexitis, which is not uncommonly seen in women with IUDs.

According to Homes even laparoscopy is not error-free for the diagnosis of salpingitis. For the diagnosis of salpingitis and its etiology examination of an endometrial specimen obtained by aspiration may complete the data yielded by laparoscopy. When there is mucopurulent cervicitis, endometritis is present in about 50% of cases in the absence of symptoms of salpingitis; endometritis has also been found in 85% of cases of clinical salpingitis confirmed by laparoscopy (and in 20% of cases of suspected salpingitis with normal laparoscopic findings). In 90% of women with salpingitis and endometritis, confirmed by biopsy, endometrial or fallopian tube infection by chlamydia or gonorrhea is found. According to Homes and coworkers, histopathological criteria allowing differentiation of *C. trachomatis* and *N. gonorrhea* endometritis can be defined.

Endometritis due to Actinomycetes. Actinomycetes are filamentous gram-positive bacteria. Their usual host is the upper respiratory tract, but these bacteria may invade the genital tract after orogenital sexual contact. The incidence on systematic cervical and vaginal smears varies widely in women with IUDs: 14.4% of cases among 428 asymptomatic women with copper IUDs (after a Papanicolaou stain) were reported by Hermet [29], but only 2.8% of cases in 350 women with inert or copper IUDs were reported by Nayar. However, it should be remembered that there are many false positives, and that only immunofluorescence tests or cultures (slow and difficult in anaerobiosis) of pus, of the IUD, or of endometrial fragments allow positive diagnosis.

According to Keith, the presence of actinomycetes in cervical and vaginal smears is not necessarily pathological, and a cause-effect relationship between IUDs and actinomycetes has not yet been demonstrated. Actinomycetes are thought to be a risk factor for endometritis and pelvic infection; women with genital actinomycosis have a 3.6-fold higher risk of pelvioperitonitis in comparison with women who do not have such bacteria. In exceptional cases this may also be true for actinomycosis abscess of the ovary. From the endometrium the germ appears to pass into the lymphatics, which explains why the infection is usually unilateral. In actinomycotic abscess of the ovary the course is usually slow, suggesting an adnexal tumor or endometriosis. Penicillin therapy ensures early cure, before the abscess stage.

After constitution of an abscess (of the ovary) surgical treatment is required. The essential question concerning the association of IUDs and actinomycetes is how to treat women with actinomycetes in their smears, who have an IUD, and are asymptomatic.

Other Disorders of the Endometrium

Hyperplasia and Polyps of the Endometrium. The occurrence of hyperplasia is exceptional in women with IUDs. Clinically, these lesions are suspected primarily in women with metrorrhagia. Routine tests, such as endometrial biopsy or even hysteroscopy or hysterography (if these are not contraindicated), may help guide the diagnosis, which can be confirmed by a pathological examination: endometrial histology is normal in women with IUDs, but the surface of the endometrium is lumpy, and there are foci of massive vessels.

Treatment of hyperplasia is based on progestins. If polyps are present, management (usually curettage) will depend on their size, number, and site.

It should be mentioned that the relationship between IUDs and endometrial carcinoma is not statistically significant.

Intrauterine Pregnancy. IUDs do not always prevent pregnancy; the incidence of intrauterine pregnancy is 0.3–2.2 per 100 women after 1 year with bioactive IUDs. How can we explain this?

In some cases the IUD may not be adjusted to the size of the uterine cavity. The best IUDs are, according to Hasson [33], those which measure 1.5 cm less than the height of the corpus uteri. The worst results are those obtained with IUDs which are longer than the height of the corpus uteri or 2 cm less than this height. Another explanation may be secondary displacement of the device due to increased uterine contractility (the effect of prostaglandins) which displaces it from the fundus uteri. Most commonly, however, the cause lies in incorrect insertion of the IUD. These seem to be the most frequent causes of failure. In these cases the endometrial injury normally induced by the IUD, together with the inflammatory response and concomitant vascular changes, are insufficient to prevent implantation of the blastocyst in the endometrium. Insufficient (or abnormal) biochemical changes normally induced by the endometrium in the presence of an IUD may also be involved. This could explain pregnancy in IUD users taking anti-inflammatory agents (antiprostaglandins).

When a woman with an IUD is pregnant (plasma HCG $\geq$ 15 IU/ml), an ectopic pregnancy must first be ruled out. Indeed, the percentage of ectopic pregnancies is known to be higher in IUD users (one ectopic pregnancy per 20–30 intrauterine pregnancies) than in women who do not use this type of contraception (one ectopic pregnancy per 300 intrauterine pregnancies). In case of pregnancy the IUD should be removed whenever possible and cultured for aerobic and anaerobic germs and for *Chlamydia*, and broad-spectrum antibiotic treatment should be initiated. Treatment should be with antibiotics that are not deleterious to pregnancy if the woman wishes to keep the baby; erythromycin, a broad-spectrum macrolide which is active against *Chlamydia*, appears to be indicated [34].

If the string is no longer visible or if the woman does not wish to have the IUD removed but nevertheless wishes to keep the baby, she should be informed of the risk of infection and, especially, the possibility of second trimester septic abortion, sometimes complicated by potentially lethal sepsis, as has been reported in the literature. In this case, and even in the absence of signs of infection [10], it is essential to prescribe broad-spectrum antibiotic therapy combining a penicillin with a β-lactamase inhibitor (Augmentin) and erythromycin.

Apart from the risk of infection entailed by an intrauterine pregnancy when the IUD remains in place, one should bear in mind the following: (a) There is a 50% risk of spontaneous abortion; this may be due to infection, abnormal implantation, or the toxic effect of the IUD. (b) The incidence of premature rupture of the membranes and of premature delivery (17%) is abnormally high. (c) According to some authors, in rats and in women, there is an increased risk of fetal malformation; in 1975, however, the WHO considered this risk nil. Should the pregnancy be terminated by induced abortion, the risk of infection is the same, and antibiotic therapy should be the same.

Conclusions

Thorough knowledge of the effects of IUDs on the endometrium is essential to understand the mechanisms of action of IUDs, to prevent and treat some adverse effects and complications of this type of contraception, and to guide research in development of IUDs (materials, shape, therapeutic agents added). The physician's role will nevertheless always be essential for proper tolerance and effectiveness of this contraceptive method.

References

1. Serfaty D (1986) Les dispositifs intra-utérins. In: Serfaty D (ed) La contraception. Doin, Paris, pp 335–361
2. Audebert A (1982) Contraception par stérilet. Rev Med Interne 18:947–969
3. Dawood MY (1985) Etiology and treatment of dysmenorrhea. Semin Reprod Endocrinol 3:283–294
4. Rozenbaum H, Papiernik-Berkhauser E (1987) Grossesse sur DIU et Interactions médicamenteuses. Encyclopédie Médico-Chirurgicale – Instantanés Médicaux. 1987, 58è Année, n°1, pp 3–4
5. Buhler M, Papiernik E (1983) Successive pregnancies in women fitted with intrauterine devices who take antiinflammatory drugs. Lancet:483
6. Serfaty D (1986) Interaction des médicaments et des dispositifs intrautérins. In: Serfaty D (ed) La contraception. Doin, Paris, pp 421–425
7. Serfaty D (1986) Le stérilet à la progestérone. In: Serfaty D (ed) La contraception. Doin, Paris, pp 395–405
8. Serfaty D (1986) Dispositifs intra-utérins au lévonorgestrel. In: Serfaty D (ed) La contraception. Doin, Paris, pp 406–416
9. Cohen J (1986) Dispositifs intra-utérins et infection génitale. In: Serfaty D (ed) La contraception. Doin, Paris, pp 385–394
10. Henry-Suchet J, Holwani N (1986) Les grossesses utérines et extra-utérines chez les femmes porteuses de stérilet. In: Serfaty D (ed) La contraception. Doin, Paris, pp 379–384

Clinical Results of a New Contraceptive Intra-uterine Device: Ombrelle 250

A. J. M. Audebert

Institut Robert B. Greenblatt 4, rue Vauban, 33 000 Bordeaux, France

Today endo-uterine contraception occupies an important place among birth-control methods, as proven by the increasing number of users throughout the world and the improvement of the performance. The number of women using an intra-uterine device (IUD) is estimated at more than 80 million. The distribution is very uneven across countries (Ketting et al. 1985) as a result of such factors as: other available methods, religious and cultural contexts, attitudes of the medical profession, and legislation regarding abortion and sterilization. The use of IUDs is high in some countries, such as China or Finland (29%), but low in the United States and Canada (5.8%); in France 14% of women between the ages of 15 and 44 use IUDs. The performance of the most recent ones (TCu-200, Nova T, ML Cu-375, TCu-380) explains the growing acceptability of this contraceptive method, both to users and to physicians. At the end of the 1st year of use the percentage of unwanted pregnancies varies between 0.4 and 1.9, the percentage of expulsions between 1.8 and 5.8, the percentage of removals because of bleeding between 5.9 and 11.4, and the percentage of continuation after 1 year between 75.7 and 85 (Table 1) (Luukkainen et al. 1983; Sivin 1981; Thierry et al. 1985).

Among the complications the most worrisome is pelvic inflammatory disease (PID) and its eventual further consequences on fertility and the risk of an ectopic pregnancy. However, the infection depends greatly on the type of sexual activity and on risk factors linked to previous history and other characteristics of the patient. This emphasizes the importance of the selection of women to receive IUDs and the influence of selection on performance (Mishell 1975). For copper IUDs,

Table 1. Results at 12 and 24 months per 100 users of modern copper IUDs

	T 200 Luukkainen et al. (1983)		MLCu 375 Thiery et al. (1985)		Nova T Luukkainen et al. (1983)		Gyne T 380 Sivin (1981)	
	12 months	24 months	12 months	24 months	12 months	24 months	12 months	24 months
Failures	1,9	3,8	0,4	1,5	0,7	1,4	0,9	1,2
Expulsions	4,2	5,2	2,4	3,2	5,5	6,9	5,8	8,2
Removals for Bleeding/pain	11.4	14.9	5.16	9.6	11.1	17.0	11.1	18.1
Continuation ratio	77.0	64.7	85.6	72.0	76.1	64.7	75.7	56.9

Female Contraception
Eds.: B. Runnebaum, T. Rabe, L. Kiesel

the device itself appears relatively low for the risk of secondary tubal sterility (Daling et al. 1985; Cramer et al. 1985).

At the price of some degree of selection copper IUDs represent an effective method of birth control, with an acceptable level of side effects and complications (Tatum 1977). Because in principle it involves insertion of a device into the uterus, the consequences associated with a vector that requires a certain degree of rigidity to ensure its retention cannot be avoided.

We felt it would be useful to devise a new vector with a low incidence of local traumatic effects, called "Ombrelle".

Description of the Ombrelle 250

With so-called active devices, such as those of copper, the vector does not play an important part in ensuring contraceptive efficacy; it must, however, be easy to insert and have a low incidence of expulsion. As for other measures of performance, the characteristics of the patient and the quality of the insertion methods play significant roles. In addition, the device must be located in the fundus of the uterine cavity (Hasson et al. 1976) and be adapted to the physiological variations of the uterine geometry; for Tatum (1977), the T shape responds the best to these two conditions. All the vectors presently used are retained because of a certain degree of rigidity and an anchoring mechanism which can create trauma to the endometrium and, if penetration occurs, sometimes to the myometrium. This trauma can explain some lack of tolerance linked to side effects of unknown mechanism. These observations have led to the development of a vector characterized by great flexibility, an ability to alter its shape, and resistance to expulsion.

The strut of Ombrelle 250 is made of polyethylene plastic (EVA 501 + EVA 571) without barium sulphate, giving it a flexible consistency. It basically consists of two parts. The first part is made of a vertical rod (measuring 31.5 mm) ending with a blunt knob to which are fastened two arms, almost horizontal, reinforced at their extremities; it is therefore roughly T shaped, with a span of 23.7 mm. The second part is made up of two vertical rods, each fastened to the middle portion of a horizontal arm; these meet at the level of a ring which slides along the vertical arm of the T; this construction forms a closed device with little available space (Fig. 1). A copper thread (99.99% pure) with a diameter of 0.3 mm is wrapped round the vertical arm, with a total area of 250 mm^2. Two monofilament guides are fastened at the extremity of the vertical arm. The device is therefore highly flexible, especially in the uterus at 37 °C, and allows its shape to alter when the ring slides to the top of the vertical arm (Fig. 2). This distortion widens the base of the device, preventing its expulsion; it also causes a tension which has a tendency to push the device toward the fundus of the uterus. Finally, it enables the apparatus to adapt, at all times, to changes in the uterine cavity.

Insertion into the uterine fundus is performed with an insertion tube placed over the vertical rod; this is done easily without mandril. No preliminary manipulation of the device is necessary. The flexibility of the IUD avoids a forceful extension of the lateral arms, which can be a cause of pain during insertion. The di-

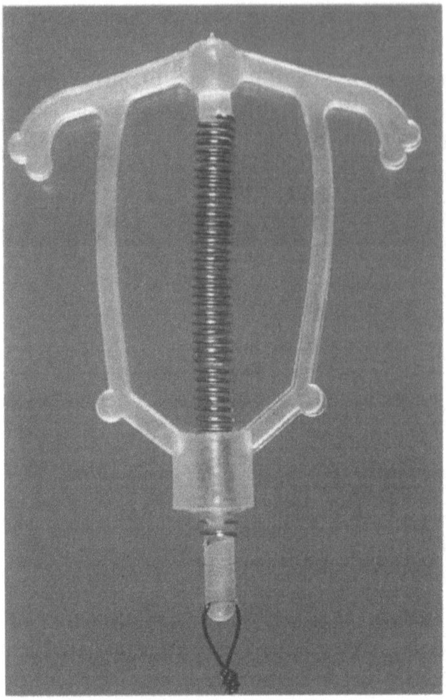

Fig. 1. The Ombrelle 250

ameter of the insertion device is slightly greater than that of the Nova T. The insertion device has been designed to be flexible; this prevents any forced manoeuvre which may risk uterine perforation, since we know that most perforations occur at the time of insertion (Audebert et al. 1980). Therefore, the patency of the cervix must be verified before insertion. The fact that the device is not completely covered during insertion does not produce an increased risk of infection.

Removal is carried out by simple traction on the thread. The horizontal arms rise, carrying the ring along, which comes into contact with the top of the vertical rod. The flexibility of the plastic makes this manoeuvre less painful.

Clinical Results

After toxicological studies regarding the materials were performed, the first clinical trials began in 1979. Today, several thousand women wear the Ombrelle 250, already marketed in France (since June 1986). The results previously published concern the pilot study (Audebert et al. 1985) and a multicentre study (Cohen et al. 1985; Cittadini and Pastore 1985). The patients included in these studies were not selected in any particular manner besides the usual contra-indications and their desire to use this mode of contraception. Their characteristics reflect those of women representing, for the French gynaecologist, those most suitable to endo-uterine contraception, i.e., over 29 years of age (77%) and seldom nulliparous (less than 10%) (Fig. 2).

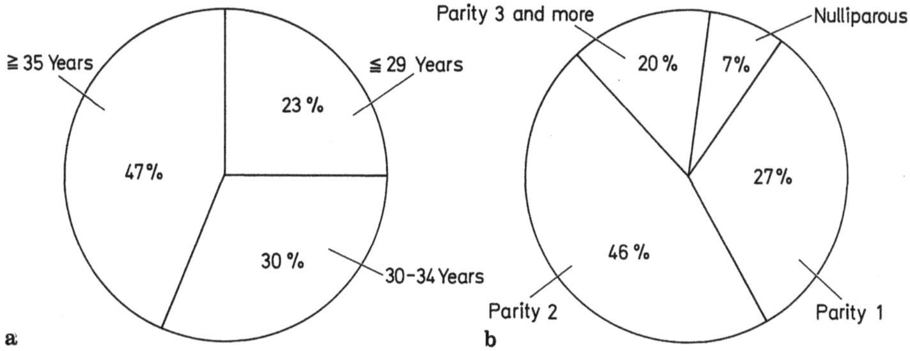

Fig. 2 a, b. Characteristics of Women included in the Present Study. **a** age distribution; **b** parity distribution

In the pilot study "high-risk" women were purposely included (25%); these had either had difficulties with another IUD previously used (Van der Pas 1985) or past events recognized as risks factors (ectopic pregnancy, cervico-isthmic incompetence). No selection was made according to the size of the uterus since the total hysterometries vary between 6 and 9.5 cm. The great majority of insertions were performed during a normal menstrual cycle, preferably during or just after menstruation. The patients were seen again or contacted 3 months after the insertion of the IUD, then regularly every 12 months. At the beginning of the study the devices were voluntarily removed after 2 years; subsequently, the time of usage was extended to 36 months. This is the reason why the continuation ratio at 36 months is artificially lowered.

Results were analysed with the help of a computer program using actuarial statistical methods advocated for this type of study (Tietze and Lewit 1973), except for the multicentre study in which only the net numbers of events are indexed. This analysis is still in progress (Tables 2 and 3).

The numbers of utilization cycles (16721 cycles at 2 years) and the low percentage of losses at follow-up make these results quite significant. Failure rates are low, both in cumulative actuarial percentages (0.9 for 100 women at 3 years) and in Pearl index (0.4). Among the pregnancies that were observed one was ectopic. These two studies showed only nine expulsions. In a group of 22 women who had previously expelled one or several other IUDs only a single expulsion was observed with Ombrelle 250 during the 12th cycle. Removals for medical reasons were infrequent (7.2% at 3 years), showing the good local tolerance of the device. Genital infection necessitated the removal of 11 devices. There was an excellent rate of continuation, respectively, 88.4% and 85.2% at 2 and 3 years. To date 437 devices have already been removed and documented without any special difficulties. Only 24 retrievals were painful or difficult (5.5%). Control biopsies of the endometrium revealed no abnormalities except in cases of removal because of complications. Of 45 patients, 34 (including 5 lost to follow-up) in whom the IUD was removed because of a desire for pregnancy did become pregnant within the next 12 months.

Table 2. Results of the pilot study (September 1986): gross cumulative rates per 100 users

Events	Duration of use			
	12 months	24 months	36 months	48 months
Unwanted pregnancies	0.3	0.7	0.9	0.9
Expulsion	0.5	0.7	0.7	0.7
Removals				
Bleeding/pain	1.6	3.4	3.5	3.9
Other medical reason	1.1	1.8	2.7	2.7
Planned pregnancies	1.4	4.4	6.1	6.4
Continuation rate	95.3	88.4	85.2	84.6
Loss of follow-up	1.4	6.7	28.6	68.2
Number of insertions	711	624	407	89
Number of Cycles	8787	16721	22985	25275

From Tietze and Lewit (1973).

Table 3. Results of the multicentre study

	12 months	Overall
Number of IUDs in situ	925	925
Unwanted pregnancies	2	6
Expulsions	4	6
Removals		
Bleeding/pain	27	45
Infection	6	11
Other medical reasons	10	18
Wanted pregnancies	16	52
Continuation (%)	92	83.5
Lost to follow-up	89	89
Number of women-months	9064	17974

From Cohen et al. (1985).

Discussion

The Ombrelle 250 offers a contraceptive protection comparable to the most effective IUDs. The most interesting fact is the excellent retention obtained with this new system, which enables a low rate of expulsion of this very flexible vector. The flexibility of the device makes its insertion and removal easy and, in addition, prevents trauma to the endometrium. Its adaptability to the variations of the uterine cavity prevents secondary lack of tolerance.

The closed configuration of passive devices has been held responsible for the risk of intestinal obstruction in cases of uterine perforation and presence of the device in the abdominal cavity, but this has never been proven statistically. In the case of a copper IUD the release of copper causes an important immediate inflammatory reaction leading to the encapsulation of the device so that the main risk is the inflammatory reaction and the penetration of a viscus, linked to the rigidity of the device, rather than the risk of obstruction, whatever the shape of the device (Larsson et al. 1981). In all cases the device must be removed as soon as the diagnosis of its position in the abdomen is made (Audebert et al. 1980). Comparative studies presently in progress will enable us to estimate the real advantages of this new intra-uterine device.

Summary

The Ombrelle 250 is a new intra-uterine copper device used for contraceptive purposes. It is characterized by the properties of a very flexible and adaptable plastic vector, enabling it to decrease the risk of endometrial trauma and to adjust itself to the variations of shape of the uterine cavity, thus preventing its expulsion. The performance of this IUD, as demonstrated by pilot studies and a multicentre study, is favorable.

References

Audebert AJM, Larue-Charlus S, Emperaire JC (1980) Considérations sur la perforation utérine complète: à propos de 11 cas. Gynécologie 31:387–396
Audebert AJM, Emperaire JC, Larue-Charlus S, Van der Pas H (1985) Clinical performance of the Ombrelle 250 – a new copper IUD. In: Zatuchni G, Goldsmith A, Sciarra JJ (eds) Intra-uterine-contraception, vol I Harper-Row, Philadelphia, pp 263–265
Cittadini E, Pastore R (1985) Esperienza clinica con un nuovo dispositivo intra-uterino: Ombrelle 250. Contraccezione-fertilità-sessulità 12:169–170
Cohen J, Audebert A, Emperaire JC, Larue-Charlus S, Cittadini E, Nahmanovici C, Erny R (1985) Multicentric study of the Ombrelle IUD. Third Annual Meeting – Society for the advancement of contraception. Bordeaux September 9–13
Cramer DW, Schiff I, Schoenbaum SC et al. (1985) Tubal infertility and the intrauterine device. N Engl J Med 312:941–947
Daling JR, Weil NS, Metch BJ et al. (1985) Primary tubal infertility in relation to the use of an intrauterine device. N Engl J Med 312:937–941
Hasson HM, Berger GS, Edelman DA (1976) Factors affecting IUD performance: I endometrial cavity length. Am J Obstet Gynecol 126:973–979
Ketting E, Van Os W (1985) IUD use in western Europe in intra-uterine contraception. In: Zatuchni GI, Goldsmith A, Sciarra JJ (eds) vol I. Harper and Row, Philadelphia, p 37
Larsson B, Astrom G, Einarsson S, Rydel L et al. (1981) The possible risks of a copper and an inert intra-uterine device situated in the abdominal cavity: an experimental study in pigs and dogs. Fertil Steril 36: 229–232
Luukkainen T, Allonen H, Nielsen NC, Nygren KG, Pyorala T (1983) Five years experience of intra-uterine contraception with the Nova-T and the copper-T-200. Am J Obstet Gynecol 147:885–892
Mishell D (1975) The clinical factor in evaluating IUDs. In: Hefnawi F, Segal S (eds) Analysis of intra-uterine contraception. North Holland, Amsterdam, p 27
Sivin I, Tatum MJ (1981) Four years of experience with the Tcu 380. An intra-uterine contraceptive device. Fertil Steril 36:159–163
Tatum MJ (1977) Clinical aspects of intra-uterine contraception: circumspection. Fertil Steril 28:3–28
Thiery M, Van der Pas H, Vankets H (1985) The MLcu 375 intra-uterine contraceptive device. Adv Contracept 1:37–44
Tietze C, Lewit S (1973) Recommended procedures for the statistical evaluation of intra-uterine contraception. Stud Fam Plann 4:35–41
Van der Pas H (1985) 9re current reporting methods of clinical UID experience up to in "intra-uterine contraception", vol 1. Zatuchni GI, Goldsmith A, Sciarra JJ (eds) Harper and Row, Philadelphia, p 115

Immunology of Female Contraception

Immunological Aspects of Fertility Regulation

G. P. Talwar and A. Gaur

National Institute of Immunology, Shahid Jeet Singh Marg, New Delhi-110 067, India

Infertility due to immunological factors is recognized in females. This can be due to the presence of either (a) antibodies reacting with sperm (Katsh 1959; Isojima et al. 1968); (b) antibodies curtailing the action of luteinizing hormone (LH) with a slightly shortened cycle; or (c) cell-mediated immune reactions resulting in recurrent abortions (Genetet et al. 1986).

A number of tests based on agglutination or immobilization of sperm help to put in evidence the presence of antisperm antibodies (Kibrick et al. 1952; Franklin and Dukes 1964; Isojima et al. 1968; Shulman et al. 1971; Friberg 1974). The manner in which these antibodies were induced in patients is not known. The response in most cases, however, is of a long-lasting duration, presumably because sperm carry a large number of auto- and isoantigens (Hekman and Rumke 1976). In males antisperm antibody formation is frequently observed in situations where the blood testis barrier is disrupted, which happens in some infections, injury or vasectomy (Wartman 1975; Goldberg 1983). In case pregnancies are desired in women having antisperm antibodies, use of condoms over a period to lower the antibody titers or therapy with corticosteroids are reported to give satisfactory results (Shulman and Shulman 1982; Hargreave and Elton 1982; Alexander et al. 1983).

Infertility by LH cross-reactive antibodies can be induced in experimental animals by immunization with β-oLH (ovine luteinizing hormone) (Thau et al. 1979; Thau and Sundaram 1980) and/or with β-HCG (human chorionic gonadotropin) and β-oLH (Talwar et al. 1986). The animals continue ovulating; the luteal cycle, however, is shortened by about 2 days, and the progesterone production capacity of the corpus luteum is reduced. Long-term safety studies (7 years of repeated hyperimmunization) have not shown any pathological consequences (Thau et al. 1986).

Couples sharing histocompatibility antigens have a higher frequency of recurrent abortions (Beer et al. 1981; Thomas et al. 1985). Transfusion of husband or donor leukocytes to the female has resulted in successful pregnancy in many cases (Taylor and Faulk 1981; Beer et al. 1986; Mowbray 1986). Intricate mechanisms are implicit in the phenomenon (Gill 1983; Johnson et al. 1985).

Birth Control Vaccines (BCVs) are a new class of vaccines. In contrast to traditional vaccines, which are directed against communicable diseases, BCVs seek to intercept a selected physiological process within the body. The rationale of these vaccines is to induce antibodies and/or sensitize cells to interfere in the action of a key reproductive hormone or a reproductive process. Theoretically a number of vaccines are possible. Present research is focussed on the following

Female Contraception
Eds.: B. Runnebaum, T. Rabe, L. Kiesel

vaccines: gonadotropin-releasing hormone (GnRH), follicle-stimulating hormone (FSH), LH, and HCG.

1. GnRH: A vaccine directed against the decapeptide GnRH is of potential use in both males and females (Fraser 1983, 1986; Talwar et al. 1984). Other applications of the GnRH vaccine may be found in the treatment of precocious puberty, carcinoma of the prostate, and breast cancer. Immunization against this hormone reduces the production of sex hormones. Bioeffective level of immunization can be achieved without Freund's complete adjuvant (Shaha et al. 1986).
2. FSH: This vaccine is being developed to control male fertility (Murty et al. 1979; Srinath et al. 1983). The vaccine is currently under evaluation in bonnet monkeys with encouraging results (Moudgal et al. 1986).
3. LH: Thau et al. (1979) have demonstrated the efficacy of immunization of rhesus monkeys with β-oLH for control of fertility. Long-term safety studies in monkeys have shown no side effects (Thau et al. 1986). In another modality β-oLH is used in combination with β-HCG (Talwar et al. 1986).
4. HCG: Vaccines against HCG are at the most advanced stage of development. These are intended to be used in females. Currently four vaccines are in phase I clinical trials; these are: (a) α-oLH-β-HCG-TT/CHB, (b) β-HCG-TT/CHB + β-oLH-TT/CHB, (c) β-HCG-TT, and (d) 37aa CTP-DT.

Broadly speaking, these fall into three categories. The CTP (carboxy terminus peptide) vaccine induces antibodies specific to HCG and is non-cross-reactive with LH (Griffin 1986). The peptide has, however, low immunogenicity and requires the use of adjuvants, emulsifiers and oily vehicle (norMDP, Arlacel A, and squalene). The antibodies are of lower affinity ($K_a = 10^9 M^{-1}$) than those generated by immunization with β-HCG ($K_a = 10^{10}$–$10^{11} M^{-1}$) (Shastri et al. 1978; Chen et al. 1980). The bioneutralization capacity of the antibodies is also lower (Louvet and Ross 1974; Ramakrishnan et al. 1979). The demand on the quantum of antibodies and their quality for effective control of fertility in humans will only be known when phase II trials with these vaccines are carried out. Immunization with β-HCG has been demonstrated to control fertility in two species of primates by three laboratories (Stevens 1976; Hearn 1979; Talwar et al. 1980). β-HCG is definitely more immunogenic and produces antibodies of high affinity (Thanavala et al. 1979) and with better bioneutralization capacity (Das et al. 1976). The immunogenicity of β-HCG is further improved by its annealing with the α subunit of oLH. The annealed antigen has a conformation akin to the native hormone and produces antibodies with an improved bioneutralization capacity (Talwar 1986). β-HCG and α-oLH × β-HCG also produce antibodies which are cross-reactive to the extent of 10%–50% with LH. This cross-reaction contributes in an additional way to the efficacy of the vaccine, as demonstrated by the extensive studies of Thau et al. (1979) and many other investigators.

Probing clinical trials with β-HCG-TT vaccines were conducted several years ago in Helsinki, Uppsala, Santiago, Bombay, New Delhi, and Bahia. In all, 63 women received the vaccine at an arbitrary dose of 80 μg of β-HCG linked to 10 Lf (limit of flocculation) of tetanus toxoid. Four fortnightly injections were given for primary immunization; 61 of these made antibodies against HCG and tetanus. Women continued ovulating, and regularity of menstrual cycles was maintained. No disturbance was observed in endocrine, haematological and metabolic functions (Kumar et al. 1976; Hingorani and Kumar 1979; Shahani et al. 1979, 1982). The antibody response in every case was reversible, and in women with good titers, it lasted between 300–500 days. The circulating antibodies were competent to recognize exogenously administered HCG and inactivate its bioactivity (Ramakrishnan et al. 1976). Follow-up of these women over 5 years has indicated no residual or latent effects of immunization and no immunopathological abnormalities have been observed (Nath et al. 1976; Nash et al. 1980).

IND status has been granted by the United States Food and Drug Administration to resume trials with β-HCG-TT vaccines at three dose levels. Approvals have also been given by the National Regulatory Agency in India to start phase I clinical trials of two additional formulations developed by us, namely, (a) α-oLH × β-HCG-TT/CHB and (b) β-HCG-TT/CHB + β-oLH-TT/CHB. Trials have started in five different centers in India. A total of 105 women will be immunized. The protocol envisages basal information and regular monitoring of various physical, hematological, and metabolic functions. The volunteers will also be monitored for regularity of menstrual cycles, hormonal profiles, and auto- and tissue cross-reactive antibodies. The kinetics of antibody response to HCG and carriers will be followed at defined intervals. Fifteen subjects will receive only the vehicle and will serve as controls. To date all the 105 subjects have been enrolled, and 62 women have completed the primary course of three injections. In every case anti-HCG antibodies have been formed. The titers started appearing in circulation after the first injection. No significant side effect has been reported nor any abnormality observed in clinical chemistry, hematology, or immunopathological reactivity of sera. Based on the levels of HCG in early phases of pregnancy, the antibody titer in every woman is distinctly higher than that required to meet the initial challenge.

While trials are in operation on the presently developed vaccines, some laboratories, including our own, have cloned genes for pituitary and placental gonadotropins which could serve eventually as alternate source material for the vaccine. These genes have also been inserted in vaccinia to develop a live recombinant dual-purpose vaccine. The two promoters in the TK region would drive the expression of the subunit genes and the hepatitis B surface antigen (Chakrabarti et al. 1987).

It is envisaged that the next generation of vaccines will be polyvalent in character, containing more than one antigen of the reproductive tract together with one or more carriers of immunoprophylactic benefit.

References

Alexander NJ, Sampson JH, Fulgham DL (1983) Pregnancy rates in patients treated for antisperm antibodies with prednisone. Int J Fertil 28:63

Beer AE, Quebbeman JF, Ayers JWT, Haines RF (1981) Major histo-compatibility complex antigens, maternal and paternal immune response, and chronic habitual abortions in humans. Am J Obstet Gynecol 141:987

Beer AE, Xiaoyu Z, Semprini AE, Quebbeman JF (1986) Pregnancy outcome in human couples with idiopathic recurrent abortions: The role(s) of female serum, mixed lymphocyte culture blocking factors, potentiating factors and local uterine immunity before and after paternal leukocyte immunization. In: Talwar GP (ed) Immunological approaches to contraception and promotion of fertility. Plenum, New York, p 393

Chakrabarti S, Moss B, Srinivasan J, Talwar GP (1987) Vaccinia virus expression vector: live polyvalent vaccine for fertility control and immunoprophylaxis. In: Talwar GP (ed) Contraception research for today and the ninety's. Springer, New York (in press)

Chen HC, Matsuura S, Ohashi M (1980) Limitations and problems of hCG specific antisera. In: Segal SJ (ed) Chorionic gonadotropin. Plenum, New York, p 231

Das C, Salahuddin M, Talwar GP (1976) Investigations on the ability of antisera produced by Pr.β-hCG-TT to neutralize the biological activity of hCG. Contraception 13:171

Frankin RR, Dukes CD (1964) Studies on sperm agglutinating antibody and unexplained infertility. JAMA 190:682

Fraser HM (1983) Active immunisation of stump tailed macaque monkeys against luteinizing hormone releasing hormone, and its effects on menstrual cycles, ovarian steroids and positive feedback. J Reprod Immunol 5:173

Fraser HM (1986) LHRH immunoneutralization: basic studies and prospects for practical application. In: Talwar GP (ed) Immunological approaches to contraception and promotion of fertility. Plenum, New York, p 125

Friberg J (1974) A simple and sensitive micro method for demonstration of sperm agglutinating activity in serum from infertile men and women. Acta Obstet Gynecol Scand [Suppl] 36:21

Genetet N, Fauchet R, Commereuc A, Villard J, Phillippe HJ, Giraud JR, Grall JY, Genetet B (1986) Maternal immune responses and recurrent spontaneous abortions in humans. J Reprod Immunol [Suppl] 154

Gill TJ (1983) Immunogenetics of spontaneous abortions in humans. Transplantation 35:1

Goldberg E (1983) Current status of research on sperm antigens: potential applications as contraceptive vaccines. In: Zatuchni GI (ed) Research frontiers in fertility regulation. Chicago, p 6 (PARFR, vol 2)

Griffin PD (1986) A fertility regulating vaccine based on a carboxyl-terminal peptide of the beta subunit of human chorionic gonadotropin. In: Talwar GP (ed) Immunological approaches to contraception and promotion of fertility. Plenum, New York, p 43

Hargreave TB, Elton RA (1982) Treatment with intermittent high dose methylprednisolone or intermittent betamethasone for antisperm antibodies: preliminary communication. Fertil Steril 38:586

Hearn JP (1979) Long term suppression of fertility by immunization with β-hCG subunit and its reversibility in female marmoset monkeys. In: Talwar GP (ed) Recent advances in reproduction and regulation of fertility. Elsevier/North-Holland, Amsterdam, p 427

Hekman A, Rumke B (1976) Auto and isoimmunity against spermatozoa. In: Miescher PA, Muller-Eberhard HJ (eds) Textbook of immunopathology, 2nd edn. Grune and Stratton, New York, p 947

Hingorani V, Kumar S (1979) Anti hCG immunization phase I clinical trials. In: Talwar GP (ed) Recent advances in reproduction and regulation of fertility. Elsevier/North-Holland, Amsterdam, p 467

Isojima S, Li TS, Ashitaka Y (1968) Immunological analysis of sperm-immobilizing factor found in sera of women with unexplained sterility. Am J Obstet Gynecol 101:677

Johnson PM, Barner RMR, Rish JM, Mollay CM, Woodrow JC (1985) Immunogenetic studies of recurrent spontaneous abortions in human. Exp Clin Immunogenet 2:77

Katsh S (1959) Immunology, fertility and infertility: a historical survey. Am J Obstet Gynecol 77:946

Kibrick S, Belding DL, Merrill B (1952) Methods for the detection of antibodies against mammalian spermatozoa. II. A gelatin agglutination test. Fertil Steril 3:430

Kumar S, Sharma NC, Bajaj JS, Talwar GP, Hingorani V (1976) Clinical profile and toxicology studies on four women immunized with Pr-β-hCG-TT. Contraception 13:253

Louvet JP, Ross GT (1974) Absence of neutralizing effect of antisera to the unique structural region of human chorionic gonadotropin. J Clin Endocrinol Metab 39:1155

Moudgal NR, Murthy GS, Rao AJ, Ravindranath N, Sairam MR, Kotagi SG, Martin F (1986) Immunization against FSH as a method of male contraception. In: Talwar GP (ed) Immunological approaches to contraception and promotion of fertility. Plenum, New York, p 103

Mowbray JF (1986) Effect of immunisation with paternal cells on recurrent spontaneous abortion. In: Clark DA, Croy BA (eds) Reproductive immunology 1986. Elsevier, Amsterdam, p 269

Murty GSRC, Rani CSS, Moudgal NR, Prasad MRN (1979) Effect of passive immunization with specific antiserum to FSH on the spermatogenesis process and fertility of adult male bonnet monkeys (Macaca radiata). J Reprod Fertil [Suppl] 26:147

Nash HA, Talwar GP, Segal S, Luukkainen T, Johansson EDB, Vasquez J, Coutinho E, Sundaram K (1980) Observations on the antigenicity and clinical effects of a candidate antipregnancy vaccine: β-subunit of human chorionic gonadotropin linked to tetanus toxoid. Fertil Steril 34:328

Nath I, Whittingham S, Lambert PH, Talwar GP (1976) Screening for auto antibodies in human subjects immunized with Pr-β-hCG-TT. Contraception 13:225

Ramakrishnan S, Dubey SK, Das C, Salahuddin M, Talwar GP, Kumar S, Hingorani V (1976) Influence of hCG and tetanus toxoid injection on the antibody titers in a subject immunized with Pr-β-hCG-TT. Contraception 13:245

Ramakrishnan S, Das C, Dubey SK, Salahuddin M, Talwar GP (1979) Immunogenicity of three C-termina synthetic peptides of the B-subunit of human chorionic gonadotropin and properties of the antibodies raised against 45 amino acid C-terminal peptide. J Reprod Immunol 1:249

Shaha S, Kaul S, Kini M, Chowdhury M, Anand R, Das C, Talwar GP (1986) Immunization against LHRH without the use of Freund's complete adjuvant. In: Talwar GP (ed) Immunological approaches to contraception and promotion of fertility. Plenum, New York, p 143

Shahani SM, Kulkarni PP, Patel KL (1979) Evaluation of immunological and safety data in women treated with Pr-β-hCG-TT vaccine. In: Talwar GP (ed) Recent advances in reproduction and regulation of fertility. Elsevier/North-Holland, Amsterdam, p 473

Shahani SM, Kulkarni PP, Patel KL, Salahuddin M, Das C, Talwar GP (1982) Clinical and immunological response with Pr-β-hCG-TT vaccine. Contraception 25:421

Shastri N, Dubey SK, Vijaya Ragh Van S, Salahuddin M, Talwar GP (1978) Differential affinity of auto Pr-β-hCG-TT antibodies for hCG and hLH. Contraception 18:23

Shulman JF, Shulman S (1982) Methyl prednisolone treatment of immunologic infertility in the male. Fertil Steril 38:591

Shulman S, Hekman A, Paun C (1971) Antibodies to spermolozoa. II. Sperm agglutination techniques for guinea pigs and human sense. J Reprod Fertil 27:31

Srinath BR, Wickings EJ, Withing C, Nieschlag E (1983) Active immunization with follicle stimulating hormone for fertility control: a four and a half year study in male rhesus monkeys. Fertil Steril 40:110

Stevens VC (1976) Perspectives of development of a fertility control vaccine from hormonal antigens of the trophoblast. In: Development of vaccines for fertility regulation. Scriptor, Copenhagen, p 93

Talwar GP (1986) Immunological approaches contraception: The need; basic premise and overview. In: Talwar GP (ed) Immunological approaches to contraception and promotion of fertility. Plenum, New York, p 17

Talwar GP, Das C, Tandon A, Sharma MG, Salahuddin M, Dubey SK (1980) Immunization against hCG. Efficacy and teratological studies on baboons. In: Anand Kumar TC (ed) Non human primate models for study of human reproduction. Karger, Basel, p 190

Talwar GP, Singh V, Singh O, Das C, Gupta SK, Singh G (1984) Pituitary and extra pituitary sites of action of LHRH-potential uses of active and passive immunization against LHRH. In: Saxena BB, Catt KJ, Birmhauma L, Martini L (eds) Hormone receptors in growth and reproduction. Raven, New York, p 351

Talwar GP, Singh O, Rao V, Sharma DN, Das C, Rao LV (1986) Enhancement of antigonadotropin response to the β subunit of ovine luteinizing hormone by carrier conjugation and combination with the beta-subunit of human chorionic gonadotropin. Fertil Steril 46:120

Taylor C, Faulk WP (1981) Prevention of recurrent abortions with leukocyte transfusions. Lancet 2:68

Thanavala YM, Hearn JP, Hay FC, Hulme M (1979) Characterization of the immunological response in marmoset monkeys immunized against hCG β-subunit and its relationship with their subsequent fertility. J Reprod Immunol 1:263

Thau RB, Sundaram K (1980) The mechanism of action of an antifertility vaccine in the rhesus monkey: Reserval of the effects of antisera to the β-subunit of ovine luteinizing hormone by medroxyprogesterone acetate. Fertil Steril 33:317

Thau RB, Sundaram K, Thornton YS, Seidman LS (1979) Effects of immunization with β-subunit of ovine luteinizing hormone on corpus luteum function in the rhesus monkey. Fertil Steril 31:200

Thau RB, Bond MG, Witkin SS, Sundaram K, Sawyer JK (1986) Lack of toxicological effects following seven years of active immunization of rhesus monkeys with the β-subunit of ovine luteinizing hormone. In: Talwar GP (ed) Immunologic approaches to contraception and promotion of fertility. Plenum, New York, p 25

Thomas ML, Harger JH, Wagener DK, Rabin BS, Gill TJ III (1985) Sharing and spontaneous abortions in humans. Am J Obstet Gynecol 151:1053

Wartman J (1975) Popul Rep [D] 2:31

Application of New Concepts in Cell-Mediated Immunity to the Development of Effective Antifertility Vaccines*

D. J. Anderson, J. A. Hill, F. Haimovici, and C. Xu

Fearing Research Laboratory, Department of Obstetrics, Gynecology and Reproductive Biology, Harvard Medical School, Boston, Massachusetts 02115, USA

A successful antifertility vaccine, based on β-HCG (human chorionic gonadotropin), sperm, or other reproductive-tissue-specific antigens, must elicit an immune response which effectively achieves an antifertility effect. A major problem facing antifertility-vaccine development is the fact that reproductive-tissue antigens are weak immunogens; most vaccine studies to date, in both animal models and human phase I clinical trials, have failed to produce a sustained antibody response and/or the desired antifertility effect.

Limited data on antibody levels in the human female reproductive tract indicate that sufficient antibody levels may not be constantly available for inactivation of reproductive processes. Based on recent evidence that cell-mediated immunological mechanisms often accompany antibody responses in infertility patients [1–3] and on data from our laboratory that soluble products of activated lymphocytes and monocytes (i.e., lymphokines and monokines) affect sperm function [4], embryonic differentiation [5], and trophoblast proliferation [6], we have proposed that local cell-mediated immunological mechanisms may be as important or even more important than antibodies in immunologic infertility. The generation of effective antifertility vaccines therefore may depend on knowledge of local cellular immune mechanisms in the reproductive tissues and on ways to manipulate them.

This chapter provides a review of cellular immunological mediators in the female reproductive tract, featuring recent studies from our laboratory which have begun to characterize immune cell types and soluble products present in the female reproductive tract and their effects on fertility. We will also speculate on how cell-mediated immunological responses may be elicited and regulated to possibly enhance the efficacy of antifertility vaccines.

Cellular Immunological Mediators in the Human Endometrium

The uterus is a mucosal organ which must defend against foreign microorganisms and must periodically both defend against and protect allogeneic tissues such as spermatozoa and the fetus. Early histologic studies of the human endometrium record the presence of lymphoid, monocytic, and granulocytic cells and a pronounced abundance of large granular leukocytes and polymorphonuclear leuko-

* This research was supported by NIH grant CA 42738 and by the Fearing Laboratory Endowment.

Female Contraception
Eds.: B. Runnebaum, T. Rabe, L. Kiesel

cytes in samples taken during predecidualization and menstrual stages of the cycle [7]. Recently, immunohistologic techniques employing antibodies specific for leukocyte subpopulation markers have enabled more precise characterization and quantification of lymphocyte, monocyte, and granulocyte populations in the human endometrium. Macrophages and both suppressor/cytotoxic and helper T-lymphocytes have been identified in the human endometrium by immunohistologic technique [8–10]. Our studies indicate that leukocytes (stained by the pan leukocyte antibody HLe1) comprise up to 20% of the total cells in the endometrial stroma; of the leukocyte population NKH-1 positive cells (natural killer cells?) are the most numerous (50%–70%), followed by macrophages (20%), helper T cells (5%), and suppressor T cells (2%). B lymphocytes are rarely found. The helper:suppressor T-cell ratio fluctuates during the menstrual cycle, with a relatively high ratio observed at periovulation due to a decreased level of suppressor cells.

Data from studies performed in experimental animals indicate that the immunological responsiveness of the uterus is different from that of other mucosal surfaces. There appears to be a poor lymphatic drainage system in the endometrium, although there is an abundance of Ia positive (antigen-presenting) cells. In rat experiments injection of soluble antigen into the uterine lumen failed to induce a primary antibody response, although the antigens primed helper T cells so that a second injection induced a secondary immune response [11]. Lymphocytic infiltration and allograft rejection, evidence of effective cell-mediated immune responses in the uterus, have also been demonstrated in experimental animals [12, 13]. There is essentially no information on the immunological responsiveness of the *human* endometrium. Our preliminary data of immunological mediators residing in the endometrium of infertility patients indicate that a number of patients had proliferating follicles of T cells within the endometrium, and two patients in this group had dramatically elevated B-lymphocyte densities. This interindividual variability suggests that the human endometrium can and does respond to foreign stimuli in some individuals.

Effects of Soluble Products of Immune Responses on Fertility

Recent studies indicate that nonantibody-soluble products of activated lymphocytes and macrophages (termed lymphokines and monokines) can affect a variety of reproductive cell functions in vitro. In initial experiments we found that supernatants from cultures of mitogen-activated lymphocytes decrease sperm motility in vitro; when we tested a panel of currently available purified lymphokines and monokines (Table 1) for effects on human sperm motility we found that the lymphokine γ-interferon and the monokine tumor necrosis factor both significantly affected sperm motility in short-term culture [4]. It has been known for some time that sperm motility is decreased in semen samples containing high numbers of leukocytes [14–16]; our study implicates specific leukocyte factors as being responsible for these effects.

Studies by Berger et al. [15] and Maruyama et al. [17] have also documented inhibitory effects of white blood cells on sperm function in the hamster egg pen-

Table 1. Summary of well characterized lymphokines

	Principal producing cell	Principal cell type affected	Effect	Molecular weight
Lymphokine				
Interleukin 2 (IL-2)	T-lymphocytes	Many cell types, notably T-lymphocytes	T-lymphocytes proliferation; cytotoxic T-cell differentiation; lymphokine-activated killer cell (LAK) activation	14500
Interleukin 3 (IL-3)	Mouse T-lymphocytes	T-lymphocytes, mast cells	T-lymphocyte proliferation; mast cell proliferation; 20 hydroxysteroid dehydrogenase induction	28000–41000
α-Interferon	Virally infected leukocytes	Virus-infected cells, tumors, other lymphocytes, endocrine cells	Cytolysis, hormone-like effects (ACTH, TSH, endorphine)	18000–20000
β-Interferon	Virally infected fibroblasts	Diverse cell populations, macrophages	Inhibition of motility and proliferation	23000
γ-Interferon	Activated T-lymphocytes	Virally infected cells, tumors, trophoblast, allografts	Enhanced phagocytosis	20000–25000
B-cell growth factor	T-lymphocytes	B cells	Induces differentiation and proliferation of B cells	17000
GM-colony stimulating factor	Leukocytes	Bone marrow, macrophage and granulocyte precursors	Induces differentiation of granulocyte and macrophage lineage cells	17000
Monokine				
Interleukin 1 (IL-1)	Macrophages (and others)	Lymphocytes, other cell types	Lymphocyte activation, enhanced antibody production, toxic to certain tumor cells, fibrosis, endogenous pyrogen	17000 (major stable form)
Tumor necrosis factor	Macrophage	Tumor cells	Toxic effect on tumor cell	17000

etration test (HEPT). Preliminary data from studies on the effects of individual lymphokines and monokines on sperm function in the HEPT indicate that low doses of γ-interferon and tumor necrosis factor also inhibit sperm function in this assay [18]. It is predicted, therefore, that soluble products of activated lymphocytes and macrophages residing in the female reproductive tract (i.e., endometrium, oviduct, peritoneal cavity) could affect sperm motility and fertilizing capabilities, contributing to the antifertility effect of local cell-mediated immune responses. Lymphokines and monokines could be induced specifically by sperm antigens or nonspecifically by, for example, infectious organisms or other inflammatory agents in the female reproductive tract.

We have also recently determined that certain lymphokines and monokines affect development of preimplantation mouse embryos in vitro [5]. The lymphokines demonstrating effects in this system were: γ-interferon, colony-stimulating factor, and B-cell growth factor. The lymphokine IL-2 and the monokines tumor necrosis factor and IL-1 did not have significant effects at physiologic doses. However, tumor necrosis factor, in addition to γ-interferon and colony-stimulating factor significantly inhibited the growth of human trophoblast cells (the choriocarcinoma cell line Jeg-3) in vitro [6]. These data suggest that activation of endometrial lymphocytes could produce an environment which adversely affects the preimplantation and implanting embryo. Endometrial lymphocytes/macrophages could become activated in certain women by sperm antigens, embryonic, or trophoblastic antigens or by nonreproductive-tissue-specific antigens such as those of infectious organisms.

Induction of Cell-Mediated Immune Responses

Adjuvants (agents that act nonspecifically to increase specific immune responses to an antigen) can be selected for vaccine administration that selectively enhance cell-mediated immune responses. The muramyle-dipeptide series adjuvants (MDP) are particularly good T-cell adjuvants [19]. Systemic immunization of sperm, trophoblast or other reproductive antigens combined with such an adjuvant could elicit a local (uterine) cell-mediated immune response with introduction of antigen locally (i.e., intercourse or pregnancy). Evidence that such cell-mediated immune responses occur naturally in infertility patients [1] suggests that feedback regulatory mechanisms prevent hypersensitization of the reproductive tissues.

Little is known specifically about the status of cell-mediated immunity in the uterus, including the presence of memory T-cells. It may be possible to enhance local cell-mediated immune responses by implanting intrauterine devices that release antigen combined with a cell-mediated immune adjuvant or specific lymphokines that enhance T-cell responses [20].

References

1. McShane PM, Schiff I, Trentham D (1985) Cellular immunity to sperm in infertile women. JAMA 253:3555
2. Nagarkatii RS, Rao SS (1976) Cell-mediated immunity to homologous spermatozoa following vasectomy in the human male. Clin Exp Immunol 26:239

3. Anderson DJ, Alexander NJ, Fulham DL, Vandenbark AA, Berger DR (1982) Immunity to tumor-associated antigens in vasectomized men. INCI 69:551–556
4. Hill JA, Haimovici F, Politch JA, Anderson DJ (1987) Effects of soluble products of activated lymphocytes and macrophages (lymphokines and monokines) on human sperm motion parameters. Fertil Steril 47:460
5. Hill JA, Haimovici F, Anderson DJ (1987) Products of activated lymphocytes and macrophages inhibit mouse embryo development in vitro. J Immunol (in press)
6. Berkowitz RS, Hill JA, Kurtz CB, Anderson DJ (1987) Effects of products of activated leukocytes (lymphokines and monokines) on the growth of malignant trophoblast cells in vitro. Am J Obstet Gynecol (in press)
7. Noyes RW, Hertig AT, Rock J (1950) Dating the endometrial biopsy. Fertil Steril 1:3–25
8. Kamat BR, Isaacson PG (1987) The immunocytochemical distribution of leukocytic subpopulations in human endometrium. Am J Pathol 127:66–73
9. Morris H, Edwards J, Tiltman A, Emms M (1985) Endometrial lymphoid tissue: an immunohistological study. J Clin Pathol 38:644–652
10. Xu C, Hill JA, Anderson DJ (1987) Identification of T lymphocyte subpopulations in normal and abnormal human endometrial biopsies. Annual Meeting for the Society of Gynecologic Investigation
11. Head JR, Billingham RE (1986) Concerning the immunology of the uterus. Am J Reprod Immunol Microbiol 10:76–81
12. Beer AE, Billingham RE (1974) Host responses to intra-uterine tissue, cellular and fetal allografts. J Reprod Fertil [Suppl] 21:59–88
13. Anderson DJ, Alexander NJ (1979) Induction of uterine leukocytosis and its effect on pregnancy in rats. Biol Reprod 21:1143–1152
14. Sokol S, Jacobson CV, Derrick FC (1975) Use of methenamine hipurate in male infertility. Urology 6:59–62
15. Berger RE, Karp LE, Williamson RA, Koehler J, Moore DE, Holmes KK (1982) The relationship of pyospermia and seminal fluid bacteriology to sperm function as reflected in the sperm penetration assay. Fertil Steril 37:557–564
16. Caldamone AA, Emilson LBV, Al-Jrburi A, Cockett ATK (1980) Prostatitis: prostatic secretion dysfunction affecting fertility. Fertil Steril 34:602–603
17. Maruyama DK, Hale RW, Rogers BJ (1985) Effects of white blood cells on the in vitro penetration of zona-free hamster eggs by human spermatozoa. J Androl 6:127–135
18. Hill JA, Cohen J, Anderson DJ (1987) Effects of activated leukocyte products (lymphokines and monokines) on human sperm function as assessed in the hamster egg penetration test. 5th World Congress on In Vitro Fertilization and Embryo Transfer
19. Allison AC (1979) Mode of action of immunological adjuvants. J Reticuloendothel Soc 26:619–630
20. Anderson DJ (1986) Immunogenetic considerations in the development of contraceptive vaccines based on testicular or sperm antigens. In: Zatuchni GI, Goldsmith A, Spieler JM, Sciarra JJ (eds) Male Contraception: advances and future prospects. Harper and Row, Hagerstown

Sperm Antigens and Antibodies*

N. J. Alexander and S. Ackerman

Section of Reproductive Immunology, Department of Obstetrics and Gynecology, Eastern Virginia Medical School, The Jones Institute, Norfolk, Virginia, USA

Introduction

Immunologic infertility as a clinical entity is based on the observations that infertile men and women often possess antisperm antibodies or higher titers of such antibodies than their fertile counterparts (Feuchter et al. 1981). Immunologic responses to sperm antigens, which occur naturally or are experimentally induced, may significantly influence spermatogenesis, sperm maturation, or gamete interaction (Haas and Beer 1986).

Antisperm antibodies of various classes and directed against multifarious sperm antigens undoubtedly have varying effects on sperm function (Bronson et al. 1984; Alexander and Anderson 1987). Since diagnostic laboratories confine their reports to the presence and titer of a polyclonal immune response to a multitude of sperm antigens, antibodies to nonfunctional sperm components discernible in high concentrations that may not impinge on the ability of sperm to succeed in reproductive processes may be recorded. Likewise, undetectable levels of antibodies may be the causative factor in some cases of infertility.

In order to address these concerns, reproductive immunologists are embracing specific and sensitive assays using monoclonal-antibody and lectin-binding technologies to delineate the integral components of sperm. These methodologies allow for: (a) the delineation of the complexities of sperm differentiation and maturation antigens thereby affording assessment of normal and pathologic aspects of these processes; (b) the characterization and isolation of specific antigens with a view to developing diagnostic assays for immunologic infertility; and (c) the development of antifertility vaccines (Anderson and Alexander 1983). In this review we will concentrate on recent investigations which have utilized either monoclonal antibodies or carbohydrate-binding lectins as probes of the molecular composition of eutherian sperm. We will summarize studies describing monoclonal antibodies which inhibit some aspect of the normal processes of reproduction.

Examination of the sequence of events at the molecular level of spermatogenesis, sperm maturation within the male reproductive tract, and sperm alterations within the female reproductive system prior to and during fertilization allows a better perception of the crucial transition stages in sperm physiology and membrane characteristics (Tesarik 1986; Wassarman 1987). Changes occur: (a) within

* Support for this project was provided by the Contraceptive Research and Development Program, Eastern Virginia Medical School under a cooperative agreement with the United States Agency for International Development (AID) (DPE-2044-A-00-6063-00). The views expressed by the authors do not necessarily reflect the views of AID.

Female Contraception
Eds.: B. Runnebaum, T. Rabe, L. Kiesel

the testis during spermatogenic development (Pelletier and Friend 1983); (b) within the epididymis during sperm maturation (Voglmayr et al. 1983; Cornwall et al. 1986); (c) after migration from the seminal plasma during capacitation (Yanagimachi 1983); (d) at contact with the zona pellucida during zona binding and the acrosome reaction (Lopez et al. 1985; Benau and Storey 1987); and (e) upon fusion of the sperm and egg membranes (Gundersen and Shapiro 1984).

Sperm Differentiation

The process of mammalian spermatogenesis involves well-defined stages of cellular differentiation. These include the mitotic division from spermatogonia to primary spermatocytes, the first meiotic division to secondary spermatocytes, the second meiotic division to spermatids, and the morphologic transformations of spermiogenesis. The appearance of unique membrane antigens on differentiating germ cells has been described in mice (Millette and Bellve 1977), rats (Tung and Fritz 1978), guinea pigs (Tung et al. 1979), and rabbits (O'Rand and Romrell 1980).

The heterogeneity of antibodies found in polyclonal antisera often precludes a definitive characterization of differentiating antigens (Bellve and Moss 1983). Therefore, monoclonal antibodies against testicular cell mixtures (Bechtol et al. 1979) and sperm from the cauda epididymis (Feuchter et al. 1981) have better defined antigens of various mouse spermatogenic cell populations. In fact, monoclonal antibodies have been used to illustrate testicular cell differentiation antigens in mice (Fenderson et al. 1984; Lee and Wong 1986), rats (Gaunt 1982), rabbits (O'Rand et al. 1984), and baboons (Isahakia 1987).

Sperm Maturation

Mammalian sperm undergo many physiologic alterations during their passage through the rete testis, efferent ducts, and epididymis, leading to increased motility and culminating in fertility (Bedford and Cooper 1978; Hinrichsen-Kohane et al. 1984). The recognized maturation changes include: (a) alterations in size and structure of the head, acrosome, and midpiece regions (Yanagimachi 1981); (b) changes in surface physiochemistry, including an increase in negative charge and modifications of membrane-bound biomolecules (Moore and Bedford 1979; Rifkin and Olson 1985); (c) acquired capacity for motility related to changes in disulfide bonding in the tail and/or the effects of "forward motility factor(s)" secreted by the epididymal epithelium (Bedford et al. 1973; Acott and Hoskins 1981); (d) ability to interact with the zona pellucida and to bind to and penetrate the egg plasma membrane (Orgebin-Crist and Fournier-Delpech 1982).

Although compositional changes in sperm surface while in the epididymis may include the loss, alteration, or unmasking of preexisting molecular components, most changes reflect the addition of new substances to the sperm membrane (Eddy et al. 1985). Monoclonal antibodies have been used to demonstrate changes in membrane antigenicity during maturation. Four sperm antigens have been found in increasingly greater concentrations in sperm from testis, caput, corpus, cauda, and vas (Feuchter et al. 1981). Sperm retained in the efferent ducts and not exposed to epididymal secretions do not acquire one of these antigens – evidence that the antigen was not intrinsically synthesized (Vernon et al. 1982). Monoclonal antibodies have defined sperm maturational antigens of epididymal origin in rats (Rifkin and Olson 1985; Gaunt et al. 1983), hamsters (Moore and Hartman 1984), and mice (Fox et al. 1982). A number of monoclonal antibodies also have been generated to human seminal plasma antigens (Shigeta et al. 1980; Paul et al. 1982; Wolf et al. 1983; Lee et al. 1984; Mettler et al. 1984).

Capacitation

Capacitation, a process occurring within the female reproductive system or in appropriate in vitro conditions, results in changed sperm motility patterns and facilitates the acrosome reaction (Moore and Bedford 1983). Although the complete molecular dynamics of capacitation are unknown, sperm membrane modifications have been observed (O'Rand 1979; Friend 1984). This process involves the loss of surface antigens (Koehler 1981; Vernon et al. 1985); redistribution of membrane macromolecules (Myles and Primakoff 1984) and intramembrane particles (Tesarik 1986); and alterations in lectin-binding patterns (Talbot and Franklin 1978; Cross and Overstreet 1987). Apparently these membrane changes involve the selective removal of seminal plasma fertilization inhibitors (i.e., decapacitating substances) (Van der Ven et al. 1982). During capacitation sperm experience a reduction in net membrane negativity, decreased free surface -SH or $-NH_2$ groups, and increased membrane permeability (Hinrichsen-Kohan et al. 1984). These seemingly dramatic changes, however, are reversible (Gulyas and Schmell 1981).

Capacitation precipitates striking changes in the binding patterns of antisperm monoclonal antibodies. In the guinea pig one monoclonal antibody binds to the posterior tail prior to capacitation but to the anterior tail after capacitation (Myles and Primakoff 1984). Following capacitation three monoclonal antibodies directed against mouse sperm change their binding site from the acrosome and become uniformly distributed over the whole sperm surface. (Lee et al. 1986) In a series of World Health Organization (WHO) workshop analyses of 66 antihuman sperm monoclonal antibodies, three (S20, S32, S37) reacted more strongly with uncapacitated sperm and one (S60) with capacitated sperm (Anderson et al. 1987). Monoclonal antibodies to sperm antigens which undergo qualitative or positional change during capacitation are important reagents that allow the interpretation of this crucial reproductive process.

Acrosome Reaction

The acrosome reaction, a series of focal fusions between the outer anterior acrosomal and plasma membranes, resulting in vesiculation of these membranes that allows release of the acrosomal matrix (Moore and Bedford 1983), is completed after sperm contact the zona pellucida (Gulyas and Schmell 1981). Enzyme release (e.g., hyaluronidase, acrosin, and other proteases) from sperm that have not yet reached the zona assists the motile sperm in dispersing the cumulus allowing acrosomal intact sperm to contact, bind and, initiate penetration of the zona pellucida (Gulyas and Schmell 1981).

Zona pellucida sperm receptors have been identified in mice (Wassarman 1987). The receptor ZP3 provides the zona with binding specificity and assists in the initiation of the acrosome reaction. ZP3 is a glycoprotein of molecular weight 83 000 with both asparagine-linked (N-linked) and serine-threonine-linked (O-linked) oligosaccharide residues. The O-linked oligosaccharides are responsible for sperm binding, suggesting why various lectins, monosaccharides, and glycoconjugates prevent binding of sperm to eggs (Shur and Hall 1982). Several sperm surface macromolecules are thought to be the sperm complement to ZP3. One of these, galactosyl transferase, presumably binds to N-acetylglucosamine of the O-linked oligosaccharide of ZP3 (Shur and Hall 1982). Some investigators suggest that a trypsin-like proteinase may be involved (Lopez et al. 1985; Benau and Storey 1987), while others postulate a glycosidase or lectin (Wassarman 1987). Identification of this component will surely advance our understanding of sperm-egg interactions and may provide the means for contraceptive manipulation of this key link in the chain of reproductive reactions.

Although only acrosome-reacted sperm can penetrate the zona, the mechanism by which zona penetration by sperm is accomplished remains uncertain (Tesarik 1986; Wassarman 1987; Gulyas and Schmell 1981). It has been postulated that the presence of acrosin, bound to the inner acrosomal membrane and exposed after the acrosome reaction, allows the sperm to enzymatically digest their way through the zona. Support for this concept is provided by the finding that trypsin inhibitors impair in vitro penetration of the zona by rabbit sperm (Stambaugh et al. 1969). Monoclonal antibodies against human acrosin may also inhibit hydrolysis of the zona by purified human acrosin (Elce et al. 1986). However, other studies do not support this hypothesis. An immunoelectron microscopy study (Huneau et al. 1984) and one employing monoclonal antibodies reactive to acrosin (Kallajoki et al. 1986) indicate that acrosin is not on the inner acrosomal membranes following in vitro induction of the acrosomal reaction. These disparate findings could be explained if zona penetration varies according to species, and that is not yet known.

Fusion of Gamete Membranes

The passage of sperm into the egg cytoplasm can arbitravily be divided into: (a) binding of sperm to egg membrane, (b) fusion of the membranes, and (c) incorporation of sperm nuclear matrix and flagellum into the egg (Moore and Bedford 1983; Hartmann 1983). Only capacitated and acrosome-reacted sperm can bind to the egg plasmalemma. Fusion begins in the equatorial region. Contrary to earlier reports of fusion initiated in the postacrosomal region, electron-microscopic evidence indicates (Moore and Bedford 1983) that the fusion of membranes and dissolution of the nuclear envelope begin within a zone of intimate contact. Fusion then proceeds posteriorly along and over the sperm's plasma membrane, covering the postacrosomal region of the head and tail, until the nuclear matrix and flagellum are gradually incorporated in the egg cytoplasm.

Unlike the binding of sperm to the zona pellucida, the attachment and penetration of sperm into the egg plasma membrane is not confined to a particular region (Moore and Bedford 1983). This is especially apparent in the zona-free hamster egg, a major model for studies of fertilization (Pavlok 1979). The degree of specificity, demonstrated at the sperm-egg interface, and the lack of protein or polysaccharide receptors on the vitellus may explain the nondifferentiated nature of the sperm-egg interface (Moore and Bedford 1983). However, blocking of gamete membrane fusion by monoclonal antibodies reactive to sperm antigens of mice (Saling et al. 1985), guinea pigs (Primakoff et al. 1987), hamsters (Moore and Hartman 1984), and humans (O'Rand and Irons 1984), argues for the interaction of antigenic ligands and receptors are involved in this process. For example, Primakoff et al. (1987) have generated a monoclonal antibody, PH-30, which inhibits fusion between zona-free guinea pig eggs and the acrosome-reacted sperm of guinea pigs. This monoclonal antibody recognizes two proteins (44 000 and 60 000 molecular weight) from the posterior head region and not from the equatorial region. Alternatively, Saling et al. (1985) produced a monoclonal antibody, M-29, which inhibits fusion of mouse sperm and eggs but does bind to the equatorial region of acrosome-reacted sperm. Whether this discrepancy between the site of the "fusion-related" antigens is associated with species differences or with the phenomenon of antigen mobility/redistribution in sperm plasma membranes (Primakoff and Myles 1983) must be addressed.

Effects of Antisperm Antibodies on Fertility

Fertility dysfunctions induced by monoclonal antibodies can be made manifest by impaired sperm motility, sperm-zona binding, acrosome reaction, zona penetration, fusion of gamete plasma membranes, or postfertilization embryonic development. Monoclonal antibodies that impede some aspect of fertilization provide elucidation of the fertilization process.

Some monoclonal antibodies to mouse sperm inhibit sperm motility while others inhibit sperm-zona binding. A monoclonal antibody specific for rabbit sperm acrosomes blocks in vitro binding to the zona pellucida (Naz et al. 1983) but apparently does not impair in vivo binding or penetration of the zona. Various other monoclonal antibodies inhibit in vitro fertilization by blocking sperm-zona attachment in hamsters (Moore and Hartman 1984), rabbits (O'Rand et al. 1984), and mice (Saling and Lakoski 1985; Lee et al. 1986).

An antigen of mouse sperm of molecular weight 220 000–240 000 participates specifically in the induction of the acrosome reaction (Saling 1986), whereas monoclonal antibody M42 inhibits fertilization without impairing sperm-zona binding. When the calcium ionophore A23187 is used to override the effects of M42, treatment of sperm with M42 does not irreversibly affect the ability of sperm to penetrate the zona, a finding that suggests M42 directly inhibits the acrosome reaction. A constituent of mouse zona pellucida ZP3 is also implicated in the initiation of the acrosome reaction (Wassarman 1987). Monoclonal antibody to the protein moiety of this glycoprotein antigen (i.e., anti-ZP3) inhibits fertilization of mouse eggs by mouse sperm both in vitro and in vivo (East et al. 1985). Anti-ZP3 does not block sperm-zona binding or the fusion of gamete membranes when zona-free eggs are used. It is postulated, therefore, that inhibition of fertilization is caused by the impaired zona penetration resulting from a direct inhibition of the acrosome reaction.

The encounter and fusion of the sperm and egg plasma membrane probably requires specific ligand/receptor interactions (Primakoff et al. 1987). It is not surprising, therefore, that antibodies to sperm antigens of infertile individuals have been shown to occasionally inhibit the penetration of human sperm into zona-free hamster eggs (Haas et al. 1980; Alexander 1984). Two recent studies have apparently corroborated this phenomenon, using monoclonal antibodies to specific sperm antigens (Primakoff et al. 1987; Saling et al. 1985).

Since sperm antigens have been found on preimplantation stage embryos, it is conceivable that antisperm immune responses may affect postfertilization embryo development. Gabel et al. (1979) report that mouse embryos exhibit a "patch" of sperm-derived membrane antigens after fusion of the gametes during the early cleavage stages. Recently, Wiley et al. (1987) reported that human sperm antigens were detected on zona-free hamster eggs after sperm penetration. Naz et al. (1986) have isolated a germ cell antigen from rabbit sperm and testes (GA-1, 63 000 molecular weight) using monoclonal antibody 8C10.5, and have demonstrated reduced fertility in both rabbits and mice actively immunized with this antigen. Interestingly, evidence suggests that the antibodies produced to GA-1 do not inhibit in vivo or in vitro fertilization rates, nor do they affect development of fertilized mouse eggs cultured in anti-GA-1 antiserum. However, when sperm are incubated in this antiserum prior to artificial insemination of rabbits, significantly fewer fertilized eggs reach the blastocyst stage compared to eggs fertilized with control serum. This finding suggests that antibodies attached to GA-1 on the sperm may enter the egg and adversely affect early embryonic development.

Distribution of Monoclonal Antibody and Lectin-Binding Patterns

The plasma membrane reflects the changing developmental and physiological states of sperm, and membrane-associated receptors are intimately involved in the initiation and control of many of these changes (Koehler 1985). Characterization of the sperm membrane surface can yield important clues to the sperm's functional capabilities. For example, changes can be observed in membrane antigenicity, lectin-binding patterns, distribution and density of intramembraneous particles, and distribution of the surface charge during differentiation, maturation, capacitation, and the acrosome reaction (Koehler 1978; Moore and Bedford 1983). The sperm membrane can be characterized according to: (a) regional differentiation into discrete structural and functional domains; (b) fluid mobility of some macromolecules within the membrane; (c) specific induction of surface modifications via intrinsic cues (e.g., genetic induction of LDH-C4 of H-Y antigens during differentiation) or by extrinsic cues (e.g., uterine factors inducing capacitation and zona factors inducing the acrosome reaction); and (d) derivation of some surface components from exogenous sources (e.g., secretory products of the epididymal epithelium).

As we have mentioned, two common approaches used to probe sperm surface determinants are analyses of binding patterns of monoclonal antibodies (Bellve

Table 1. Anti-sperm monoclonal antibody bindings sites

Sperm source	Investigators	Monoclonal antibody	Binding site
Mouse	Schmell et al. (1982)	SMA-1	AA
		SMA-2	PA+M
		SMA-3	H
		SMA-4	M+T
	Saling et al. (1983)	AMS IV-25	Mostly M (diffuse H+T)
		AMS IV-33	A
		AMS IV-54	M+T
		AMS IV-76	M+T
	Lee and Wong (1986)	M29	Eq
	Feuchter et al. (1981)	27 MAB clones	A
		17 MAB clones	H
		7 MAB clones	PA
		4 MAB clones	M+T
		1 MAB clones	T
Rat	Gaunt et al. (1983)	1B6	PA
		2D6	WS
		2B1	T+CD
Hamster	Moore and Hartman (1984)	18 MAB clones	AA
		10 MAB clones	A
		9 MAB clones	WS
		2 MAB clones	A+M
		1 MAB clones	T
Guinea pig	Primakoff and Myles (1983)	HM 3.10	H
		HM 5.8	T
		HM 9.0	M
		HM 2.0, HM 1.0	H+T
Rabbit	O'Rand et al. (1984)	A.F. 1	Mostly H (+M)
Human	O'Rand and Irons (1984)	A.F. 1	Mostly M (diffuse H+T)
	Lee et al. (1982)	HS-206-1	A
		HS-206-2	A
	Anderson et al. (1987)	9 MAB clones	A
		11 MAB clones	WS

A, acrosome; AA, anterior acrosome; CD, cytoplasmic droplet; Eq, equatorial region; H, head; M, midpiece; PA, postacrosomal; T, tail; WS, whole sperm.

and Moss 1983) or lectins (Ahuja 1985). Since sperm membranes are vulnerable to damage by manipulation and fixation, which may result in either the loss of integral membrane components or the artificial exposure of subsurface moieties (Cross and Overstreet 1987), one must evaluate with caution the results reported by different investigators. Membrane components may become mobile and/or shed after placement in various in vitro conditions or after attachment of a probe (Gaunt et al. 1983; Myles et al. 1984). Finally, regionality of surface antigens and lectin-receptors demonstrate species-specificity and differentiate stage-specificity (Holt 1982). Should these latent problems be addressed appropriately, elucidation of the molecular architecture of the sperm's surface can provide insight into the molecular control of sperm action.

We have compiled a list of monoclonal antibody binding sites reported in several recent studies (Table 1). It is intended that this representative sample illustrates the diversity of antigen distribution patterns in various species of sperm. Of 65 monoclonal antibodies generated to mouse sperm antigens by four groups of investigators, 38 were reactive to acrosomal antigens. In a recent study of 66 monoclonal antibodies to human sperm submitted by 29 laboratories to a WHO workshop, the most common binding site was again the acrosome region (Anderson et al. 1987). Likewise, a predominance of antiacrosomal specificity was reported by Primakoff and Myles (1983).

Contraceptive Vaccine Potential

The possibility of controlling fertility through immunization with unique antigens is enticing but depends on identification of physiologically active moieties specific to the human reproductive tract. The principle governing any contraceptive vaccine is that circulating antibodies will combine with reproductive-tract or pregnancy-specific antigens inhibiting the biological action of the target cell. Antibodies can impede reproductive functions in many ways, including: causing conformational changes in surface antigens by blocking binding sites; affecting motility or cellular interaction; or inducing cell death (complement-mediated cytotoxicity). Since reproductive cycles are episodic in women, it seems more likely that vaccines will be developed for use in women, even if the antigen is derived from men. Antibodies against spermatozoa may hold a greater promise of reversal in women; in men they could possibly destroy the germinal epithelium and thus cause irreversible sterility.

Many theoretical problems are associated with contraceptive vaccine development. A major concern, and one that must be addressed, is the possibility that the antigen may not cross-react and cause damage to other tissues. Many antigen determinants found in the reproductive tract have both normal tissue constituents and their products in common. Many antigens in seminal plasma are also found in other body fluids. In a recent evaluation of antisperm monoclonal antibodies by the WHO, only three were found to be relatively sperm-specific. Many monoclonals developed to human sperm are directed against antigens from the seminal plasma. However, an antibody to seminal plasma is not in and of itself inappropriate if the antigen is unique to the male reproductive tract.

Because individual responses to antigens vary considerably, some individuals will show a heightened immune response to a vaccine and others will not. Patients will probably require repeated exposure to contraceptive vaccines; only certain viruses to which we are exposed during childhood provide life-long immunity. Although there is of yet no evidence, researchers have frequently expressed the hope that use of sperm antigens in a vaccine would allow sexual intercourse itself to provide a booster.

The variability inherent in the immune response coupled with the need to use powerful adjuvants to achieve high antibody titers, have impeded the development of a reliable and acceptable form of immunologic contraception for human use. Since we do not completely understand the maternal fetal immune relationship, the possibility exists that incomplete effects of contraception will result in abortion or teratogenesis or in a higher incidence of neoplasms. Testing a vaccine approach therefore will be a prodigious, expensive, and time-consuming task.

References

Acott TS, Hoskins DD (1981) Bovine sperm forward motility protein: binding to epididymal spermatozoa. Biol Reprod 24:234–240
Ahuja KK (1985) Carbohydrate determinants involved in mammalian fertilization. Am J Anat 174:207–223
Alexander NJ (1984) Antibodies to human spermatozoa impede sperm penetration of cervical mucus or hamster eggs. Fertil Steril 41:433–439
Alexander NJ, Anderson DJ (1987) Immunology of semen. Fertil Steril 47:192–205
Anderson DJ, Alexander NJ (1983) A new look at antifertility vaccines. Fertil Steril 40:557–571
Anderson DJ, Johnson PM, Alexander NJ, Jones WR, Griffin PD (1987) Monoclonal antibodies to human trophoblast and sperm antigens. Report of two WHO-sponsored Workshops June 30, 1986 – Toronto, Canada. J Reprod Immunol 10:231–257
Bechtol KB, Brown SC, Kennett RH (1979) Recognition of differentiation antigens of spermatogenesis in the mouse by using antibodies from spleen cell-myeloma hybrids after syngeneic immunization. Proc Natl Acad Sci USA 76:363–367
Bedford JM, Cooper GW (1978) Membrane fusion events in the fertilization of vertebrate eggs. In: Poste G, Nicolson GL (eds) Membrane fusion. Elsevier, Amsterdam, pp 65–125
Bedford JM, Calvin H, Cooper GW (1973) The maturation of spermatozoa in the human epididymis. J Reprod Fertil [Suppl] 18:199–213
Bellve AR, Moss SB (1983) Monoclonal antibodies as probes of reproductive mechanisms. Biol Reprod 28:1–26
Benau DA, Storey BT (1987) Characterization of the mouse sperm plasma membrane zona-binding site sensitive to trypsin inhibitors. Biol Reprod 36:282–292
Boettcher B, Hjort T, Rumke P, Shulman S, Vyazov OE (eds) (1977) Auto- and iso-antibodies to antigens of the human reproductive system. I. Results of an international comparative study. Clin Exp Immunol 30:173–180
Bronson R, Cooper G, Rosenfeld D (1984) Sperm antibodies: their role in infertility. Fertil Steril 42:171–183
Bronson R, Cooper G, Hjort T, Ing R, Jones WR, Wang SX et al. (1985) Anti-sperm antibodies, detected by agglutination, immobilization, microcytotoxicity and immunobeadbinding assays. J Reprod Immunol 8:279–299
Cornwall GA, Smyth TB, Vindivich D, Harter C, Robinson J, Chang TSK (1986) Induction and enhancement of progressive motility in hamster caput epididymal spermatozoa. Biol Reprod 35:1065–1074
Cross NL, Overstreet JW (1987) Glycoconjugates of the human sperm surface: distribution and alterations that accompany capacitation in vitro. Gamete Res 16:23–35
Davajan V, Nakamura RM, Bernstein GS (1986) Role of immunology in infertility. In: Mishell DR Jr, Davajan V (eds) Infertility, contraception, and reproductive endocrinology. Medical Economics, Oradell, pp 521–530
East IJ, Gulyas BJ, Dean J (1985) Monoclonal antibodies to the murine zona pellucida protein with sperm receptor activity: effects on fertilization and early development. Dev Biol 109:268–273
Eddy EM, Vernon RB, Muller CH, Hahnel AC, Fenderson BA (1985) Immunodissection of sperm surface modifications during epididymal maturation. Am J Anat 174:225–237
Elce JS, Graham EJ, Zboril G (1986) Monoclonal antibodies to bovine and human acrosin. Biochem Cell Biol 64:1242–1248

Fenderson BA, O'Brien DA, Millette CF, Eddy EM (1984) Dev Biol 103:117–128
Feuchter FA, Vernon RB, Eddy EM (1981) Analysis of the sperm surface with monoclonal antibodies: topographically restricted antigens appearing in the epididymis. Biol Reprod 24:1099–1110
Fox N, Damjanov I, Knowles BB, Solter D (1982) Teratocarcinoma antigen is secreted by epididymal cells and coupled to maturing sperm. Exp Cell Res 137:485–488
Friend DS (1984) Membrane organization and differentiation in the guinea-pig spermatozoon. In: Blerkom JV, Motta PM (eds) Ultrastructure of reproduction. Nijhoff, pp 75–85
Gabel CA, Eddy EM, Shapiro BM (1979) After fertilization, sperm surface components remain as a patch in sea urchin and mouse embryos. Cell 18:207–215
Gaunt SJ (1982) A 28K-dalton cell surface autoantigen of spermatogenesis: characterization using a monoclonal antibody. Dev Biol 89:92–100
Gaunt SJ, Brown CR, Jones R (1983) Identification of mobile and fixed antigens on the plasma membrane of rat spermatozoa using monoclonal antibodies. Exp Cell Res 144:275–284
Gulyas BJ, Schmell ED (1981) Sperm-egg recognition and binding in mammals. In: Bioregulators of reproduction. Academic, New York, pp 499–519
Gundersen GG, Shapiro BM (1984) Sperm surface proteins persist after fertilization. J Cell Biol 99:1343–1353
Haas G Jr, Sokoloski JE, Wolf DP (1980) The interfering effect of human IgG antisperm antibodies on human sperm penetration of zona-free hamster eggs. Am J Reprod Immunol 1:40–43
Haas GG Jr, Beer AE (1986) Immunologic influences on reproductive biology: sperm gametogenesis and maturation in the male and female genital tracts. Fertil Steril 46:753–765
Hartmann JF (1983) Mammalian fertilization: Gamete surface interactions in vitro. In: Hartmann JF (ed) Mechanism and control of animal fertilization. Academic, New York, pp 325–364
Herr JC, Eddy EM (1980) Detection of mouse sperm antigens by a surface labeling and immunoprecipitation approach. Biol Reprod 22:1263–1274
Hinrichsen-Kohane AC, Hinrichsen MJ, Schill W-B (1984) Molecular events leading to fertilization – a review. Andrologia 16:321–341
Holt WV (1982) Functional development of the mammalian sperm plasma membrane. Oxford Rev Reprod Biol 4:195–240
Huneau D, Harrison RAP, Flechon J-E (1984) Ultrastructural localization of proacrosin and acrosin in ram spermatozoa. Gamete Res 9:425–440
Isahakia MA (1987) Characterisation of baboon testicular antigens using monoclonal antisperm antibodies. (in press)
Kallajoki M, Virtanen I, Suominen J (1986) The fate of acrosomal staining during the acrosome reaction of human spermatozoa as revealed by a monoclonal antibody and PNA-lectin. Int J Androl 9:181–194
Kay DJ, Boettcher B (1985) Common Specificities of Auto- and Iso-Antibodies to Human Spermatozoa. Am J Reprod Immunol Microbiol 8:10–14
Koehler JK (1978) The mammalian sperm surface: studies with specific labeling techniques. Int Rev Cytol 54:73–105
Koehler JK (1981) Surface alterations during the capacitation of mammalian spermatozoa. Am J Primatol 1:131–141
Koehler JK (1985) Introduction. Am J Anat 174:205
Lee C-YG, Huang Y-S, Huang C-H, Hu P-C, Menge AC (1982) Monoclonal antibodies to human sperm antigens. J Reprod Immunol 4:173–181
Lee C-YG, Wong E (1986) Development studies of sperm surface antigens using sperm-specific monoclonal antibodies. J Reprod Immunol 9:275–287
Lee C-YG, Wong E, Richter DE, Menge AC (1984) Monoclonal antibodies to human sperm antigens II. J Reprod Immunol 6:227–238
Lee C-YG, Wong E, Zhang J-H (1986) Inhibitory effects of monoclonal sperm antibodies on the fertilization of mouse oocytes in vitro and in vivo. J Reprod Immunol 9:261–274

Lopez LC, Bayna EM, Litoff D, Shaper NL, Shaper JH, Shur BD (1985) Receptor function of mouse sperm surface galactosyltransferase during fertilization. J Cell Biol 101:1501–1510

Mettler L, Paul S, Baukloh V, Feller AC (1984) Monoclonal sperm antibodies: their potential for investigation of sperms as target of immunological contraception. Am J Reprod Immunol 5:125–128

Millette CF (1979) Cell surface antigens during mammalian spermatogenesis. In: Moscona AA, Monroy A (eds) Current topics in development biology. Academic, New York, pp 1–29

Millette CF, Bellve AR (1977) Temporal expression of membrane antigens during mouse spermatogenesis. J Cell Biol 74:86–97

Moore HDM, Bedford JM (1979) Net surface-charge of mammalian spermatozoa as determined by isoelectric-focusing changes following sperm maturation, ejaculation, incubation in the female tract, and after enzyme treatment. Int J Androl 2:449–462

Moore HDM, Bedford JM (1983) The interaction of mammalian gametes in the female. In: Hartmann JF (ed) Mechanism and control of animal fertilization. Academic, New York, pp 453–497

Moore HDM, Hartman TD (1984) Localization by monoclonal antibodies of various surface antigens of hamster spermatozoa and the effect of antibody on fertilization in vitro. J Reprod Fertil 70:175–183

Myles DG, Primakoff P (1984) Localized surface antigens of guinea pig sperm migrate to new regions prior to fertilization. J Cell Biol 99:1634–1641

Myles DG, Primakoff P, Koppel DE (1984) A localized surface protein of guinea pig sperm exhibits free diffusion in its domain. J Cell Biol 98:1905–1909

Naz RK, Saxe JM, Menge AC (1983) Inhibition of fertility in rabbits by monoclonal antibodies against sperm. Biol Reprod 28:249–254

Naz RK, Poffenberger RJ, Menge AC (1986) Reduction of fertility in female rabbits and mice actively immunized with a germ cell antigen (GA-1) from the rabbit. J Reprod Immunol 9:163–173

O'Rand MG (1979) Changes in sperm surface properties correlated with capacitation. In: Fawcett DW, Bedford JM (eds) The spermatozoon: maturation, motility, surface properties and comparative aspects. Urban and Schwarzenberg, Munich, pp 195–204

O'Rand MG, Irons GP (1984) Monoclonal antibodies to rabbit sperm autoantigens. II. Inhibition of human sperm penetration of zona-free hamster eggs. Biol Reprod 30:731–736

O'Rand MG, Romrell LJ (1980) Appearance of regional surface autoantigens during spermatogenesis: comparison of anti-testis and anti-sperm autoantisera. Dev Biol 75:431–441

O'Rand MG, Irons GP, Porter JP (1984) Monoclonal antibodies to rabbit sperm autoantigens. I. Inhibition of in vitro fertilization and localization on the egg. Biol Reprod 30:721–729

Orgebin-Crist M-C, Fournier-Delpech S (1982) Evidence for maturational changes during epididymal transit. J Androl 3:429–433

Paul S, Baukloh V, Baillie M, Mettler L (1982) Generation of monoclonal antibodies against human spermatozoa and seminal plasma constituents. Clin Reprod Fertil 1:235–240

Pavlok A (1979) Interspecies interaction of zona-free ova with spermatozoa in mouse, rat, and hamster. Anim Reprod Sci 2:395–402

Pelletier RM, Friend DS (1983) Development of membrane differentiations in the Guinea pig spermatid during spermiogenesis. Am J Anat 167:119–141

Primakoff P, Myles DG (1983) A map of the guinea pig sperm surface constructed with monoclonal antibodies. Dev Biol 98:417–428

Primakoff P, Hyatt H, Tredick-Kline J (1987) Identification and purification of a sperm surface protein with a potential role in sperm-egg membrane fusion. J Cell Biol 104:141–149

Rifkin JM, Olson GE (1985) Characterization of maturation-dependent extrinsic proteins of the rat sperm surface. J Cell Biol 100:1582–1591

Saling PM (1986) Mouse sperm antigens that participate in fertilization. IV. A monoclonal antibody prevents zona penetration by inhibition of the acrosome reaction. Dev Biol 117:511–519

Saling PM, Lakoski KA (1985) Mouse sperm antigens that participate in fertilization. II. Inhibition of sperm penetration through the zona pellucida using monoclonal antibodies. Biol Reprod 33:527–536

Saling PM, Raines LM, O'Rand MG (1983) Monoclonal antibody against mouse sperm blocks a specific event in the fertilization process. J Exp Zool 227:481–486

Saling PM, Irons G, Waibel R (1985) Mouse sperm antigens that participate in fertilization. I. Inhibition of sperm fusion with the egg plasma membrane using monoclonal antibodies. Biol Reprod 33:515–526

Schmell ED, Yuan LC, Gulyas BJ, August JT (1982) Identification of mammalian sperm surface antigens. I. Production of monoclonal anti-mouse sperm antibodies. Fertil Steril 37:249–257

Shigeta M, Watanabe T, Maruyama S, Koyama K, Isojima S (1980) Sperm-immobilizing monoclonal antibody to human seminal plasma antigens. Clin Exp Immunol 42:458–462

Shulman S, (1986a) Sperm antigens and autoantibodies: Effects on fertility. Am J Reprod Immunol Microbiol 10:82–89

Shulman S (1986b) Infertility as caused by sperm antibodies. Gynecol Obstet Invest 22:113–127

Shur BD, Hall NG (1982) A role for mouse sperm surface galactosyltransferase in sperm binding to the egg zona pellucida. J Cell Biol 95:575–579

Stambaugh R, Brackett BG, Mastroianni L (1969) Inhibition of in vitro fertilization of rabbit ova by trypsin inhibitors. Biol Reprod 1:223–227

Talbot P, Franklin LE (1978) Surface modifiction of guinea pig sperm during in vitro capacitation: an assessment using lectin-induced agglutination of living sperm. J Exp Zool 203:1–14

Tesarik J (1986) From the cellular to the molecular dimension: the actual challenge for human fertilization research. Gamete Res 13:47–89

Tung KS, Han LP, Evan AP (1979) Differentiation autoantigen of testicular cells and spermatozoa in the guinea pig. Dev Biol 68:224–238

Tung PS, Fritz IB (1978) Specific surface antigens on rat pachytene spermatocytes and successive classes of germinal cells. Dev Biol 64:297–315

Van der Ven H, Bhattacharyya AK, Binor Z, Leto S, Zaneveld LJD (1982) Inhibition of human sperm capacitation by a high-molecular-weight factor from human seminal plasma. Fertil Steril 38:753–755

Vernon RB, Muller CH, Herr JC, Feuchter FA, Eddy EM (1982) Epididymal secretion of a mouse sperm surface component recognized by a monoclonal antibody. Biol Reprod 26:523–535

Vernon RB, Hamilton MS, Eddy EM (1985) Effects of in vivo and in vitro fertilization invironments on the expression of a surface antigen of the mouse sperm tail. Biol Reprod 32:669–680

Voglmayr JK, Fairbanks G, Lewis RG (1983) Surface glycoprotein changes in ram spermatozoa during epididymal maturation. Biol Reprod 29:767–775

Wassarman PM (1987) The biology and chemistry of fertilization. Science 235:553–560

Weil AJ, Kotsevalov O, Waten L (1956) Antigens of human seminal plasma. Proc Soc Exp Biol Med 92:606–610

Wiley LM, Obasaju MF, Overstreet JW, Cross NL, Hanson FW, Change RJ (1987) Scientific Program and Abstracts for the Society for Gynecologic Investigation. 34th Annual Meeting, March 18–21, Atlanta (Abstract #106P)

Wolf DP, Sokoloski JE, Dandekar P, Bechtol KB (1983) Characterization of human sperm surface antigens with monoclonal antibodies. Biol Reprod 29:713–723

Yanagimachi R (1981) Mechanisms of fertilization in mammals. In: Mastroianni L Jr, Biggers JD (eds) Fertilization and embryonic development in vitro. Plenum, New York, pp 81–182

Yanagimachi R (1983) Fertilization. In: Crosignini PG, Rubin BL (eds) In vitro fertilization and embryo transfer. Academic, London, Grune and Stratton, New York, pp 65–100

Postcoital Contraception

Post-coital Interception

A. A. Haspels

Academisch Ziekenhuis, Department of Obstetrics and Gynaecology,
University of Utrecht, 3511 GV Utrecht, Netherlands

Introduction

Sexarche – the age of the first coitus – is happening earlier nowadays as ever younger adolescents engage in intercourse. Rarely is a good method of contraception used in the beginning of sexual experimenting, and this results in a high demand for emergency counselling. In the Netherlands many women use a post-coital method of contraception in "emergency" situations. Some of these methods may also be used as an "ongoing" contraceptive method.

The incidence of induced abortions is only 15000 in Dutch women, as compared to 180000 live births – the lowest incidence in the world. The position of the Netherlands is the same regarding the incidence of pregnancy in teenagers: 14 per 1000 in the Netherlands [1] and, for example, 45 per 1000 in England and Wales; the United States had the highest rate of teenage pregnancy in the Western world with 96 per 1000. The suggestion that an enlightened attitude towards sex is associated with a much lower rate of teenage pregnancy, abortion and child-bearing emerges from a study of rates of teenage pregnancy in 36 Western nations. The low rate of teenage pregnancy in the Netherlands may be based on the matter-of-fact acceptance of the reality of teenage sexuality, formal and informal sex education, and readily accessible contraceptive services. Ketting [1] compared the romantic view of sex in the United States, which leads young people to believe that mutual attraction sweeps people wordlessly off feet and into bed, with the open discussion that occurs in Holland and the resultingly responsible use of postcoital interception and contraception.

Awareness that sexuality is not only bound to reproduction but is a pleasure in itself is observed in all social classes and all age groups. Many doctors believe that the material wealth of our society leads to permissiveness. Others have questioned just how comfortable some teenagers are with their decision to engage in sexual intercourse. The devastating effects of teenage pregnancies are of great concern in many countries. In the Netherlands psychosexual enquiries were conducted in 1968 and in 1981; interesting changes in this relatively short time span were evident. In 1968 Dutch women were more conservative than men; in 1981 there are few differences. For example the question "Are adolescents permitted to use contraceptives?" was answered affirmatively by 39% of women in 1968 and by 84% in 1981. The resistance towards induced abortion declined over this period from 32% to 19% in men and from 44% to 26% in women.

In industrialized countries, over half of all pregnancies are unplanned. Some 60% of the first sexual exposures among youngsters are unprotected [2]. In view

Female Contraception
Eds.: B. Runnebaum, T. Rabe, L. Kiesel

Table 1. Rate of induced abortions in the Netherlands and Sweden in 1982

	Netherlands	Sweden
Live births	172000	85000
Postcoital contraception	35000	seldom used
Induced abortions	15000	35000

of the medical, social-psychological and financial hazards of induced abortion it has become evident that these procedures, while offering possible solutions, are certainly far from ideal [3]. Postcoital contraception (PCC) in women was developed in the 1960s in the United States when Morris and van Wagenen [4] started using diethylstilbestrol and in Europe when Haspels [5, 6] started using ethinylestradiol (EE) in high dosage. This resulted in substantial social implications, for PCC services have now been offered to women in the Netherlands since the 1960s. In some countries, e.g., Sweden, PCC is not yet commonly used, and, thus, the rate of induced abortion is high (Table 1).

PCC services usually result in using a PCC method once, followed by a continuing method of contraception; only 8% report a second PCC. However, prevention is preferable to treatment. Postovulatory interceptive methods are invaluable in cases of rape, incest, intoxication, and when mechanical contraceptives fail, as in rupture or displacement of condoms or diaphragms. Moreover, it provides a method for women who engage in unprotected coitus and who later reject the idea of a possible pregnancy and fear an abortion.

Hormonal Methods

In 1964 the Amsterdam police brought to our department a girl of 13 who had been raped by three men. She was in mid-cycle, and we asked a veterinary doctor about the estrogen dose used for dogs after unwanted mating; we then administered postcoital EE in a similar fashion. This method has become popularly known as the "morning-after pill." A peak consumption of 55000 was reached in the Netherlands in 1975. The fact that the postcoital administration of large doses of estrogens interferes with pregnancy in animals had been known for some time [7]. Monkeys differ in this respect in that estrogens have no abortifacient effect once nidation has occurred [8].

In humans, too, once the ovum is implanted, the administration of large doses of estrogens does not interfere with pregnancy. The administration of such large doses shortly after unprotected intercourse, however, is highly efficient in preventing pregnancy. Although this is not to be regarded as a routine method of contraception, it appears to be a useful method in cases of emergency where unprotected intercourse could otherwise lead to pregnancy.

An ongoing survey in Dutch abortion clinics reveals that 25% of all abortion patients became pregnant at the time of their first intercourse. In our series of over 4000 patients the pregnancy rate was 0.15.

Side Effects

In our study [6] on 3016 women the following side effects were reported: nausea in 54%, vomiting in 24%, tender breasts in 23%, and menorrhagia in 11%. In cases where vomiting occurred within 1 h after ingestion of the tablet, an additional dose was to be taken 30 min after an antiemetic. In a few cases where all tablets were vomited on the 1st day, estrogens were injected using 30 mg estradiol benzoate per day for 5 days. Changes in the length of the menstrual cycle were reported by 24% of the users. In 11% menstruation occurred 5 or more days sooner, and 13% showed a cycle 5 or more days longer than usual.

These side effects are substantial, and together with the availability of morning-after counselling, these may have motivated patients to use a dependable method of contraception after PCC.

Mechanism of Action

Concerning the mechanism of action several hypotheses are proposed. Endometrial biopsies disclosed evidence of a retarded hyperplasia. Basal vacuoles, usually not found after the 4th day of the secretory phase, remained visible throughout the remainder of the cycle under this treatment. A study in six volunteers at our department demonstrated this effect clearly [9].

Several points of impact may be postulated, such as an accelerated or a slowed tubal passage of the ovum, changes in the blastocyst or its "stickiness," retarded endometrial growth, metabolic and histochemical changes in the endometrium, and interference with luteinizing hormone (LH) secretion, with progesterone production or (in some cases) inhibition of ovulation. There are enough reasons to assume that the administration of large doses of estrogens disturbs the "implantation interaction" between the ovum, tubes, and endometrium, resulting in the prevention of nidation. Important may be, in this respect, the drop in the level of endometrial carbonic anhydrase induced by a high dose of estrogens, an indispensable nutrient to the blastocyst.

During the transport of eggs from the tubes to the uterus, the latter undergoes certain developmental changes which are essential for the survival and implantation of the embryo. The progestational reaction of the endometrium should be in line with the stage of the fertilized ovum to ensure proper implantation. A later ovum or an early endometrium creates unfavorable conditions for the egg. A close phase relationship is required; early or later arrival by more than 1 day results in nidation failure [10]. As early as 1950 asynchronization of blastocyst and endometrium was suggested as a cause of ova perishing and making implantation of an intact ovum impossible.

The endometrium is controlled by estrogen in the proliferative stage and, after the LH surge, also by estrogen and progesterone. As described by Noyes [10], the endometrium changes every day with the menstrual cycle, which is reflected in the histological epithelial pattern. High doses of estrogen interfere in this daily sequence of alterations, as was shown by a study carried out at our department [9]. The proliferative stage is extended by the use of estrogens. Biopsies from patients taking 5 mg EE per day on postovulatory days show a standstill at an early stage of secretion. The retronuclear vacuoles, containing glycogen meant for apical secretion, on the 6th postovulatory day remain at the basal level.

In our patients, carefully dated, biopsies were taken on day 13 after ovulation. Glands should have collapsed. Predecidual changes starting as mantles around the vessels on the 10th day appear not to have occurred. The earliest signs of corpus luteum regression, which can be seen in the physiological cycle as shrinkage of the endometrial epithelium, are completely lacking. An attempted dating is day 6 or 7. Stroma is compact; no edema is found. The nuclei are rounded, returning to their basal positions. At higher magnification vacuoles are found at the apical rim of the cell. A retardation of about 6 days is established. This results in suppression of the uterine enzymes of pregnancy, e.g., carbonic anhydrase and monoamina oxidase (MAO), and, consequently, prevention of implantation. More or less the same discrepancy was observed in other patients. Other mechanisms may be involved. Prostaglandin $F_{2\alpha}$ administered postcoitally in rabbits inhibits implantation of the blastocyst. The mechanism of action of prostaglandins is not yet clear; they may interfere with tubal function or may disrupt ovarian hormone synthesis. The interactions between ovarian hormones, adrenergic drugs, and prostaglandins are complex. Combinations of antiprogestogens and prostaglandins seem promising as future postovulatory interceptives and abortifacients.

Endocrine Effects of 25 mg Ethinylestradiol

Blood samples could be taken from the volunteers mentioned above in control and experimental cycles. The blood levels of EE taken at a dosage of 5 mg per day increased to 3319 pmol/l on the 1st day and to 4802 pmol/l on the 5th day. It took 13 days to normalize EE in plasma. Prolactin levels increased up to 48 ng/ml in normoprolactinemic women, parallel to the increase in the EE levels. The mean decrease in plasma antithrombine III level was 17% of the pretreatment value. This is caused by hemodilution due to water and salt retention rather than by a decreased synthesis or increased consumption [11]. Our study, in which control antithrombine III levels were used, did not conform these results.

Complications

In view of the high dosages of estrogens, thromboembolism could be expected but has not been reported. One case of nonfatal pulmonary edema was reported [8]. In one patient we observed a weight gain of 8 kg in 5 days, rapidly returning to normal after cessation of treatment. The main complication is ectopic pregnancy, the incidence of which is increased to about 10% of pregnancies occurring after failure of EE therapy. We reported three cases of pregnancy continuing to term after failure of estrogen therapy. No teratogenic effect was observed in these few cases. Moreover, this is not expected since estrogens are administered before the implantation and 34 days before organogenesis of the reproductive organs.

Recent Postcoital Contraceptive Combinations

A combination of 50 µg EE and 250 µg levonorgestrel (Neogynon) are given in a dose of two pills immediately and two tablets 12 h later. This method, advocated by Yuzpe [12], has the advantage of a low dose of hormone administration compared to our original method of 5 mg EE for 5 days. Therefore [13] a double-blind randomized study was conducted in our department on these two above-mentioned regimens. Contraceptive efficacy was excellent in both groups. No significant difference between pregnancy rates was observed. As a result of this study we now advocate the use of the Yuzpe regimen. Contrary to our expectations side effects were about the same as mentioned for the high-estrogen regimen. In the combination regimen we found 46% with nausea and 13% with vomiting. As the amount of hormones prescribed is much less, and treatment is reduced from 5 days to 1 day, only the alternative morning-after pill is the pill of choice.

Postcoital Insertion of an Intrauterine Device (IUD)

The postcoital use of an IUD to prevent pregnancy was proposed by Tatum and Lippes [14]. It can be used as an alternative to the hormonal method either if the woman presents more than 72 h after intercourse, or if she would like to use the IUD as an ongoing method of contraception [15]. In all patients in whom estrogens are contraindicated, such as with a history of previous thromboembolism, hepatic disease or mammary cancer, postcoital IUD insertion provides a good nonhormonal alternative in preventing pregnancy.

A major disadvantage of postcoital IUD use is that IUD insertion can produce serious complications if a patient has a vaginal or venereal infection, an asymptomatic cervicitis, or even pelvic inflammatory disease (PID). After proper physical examination suitable patients are selected from among those requesting postcoital treatment. Cases involving rape are mostly excluded from these services; however, if they present early, proper work-up and treatment can be performed within the 7 days available for this method, and it will still be possible to fit a postcoital IUD [16].

The potential risk of future infertility should be considered, as PID rates in nulliparous IUD users are up to 7 times higher than in nonusers. Young nulliparous, sexually active women – especially of lower socioeconomic strata – are identified as high-risk patients. Over 70% of women requesting interception are nulliparous. Clients asking for postcoital insertion should be informed of its potential risk, as women under 25 years of age are more prone to infection. The risk of septic abortions exists if an IUD is inserted into a gravid uterus, due to pregnancy resulting from unreported previous sexual intercourse. Septic abortion is a life-threatening condition.

Mechanism of Action

Spermatozoa proceed rapidly through the uterus to the tubes after sexual intercourse. Within 5–30 min after deposit of semen at the cervical mucus numerous spermatozoa reach the fimbrial part of the fallopian tube. No interceptive action is expected from the sperm-destroying effect of the IUD. An IUD does not prevent either ovulation or capacitation. IUDs do not alter the endometrium during the menstrual cycle or interfere with daily changes. Luteolysis occurs in sheep by the mediation of prostaglandin $F_{2\alpha}$ liberated by laceration of the endometrial surface. Enhanced tubal motility through prostaglandin mediation causes the oocyte to arrive in the uterine cavity too early, in asynchrony with the endometrium, thus causing the ovum to die.

Insertion of an IUD contaminates the uterine cavity at a much higher rate than previously assumed. Upon laparotomy fundal removals of an IUD proved 75% bacterial contamination. Cultures and identification of strains measured by the same methods show positive endometrial cultures in 58%. This incidence is significantly lower in transfundal studies. Sterile uterine cavities are demonstrated as early as 24 h after insertion and 40 h after insertion; the uterine cavity is sterile in 80% of cases. Bacterial clearance is demonstrated within 4 weeks. In nulliparous women 100% contaminated IUDs were found upon removal after 2–72 months of use, while 13% multiparous women had sterile IUDs. Postinsertion endometritis or endoparametritis is as frequent as 3%. The blastocidal effect of bacterial infection or the reactions to it are potential mechanisms of action of the postcoital IUD. In continuing contraception with IUDs, however, inflammatory reactions are not a mechanism of action of the IUD.

Effect of Copper

The copper dispersion in the 1st month of use is important for postcoital use. In the mouse it was estimated in vitro that a concentration of 2.5×10^{-5} mol/l is embryotoxic. Copper IUDs with a clean 200-mm^2 copper surface cause a concentration of 9×10^{-4} mol/l in the uterine cavity by the release of copper ions. Copper release is highest during the 1st month after insertion. The high efficacy of the postcoital copper IUD may be due to this high embryotoxic copper ion concentration in the uterus, in contrast to inert IUDs with their maximum pregnancy rates in the first months of use [16].

Method

Traditionally many young girls call at the Utrecht University Hospital for postcoital interception counselling. Our study [15] included 55 clients, but our ongoing study concerns over 100 patients at the moment. Initially Copper 7 and Copper-T IUDs were used. One client had an unnoticed partial expulsion of a Copper 7 IUD and was found to be pregnant at a postinsertion check 6 weeks later. By repeated ultrasound it was proven that her conception occurred in the 2nd month after insertion. Thereafter the Multiload Copper 250, later ML 375, was used exclusively, as a high copper ion concentration has a blastocidal effect, and the ML has a low expulsion rate. In our series no pregnancies occurred in the month of insertion of the IUD; a 100% follow-up was achieved.

Postcoital IUD insertion is a means of interception after the time for postcoital hormonal methods has passed, up to 7 days after unprotected intercourse.

Recent Developments

Anti-implantation drugs

Drugs that interfere with the normal physiology of early embryonic development and implantation could constitute an effective approach to contraception. As yet no selective anti-implantation agents for widespread clinical use are available. This deficiency is undoubtedly related to our incomplete understanding of these processes in humans. Extrapolation of animal data is often hazardous and may lead to false assumptions.

The history of clomiphene is a case in point. Hailed as a potent anti-implantation agent on the basis of studies in the rat, this drug remains to this day one of the most successful medical treatments of infertility. Such seemingly contradictory effects are probably the result of interspecies differences in the hormonal requirements for implantation.

To examine the role of estrogen during the peri-implantation period, in vivo studies in monkeys are being conducted: the first involves the reduction of endogenous estrogen production by passive immunization against LH. Immunoneutralization of LH on day 30 of the cycle – day 16–18 after conception – by intramuscular injection of an antiserum raised against the β subunit of ovine LH results in a rapid decline of peripheral levels of progesterone and estradiol and termination of pregnancy within 2–3 days. However, if the fall in circulating levels of progesterone is prevented by supplementing the antiserum treatment with exogenous progesterone in a decreasing dosage regimen, abortion does not occur despite the decline of estradiol to low, albeit still detectable, values in these animals. The second study involves inhibition of the effects of endogenously produced estrogen by the administration of an antiestrogen such as tamoxifen.

In Shanghai the chemical synthesis and biological testing of anordrin and anordrin-analogues has for many years been a major area of interest. This derives from the fact that orally administered anordrin is a commonly used, highly effective anti-implantation agent when used in a "vacation pill" regimen – 7.5 mg every other day over a 20-day period. The World Health Organization places high priority on comparative studies of bioavailability and pharmacokinetics of these compounds.

Antiprogestational Drugs

In most mammalian species the establishment and maintenance of pregnancy is critically dependent upon the presence of progesterone. Consequently, a variety of techniques are being explored that prevent progesterone action, either by inhibiting synthesis of the hormone or by interfering with its effects on target organs.

Recently a novel steroidal antiprogestin, RU 486-mifepristone, was made available for a study of its antifertility activity in early pregnancy and as a late postcoital interceptive. The study is still going on. Preliminary results have been published [17] and are in press [18–20]. A total of 80 women with amenorrhea of

55 days or less were treated with 100 or 200 mg mifepristone daily for 4 consecutive days. All patients started to bleed during the treatment. Clinical efficacy of the treatment in terms of frequency of complete abortion was 83%; the success-rate in nulliparous women was even 92%. Most patients experienced only minor side effects (mild uterine pain), but two women suffered from heavy bleeding requiring blood transfusion and curettage. Cortisol concentrations increased during treatment, but the levels remained within the normal range. Taken together these results indicate that treatment with mifepristone causes fewer gastrointestinal side effects and less uterine pain but is also less effective than currently available prostaglandin analogues. For 6 months our results have improved by using 0.250 mg sulprostone, a prostaglandin E_2 analogue, on day 5 if the abortion has not been completed with mifepristone [21].

This antiprogestin may also be used regularly on a once monthly basis from day 27–30 of each cycle. Preliminary results are disappointing, as cycle disturbances follow administration, making regular administration difficult. However, promising is the use of mifepristone as a late morning-after pill [22] for emergency use from day 27–30 of a particular cycle in a dosage of 100 mg daily. In all, 55 patients were treated. All women but one started to bleed on the 2nd or 3rd day of treatment and observed a normal menstrual period. One woman remained amenorrheic for 2 months. She was not pregnant but had an anovulatory cycle with a low progesterone level. No side effects were observed. At present a pharmacokinetic study on intravaginal administration of mifepristone is being performed in our clinic.

Luteinizing Hormone-Releasing Hormone Analogues

Studies on luteinizing hormone-releasing hormone (LHRH) analogues as fertility-regulating agents are, to a certain extent, a high-risk venture. Animal and clinical studies employing various analogues have produced conflicting results.

Ethical Considerations

The consensus of legal opinion is that a miscarriage cannot be procured until implantation has taken place. Some pressure groups equate postcoital interception with abortion; they believe that pregnancy exists as soon as fertilization takes place. This opinion was still mentioned in an editorial of the *British Journal of Family Planning* in 1983 as being important [23]. Other fears to be allayed are those with moral and ethical overtones. Arguments that widespread availability of PCC will encourage irresponsible behavior and abandonment of regular contraceptive use are well-countered in the same article.

In this context it is important to bear in mind that failure to implant frequently occurs spontaneously. The legal expression "procure a miscarriage" cannot therefore be construed to include the prevention of implantation. As mentioned earlier, three women continued pregnancies to term after failure of estrogen therapy. No teratogenic effect was observed in the three children born. As the postcoital treatment occurs long before organogenesis, an increased number of genital abnormalities is not expected. However, Rowlands and Guillebaud [24] advise early abortion in these cases, as the possibility of congenitally malformed babies cannot be completely excluded. Some form of congenital malformation is present in 2.5% of all babies. The birth of such a baby subsequent to hormone treatment might induce guilt in the mother, even if she could be assured that her child's type of malformation was an unlikely result of treatment.

An open discussion is advocated. We do not agree with Rowlands and Guillebaud that postcoital treatment is not appropriate for those with a moral or religious objection to abortion. IUD insertion would raise the same moral objection as a postcoital hormonal regimen. Postcoital interception using mifepristone on day 27–30 of the cycle must be seen as a possible interruption of early pregnancy. Patients who object to methods available after implantation has taken place should not use this method on ethical grounds.

Postcoital methods spare the women an anxious wait for her next period and will almost always be effective. They are cheap, and preferable to and more acceptable than abortion, both from a physical as well as a psychological point of view.

Conclusion

At present there seems to be a need for postcoital contraception, as much of the psychic trauma experienced by a woman who has had unprotected coitus while awaiting the onset of her next menses could be avoided with the use of an effective post-coital pill.

Countries with good health services – including availability of postcoital contraception – have low abortion rates.

Postcoital interception can be designed for two categories of women. In the first it can be used as an emergency method where unprotected intercourse has occurred due to an isolated incident. In the second it can be designed as an ongoing contraceptive regimen. For this second category, only women who have infrequent intercourse would be suitable, whereas women who engage in sexual intercourse frequently would be better advised to use an ongoing method of contraception such as a combined oral contraceptive, which would give a much lower total hormonal load per cycle compared with the doses used in postcoital interception.

Postcoital progestagens could well be used if intercourse is infrequent. However, progestagen therapy may cause menstrual upset and irregular bleeding. For emergency use estrogen alone or estrogen-progestagen combinations are suitable, but they must be given soon after exposure.

For the woman who has presented late – between 72 h and 7 days after coitus – insertion of a copper-bearing IUD may seem appropriate. A new development is the administration of an antiprogestagen pill from day 27–30 of the cycle. Side effects are minimal, and the success rate is high.

Postcoital interception has a definite place in family planning and fertility regulation. Careful assessment of individual needs would help to decide which is the method of choice.

References

1. Adolescent Sex (1985) The Lancet 1114–1115
2. Bauman KE (1971) Selected aspects of the contraceptive practices of unmarried university students. Am J Obstet Gynec 108:203
3. Aref I, Hafez ESE (1977) Post coital contraception. Obst Gynec Surv 32:417
4. Morris JM, Van Wagenen G (1966) Compounds interfering with ovum implantation and development. Role of estrogens. Am J Obstet Gynec 96:804
5. Haspels AA (1969) The morning-after pill: a preliminary report. IPPF Med Bull 3:6
6. Haspels AA (1976) Interception, Post coital estrogens in 3016 women. Contraception 14:275
7. Parkes AS, Dodds EC, Noble R (1938) Interruption of early pregnancy by means of orally active estrogens. Br Med J II:557
8. Morris JM, Van Wagenen G (1973) Interception: the use of post-ovulatory oestrogens to prevent implantation. Am J Obstet Gynec 115:101
9. Van Santen MR, Haspels AA (1980) Interfering with implantation by post coital estrogen administration. In: Hubinont P (ed) Progr Reprod Biol 7:310, Karger, Basel
10. Noyes RW, Hertig AT, Roch J (1950) Dating the endometrial biopsy. Fert Steril 1:3
11. Weenink GG, ten Caten JW, Kahle LH (1983) "Morning-after pill" and Antithrombine III. Acta Obstet Gynec Scand 62:359
12. Yuzpe AA, Lancee WJ (1977) Ethinyl-estradiol and dl-norgestrel as a post coital contraceptive. Fertil Steril 28:932
13. Van Santen MR, Haspels AA (1982) Comparative randomized double-blind study of high dosage ethinyl estradiol versus ethinyl estradiol and norgestrel combination in post coital contraception. Acta Endocrin Suppl 246:2
14. Tatum HJ, Lippes J (1975) Fellows succeed in IUD work. Am Coll Obstet Gynec Newsl 19:6
15. Van Santen MR, Haspels AA (1981) Interception by post coital IUD insertion. Contracept Deliv Syst 2:189
16. Van Santen MR, Haspels AA (1982) Interception by post coital insertion of an IUD. In: Progress in Contraceptive Delivery Systems. IUD Technology, vol 4:65, MTP Press Ltd
17. Haspels AA (1985) Interruption of early pregnancy by the antiprogestational compound RU 486. In: The antiprogestin steroid RU 486 and human fertility control. Plenum, New York, pp 199–209
18. Haspels AA (1985) Interruption of early pregnancy by an anti-progestational compound – RU 486. Eur J Obstet Gynecol Reprod Biol (in press)
19. Vervest HAM, Haspels AA (1985) Preliminary results with the antiprogestational compound RU 486 (mifepristone) for interruption of early pregnancy. Fertil Steril (in press)
20. Vervest HAM, Haspels AA (1985) Interruptie vroege zwangerschap met RU 486. Ned Tijdsch Geneeskd (in press)
21. Haspels AA, van Santen MR (1985) Post coital interception by an antiprogestational compound RU 486 (Abstr). 11th World Congress on Gynecology and Obstetrics, Berlin
22. Haspels AA, Vervest HAM (1985) Interruption of early pregnancy by an antiprogestational agent – RU 486 (Abstr). 11th World Congress on Gynecology and Obstetrics, Berlin
23. Editorial (1983) Post coital contraception. Br J Fam Plann 9:41
24. Rowlands W, Guillebaud J (1981) Post coital contraception. Br J Fam Plann 7:3

Endometrial and Myometrial Effects of Progesterone Antagonists in Pregnant Guinea Pigs

W. Elger[1], M. Fähnrich[1], S. Beier[1], S. Shao-Qing[2], and K. Chwalisz[1]

[1] Research Laboratories of Schering, Berlin-Bergkamen, FRG
[2] National Research Institute for Family Planning, Beijing, China

Antiprogestins of the RU 486 type (RU 486, ZK 98 734, ZK 98 299) were studied at different stages of pregnancy in the guinea pig. Treatment starting on day 4 postconception was able to prevent nidation completely, all compounds had comparable inhibitory potency. Treatment after nidation, starting on day 8 postconception induced decidual collapse and bleeding; however, embryonic tissue was retained in nidation sites. Luteolysis, as opposed to animals in nonfertile cycles, was not induced, indicating a lack of ability of antiprogestins to induce uterine prostaglandin synthesis/liberation. On day 43 postconception there was marginal abortifacient activity of RU 486. The other compounds induced expulsion more rapidly and at a higher rate. The comparatively pronounced antiglucocorticoid activity of RU 486 may account for this difference. High uterine prostaglandin sensitivity and a cervical ripening were induced consistently; fast, spontaneous labor, on the other hand, occurred after several days if at all. Complete uterine evacuation was induced within hours by otherwise inactive doses of Sulprostone in various combinations with ZK 98 299 and RU 486, but surprisingly not with ZK 98 734. A single dose of ZK 98 299 induced an approximately 30-fold increase in uterine prostaglandin sensitivity within 24 h, exceeding that present preterm, but no spontaneous labor.

This is evidence that endogenous prostaglandins were not activated, in analogy to perinidation stages. Observation of antiluteolytic activity of antiprogestins in nonpregnant animals is considered of major theoretical importance in this context. It seems that inhibition of progesterone leads to a paralyzed uterine prostaglandin liberation. The same effect in pregnancy could explain the inability of the uterus to expel a seriously compromised conceptus.

In conclusion, we suggest that progesterone is a stimulator rather than a depressor of uterine prostaglandins in late luteal phase and pregnancy. The capability of the conceptus to neutralize this stimulatory action of progesterone is considered to be essential for the rescue of the corpus luteum and uterine motor quiescence in the guinea pig. The clinical significance of this is that high frequency of incomplete abortions and protracted, in part, heavy bleedings in pregnant women treated with RU 486 may reflect decidual compromise and simultaneous uterine prostaglandin deficiency, as found in our animal model after progesterone blockage.

Female Contraception
Eds.: B. Runnebaum, T. Rabe, L. Kiesel

Politics and Religion in Contraception

The Role of Public Sector Agencies in Contraceptive Research and Development

G. Benagiano[1], G. Perkin[2], and M. Potts[3]

[1] First Institute of Obstetrics and Gynecology, University la Sapienza, Rome, Italy
[2] Programme for the Introduction and Adaptation of Contraceptive Technology, 4 Nickerson Street, Seattle, Washington, United States
[3] Family Health International, Research Triangle Park, North Carolina, United States

Introduction

Until recently, contraceptive product development, the translation of a research finding into a final product, was successfully carried out by profit-making, commercial pharmaceutical companies. Interaction between commercial companies, scientists, and drug-regulatory agencies has defined the steps necessary for development of a safe, acceptable, and economically feasible product. Expected financial returns from sales of the final product have driven the development process.

During the past 10–15 years, however, the pharmaceutical industry has played a reduced role in contraceptive development. Various factors, including more time-consuming preclinical requirements and aggressive campaigning against some methods by consumer advocates, have made contraceptive development a much more costly undertaking. Many companies have withdrawm from the market after concluding that the high risk associated with developing new methods is not properly compensated by financial returns or by an improved image of the company with the public at large.

The major reasons for the reduced role of profit-making companies in contraceptive development are:

- Increasingly, contraceptive users (mostly young, healthy women) are unwilling to take even the smallest health risk, while at the same time expecting a method that provides full protection.
- Consumer-advocate groups have attacked a number of contraceptive products. The example of Depo-Provera, where scientific arguments were overshadowed by emotional rhetoric, has had a major impact on the industry.
- Research leads for completely new products are scarce due to the lack of investment by private industry and limited resources available from governments and donor agencies. Consequently, development activities often are limited to refining an existing product – lowering the dosage or improving the administration schedule – rather than working on new products.
- Leading drug-regulatory agencies require time-consuming and costly preclinical testing for new contraceptive drugs and devices. Their standards can be extraordinarily stringent. They frequently have taken the view that if any adverse effect surfaces, the product is unacceptable, even if this effect occurs only when exposure is at 50 or even 100 times the normal dose.
- Presently available methods seem to be satisfactory for a relatively large proportion of women in industrialized countries, representing the bulk of the market for most companies. Developing countries, where new and improved

Female Contraception
Eds.: B. Runnebaum, T. Rabe, L. Kiesel

methods more acceptable to users are needed, do not generally have appeal as potential markets.

Given these realities, how can it be assured that new, safe, culturally appropriate contraceptive methods are developed and made widely available, particularly in developing countries where the need is most acute? It is clear that public-sector agencies will have to take the lead, working together with regulatory agencies, commercial manufacturers, and academic institutions to produce the best new methods.

Meeting Future Contraceptive Needs

The need for new, safe, and appropriate contraceptive methods is critical. Every 5 days the world's population increases by about 1 million; every minute a woman dies in childbirth, commonly due to a pregnancy she did not know how to postpone or control. In developing countries approximately half the women of fertile age, while stating that they do not want more children, do not use effective contraceptive methods [1]. Over the next few decades there will be some one-half billion new potential contraceptive acceptors, mostly in developing countries [2].

Most present contraceptive technology is not adapted to the needs, social structures, or financial resources of developing societies. The relatively costly, high-technology methods presently available through international donor agencies may become increasingly difficult to supply as sources dwindle and costs rise. What is needed are relatively inexpensive, easy-to-use methods that can be made widely available in developing countries and, in some cases, manufactured in these countries. Possible methods include once-a-month injectables, new spermicides, and subdermal, long-acting steroid pellets.

New methods will have to be tailored to the preferences of people in developing countries, regardless of potential economic returns. In the past, researchers have attempted to develop new products by applying the best scientific knowledge and have left the task of convincing people to use the method to the marketing force. Today, however, what is known about users' preferences must be a major factor in deciding research and development priorities [3]. Public-sector agencies must refer to psychosocial studies of future users and their societies to ensure that local requirements are met, and that technologies are well adapted to existing cultural values [4]. This new dimension in product research and development was clearly defined by the International Conference on Family Planning held in Jakarta in 1981. The conference underlined the necessity of developing workable techniques for identifying people's needs, problems, and preferences, and of incorporating this information into the design of new or improved contraceptive methods [5].

The Process of Research and Development

Producing a new contraceptive method encompasses all activities from identification of a potential new contraceptive substance or device to the process of making a new product available to programs throughout the world.

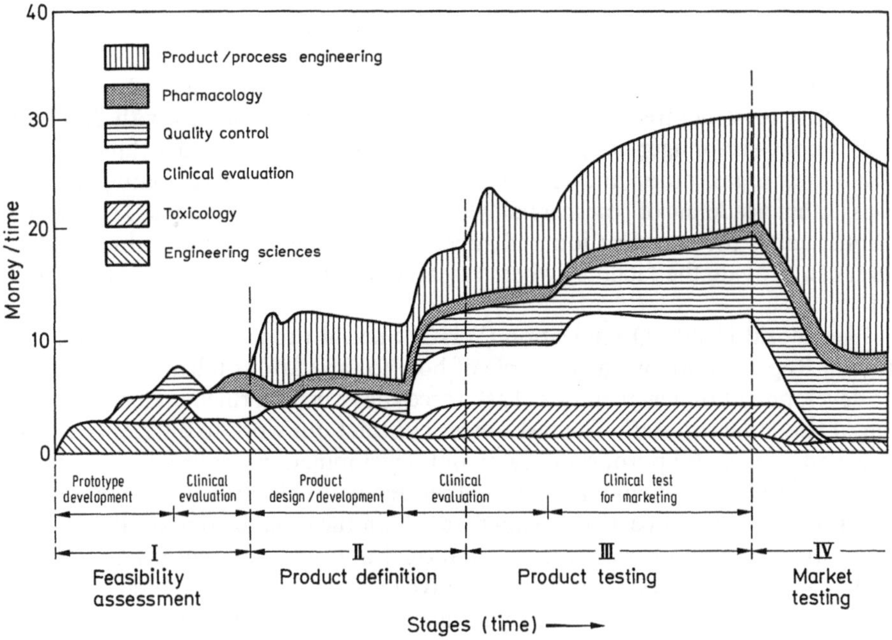

Fig. 1. Relative time and cost estimates associated with the four stages of product development

Agencies and institutions embarking on this endeavour must recognize the interactive nature of the process, its complexity and inherent risks, and the resources required for its successful completion. Product development must be considered as a series of interrelated, increasingly complex and costly stages. Following completion of each stage, a careful assessment is mandatory in order to permit optimal decision making in terms of programming opportunities and allocation of funds.

In a paper prepared for the Program for the Introduction and Adaptation of Contraceptive Technology (PIACT) [6] Richard Buckles defined the development process as encompassing four reasonably distinct stages:

1. *Feasibility assessment*, where scientists advising the agency developing a new method conclude that an idea warrants further investigation.
2. *Product definition*, where the product is extensively defined so that scientists are convinced that the idea is sound but are uncertain as to how well it will perform under field conditions.
3. *Product testing*, the point at which the specifically described product is manufactured, initially as a prototype but later on a large scale. During this stage the product must also undergo satisfactory toxicological testing followed by extensive clinical trials to ascertain how well it works.
4. *Market testing*, when studies are undertaken to evaluate local acceptability and the extent of side effects, and when support materials are prepared for the method's introduction and adaptation to specific populations. Buckles developed a chart (shown in Fig. 1) detailing the relative time and costs associated with each stage.

Managing and Coordinating Product Development

An agency wishing to organize the development of new contraceptive drugs or devices must be structured so that it can draw upon professionals with different skills. Public-sector agencies generally do not have all the required technical skills within their organization and so must contract with outside participating institutions, either academic or commercial, when developing new methods. These institutions, under the coordination and supervision of the agency's product leader, often can provide the facilities where research and development work is carried out.

The World Health Organization (WHO) Special Programme of Research in Human Reproduction is one example of how to tap various talents and skills in the development of new methods. Task forces have been formed under the direction of headquarters staff. The task forces contract out work to different institutions and, wherever appropriate, carry out development work as a joint venture with a pharmaceutical company or another agency. This strategy fully compensates for any lack of a particular expertise within the organization itself.

Frequently a number of different national and international agencies must work together to develop a new contraceptive method. There are several examples of successful cooperation between national and international agencies; this has confirmed the view that all major groups *can* and *must* work together, without losing their identities, specific skills, or even their structural differences. More and more, leading agencies tend to concentrate efforts in those areas in which they possess specific expertise and appropriate manpower. This avoids duplication of effort and at the same time improves the prospects of producing new contraceptive methods properly adapted to the needs of the developing world.

An example of this new attitude is shown by the collaboration between the Population Council, Family Health International (FHI), and the Program for the Introduction and Adaptation of Contraceptive Technology (PIACT) in the development, testing, and introduction of Norplant, a multiple, non-biodegradable, subcutaneous delivery system for levonorgestrel that provides protection for 5 years. Norplant was developed by the Population Council over a 15-year period. Following successful clinical testing it was approved for use by family planning programs throughout the world [7]. Realizing the specific expertise of PIACT, the Population Council turned to that organization to plan and execute the introduction of Norplant. The result of this interagency collaboration was a joint marketing strategy that produced special instruction manuals for users and implementors [8]. Currently FHI has ongoing clinical trials in Asia, Africa, and the Caribbean that involve about 4000 users. Norplant has been approved for marketing in six countries and the Population Council is working toward United States Food and Drug Administration (USFDA) approval before the end of this decade.

Another outstanding example of a coordinated, international, and interagency research and development effort by academic, national, and international entities is the WHO-sponsored Long Acting Steroid Coordinating Group which has led to the development of a number of promising compounds. The Group sought the advice of leading steroid chemists before designing the synthesis protocols and took advantage of excellent chemical facilities available at academic institutions in developing and developed countries in carrying out the synthetic work [9, 10]. It then turned to schools of pharmacy in the industrialized world for quality control and purification of the new substances and for formulation into either microcrystalline suspensions or oily solutions [10, 11]. The subsequent step, biological testing in suitable animal models, required facilities generally available only within commercial companies. In view of this, WHO turned to the Center for Population Research of the United States National Institutes of Health (NIH), which had an ongoing program for the screening of new contraceptive drugs [12].

Promising New Directions

As the previous section suggests, some of the most promising new methods that public sector agencies should investigate are various long-acting steroids. They are financially and practically feasible because they involve USFDA approved compounds, most of which have been in human use so long that their patents have expired. Also, the decision by the USFDA to permit cross-referencing to existing teratological and toxicological data when developing new steroid formulations saves time and money when developing new methods.

As discussed, the long-acting steroidal method Norplant has been developed by the public sector, and the method will likely be granted USFDA approval within a few years.

Another long-acting steroid likely to receive USFDA approval is the 90-day PolyNET intramuscular injectable. The technology has been perfected by the Stolle Corporation. Initial clinical trials were supported by the Program for Applied Research on Fertility Regulation (PARFR), and in January 1987 FHI received USFDA approval to begin phase III clinical trials. If these trials are without untoward events, FHI expects to submit materials for USFDA approval in 1990.

Work also is ongoing on monthly injectable contraceptives. WHO and FHI have collaborated on phase III clinical trials of two-monthly formulations of a progestogen and an estrogen. The protocol calls for testing of 200 women and will be completed and ready for analysis during 1987.

Perhaps the most promising and versatile long-acting steroid is the subdermal NET pellet, which gives 1-year protection against pregnancy, is biodegradable, and yet can be removed if the user does not like the menstrual irregularities associated with most long-acting steroids during the first 6 months of use.

A number of new spermicidal agents that may be useful in developing countries are currently being investigated. FHI has developed a unique strategy of systematically exploring the number of possible spermicidal agents among chemical entities already approved by USFDA. The most intriguing of these is the possibility of using Propranolol, the beta blocker used in the treatment of hypertension, as a spermicide. Propranolol was at one time the fifth most widely prescribed drug in the United States and its toxicology and teratology are well understood.

Another interesting new direction is in the field of immunocontraception. While there are at least three research leads that could result in a contraceptive vaccine, all of them are in the relatively early stages of research. As currently funded none of them is likely to lead to a widely used product in this century. Additional funding – another $5–$10 million – made available in the 1990s would most certainly bring major research results that could lead to human clinical trials of this potentially important new method.

Making New Methods Available in Developing Countries

Making new methods available in developing countries demands different strategies, depending upon the method. International donor agencies will probably always play a major role in supplying relatively high-technology methods. It may be possible, however, to supply some effective lower technology methods through local manufacture and distribution, thereby increasing the likelihood that the method will be available on a long-term basis.

Many high technology drugs, such as pills, IUDs, condoms, injectables, the new NET microspheres, and probably Norplant, require sophisticated manufacture and a high degree of quality control. They are likely to be expensive drugs and, therefore, if they are to be used widely in developing countries, are almost certain to require subsidy. Most will have to be provided by donor agencies.

The United States Agency for International Development (USAID) has been a leader in purchasing contraceptive commodities and supplying them to developing countries – in 1986 USAID spent $ 30.4 million on commodities. On the whole, other agencies have not been as farsighted as USAID. The Swedish International Development Authority (SIDA) was the first international agency to buy contraceptives but has partially pulled out of the field. The Japanese buy some condoms and spermicides. The United Nations Fund for Population Activities (UNFPA) and International Planned Parenthood Federation (IPPF) do what they can, but their sources of funds have not grown as rapidly as the need.

In short, it may be that by the second half of the 1990s it will be increasingly difficult for donor agencies to meet the need for various methods of contraception. Since the countries in greatest need often are those with the weakest foreign exchange situation, it also is highly unlikely that these countries will be able to spend millions of dollars to purchase high-technology contraceptives themselves.

Therefore, in some cases it may be crucial that a decision be made early in development of a method to pursue the manufacture and testing of the method in a developing country. Within this scenario, clinical testing can be planned to meet the developing country's licensing requirements, and manufacture and distribution can be carried out according to the country's needs.

Experience over the past 20 years has shown that if drugs are developed and approved for manufacture and distribution within the country, then, assuming they are valid, useful, and affordable methods, they can be made widely available. About 1 million doses of monthly contraceptives are manufactured and sold in Mexico each year, and the method is also available in most countries of Latin America. The current formulation was pirated from a monthly contraceptive that Squibb began developing in the late 1960s and early 1970s. The drug was never submitted to any kind of careful clinical trial. It is not endorsed by the WHO Toxicology Panel, and its availability in some countries is of sufficient concern to national family planning programs that they have not felt able to endorse it. Yet neither has there been sufficient evidence to remove it from the market. A new monthly contraceptive tested to modern standards and, it is hoped, approved by WHO could be available before the end of this decade and could make a major impact by replacing the present unsatisfactory product in Latin America and by providing a new method in countries such as Egypt, the Philippines, Indonesia, Bangladesh, India, and Pakistan.

The Role of the United States Food and Drug Administration

To date the widespread use of most new contraceptive methods has been tied to United States requirements for drug and device testing. The USFDA requirements are uniquely stringent. USFDA staff, while highly professional, are influenced by a variety of political forces. Occasionally they must deal with a powerful manufacturer and, more commonly, with well-organized consumer advocates. The failure of the USFDA to approve Depo-Provera is an example of non scientific decision making being strongly influenced by political forces.

The United States, through its wealth and scientific leadership, has an important contribution to make to international contraceptive development. At the same time, however, the USFDA has explicitly said that it does not wish to be the world's guardian, and that the needs and circumstances of other countries may lead to differing patterns of drug regulation. Agencies working on developing new methods should bear in mind that the USFDA does not necessarily have to be the standard by which drug and device development is judged.

Conclusions

Development of new contraceptive methods for the developing world will largely be the task of public-sector agencies. Research and development activities aimed at producing a new, viable product must focus upon the real needs of the developing world, respectful of social and cultural conditions. At the same time, new methods must be technically advanced, and high-quality products with large safety margins must be produced.

In order to achieve these goals, various public-sector agencies with different areas of expertise must work together to plan for the development, clinical testing, manufacture, and introduction of selected new methods. Development should either be in parallel but on a fast track in relation to USFDA-approved studies or should proceed without submitting the product to USFDA for approval.

References

1. Editorial (1980) Key findings highlight diversity. People 7:5
2. Atkinson L, Schearer SB, Harkavy O (1980) Prospects for improved contraception. Fam Plann Perspect 12:173

3. Wahren C (1984) The role of industry, agencies and governments in research on fertility regulation: past experience and future prospects. In: Diczfalusy A, Diczfalusy E (eds) Research on the regulation of human fertility. Scriptor, Copenhagen
4. UN General Assembly (1981) The least developed countries in the 1980s. UN conference on the least developed countries, A/CONF. 104/4 Add.1
5. UNFPA (1981) Family planning in the 1980s: challenges and opportunities. Report of the International Conference on Family Planning in the 1980s, Jakarta. New York: Population Council, New York
6. Buckles RG (1979) Contraceptive product development in public-sector programmes. PIACT paper 3
7. Population Council (1983) Stud Family Plann [Special issue] 14:159–193
8. PIACT. NORPLANT® (1981) Instructions for clinicians
9. Crabbe P, Archer S, Benagiano G (1983) Design of the WHO chemical synthesis programme. Steroids 41:243
10. Matlin SA, Chan L, Hordjigeogiou P (1983) Analysis and purification of steroid esters. Steroids 41:359
11. Enever RP, Lewis GA (1983) The influence of pharmaceutical formulation upon biological activity of esters of norethisterone. Steroids 41:359
12. Bialy G, Blye RP, Enever RP (1983) Structure activity relationships in a series of norethisterone and levonorgestrel esters. Steroids 41:419

Jewish Law and Contraceptive Practice

J. G. Schenker

Department of Obstetrics and Gynecology, Hadassah University Hospital, Jerusalem, Israel

Support for regulation of individual fertility has been evident in all cultures and at all times, even in those societies in which social and religious rules have favored the abundant production of children. The oldest recorded medical recipes to prevent conception are found in ancient Egyptian papyri from 1850 B.C. Contraceptive knowledge had a written basis from the works of Aristotle in the fourth century B.C. through a variety of Greek and Roman medical writings. The scientific basis for contraception up to the late seventeenth century was spread through Europe by Islamic physicians. Dissemination of birth control methods did not begin until the twentieth century.

The problem entailed by the rapid increase of world population and the need for birth control measures to be applied by national and regional authorities was first discussed internationally by the United Nations Population Committee in 1947. The United Nations General Assembly in 1968 affirmed family planning as a basic human right. Population control can be achieved by individual voluntary measures or by involuntary ones provided by governmental policy. Both types of measures, the voluntary and especially the involuntary, raise several ethical, religious, and political issues.

Religion and medicine have been interrelated since the beginning of human history. The partnership of religion and medicine has not always been either holy or healthy. Medicine for its part is related to religion in its emphasis on the supreme values of human life and health and through its assistance in the development of medical services. On the other hand, through the various fields of medicine, and especially that of reproduction and its control, it was medicine that payed the higher price for the partnership with traditional religious views.

Historically, medicine and halakah (Jewish law) have been closely interwoven in Jewish thought. Halakah is derived from the Hebrew verb "to go," in the sense of traditional practice or rule of conduct. It consists of laws and prescriptions that have evolved since biblical times, and that regulate religious observations and the day-to-day life and conduct of Jewish people. Quite distinct from the Jewish law written in the Bible, halakic purpose is to preserve and represent oral traditions handed down since the revelation on Mount Sinai. The oral traditions were recorded in the Mishna, the Talmund, and other rabbinical writings. For thousands of years the halakah has been the main legal and ritual source of the religion and ethical life of Jews. As their circumstances have changed, it has been reinterpreted and made relevant to current science. Although Judaism acknowledges the continuous development of the halakah, interpretation and discussion are still being pursued by rabbinical studies. On the one hand, Jewish law regards both the study

Female Contraception
Eds.: B. Runnebaum, T. Rabe, L. Kiesel

and practice of medicine as a duty and a religious obligation. On the other hand, from a practical point of view conflicts occasionally arise between halakah and medicine. When such conflicts arise, medical halakah must be analyzed and discussed on the basis of legal precepts and Responsa literature (written opinions given to questions on aspects of Jewish law by qualified authorities).

In this paper we shall look at the orthodox halakic principles and their relation to the practice of birth control methods.

Religious Attitudes to the Practice of Contraception

The major religious opponents to the practice of birth control methods are the following:

Roman Catholic Church. In Roman Catholic doctrine the primary purpose of marriage is procreation. Procreation is a natural result of coitus, and therefore the practice of contraceptive methods opposes natural law. Abstinence and the rhythm method have been approved by the pope. These can be practiced for a number of medical, eugenic, economic, and social indications.

Eastern Orthodox Church. According to the Eastern Orthodox view, interference with any phase of reproduction is forbidden. Parenthood is a duty, and economic and social problems of the couple should be solved by governments and other social institutions. Abstinence is the only method permitted.

Protestant Church. Protestant doctrine has recently permitted the practice of birth control. It was approved by the Lamberth Conference and Anglican bishops in 1958. The Methodist conference in 1939 accepted the practice of contraception. The World Council of Churches in 1961 committed itself to cooperate with the United Nations on demographic tasks.

Islam. Islamic law has advocated marriage and procreation, but the Koran does not prohibit the practice of birth control. Islamic physicians in the tenth century offered many remedies to prevent conception. In 1937 the grand mufti of Egypt declared that there is no objection to the use of methods preventing gestation. Birth control methods are practiced in various Islamic countries. However, there is no clear religious consensus about its application. Some religious authorities opposed limitations on family size through legislative action.

Hinduism. According to Hinduism, women were created in order to give birth, especially to sons. There is no specific religious prohibition to the use of contraceptives.

Buddhism. Buddhist doctrine does not put a stress on procreation. Therefore birth control methods can be applied.

Judaism. The Jewish faith is greatly concerned with the problem of reproduction. Therefore, aspects of the Jewish attitude to contraception are to be found in the Talmud and commentaries, law codes and their commentaries, the mystic literature, moral tracts and above all in the rabbinical literature (Responsa).

The duty of procreation – "Be fertile, multiply, and fill the earth (Genesis 1:27) – is a mitzvah, a charitable deed. It is the first biblical commandment that was given to men, and through it all other commandments which were given to men and not to angels may be fulfilled. This commandment considers any interference with the act of procreation as morally wrong and prohibits the use of birth control. According to biblical definition, the duty of procreation is defined as the birth of one son and one daughter – "Male and female created He them" (Genesis 1:27). According to the Talmud and the later Responsa literature, the biblical obligation of giving birth to one son and one daughter is the minimal obligation, and therefore a man is obliged not to desist from procreation while he yet has strength.

All rabbinical rulings permit the use of contraceptives when medical indication exists to prevent conception. Economic difficulties and inconveniences of children raising are no indications for birth control practice. The talmudic ruling permits or even requires that women who are minors, pregnant, or lactating should insert a tampon during intercourse in order to prevent conception which may endanger the life of the mother and/or the fetus or prevent the mother from nursing. The practice of contraceptive methods was frequently discussed in the Responsa literature. Rabbi Luria in the sixteenth century and Rabbi Enger in the eighteenth century approved the practice of mechanical methods in order to control birth. Several rabbis in the present century have even approved the method of female sterilization. The Jewish attitude to marriage is largely contrary to the Roman Catholic attitude, in which the primary purpose of marriage and sex is procreation, and all forms of contraception are prohibited except abstinence and the "safe period." According to Judaism, marriage is a basic mitzvah, and procreation is only one of its objectives. It also includes the separate mitzvah of *onah* (conjugal duties; Exodus 21:10). *Onah* rests upon the basis that besides procreation the sexual act is to fulfill the wife's desire. The mitzvah of *onah*, according to Talmud teaching, is not only limited to the obligation of the husband to have intercourse, but the man is required to give joy to his wife. In Jewish marriage the goals are also maintaining harmony and domestic peace.

Jewish Attitude to Different Methods of Contraceptive Practice

According to Judaism, any method of contraception employed by the man is prohibited: Abstinence is prohibited since it is against the commandment "be fruitful and multiply," and since it also fails to fulfill the wife's conjugal rights (the mitzvah of *onah*). Coitus interruptus is forbidden, based on the prohibition of improper emission of sperm, as first mentioned in the Bible in Genesis 38, by Er and Onan. Condoms are opposed in the talmudic and rabbinical literature, based on the prohibition of the destruction of the seed (*hashatat zera*) and improper emission of it. Male hormonal preparations are also forbidden.

The contraceptive methods that are allowed for use by the woman in cases of medical indications are discussed in the Talmud. These include those of the "safe" period and of bodily movements following intercourse to spill the husband's sperm. The use of "cup roots" in order to prevent conception or to induce sterilization was practiced in the talmudic period and was recommended by Mamonides, Karo's Codes, and later by various rabbis. Recent Responsa literature finds analogy between hormonal contraceptive preparation (for example, in the pill) and the practice of "cup roots", therefore no halakic objection exists to the use of the pill. It should be mentioned that the use of oral contraception may cause spotting or breakthrough bleeding which would render the pill unsuitable for Jewish women because of the *nidah* state (the 7-day period from onset of menstruation until the wife immerses herself in the *mikve*, the ritually blessed water).

The approval of barrier methods – diaphragm and cervical cap – is based on the talmudic statement that has been called "The *Beraita* of Three Women." The use of *moch*, an absorbent material inserted into the vagina during intercourse, was allowed for minors and for pregnant and lactating women. The use of barrier methods is broadly discussed in Responsa literature. The most liberal view was expressed in the sixteenth century by Rabbi Luria, who allowed the application of a tampon before intercourse if there was a hazard to the health of the woman. Also theoretically approved for the woman is the intrauterine device (IUD), the biologic contraceptive action of which is obscure. If medical indication for birth control exists, an IUD can be employed. The use of an IUD is often accompanied by intermenstrual spotting, which affects the *nidah* state of Jewish woman. And, finally, a major ruling has permitted the use of spermicides. This is even preferred over barrier methods since it does not block passage of sperm, and coitus is in the normal manner.

According to views based on the halakah, if there is indication for birth control practice, the order of the contraceptive methods according to preference is as follows: Oral contraceptives, IUD, tampon or douche, spermicides, diaphragm.

Castration and Sterilization

According to Jewish law, it is forbidden to impair the reproductive organs in man (except for urgent medical indications), domestic animals, and birds. Such a religious prohibition is not endorsed by other religions such as Christianity, Islam, Buddhism, and Confucianism.

The practice of castration for reasons such as punishment, service in harems, service to God, political motives, and even to preserve the soprano voice have been employed in history from the time of Babylon to the 19th century. Based on the prohibition of this in Jewish law, the practice of vasectomy is prohibited. According to talmudic views, man is not permitted to drink the "cup of roots" in order to become sterile. This statement also stresses that the male hormonal preparations for contraceptive use are prohibited.

Sterilization of females is permissible on strictly medical grounds. The opinion of some rabbis is that even upon medical indications sterilization should not be employed without the consent of the husband. On the other hand, some rabbis state that in cases of a threat to the wife's life it can be performed without the husband's consent.

Induced Abortions

About 50 million induced abortions take place yearly throughout the world as a result of the couple's desire to space or limit the number of their children due to social or economic situations. The practice of criminal abortion is well-known and well-recorded in human history. There are laws in all countries restricting the termination of pregnancies. Over the past four decades a movement to legalize abortions on all or some grounds has gained vehement support from the feminist movements and as a result of problems related to the population explosion and the very high maternal death rate associated with illegal abortions. In most communist countries, the United States, United Kingdom, and Japan a woman is entitled to an abortion on demand in the first trimester of pregnancy.

Most religions have condemned the practice of induced abortion. Induced abortions are not discussed in the Bible, Talmud, the Codes, or the Responsa literature prior to the seventeenth century. Contrary to the Catholic Church, which has considered as murder the killing of any human fetus from the moment of conception, the position of Jewish law is that killing an unborn fetus is not considered as murder punishable by death. The basic halakic principles governing abortion practice are recorded in the mishna: (a) The point at which the fetus reaches the status of a living being (*nefesh*) and is of equal value to that of any other person is when the head during birth has emerged from the birth canal. (b) The mother's life has priority over the fetus' life. (c) The embryo is considered to be "mere water" during the first 40 days of gestation. Based on these principles, abortion and even embryotomy are indicated in any situation that endangers the mother's life. The rabbinical court of Jerusalem is inclined to permit an abortion to a Jewish mother even in the absence of any actual danger to her life, provided that there is a serious medical indication, either physical or mental, or in cases of rape, incest, or a defined risk that the child may be born physically or mentally handicapped. Such abortions should preferably be carried out within the first 40 days of pregnancy or, at least, within the first 3 months. The above indications for abortion, as stated by the Jerusalem Rabbinical Court, are not always approved by other Jewish religious authorities.

Population Control

The tremendous explosion of world population has caused political leaders to look upon national and regional birth control projects as vital. It should be pointed out again that the philosophy of the halakah is clearly opposed to any limitation of global or national population or of family size. All Jews and non-Jews should procreate: "God is praised for providing sustenance for all his creatures" (Psalms 145). Rabbis may, as discussed in the Responsa literature, under specific conditions permit the use of some birth control methods. Any permission is granted to a specific couple with a specific query. This permission, however, cannot be transferred or extended. According to Jewish religious authorities, Jewish couples have never been in a situation in which they might aggravate the problem of the world population explosion. On the contrary, during the 2000 years of the diaspora the Jewish community very often feared extinction after a pogrom or exile. In our own generation the world Jewish population before the Second World War was nearly 17 million, while at present it is only 14 million; 6 million Jews were killed during the Second World War. According to Jewish orthodox religious authorities, a Jew must reject the suggestion of limiting the size of his family. Contraceptive practice may be applied only in cases of medical indications, physical or mental, or in other special situations.

Epidemiology and AIDS in Contraception

Epidemiology and Sexually Transmitted Diseases

D. Serfaty

Birth Control Centre, St. Louis Hospital, 40 rue Bichat, 75010 Paris, France

Introduction

Sexually transmitted diseases represent a worldwide problem for public health. They are occurring with increasing frequency. Table 1 shows the annual incidence of the most important sexually transmitted diseases in the USA according to M. Guinan and W. Cates of the Center for Disease Control, Atlanta (quoted in [1]).

The high number of cases of *Chlamydia* infection, the most frequent venereal disease in the world, is particularly striking. In the USA, only gonorrhoea and syphilis are notifiable. Consequently, the figures shown probably underestimate the real incidences of the diseases. While the frequency of syphilis seems to be decreasing (except for congenital syphilis), the number of cases of gonorrhoea is increasing again. Additionally, there are more and more cases of penicillinase-positive gonococcus infection.

According to R. Barasso (quoted in [2]), 65% of the male sexual partners of women infected by the papilloma virus, some types of which are oncogenic, carry the virus themselves.

According to a recent publication by Henry-Suchet [2a], one in every three extrauterine pregnancies is a result of *Chlamydia* infection. This is the reason for the particular interest in *Chlamydia*, research being done by taking smears from the pelvic region during operations, by serological examinations, and by studies of the treatment of *Chlamydia* infection when terminating an extrauterine pregnancy.

"Venereal diseases occur in all races, in all social classes, religions and age groups" (A. Siboulet). In 1988, venereal diseases are no longer only the respon-

Table 1. Annual incidence of sexually transmitted diseases in the USA (1985) [1]

Chlamydia trachomatis infection	3 million
Gonorrhoea	910000
Herpes (new cases)	200000–500000
Trichomonas infection	1 million
Genital condylomata	1 million
Syphilis	68000
AIDS	29000 and 2 million HIV^+
Salpingitis	1 million, 10% leading to sterility

Female Contraception
Eds.: B. Runnebaum, T. Rabe, L. Kiesel

sibility of dermatologists and venerologists, but all other doctors are also involved. The emergence of AIDS since 1980 is an additional important reason for becoming conscious of venereal diseases and for attempting to fight against their increase. There is, of course, a very close relationship between contraception, sexuality and venereal disease. The risk of infection, however, is not equally high for every method of contraception. Certain methods may favour or aggravate venereal diseases, whereas others may protect their users against venereal diseases and their consequences. Nevertheless, it has to be stated that there is no agreement about the influence of various contraceptive methods on the frequency of venereal diseases.

Contraceptive Methods Favouring or Aggravating Venereal Diseases

Intrauterine Devices (IUDs)

Of all cases of pelvic infection, 25%–35% occur in women who use either inert or copper-medicated IUDs (R. Herion, quoted in [3]). Sometimes the IUD has been inserted during a pre-existing cervical infection (e.g. by gonococci or *Chlamydia trachomatis*) which had not been diagnosed. IUDs can also favour ascending infections (vagina – cervix – endometrium – ovaries – peritoneum) due to the IUD tail because of the loss of the endocervical barrier that protects the uterus. It is noteworthy that an ascending infection can be sexually transmitted.

Salpingitis and Pelvic Peritonitis in IUD Users

Infections (endometritis, salpingitis, pelvic peritonitis, and in some rare cases even endocarditis) [4] are the most severe complications of IUD use. Among all contraceptive methods, the IUD is associated with the highest risk of salpingitis and pelvic peritonitis (Table 2) [5].

Table 2. Risk of salpingitis and pelvic peritonitis with various contraceptive methods [5]

Contraceptive method	No. of cases of salpingitis or pelvic peritonitis	No. of patients tested	Relative risk
Oral contraceptives	127	830	0.5 (0.4–0.8)
Barrier methods	60	439	0.6 (0.4–0.8)
All IUDs	185	337	1.9 (1.5–2.4)
Dalkon Shield	35	15	8.3 (4.7–14.5)
Other IUDs	150	322	1.6 (1.2–2.0)
No contraception	250	763	1 (reference value)
Total	622	2369	

Table 3. Severity of acute salpingitis in relation to method of contraception in 546 women (new cases). (From Svensson, quoted in [7])

Severity of salpingitis	Neither IUD nor OC	IUD	OC
Low	51.3%	54.6%	73.5%[a]
Moderate	34.6%	29.7%	17.1%[a]
High	24.1%	15.7%	9.4%[a]

[a] Significant difference; OC, oral contraceptives.

Statistical estimates of the risk of salpingitis vary. Approximately 2% of women that use inert or copper-medicated IUDs have pelvic infections during the first year of use [6].

According to Senanayake and Burkman (quoted in [7]), the risk of acute salpingitis in IUD users is 2.7- to 7.3-fold higher than in women using no contraception, and 1.8- to 9.3-fold higher than in women using contraceptive methods other than IUDs.

Lars Westrom from Sweden and co-workers [8] found that 24.3% of 515 women with acute salpingitis (proven by laparoscopy) were IUD users, whereas only 9.7% of a control group of 741 sexually active women of the same age and with the same socio-economic background were users of IUDs. From these data it can be concluded that the average risk of acute salpingitis in IUD users is 3 times as high as in non-users.

Besides a risk of acute salpingitis, there is also a risk of subclinical salpingitis, which can rapidly become chronic, although the real incidence of this is unknown [7]. In addition, the frequency of salpingitis is not only higher in IUD users than in women taking oral contraceptives, but it also occurs in more severe forms (see Table 3). Finally, according to Stadel and Schlesselman [9] the risk of severe salpingitis that has to be treated surgically increases considerably when the IUD has been used for more than 5 years.

Bacteriological examination of salpingitis during IUD use shows the following distribution [7]: gonococci, 10%–20%; *Chlamydia trachomatis*, 45%–60%; mycoplasms, 10%–30%; aerobic and anaerobic bacteria, 10%–40%. It must be noted that the main causes of salpingitis (in users of IUDs) are sexually transmitted organisms (60% according to Siboulet [3], 70%–80% according to Henry-Suchet [7]).

Whatever germ triggers salpingitis, which has become more and more frequent recently, it will be superinfected by aerobic and anaerobic saprophytic flora. Siboulet [3] has emphasized that *Chlamydia trachomatis*, gonococci, and anaerobic germs often exist in association, this requiring treatment with a combination of several antibiotics (Vibramycin, Gentalline, imidazol derivatives).

The risk of salpingitis in IUD users is unmistakable, a fact that has to be kept in mind when choosing and surveying this method of contraception. On the other hand, there is not the same risk of salpingitis for all users of IUDs. Some IUD users have a high risk of pelvic infection.

Acute Salpingitis in Nulligravidae Using IUDs

In nulliparae the risk of acute salpingitis due to the IUD seems to be higher than in parous women. According to Westrom et al. [8], the risk of acute salpingitis is 7-fold higher in nulliparae using an IUD, whereas the risk for IUD users who have had children was only 1.7-fold higher than in women not using an IUD. This increased risk of salpingitis in nulliparae using IUDs has been confirmed by Eschenbach et al. [10]. However, Larsson et al. [11] in a prospective study over 4 years could not demonstrate an increased frequency of salpingitis when different methods of contraception were compared.

Acute Salpingitis in IUD Users under 25 Years of Age

The risk of acute salpingitis seems to be increased in younger women, according to Westrom et al. [8]. This has been confirmed by other authors. The relative risk of acute salpingitis in IUD users according to Burkman et al. [12] is 3.1-fold higher in women under 25 and only 1.9-fold higher in women above 25 when compared to women who do not use IUDs.

Larsson et al. [11] could not confirm the increased risk of pelvic infection in younger IUD users. Despite this, it is my opinion that young nulliparae have to be considered as a group with a high risk of salpingitis, even though this view is not unanimous. Since a pelvic infection can have severe consequences for the fertility of women without children, even if some authors have not confirmed the increased risk in this group of women, I believe that, with some exceptions, IUDs should not be inserted in young nulliparae.

Acute Salpingitis and Material of the IUD

Neither the material of the IUD, either polyethylene or copper, nor the type of IUD seems to be of importance [13, 8, 12], with the exception of the Dalkon Shield (see Table 2), to which a risk of infection 5-fold higher [5] than that with other IUDs has been attributed (possibly because of its string consisting of several fibres), and which for that reason is no longer commercially available. However, IUDs that release progesterone or other synthetic gestagens seem to have a lower risk of pelvic infections.

Progesterone-Medicated IUD. Progesterone which is released locally by a progesterone-medicated IUD (Progestasert) seems to protect its user from salpingitis. Richard Soderstrom from Seattle (quoted in [14]) found, during sterilizations, histologically detectable salpingitis by ovary biopsies in 49% of women who had not been using a progesterone-medicated IUD. Considering that the inflammation predisposes the tissue to a microbial infection, it seems correct to conclude that women using progesterone-medicated IUDs have a lower risk of a utero-ovarian infection than those using other IUDs.

Additionally, Lukkainen (quoted in [14]) found that the rate of pelvic infection in pluriparae observed over a period of 12 months was 1 infection in 556.5 months of use (27 infections in 15299 months of use). The frequency of pelvic infections with progesterone-medicated IUDs was 1 infection in 1086.7 months of use (76 infections in 82592 months of use).

Levonorgestrel-Medicated IUD. This IUD, which is not yet commercially available, has the shape of the Nova-copper-T, the vertical segment, however, containing a hormone reservoir instead of the copper coil. This reservoir contains 43 mg levonorgestrel (LNG) in a Silastic bar surrounded by a membrane, which provides a constant and very low rate of LNG release of 20 μg per day over a period of approximately 7 years [15]. In 3 years of use, there has been no removal for pelvic infection.

According to Lukkainen (quoted in [15]), there were only three cases of endometritis and two cases of pelvic infection in 25000 months of use of the LNG-medicated IUD. This "anti-infection" effect of hormone-releasing IUDs could be very valuable, but needs further confirmation by other studies. This effect seems to be related to the decrease of the severity of bleedings, the increase of mucus viscosity, which makes the ascent of spermatozoa and genital infections more difficult, and, possibly, to a reduction of uterine contractions. For these reasons, hormone-medicated IUDs should be chosen for multiparae who have a high risk of pelvic infection but who nevertheless have to use an IUD.

IUDs, Pelvic Infection, and High Risk of Sexually Transmitted Diseases

Users of IUDs who have a high risk of sexually transmitted disease (main reason: 70%–80% [7] of cases of acute salpingitis) form the group that is most at risk of pelvic infection. These are:
- Women with many sexual partners (and women with a single sexual partner, who, in turn, has many sexual partners)
- Women with a new partner for occasional sexual intercourse
- Women with many changing sexual partners
- Women whose sexual partner had urethritis previously
- Women who had sexually transmitted diseases before

Many authors consider there to be a close relation between the risk of a pelvic infection and sexuality. Cohen [16]: "Two factors favour genital infection in the female: sexually transmitted disease in the partner and the number of sexual partners." These factors are found more often in the group of women under 25, and within this group, the risk for IUD users seems to be higher than for those women using oral contraceptives or local methods of contraception. Numerous publications, including those by Rubin et al. [17] and Burkman et al. [12], confirmed the increased risk of pelvic infection when there is a higher number of sexual partners and a higher frequency of sexual intercourse. In the group of women at high risk for sexually transmitted diseases and salpingitis should be included those women who had adnexitis, tubal plastic or previous pelvic surgery (even a minor operation like curettage or aspiration) with postoperative pelvic infection. Prior to insertion of an IUD, patients should be questioned in detail about these.

Pelvic Infection in Women with Diabetes Mellitus using an IUD

Under two conditions the risk of an infection when using an IUD does not seem to be higher in women with diabetes than in women without diabetes (J. Wiese,

S. Skouby, and M. Pawless; M.P. Vessey, K. Kunz, and D. Buchsenschutz; quoted in [18]):

- When diabetes is under good control (fasting glucose between 0.8 and 1 g/l, and glucose 1.5 h after eating under 1.40 g/l; G. Cathelineau, quoted in [18]). It is now firmly established that phagocytic activity of leucocytes is diminished during hyperglycaemia, which may explain the frequency and severity of infections in women with diabetes and poorly controlled blood glucose.
- When women with diabetes who use an IUD are under good surveillance. To be more precise, each leucorrhoea and each metrorrhagia must be examined immediately and systematically and full microbiological screening must be carried out. In diabetics with persisting metrorrhagia who use IUDs the device must be removed even though the women might not have any pain.

Infectious Complications in IUD Users with Immunosuppressives

In 1983, Smith et al. [19] reported four deaths in IUD users, one of which was caused by peritonitis and sepsis 2 days after the insertion of an IUD. This was in a 42-year-old patient who had been treated for rheumatic disease with corticoids for 4 years. These authors consider any corticoid therapy or any other immunosuppressive drug a contraindication for the insertion of an IUD. This is particularly the case in two not unusual circumstances:

- Women with lupus erythematosus disseminatus (LED): except for minor forms of LED that are not treated with corticoids or other immunosuppressive drugs, and during remission of the disease, the IUD must not be used because of the already increased risk of infection due to the immunosuppressives [20].
- Women with kidney transplants: logically, IUDs are not indicated in patients with kidney transplants, who mostly have to take corticoids and immunosuppressives daily. According to Pelissier [21], there are two reasons for this: the risk of infection that a woman with diminished immune response should not run, and the lower efficiency of the IUD during this type of treatment.

IUD and Risk of Pelvic Infections in Pregnancy

Numerous trials (Tatum, Preston, Christian; quoted in [16]) have demonstrated the possible dangers of pregnancies in IUD users. Very severe and sometimes fatal cases of sepsis (13 deaths in 242 registered cases) can occur. The Dalkon Shield is not the only IUD that can be responsible for this: other IUDs have also been related to this kind of complication. Hence, it must be considered that pregnant IUD users run a high risk of infection. Whatever the type of IUD, it must be removed and treatment with antibiotics started. The removal itself does not represent any problem as long as the IUD tail is visible. If this is not the case and if the woman wishes to continue her pregnancy, further treatment will have to be even more delicate.

Prevention of Salpingitis and Pelvic Peritonitis in IUD users

Prevention of salpingitis and pelvic peritonitis in IUD users consists mainly in recognizing those women who have an increased risk of pelvic infections. The following measures are required:

- In users of the Dalkon Shield the IUD must be removed
- In pregnant IUD users it must first be removed, and then treatment with antibiotics should follow
- In patients taking immunosuppressive drugs it is necessary to remove the IUD and to recommend another method of contraception

Generally speaking, one has to suggest a different method of contraception to women with a high risk of pelvic infections. If the user insists on the IUD and if she is a multipara who has no absolute contraindication against this type of contraception, several precautions are absolutely necessary before fulfilling the patient's wish:

- It must be ensured that there is no pre-existing sexually transmitted disease (normal clinical examination and a normal microbiological examination of the genital tract)
- One must make sure that there is no infection of the tubes (normal clinical examination, NFS examination, VS examination, and perhaps hysterosalpingography, if not contraindicated)
- The insertion of the IUD must be performed under particularly strictly aseptic conditions (perhaps under systemic treatment with antibiotics)

Once the IUD is inserted, the regular use of a chemical vaginal contraceptive (e.g. ovula, foam or tablets based on benzalkonium chloride, or nonoxynol-9 ovulum) before sexual intercourse must be recommended. This should be done to increase the efficiency of the IUD and to prevent certain sexually transmitted diseases (see the following).

Endometritis

Besides the risk of salpingitis or pelvic peritonitis, possibly caused by one or several carriers of a sexually transmitted disease, there is the additional risk of endometritis in IUD users. This can be of different degrees, acute, or chronic, and occurs at a frequency of between 10% and 20%. From a bacteriological point of view, all germs can exist simultaneously, including *Chlamydia trachomatis* and gonococci (a number of authors have demonstrated the frequency of endometritis caused by gonococci in users of copper-medicated IUDs). Without proper diagnosis and therapy, this endometritis can lead to a Douglas' abscess or an ovarian abscess but, above all, it can lead to salpingitis. There is a 25% incidence of chronic salpingitis in patients with chronic endometritis who use an IUD. Endometritis was found in 85% of patients with salpingitis (proven by coelioscopy; according to K. Holmes et al., quoted in [22] and in 20% of cases of suspected salpingitis with normal results on coelioscopy). The same authors hold that:

- A diagnosis by vacuum smear of the endometrium can complete the coelioscopic results, as far as the diagnosis and an etiology of the salpingitis are concerned.
- There is endometritis in 50% of cases of muco-putrid catarrh of the cervix, even if no symptoms of salpingitis can be found.
- In 90% of women with salpingitis or endometritis confirmed by biopsy, endometrial or tubal infection caused by *Chlamydia trachomatis* can be found.
- There are histological criteria which make distinction between endometritis caused by *Chlamydia trachomatis* and *Neisseria gonorrhoeae* possible.

Conclusion

To come to an end of this section on the risk of pelvic infection whilst using IUDs, it seems appropriate to quote David A. Grimes from the University of Southern California School of Medicine and Nancy C. Lee from the Center of Disease Control's Division of Reproductive Health in Atlanta [35]:

1. The risk of pelvic infections whilst using IUDs (with the exception of the Dalkon Shield) has probably been overestimated.
2. To be able to correctly evaluate the risk of infection, comparisons must be made with women who do not use any method of contraception. However, the latter usually do not have the same sexual habits. Generally speaking, they live in a stable partnership, are sexually inactive, or are trying to become pregnant.
3. The risk of a pelvic infection whilst using IUDs depends more closely on the way of life and the sexual habits of the IUD users and, above all, on their male sexual partners than on the IUD itself. Hence, the IUD seems to be a good method of contraception for those women who live in mutual monogamy.

It would seem that a re-evaluation of the risk of pelvic infections with IUD use is absolutely necessary on the basis of these data. In the case of "good sexual habits" the risk of pelvic infections in IUD users should not be significant, except in individual cases. However, there is unanimity on the fact that, unlike oral and vaginal contraceptives, the IUD cannot protect from the risk of a pelvic infection.

Oral Contraceptives

Genital mycosis is more frequent when oral contraceptives are used than with other methods of contraception or when no contraceptive methods are used. *Chlamydia trachomatis* infection (alone or in combination with other sexually transmitted diseases) occurs more often in women who use oral contraceptives than in women who do not according to several authors including Kinghorm and Waugh (quoted in [3]). Washington et al. of the Center for Disease Control, Atlanta [36] have investigated the relation between oral contraception and *Chlamydia trachomatis* in the vaginal mucosa. Of the 14 studies performed by these authors, 12 showed an increased occurrence of *Chlamydia trachomatis* in the vaginal mucosa of women using oral contraceptives. The most likely hypothesis suggested was that infections caused by *Chlamydia trachomatis* are more frequently detected with a cervical ectropion and that this is also more frequent in users of oral contraceptives. These authors, based on animal experiments, state that contraceptive steroids and particularly gestagens favour infections by *Chlamydia trachomatis*.

In the opinion of Grimes and Lee [35], the increased risk of cervical infection does not mean that there is an increased risk of salpingitis or pelvic peritonitis (and their sequelae), which in fact represent the main risks of sexually transmitted disease in women who use contraceptives. They also say that there is no reason to assume that the use of oral contraceptives increases the risk of salpingitis caused by *Chlamydia trachomatis*.

Contraceptive Methods with a Preventive Effect on Sexually Transmitted Diseases or Their Sequelae

Oral Hormonal Contraceptives

Genital herpes recurs less frequently when oral contraceptives are used [3]. Oral contraceptives diminish the risk of salpingitis by 50% (Table 2; [5]). According to a Swedish study by Wolner-Hanssen et al., this protective effect applies to both salpingitis caused by gonococci and salpingitis caused by *Chlamydia trachomatis* [23]. This is an important beneficial effect of oral contraceptives which has not been emphasized sufficiently. According to Henry-Suchet [7], the protective effect of oral contraceptives can be explained by the suppression of cervical mucus, which is no longer penetrable by bacteria or spermatozoa, and by the diminished activity of the myometrium, the increase of the serum concentrations of protease inhibitors such as α_1-antritrypsin and α_2-macroglobulin, and an inhibiting effect on proteolytic enzymes which are normally released during an infection.

However, in theory, not all oral contraceptives should have a protective effect against ascending infections. Phasic pills with high doses of oestrogens are associated with oversecretion of mucus which, instead of inhibiting the ascent of the germs, should, in theory, favour it.

The protective effect of oral contraceptives against pelvic infections has not been confirmed by all authors. Washington et al. [36], who carried out a critical investigation about epidemiological studies which are in favour of this positive effect of oral contraceptives, remarked that this protective effect at the moment seems only valid for the severe forms of pelvic infection where a hospitalization (in only 25% of the cases) is required, and for salpingitis caused by gonococci. These authors find that conclusions concerning the protective effect of the pill against pelvic infections (above all *Chlamydia trachomatis*) are premature.

Cramer et al. [37], who investigated the previous methods of contraception of 283 nulliparae with tubal sterility and 3833 fertile women recently demonstrated that previous use of oral contraceptives neither increases nor decreases the risk of tubal sterility. However, in this regard not all oral contraceptives are to be judged equally. Those pills with a high oestrogen content ($\geqq 75$ µg ethinyloestradiol), all phasic pills and pills that contain norethisterone acetate or ethinyldiacetate (even if they contain less than 50 µg ethinyloestradiol) seem to increase slightly the risk of tubal sterility. All other oral contraceptives do not seem to have any influence on this risk.

Vaginal Contraception

Kelaghan et al. [23] reported that the ratio of the risk of hospitalization on account of adnexitis between women who use barrier methods and women who use another method or no method was 0.6 (Table 4). There was no statistically significant difference between mechanical or chemical barrier methods.

The prevention of pelvic infection by vaginal contraceptives (and thereby the prevention of the consequences, such as sterility or extrauterine pregnancy) has

Table 4. Distribution of current contraceptive methods used by women with pelvic inflammatory disease (PID) and control subjects [23]

Current contraceptive method	Women with PID (%) ($n=306$)	Control subjects (%) ($n=1175$)	Relative risk
Barrier method	19.3	36.5	0.6 (0.4–0.9)
None	80.7	63.5	1.0 (reference)

Limited to women who reported no past history of PID. Contraceptive method used in the 3 months prior to interview. Limited to current users of barrier methods and women not currently using a contraceptive. Relative risk adjusted for education and previous history of gonorrhoea: 95% confidence interval in parentheses.

Table 5. Distribution of current contraceptive methods used by women with pelvic inflammatory disease (PID) and control subjects

Current contraceptive method	Women with PID (%) ($n=306$)	Control subjects (%) ($n=1175$)	Relative risk
Condom	10.5	18.1	0.6 (0.4–0.9)
Diaphragm	4.6	12.4	0.4 (0.2–0.7)
Spermicidal foam jelly or creme	4.2	6.0	0.7 (0.4–1.4)
None	80.7	63.5	1.0 (reference)

Limited to women who reported no past history of PID. Contraceptive method used in the 3 months prior to interview. Limited to current users of barrier methods and women not currently using a contraceptive. Relative risk adjusted for education and previous history of gonorrhoea: 95% confidence interval in parentheses.

been confirmed by other authors, especially N. C. Lee (quoted in [24]) and Cramer [37]. The prophylactic properties of these methods of contraception can be explained by their actions against sexually transmitted diseases, the mechanisms of these actions varying according to the method used and depending on use of a "barrier" with or without a spermicide.

Condoms

As early as in the 16th century Gabriel Phallope in his essay "De Morbo Gallico" (1564) reported on a very thin cover made of linen that was originally used as a protection against syphilis [25]. Condoms protect women from direct contact with semen [and the microorganisms that may be contained in it: gonococci, *Chlamydia trachomatis*, hepatitis B virus, HIV (AIDS virus), *Trichomonas vaginalis, Mycoplasma hominis, Ureaplasma urealyticum* and streptococcus B], from the male

Table 6. Efficacy of condom use in preventing sexually transmitted diseases [26]

Study	Study design	Study population	Outcomes	Measures of effect	95% confidence intervals
Premberton et al. (1972)	Cross-sectional	Males, STD clinic, Belfast	Urethral gonorrhoea,	0.51	0.33–0.80
			non-gonococcal urethritis	1.20	0.90–1.59
McCormack et al. (1973)	Cross-sectional	Male college volunteers, USA	Urethral *T. mycoplasma* colonization	0.99	0.16–0.68
Darrow (1973)	Cohort	STD clinic, California	Urethral gonorrhoea	0.34	0.10–1.19
Hart (1974)	Cohort	Australian soldiers, Vietnam	Self-reported venereal diseases	0.00[a]	
Barlow (1977)	Cross-sectional	Males, STD clinic, London	Urethral gonorrhoea,	0.25	0.11–0.59
			non-gonococcal urethritis	0.85	0.69–1.07
Hooper et al. (1978)	Cohort	Naval crewmen, Far East	Urethral gonorrhoea	0.00[b]	
Kelaghan et al. (1982)	Case control	Hospitalized women, USA	Pelvic inflammatory disease	0.6	0.4 –0.9
Austin et al. (1984)	Case control	Females, STD clinic, Alabama	Cervical gonorrhoea	0.87	0.64–1.19
Syrjanen et al. (1984)	Case control	Females, obstetrics and gynaecology clinic, Finland	Cervical human papilloma virus infection	1.35	0.72–2.78

[a] $p<0.0001$; Fisher's exact test (none of 55 condom users was infected: 26 of 96 using no prophylaxis were infected).
[b] $p<0.1$; Fisher's exact test (none of 29 condom users was infected: 51 of 498 non-users were infected).

urethral secretions, and from lesions of the penis. At the same time, the condom protects the male user from direct contact with the genital secretions or lesions of his female partner (Table 6).

In vitro the condom has proven to be an effective barrier against *Chlamydia trachomatis*, HIV (see later), type 2 herpes simplex virus, and cytomegaloviruses [26]. Several clinical studies performed by Stone from Atlanta [27] demonstrated that the condom protects women and men from many sexually transmitted diseases: from urethral and cervical gonorrhoea, most probably from urethritis caused by *Ureaplasma urealyticum* in men, and from salpingitis and pelvic peritonitis (and probably cancer of the cervix, see later) in women.

So far, no protective effect of condoms against non-gonococcal urethritis in men or against cervical herpes or cervical infection by papilloma virus has been proved [28].

In order to have this protective effect, condoms must be used always and correctly and must remain intact. The importance of information, particularly for adolescents, about sexually transmitted diseases and their prevention must be kept in mind.

Results are encouraging, but they must be interpreted with caution because in most clinical trials important factors have not always been taken into account: frequency of sexual intercourse, frequency of sexual intercourse with infected partners, frequency of certain sexual methods associated with a higher risk of a sexually transmitted disease, correct or incorrect use of condoms, etc. However, we must always remember the important protective effect of the condom against sexually transmitted diseases, an effect which can only be enhanced when condoms with incorporated spermicides or additional vaginal spermicides are used.

Diaphragms

A diaphragm of adequate size and correctly inserted is a mechanical barrier covering the cervix, which otherwise is open to penetration by germs and, hence, frequently the site of infection. The use of spermicides in combination with a diaphragm provides additional chemical protection (Table 7). Several studies mentioned by Stone [26] showed that barrier methods such as the diaphragm diminish the risk of gonococcal cervicitis, of salpingitis [24] and of cervical dysplasia [34]. This protective effect persists even when the diaphragms are consid-

Table 7. The effect of the diaphragm against STDs. (From [26])

Mode of action	Efficiency
Mechanical barrier covering the cervix	The protective effect of a diaphragm against STD when used on its own has not been studied
Use in combination with spermicides which have an additional protective effect against STD	Seems to diminish the frequency of gonococcal cervicitis, cervical dysplasia and salpingitis

ered in comparison with other barrier methods of contraception. On the other hand, Austin et al. (1984) found no statistically significant effect of this barrier method. The prophylactic effect of the diaphragm against other sexually transmitted diseases such as genital herpes has not been investigated. It seems possible, however, that the diaphragm would diminish but not completely suppress the risk of an infection by that virus.

The diaphragm, like the other barrier methods of contraception, in combination with spermicides probably protects against a certain number of sexually transmitted diseases. This is likely to be one of the reasons for the increasingly frequent use that has been found in recent years [28a].

Spermicides

Spermicides act as a chemical barrier against spermatozoa on one hand and, on the other hand, against a great many sexually transmitted diseases. In vitro, a number of laboratory studies (summarized in [26]) have shown that the active principles of spermicides are effective against a great number of organisms causing sexually transmitted diseases: gonococci, *Trichomonas, Ureaplasma urealyticum, Treponema*, herpes virus and HIV. From an epidemiological point of view, there are several studies (quoted in [26]) suggesting that vaginal spermicides can reduce the risk of gonococcal cervicitis and the frequency of hospitalization with salpingitis when women using spermicides are compared with women who use no method of contraception. They can also reduce the risk of *Chlamydia trachomatis* infection and possibly also of cervical cancer.

The spermicide that has been investigated most often is nonoxynol-9, which is an anionic surfactant. It is the world's most frequently used spermicide. The Food and Drug Administration (FDA; in a report published 12 December 1980) at present has only approved three types of spermicides for their safe use and sufficient efficacy: nonoxynol-9, Menfegol, octoxynol. In France nonoxynol-9 is commercially available in Patentex ovula with 0.075 g nonoxynol-9 and as Semicid ovula with 0.1 g nonoxynol-9 per ovula.

The results of clinical studies such as that of Handsfields et al. [28b] concerning *Chlamydia trachomatis* are very instructive. The rate of infection by *C. trachomatis* is approximately 3 times lower in women using spermicides or a barrier method of contraception than in users of oral contraceptives or IUDs or women who do not use any type of contraception.

As to benzalkonium chloride, several studies have demonstrated its antibacterial effect. Benzalkonium chloride is a cationic surfactant, and it is the spermicide most frequently used in France, applied mainly as foam ovula and as Pharmatex sponges and as Alpagelle creme. In the USA benzalkonium chloride has been approved by the INDA (Investigation New Drugs Approvement) since 1985.

In 1986, at the Second International Congress of the WHO on sexually transmitted disease in Paris, Catalan demonstrated the efficiency of spermicides in vitro against *C. trachomatis* (bacteriostatic activity at a concentration of 0.002%), type 2 herpes simplex virus, *Neisseria gonorrhoeae, Staphylococcus aureus*, vaginal *Trichomonas*, and, to a lesser degree, against *Gardnerella vaginalis* and *Candida albicans*.

In 1984, M. Todd and F. Ashton of the Bureau of Epidemiology and Microbiology (Laboratory Center for Disease Control) demonstrated an inhibitory effect against *Neisseria gonorrhoeae* of four vaginal contraceptives, one of which was based on benzalkonium chloride, two on nonoxynol-9, and the fourth on *p*-diisobutylphenoxypolyethoxyethanol.

In 1985, M. Laverdiere and L. Seguin of the Maisonneuve-Rosemont Hospital in Montréal (Dossier of the Pharmelac Laboratories) showed that the concentration of benzalkonium chloride contained in Pharmatex contraceptive tampons is sufficient to almost completely destroy a concentrated suspension of *Staphylococcus aureus* in vitro and furthermore to prevent their proliferation over at least 48 h. According to the same authors and during the same study, these tampons had no or very little effect on *Escherichia coli* and *Pseudomonas aeruginosa* and showed fungicidal activity against *Candida albicans*, although this was difficult to evaluate.

This high efficacy of benzalkonium chloride in vitro against *Staphylococcus aureus* was confirmed by J. Breuillard (Toulouse; Dossier of Pharmelac Laboratories), which should help to reassure women and doctors as far as the possible risk of toxic shock syndrome in users of the benzalkonium chloride containing tampon Pharmatex is concerned.

M. Poitevin and P. Collart (WHO Centre for Sexually Transmitted Diseases in Paris) in 1986 demonstrated by experiments in hares that benzalkonium chloride (under the concentration conditions of the IPPF test) is a treponemicide (*Treponema pallidum)* in 100% of cases (Dossier of Pharmelac Laboratories).

In June 1986, during the second international congress on sexually transmitted diseases (Paris), Siboulet demonstrated, in a 6-month clinical study on vaginal suppositories containing 0.025 g benzalkonium chloride, administered to 137 women with a higher risk of sexually transmitted disease (multiple sexual relations, changing sexual partners) who had been treated for at least three such diseases during the preceeding 6 months, that the number of venereal diseases could be reduced by 43.5% (74.3% gonococci, 75% *Treponema* and 66.7% *Gardnerella*).

Definitive conclusions regarding the effect of spermicides in preventing sexually transmitted diseases are not yet possible. Nonetheless, this effect seems to be very likely. On the other hand, this effect is certainly present if the spermicides are used in combination with condoms, diaphragms or with cervical caps, since these local methods have demonstrated their protective effect against sexually transmitted diseases independently of any spermicides.

This was also demonstrated in the recent publication by Cramer [37] that shows the significant reduction (0.6) of the risk of tubal sterility in users of a barrier method of contraception. Additionally, women using a diaphragm or a condom *plus* spermicides have a lower risk of tubal sterility in comparison to those using a condom or a spermicide on its own.

Prevention of AIDS by Condoms and Spermicides

In the absence of an adequate curative treatment for and vaccines against AIDS, the only way to fight against it is by means of prevention. Do barrier methods protect from infection by HIV during sexual intercourse (>70% of all cases of AIDS)?

AIDS and Condoms

Conant et al. [29], investigated five different condoms and showed that in vitro retroviruses (mouse retrovirus and ARV-2 – AIDS associated retrovirus) cannot penetrate the walls of these condoms. Fischl [38] reported that out of 45 female partners of heterosexual men with AIDS, who were serologically HIV negative at the beginning of the study, 14 did not use condoms and, as a result, 12 of the women were serologically positive after 18 months. Seroconversion was much rarer in women who had regularly used a condom (10%). Yet, it must be stated that always using condoms significantly reduces the risk of infection with HIV in heterosexuals, though it cannot completely eliminate it. By the way, mishaps with condoms during the study were no exceptions. Of course, the results of these in vitro and clinical studies will have to be confirmed before a final judgement on the preventive action of condoms against AIDS can be made. Is there, on the other hand, sufficient protection against AIDS by standard condoms and during anorectal intercourse?

Numerous companies that were initially trying to produce condoms with higher "sensitivity" have shifted their central interest to research on solid condoms particularly appropriate for the prophylaxis of sexually transmitted diseases. In the Netherlands some companies have put condoms on the market that are 1 ½ times as thick and 3 times as solid as normal: "AIDS specials". In addition, these condoms have to be used with a sufficient amount of spermicidal gel or creme or an aqueous lubricant, and not with lubricant containing organic solvents.

Theoretically, the condom failures that are feared in the prevention of AIDS will mainly be caused by an incorrect use of the condom. Information campaigns on AIDS and its prevention should continuously remind people of the "rules" for the use of condoms such as those that have been formulated by Verdoux [30]. A worldwide boom in condoms has at any rate been induced by the emergence of AIDS. Since 1980, sales of condoms in the USA have doubled (1 billion at the moment). After the abolition of the prohibition of advertising of condoms by the Ministry of Health in France, sales by Profilex (one of the most important producers of condoms) of condoms rose by 15% within 1 month.

Only 7% of the French use condoms (in comparison to 37% of the British and 68% of the Japanese). These figures demonstrate that it will still take quite an effort to provide an expansion of the use of condoms in France.

AIDS and Spermicides

AIDS and Nonoxynol-9. Hicks et al. [31] have shown that nonoxynol-9 inactivates HIV in vitro at concentrations of 0.05% and above. Still in vitro and at a concentration of 1% and above, nonoxynol-9 significantly reduces the virulence of HIV for human lymphocytes. In addition, the inactivation of HIV by nonoxynol-9 is, according to Voeller [32], very fast (less than 60 s). If the in vitro effect of nonoxynol-9 could be proven clinically (in vivo), the speed of inactivation would be quite an important element in the prevention of sexually transmitted AIDS. It should be mentioned that nonoxynol-9-based vaginal contraceptives that are commercially available at the moment contain between 1% and 5% of these spermicides.

AIDS and Benzalkonium Chloride. Lionel Resnick et al. [32a] have demonstrated that HIV was completely inactivated within 10 min by a combination of quaternary ammonium chlorides (at a concentration of 0.08%) which contained, above all, dimethylalkylbenzylammonium (= benzalkonium) chloride.

Chermann of the Pasteur Institute in a study that was terminated in 1986 has proven that 10 min contact of the spermicide Pharmatex in a 1% solution (corresponding to 0.012 g benzalkonium chloride) at 37 °C is sufficient to completely inactivate HIV, whether the virus be searched for by the activity of its reverse transcriptase (the enzyme which indicates the replication of the retrovirus in culture) or by its virulence for normal human lymphocytes.

Prophylaxis of AIDS by condoms and/or spermicides concerns only those cases where HIV is transmitted by sperm during sexual intercourse. Good sexual habits in combination with the use of condom and/or a spermicide cannot but improve prevention of AIDS and slow down its expansion on a national or even international level.

Condoms, Diaphragms, and Cervical Carcinoma

Cervical carcinoma is epidemiologically comparable to a sexually transmitted disease. Several studies have demonstrated that women using condoms or diaphragms have a lower risk of getting cervical carcinoma or precancerous lesions of the cervix.

Harris et al. [34] demonstrated that cervical abnormalities decrease with increasing duration of use of condom or diaphragm; it is the reduction of the relative risk of severe dysplasia (from 1 to approximately 0.2 after 10 years' use of these barrier methods) which is the most significant (Table 8). These results can be confirmed even if the number of sexual partners is taken into account. Another study in England (Wright et al. 1978, quoted in [27]) also demonstrated a significant reduction of the relative risk (0.2) of cervical carcinoma in women using diaphragms.

Is the possible protective effect of condoms or diaphragms against the development of cervical carcinoma or precancerous lesions of the cervix caused by the anti-herpes simplex type 2 effect of these barriers or by their anti-human papilloma virus effect (not yet proven)?

The importance of the sexual life as a risk factor for cervical carcinoma is well known. Sensible sexual activity can equally well contribute to the prophylaxis of precancerous lesions and invasive lesions of the cervix.

Table 8. Relative risk of cervical abnormalities with barrier methods of contraception

Duration of use of diaphragm or condom (years)	Moderate dysplasia ($n = 44$)	Severe dysplasia ($n = 81$)	Carcinoma in situ ($n = 65$)
Never	1.00 (8)	1.00 (30)	1.00 (18)
5	1.55 (19)	0.86 (35)	1.14 (27)
5–9	2.32 (10)	0.38 (8)	1.43 (13)
10	0.59 (7)	0.17 (8)[a]	0.52 (7)

[a] Statistically significant. (From [34]).

Conclusion

When a certain method of contraception is chosen, the consequences of this method on sexually transmitted diseases is an important element to be taken into account. The prevention of sexually transmitted diseases should be systematically combined with contraception, particularly in young people. As long as there are no effective vaccines against sexually transmitted diseases, immediate postcoital miction and washing of the genital organs after sexual intercourse are still to be recommended even if the efficacy of these methods has never been demonstrated definitively.

In the first place, good sexual habits will have to be promoted with the aid of "high-quality" information on sexually transmitted diseases, particularly to young people (essentially by recommending limiting the number of sexual partners, avoiding sexual intercourse with unknown people or persons who have numerous sexual partners or a sexually transmitted disease, and finally carefully questioning the potential sexual partners). In addition, the systematic use of vaginal contraceptives (condoms, diaphragms, spermicides) should be recommended to persons who are at high risk of sexually transmitted disease, even independently of their contraceptive effect. These barriers definitely act preventively against many sexually transmitted diseases and so protect users from their complications, e.g. salpingitis, extrauterine pregnancy, sterility in men and women, and most probably from cervical carcinoma.

As to sexually transmitted AIDS, prevention based on a change of sexual habits and systematic use of adequate condoms, possibly in combination with spermicides, is at the moment the only weapon in the fight against this epidemic. Prevention is necessary in persons that are at high risk of AIDS (homosexual and/or bisexual men, drug addicts who inject drugs intravenously, haemophilics, prostitutes, and partners of people in these risk groups).

The aim of individual prophylaxis of sexually transmitted diseases and choosing a method of contraception which is adapted to the risk of a sexually transmitted disease in individual patients is not to put sexuality aside, but to find a way that guarantees safe sexuality which makes it possible to make love without fear.

References

1. Goldsmith MF (1986) La constante progression des MST va-t-elle remettre en cause la „révolution sexuelle"? JAMA [Suppl] 11(133):15–19
2. Siboulet A (1986) Maladies sexuellement transmissibles: un problème majeur de santé publique. JAMA [Suppl] 11(133):1–2

2a. Henry-Suchet J (1987) Presse Med 16(32):10–17

3. Siboulet A (1986) MST et contraception. In: Serfaty D (ed) La contraception. Doin, Paris
4. Serfaty D (1986) Complications infectieuses des dispositifs intra-utérins: les femmes à haut risque. Actual Gynecol 17:173–182
5. Lee NC, Rubin GL, Ory HW, Burkman RT (1983) Type of intrauterine device and the risk of pelvic inflammatory disease. Obstet Gynecol 62(1):1–6
6. Kleinman RL (1977) Intrauterine contraception, 4th edn. International Planned Parenthood Federation
7. Henry-Suchet J (1986) Contraception et salpingites. In: Serfaty D (ed) La contraception. Doin, Paris
8. Westrom L, Bengtsson LP, Mardh PA (1976) The risk of pelvic inflammatory disease in women using intrauterine contraceptive devices as compared to non-users. Lancet 221–224
9. Stadel BV, Schlesselman S (1984) Extent of surgery for pelvic inflammatory disease in relation to duration of intrauterine device use. PID surgery and IUD use. Obstet Gynecol 2:171–178
10. Eschenbach DA, Harnisch JP, Holmes KK (1977) Pathogenesis of acute pelvic inflammatory disease. Role of contraception and other risk factors. Am J Obstet Gynecol 128:883–850
11. Larsson B, Rodau S, Patek E (1981) IUD pathology. Pelvic inflammatory disease among women using copper IUDs, Progestasert, oral contraceptive pills or vaginal contraceptive pills. A 4 years prospective investigation. Contracept Deliv Syst 2:237–242
12. Burkman RT, and the Women's Health Study (1981) Association between intrauterine device and pelvic inflammatory disease. Obstet Gynecol 57(3):269–276
13. Edelman DA, Berger GS, Keith L (1979) IUDs and their complications. Halland, Boston
14. Serfaty D, Levrier M (1986) Le stérilet à la progestérone. In: Serfaty D (ed) La contraception. Doin, Paris
15. Serfaty D (1986) Dispositif intra-utérin au lévonorgestrel. In: Serfaty D (ed) La contraception. Doin, Paris
16. Cohen J (1986) Dispositifs intra-utérins et infection génitale. In: Serfaty D (ed) La contraception. Doin, Paris
17. Rubin GL, Ory HW, Layde PM (1982) Oral contraceptives and pelvic inflammatory disease. Am J Obstet Gynecol 144(6):630–635
18. Serfaty D (1986) Les DIU chez les femmes diabétiques. In: Serfaty D (ed) La contraception. Doin, Paris
19. Smith PA, Ellis CJ, Sparks RA, Guillebaud J (1983) Death associated with intrauterine contraceptive devices in the United Kingdom between 1973 and 1983. Br Med J 287:1537–1538
20. Musson P, Serfaty D, Puissant A (1986) Contraception chez les femmes atteintes de lupus érythémateux disséminé. In: Serfaty D (ed) La contraception. Doin, Paris
21. Pelissier-Langbort C (1986) La contraception des insuffisantes rénales. In: Serfaty D (ed) La contraception. Doin, Paris
22. Goldsmith MF (1986) Recherches sur les MST: un vaccin contre les gonocoques. JAMA [Suppl] 11 (133):19–20
23. Wolner-Hanssen, et al. (1986) JAMA, May 30
24. Kelaghan J, Rubin GL, Ory HW, Layde PM (1982) Barrier method contraceptives and pelvic inflammatory disease. JAMA 248(2):184–187

25. Netter A, Rozenbaum H (1986) Histoire illustrée de la contraception. De l'Antiquité à nos jours. Dacosta, Paris
26. Stone KM, Grimes DA, Magder LS (1986) Primary prevention of sexually transmitted disease. JAMA 255(13):1763–1766
27. Stone KM, Grimes DA, Magder LS (1986) Personnal protection against sexually transmitted disease. Am J Obstet Gynecol 155(1):180–188
28. Syrjanen K, Vayrynen M, Castren O, et al. (1984) Sexual behavior of women with human papillomavirus (HPV) lesions of the uterine cervix. Br J Vener Dis 60:243–248
28a. Pratt, et al. (1984) Popul Bull 39:20–24
28b. Handsfields HH, et al. (1986) JAMA 255(13):1730–1734
29. Conant M, Hardy D, Sterntinger J, et al. (1986) Condoms prevent transmission of AIDS-associated retrovirus. JAMA 255(13):1706
30. Verdoux C (1986) Les préservatifs masculins. In: Serfaty D (ed) La contraception. Doin, Paris
31. Hicks DR, Martin LS, Getchelle JP (1985) Inactivation of HTLV-III/LAV-infected cultures of normal human lymphocytes by nonoxynol-9. Lancet II:1422–1423
32. Voeller B (1986) Nonoxynol-9 and HTLV-III. Lancet I:1153
32a. Resnick L, et al. (1986) JAMA 255(4)
33. Henin Y, Marechal V, Barre-Sinoussi F, Chermann J (1987) HIV inactivation by spermicide-containing benzalkonium chloride. AIDS Forschung (in press)
34. Harris RWC, Brinton LA, Cowdell RH, et al. (1980) Characteristics of women with dysplasia or carcinoma in situ of the cervix uteri. Br J Cancer 42:359–369
35. Grimes DA, Lee NC (1987) Data on contraception, PID risk is good news for IUD, pill users. Contracept Technol Update, February:19–20
36. Washington AE, Gove S, Schachter J, Sweet RL (1985) Oral contraceptives, chlamydia trachomatis infection and pelvic inflammatory disease. A word of caution about protection. JAMA 253(15):2246–2250
37. Cramer WA, Goldman MB, Schiff I, Belisle S, Albrecht B, Stadel B, Gibson M, Wilson E, Stillman R, Thompson I (1987) The relationship of tubal infertility to barrier method and oral contraceptive use. JAMA 257(18):2446–2450
38. Fischl M (1987) Condoms not always successful in preventing AIDS transmission. Contracept Technol Update, April:53

The World Health Organization Special Programme

The World Health Organization Special Programme of Research, Development and Research Training on Human Reproduction: The Past 15 Years and the Next Decade

E. Diczfalusy

Karolinska Institute, Reproductive Endocrinology Research Unit. Box 60500
Karolinska Sjukhuset, 10401 Stockholm, Sweden

In his inimitable way Goethe says somewhere that „In der Beschränkung zeigt sich erst der Meister," and I regret very much that the master could not be asked to write this paper. Given the multifaceted character of the Special Programme and the complex international environment in which it operates, a condensed presentation such as the present one can hardly do complete justice to it, and the interested reader is referred to a more comprehensive review published recently (Diczfalusy 1986a).

Demographic Background

It took mankind a very long time, several hundreds of thousands of years, to reach the first billion in population; there is universal agreement that this took place some time between 1800 and 1850, probably in about 1807 (United Nations Population Division 1984; Demény 1985; World Development Report 1984, 1986). Decade estimates between 1920 and 1950 and quinquennial estimates thereafter indicate that it took some 120 years to reach the second billion around 1927; it then took only 33 years to reach the third billion in 1960, only 14 years to reach the fourth in 1974, and then only 13 years to reach the fifth billion, which happened some time early this year. Hence, my own generation has witnessed the birth of a new world, equal in numbers, aspirations, hopes and demands. And where do we go from here?

A great deal of thought has been given to various models for the proper extrapolation of available data; the balance of evidence strongly suggests that the world population will continue to grow, albeit at a progressively slower pace, for another 100–150 years. According to the medium-variant projections, the world is expected to have 6 billion people in 1999, 7 billion in 2010, and 8 billion in 2022 (United Nations Population Division 1986). The global population is expected to stabilize at between 10 and 11 billion people around the end of the twenty-first century (Demény 1985; United Nations Population Division 1984; World Population Report 1984); approximately 90% of this future population growth will take place in developing countries. In view of this situation, developing countries are increasingly facing a major challenge in their attempts to optimize the complex relationships between growing population, resources, environment and development.

Female Contraception
Eds.: B. Runnebaum, T. Rabe, L. Kiesel

lance studies with newly developed injectable, implantable and vaginal contraceptives, intrauterine devices and postovulatory methods, and the assessment of the interaction of various methods of contraception with HIV infection and AIDS.

Behavioural and Social Determinants of Fertility Regulation

A number of large-scale studies have been conducted on the psychosocial aspects of fertility regulation, including those on family formation patterns and health, patterns and perceptions of menstruation, user preferences in different developing countries and illegal abortions.

Among the most important ongoing studies are those concerned with the various factors affecting the choice and continuation of use of various methods of fertility regulation in developing countries and those concerned with the community barriers which impede access to family planning. Other studies address the changing roles of men and women with regard to reproductive health and adoption of different fertility-regulating methods as well as the economic, social and psychological costs and benefits of fertility regulation to couples living under various socioeconomic conditions.

Service Research

Several studies on the service aspects of fertility regulation were conducted; a number of member nations (e.g. India, Indonesia, Kenya, Pakistan, Philippines, Thailand, Turkey) have made important changes in their service delivery and national family planning programmes or even legislation, as a result of the findings and recommendations arising from these projects conducted in over 30 developing countries (cf. Diczfalusy 1986a).

Development of New and Improved Methods

Six Task Forces are entrusted with the special responsibility for developing new and improved methods: those on Long-acting Systemic Agents, Postovulatory Methods, Vaccines for Fertility Regulation, Methods for the Regulation of Male Fertility, Methods for the Natural Regulation of Fertility, and Plants for Fertility Regulation. The extent of the various clinical studies is revealed by the fact that more than 180 multicentred multinational trials were carried out. These involved more than 185000 subjects in 150 centres in 53 countries. Furthermore, a large number of single-centre clinical-pharmacological studies have been conducted. The Programme has access to records on approximately 200000 subjects.

For the conduct of the various clinical and preclinical studies contracts have been awarded to almost 500 institutions in 65 countries.

Long-Acting Systemic Agents. The Programme has developed a variety of long-acting systemic agents, which will be ready for introduction into family planning programmes by 1995 or earlier.

Four once-a-month injectable formulations, which have reached the stage beyond large-scale- (phase III) clinical trials, are indicated in Table 2. Two of the formulations (HRP-102 and Cycloprovera) have been developed by the Pro-development and research training in human reproduction, with a special emphasis on the needs of developing countries, became a reality 15 years ago in 1972.

The Special Programme and its Philosophy

Although initially it was the concern about demographic development that stimulated interest in family planning, it was rapidly realized that the health aspects of family planning are at least as important, if not more important. Indeed, WHO does not have any population policy; it is up to the governments of member states – if they so wish – to formulate their own policies in this respect. However, WHO has – and has always had – a global health policy. It has been recognized by the Special Programme from its inception that the impact of family planning and fertility regulation goes far beyond the issues of population growth and development.

Fertility regulation represents a very important tool to improve the general health status of populations, especially in developing countries. Indeed, the effective use of family planning will delay the age at first pregnancy and space further births; when integrated into primary health care, both of these will lower infant, child and maternal morbidity and mortality and significantly reduce illegal abortions and their health hazards. Children born less than 1 year after the end of their mother's last pregnancy are more than twice as likely to die than children born after an interval of 2 years or more. Furthermore, 85% of the world's births, 95% of the world's infant deaths, and 99% of the world's maternal deaths take place in developing countries. In fact, around 1983 only 55% of births occurring in the world were attented by trained personnel: 48% in developing countries and 98% in developed countries. It is estimated that some 500000 die each year from pregnancy-related causes (most of them preventable); among these are 200000 from illegal abortions (WHO 1985).

Prevalence of Contraceptive Use

A number of estimates have been published recently regarding the prevalence of contraceptive use (Population Crisis Committee 1985; Mauldin and Segal 1986; WHO 1987). It is clear from the various figures that – as a global average – more than 50% of eligible couples are still not using any modern method of fertility regulation. The proportion of married women of reproductive age in the world using contraception in 1980–1981 is presented in Table 1. These data indicate that one-third of these women living in developed countries and two-thirds of those living in developing countries did not use any contraception at the beginning of the present decade.

Past and Present Needs

To quote a scientist from a developing country, Fathalla (1983), the number of unwanted births, the high discontinuation rates and the number of induced abor-

Table 1. Married women of reproductive age in the world using contraception in 1980–1981

Area	percentage
World, total	45
Total excluding China	38
Developing regions, total	38
Total excluding China	24
Africa	11
Asia	42
East Asia	69
South Asia	24
Latin America	43
Developed regions, total	68

Source: WHO (1987).

tions convincingly indicate that available methods and services of family planning fail to meet the demand of developing countries. Hence, similar to the situation in 1972, 15 years later in 1987 there is still an enormous need for a wide variety of safe and effective methods that will suit the individual situation, the socioeconomic condition and the cultural and religious values of different couples. Furthermore, there is an even more urgent need for a substantial increase in social, behavioural and service research to better understand the factors influencing the acceptability and continuation rates of various methods and the interaction between users and providers of services. The WHO Special Programme of Research, Development and Research Training in Human Reproduction has been created to meet the above needs in a truly global context.

The Mandate

The Special Programme is the main instrument of the United Nations system for conducting, promoting, evaluating and coordinating international research on human reproduction, fertility regulation and family planning, with special emphasis on the needs of developing countries. Indeed, the mandate explicitly states that all activities should be oriented towards the needs of developing countries. To fulfil its role the Programme has a broad mandate to carry out research and development, expand and improve resources for research, to initiate, facilitate, evaluate and coordinate research, and to carry out a number of special responsibilities. A detailed description of these activities has been published elsewhere (Diczfalusy 1986a); a brief summary of the main achievements is presented below.

Research and Development

The research and development activities of the Programme can be discussed along five main lines: the safety and efficacy of fertility-regulating methods, behavioural and social determinants of fertility regulation, service research, the development of new and improved methods, and the prevention and management of infertility. These activities are carried out by a number of unique multinational and multidisciplinary collaborating mechanisms – the Task Forces. Each Task Force is composed of scientists from all over the world, who are doing research under the auspices of the Programme and of the Steering Committee. The latter group of scientists are responsible for maintaining an updated strategic plan and for eliciting and assessing the project proposals within the research lines of the strategic plan. The membership of Steering Committees is truly international, with adequate representation of women and of scientists from developing countries.

Safety and Efficacy of Fertility-Regulating Methods

A number of fertility-regulating agents have been available for several decades, and research on these methods is now moving toward epidemiological studies of long-term risks and benefits and to the assessment of rare adverse reactions. However, the bulk of available information originates from developed countries, and few, if any, data have been published from developing countries. Hence the Programme had – and still has – a unique mission when it comes to the short- and long-term assessment of the safety and efficacy of various fertility-regulating agents in the settings of different developing countries. Indeed, since its inception the Programme has conducted multinational epidemiological studies on virtually all existing fertility-regulating agents and methods. A number of studies have been published, including those on oral and injectable contraceptives and the risk of genital and breast cancer, on oral contraceptives and the risk of cardiovascular disease, on injectable contraceptives and the risk of pelvic inflammatory disease, and on intrauterine devices and the risk of ectopic pregnancies and of pelvic inflammatory disease (WHO Collaborative Study on Neoplasia and Steroid Contraceptives 1984, 1985a–c; WHO Task Force on Intrauterine Devices 1985). Other studies have addressed issues such as the relative safety of different methods of female sterilization, the sequelae of induced abortions, and the possible sequelae of vasectomy (WHO Task Force on Sequelae of Abortion 1979, 1984a, b; WHO Special Programme of Research, Development and Research Training in Human Reproduction 1982; WHO Task Force on Female Sterilization 1982 a–c).

The Programme has conducted multicentre studies with intrauterine devices (IUD) providing more than 500000 woman-months of experience. As a result of these studies it has been established that the newer copper devices (e.g. 220 C, 380 A, 380 Ag, Nova-T, Multiload) are significantly better in preventing pregnancy than the earlier copper devices (Cu 7, T Cu 200); the inert (plain) devices are no longer considered acceptable. The Programme has also established that – in contrast to insertion after second trimester abortion – insertion following first trimester abortion is as safe and effective as interval insertion.

Ongoing investigations include, for example, a study of the interaction of oral contraceptives with diseases prevalent in developing countries and/or the drugs used in their treatment, an investigation of the effect of injectable and implantable contraceptives on the progeny in utero and during lactation, health-risk surveillance studies with newly developed injectable, implantable and vaginal contraceptives, intrauterine devices and postovulatory methods, and the assessment of the interaction of various methods of contraception with HIV infection and AIDS.

Behavioural and Social Determinants of Fertility Regulation

A number of large-scale studies have been conducted on the psychosocial aspects of fertility regulation, including those on family formation patterns and health, patterns and perceptions of menstruation, user preferences in different developing countries and illegal abortions.

Among the most important ongoing studies are those concerned with the various factors affecting the choice and continuation of use of various methods of fertility regulation in developing countries and those concerned with the community barriers which impede access to family planning. Other studies address the changing roles of men and women with regard to reproductive health and adoption of different fertility-regulating methods as well as the economic, social and psychological costs and benefits of fertility regulation to couples living under various socioeconomic conditions.

Service Research

Several studies on the service aspects of fertility regulation were conducted; a number of member nations (e.g. India, Indonesia, Kenya, Pakistan, Philippines, Thailand, Turkey) have made important changes in their service delivery and national family planning programmes or even legislation, as a result of the findings and recommendations arising from these projects conducted in over 30 developing countries (cf. Diczfalusy 1986 a).

Development of New and Improved Methods

Six Task Forces are entrusted with the special responsibility for developing new and improved methods: those on Long-acting Systemic Agents, Postovulatory Methods, Vaccines for Fertility Regulation, Methods for the Regulation of Male Fertility, Methods for the Natural Regulation of Fertility, and Plants for Fertility Regulation. The extent of the various clinical studies is revealed by the fact that more than 180 multicentred multinational trials were carried out. These involved more than 185000 subjects in 150 centres in 53 countries. Furthermore, a large number of single-centre clinical-pharmacological studies have been conducted. The Programme has access to records on approximately 200000 subjects.

For the conduct of the various clinical and preclinical studies contracts have been awarded to almost 500 institutions in 65 countries.

Long-Acting Systemic Agents. The Programme has developed a variety of long-acting systemic agents, which will be ready for introduction into family planning programmes by 1995 or earlier.

Four once-a-month injectable formulations, which have reached the stage beyond large-scale- (phase III) clinical trials, are indicated in Table 2. Two of the formulations (HRP-102 and Cycloprovera) have been developed by the Pro-

Table 2. Once-a-month injectables beyond large-scale (phase III) clinical trials

Preparation	Progestogen	Oestradiol ester
Injectable no. 1 (China)	17-Hydroxyprogesterone caproate (250 mg)	Valerate (5 mg)
Perlutal (Mexico)	16,17-Dihydroxyprogesterone acetophenide (150 mg)	Oenanthate (10 mg)
HRP-102 (WHO)	Norethisterone oenanthate (50 mg)	Valerate (5 mg)
Cycloprovera (WHO)	Depomedroxyprogesterone acetate (25 mg)	Cypionate (5 mg)

Table 3. Progestogen-only injectable contraceptives at or beyond large-scale (phase III) clinical trials

Progestogen and dose	Preparation	Expected duration (months)
Norethisterone oenanthate (200 mg)	Oily solution	2
Medroxyprogesterone acetate (150 mg)	Microcrystalline suspension	3
Norethisterone (100 mg)	Biodegradable microcapsules	3
Levonorgestrel butanoate (12.5 mg)	Microcrystalline suspension	2–3

gramme in collaboration with two pharmaceutical companies. The pharmacokinetic and pharmacodynamic profiles of both products are very favourable. In a large comparative trial after 1 year of use in 1167 subjects Cycloprovera showed a Pearl index of 0.0, and in 1152 subjects HRP-102 gave a Pearl index of 0.2. The discontinuation for bleeding in the two groups was 6.4% and 7.4%, respectively – much less than reported with progestogen-only formulations, such as depomedroxyprogesterone acetate and norethisterone oenanthate (14%–15%).

Four new progestogen-only injectable contraceptives which are at or beyond large-scale (phase III) clinical trials are shown in Table 3. The available clinical data seem to suggest that the levonorgestrel butanoate microcrystalline suspension, which has been developed by the Programme in collaboration with the Contraceptive Development Branch of NICHD, Bethesda, Maryland, in the United States provides a 2- to 3-month duration of contraceptive effect when administered in a dose as small as 12.5 mg.

Furthermore, the Programme has developed, tested and submitted for registration a new vaginal delivery system, which provides constant blood levels and a contraceptive effect for a minimum of 3 months by releasing as little as 20 μg levonorgestrel per day. In addition, in collaboration with the Population Council in New York clinical studies are in progress with vaginal rings releasing natural progesterone in daily doses of 5–10 mg. These rings are intended for contraceptive use in the postpartum period.

Table 4. Interruption of early pregnancy with an antiprogestin and a prostaglandin analogue, success rate and side effects

Treatment	(Percentage of subjects)		
	RU-486 alone (Kovacs et al. 1984)	16-Phenoxy-PGE_2 alone (Bygdeman et al. 1983)	Sequential combination (Swahn and Bygdeman 1986)
Complete AB	61	94	96
Gastrointestinal side effects	0	55	0
Uterine pain requiring analgesics	0	56	13
Excessive bleeding	6	0	0

Source: Swahn and Bygdeman (1986).

A biodegradable implantable contraceptive (developed in collaboration with the Contraceptive Development Branch of NICHD) and a 6-monthly vaginal delivery system for levonorgestrel have reached the stage of clinical evaluation; by 1995 latest, the suitability of these systems should have been evaluated by large-scale clinical trials.

Postovulatory Methods. In comparative trials involving more than 15000 volunteers the Programme has established which prostaglandin analogue, dose regimen, formulation and route of administration is the most suitable in different clinical situations. Furthermore, the Programme has developed improved and safe procedures for the medical termination of first and second trimester pregnancy, generated a large body of clinical pharmacological data for registration of several products, and negotiated agreements with three manufacturers for the supply of their products for distribution in the public sector at concessionary prices.

Recent studies supported by the Programme led to the establishment of an important synergistic effect between the antiprogestin RU-486 and very small amounts of 16-phenoxyprostaglandin E_2 administered sequentially (Swahn and Bygdeman 1986). As indicated by the data of Table 4, the success rate of the sequential combination is much higher than that of RU-486 alone, whereas the side effects are much lower than those of the prostaglandin analogue alone, used previously in higher doses.

Large-scale clinical studies are also in progress to evaluate the feasibility of progestogen-only postcoital contraception with relatively large doses of levonorgestrel.

Vaccines for Fertility Regulation. The Programme has developed and brought into phase I clinical trials an almost totally synthetic birth control vaccine after obtaining permission from both the United States Food and Drug Administration (FDA) and the Australian Drug Regulatory Authority. The vaccine consists of a synthetic carboxy-terminal 109–145 amino acid region of the β-subunit of human chorionic gonadotropin conjugated to diphtheria toxoid as the carrier administered with muramyl dipeptide adjuvant in a squalene-arlacel vehicle. The development of a second generation vaccine is also in progress.

Methods for the Regulation of Male Fertility. Few advocates for the regulation of male fertility seem to realize that to develop a male contraceptive is a formidable task, because it is very difficult to inhibit spermatogenesis without interfering with testicular androgen secretion, and because it is equally difficult to invariably achieve long-term *reversible* azoospermia and not only a severe degree of oligospermia. Hence, the Programme has not yet developed a safe and effective "pill for men," nor has any other agency or organization. Nevertheless, the Programme has made and is making a number of significant contributions to the field, as indicated below.

A number of multicentre clinical studies were conducted with the aim of assessing the feasibility of using antiandrogens, or progestogen-androgen combinations as male antifertility agents. The latter studies revealed the necessity of developing much longer acting androgens than those available today. A series of novel testosterone esters have been synthesized and patented by the Programme. A single injection of one of these was shown to maintain physiological testosterone levels in castrated male monkeys for months.

Among the studies presently in progress are the following: a multicentre clinical trial on the contraceptive efficacy of very severe oligospermia induced by long-acting androgens, studies on the safety and efficacy of transdermal chemical vas occlusion, clinical-pharmacological studies on the combined administration of a luteinizing hormone-releasing hormone (LH-RH) antagonist and a long-acting androgen, a synthesis and screening programme on gossypol analogues to explore their spermicidal and virucidal activity (with special emphasis on their effect on HIV), studies on "post-testicular" fertility control with new agents of plant origin, especially those recently isolated from extracts of *Tripterygium wilfordii* Hook.f. (Celastraceae) (Qian 1986), and preclinical studies on the potential of a variety of follicle-stimulating hormone (FSH) inhibitors in male fertility control.

Methods for the Natural Regulation of Fertility. The first impartial international assessment of the cervical mucus (ovulation) method of natural family planning was undertaken by the Programme in a five-country study. A high method-effectiveness but very low use-effectiveness was found. Ironically, these findings are quoted by both protagonists and antagonists of natural family planning in support of their diametrically opposite viewpoints; the former point out the high method-effectiveness, the latter the low use-effectiveness.

Furthermore, a ten-country multicentre study (the largest of its kind ever conducted) provided more precise information than was previously available on the temporal relationships between peripheral hormone levels and the time of ovulation as determined by direct visualization and histological evaluation. In other studies a large number of potential indices of the fertile period were critically as-

Table 5. Diagnoses reached in 5857 women of the 8546 couples studied

Diagnoses	Count	% Diagnoses	% Cases
Tubal anormalities	2380	31.4	40.6
Endocrine causes	2205	29.1	37.6
No demonstrable cause	2058	27.2	35.1
Endometriosis	343	4.5	5.9
Acquired ovarian, uterine or cervical abnormalities	285	3.8	4.9
Sexual dysfunction	103	1.4	1.8
Congenital abnormalities	85	1.1	1.5
Systemic causes	50	0.7	0.9
Iatrogenic causes	34	0.4	0.6
Endometrial tuberculosis	27	0.4	0.5
Total	7570	100.0	129.2

sessed, and on the basis of the findings simple techniques were developed for the determination of the fertile period. As a next step, it is expected that by 1995 or earlier the Programme should have evaluated in large-scale multinational trials the efficacy of self-assessment of the fertile period by "do-it-yourself" kits.

It should also be borne in mind that even today lactation prevents more births than all modern methods of fertility regulation together. Therefore, the Programme conducts large-scale multinational studies to assess the determinants of lactational amenorrhoea in different populations. It is expected, on the basis of these ongoing studies, that by the mid-1990s at the latest the Programme will have developed guidelines for the optimization of spacing by lactation.

Plants for Fertility Regulation. A network of collaborating centres, predominantly in developing countries (Chicago, Hong Kong, Lucknow, Peradeniya, Seoul, Shanghai, and Wuhan), collected, extracted and evaluated in animal tests some 300 plant species with alleged antifertility effects, identified by an intensive literature search. Several new chemical entities possessing antifertility activity in rodents have been isolated and subsequently synthesized for subhuman primate studies. Examples of such new chemical entities possessing anti-implantation activity include yuehchukene (Kong et al. 1985) and pseudolaric acid B (Zhou et al. 1983). Whether or not these compounds can be tested clinically depends on the outcome of their preclinical safety assessment.

Prevention and Management of Infertility

Infertility is a major medical and social problem of global dimensions; epidemiological studies carried out by the Programme indicate that up to 15% of couples of reproductive age, perhaps as many as 50–80 million couples, may have infertility problems. Therefore, the Programme has conducted a standardized investigation of the infertile couple, which involved more than 8500 couples in 33 centres in 25 countries. This systematic study (the largest of its kind) revealed the most frequent causes of infertility both in women (Table 5) and in men (Table 6). The data of Table 5 indicate that the most common diagnoses in women were tubal

Table 6. Diagnoses reached in 6407 men of the 8546 couples studied

Diagnoses	Count	% Diagnoses	% Cases
No demonstrable cause	3127	46.8	42.8
Varicocele	806	12.1	12.6
Primary idiopathic testicular failure	717	10.7	11.2
Male accessory gland infection	441	6.6	6.9
Abnormal sperm morphology	376	5.6	5.9
Other seminal fluid abnormality	273	4.1	4.3
Low sperm motility	252	3.8	3.9
Suspected immunological factors	193	2.9	3.0
Congenital abnormalities	138	2.1	2.2
Sexual dysfunction	127	1.9	2.0
Systemic or iatrogenic causes	127	1.9	2.0
Obstructive azoospermia	64	1.0	1.0
Endocrine causes	41	0.6	0.6
Total	6682	100.0	104.3

abnormalities and endocrine causes. However, the group "no demonstrable cause" included women who did not have laparoscopy to exclude endometriosis, pelvic adhesions and tubal abnormalities. The data of Table 6 indicate that "no demonstrable cause" is by far the most common diagnosis in the male, reflecting probably our incomplete comprehension of the reproductive physiology and pathology of the male.

Ongoing or recently initiated studies include investigations on the principal causes of infertility in various communities, an assessment of the impact of sexually transmitted diseases on female and male fertility in different populations, a screening programme of spermicidal agents for anti-HIV virucidal activity, and the development of improved barrier methods of contraception, which also provide a high degree of protection against HIV.

Expansion and Improvement of Resources for Research

Almost one-third of the budged of the Programme is spent on the expansion and improvement of the resources for research in developing countries. Initially a global network of *clinical research centres* was established to conduct coordinated multicentre clinical trials, using common protocols and carefully standardized diagnostic methods and laboratory techniques. The network – 80% of which is situated in developing countries – represents a unique international health-research resource available to all interested parties. However, since the promotion of national self-reliance for research in family planning is a very important objective and integral part of the Programme, more and more effort has been devoted to the provision of resources for research on relevant local problems, as viewed by the developing countries themselves.

Thus, major efforts have been made to strengthen the *institutional resources* in a number of countries (e.g. Kenya, India, Indonesia, and the People's Republic of China). As an example, more than US$3.5 million worth of equipment, research training and consultant assistance has been provided to the Nairobi Centre for Research in Reproduction in Kenya, and the assistance provided to the eight large Chinese centres exceeds US$13 million, of which approximately half was contributed by the United Nations Fund for Population Activities (UNFPA). In addition, several centres received substantial assistance from the Programme and/or from the UNFPA in projects executed by the WHO for the strenghtening of research capacities (cf. Cotonou, Dakar, Hanoi, Tunis, Yaoundé).

The Programme has awarded *Research Training Grants* to 980 scientists from 60 countries, *Visiting Scientists Grants* to 163 senior scientists from 36 countries, and *"re-entry" grants* to 80 scientists from 31 countries (representing a total value of more than US$13 million). More than 900 of these grants were awarded to scientists from developing countries. In addition to 125 *training courses* held in collaboration with ministries of health, the Programme organized 35 *seminars*, 56 *workshops* and 39 *symposia* – altogether 130 major scientific events in some 40 countries. *Matched reagents* are currently distributed to some 80 laboratories in 40 countries, and an additional 90 laboratories participate in the *External Quality Assessment*. The number of publications based on the use of these reagents exceeds 500.

The total value of equipment, supplies and reagents provided to developing country centres exceeds US$33 million, corresponding to 16% of the total income of the Programme since its inception; this includes small supplies distributed to 120 institutions in 34 countries and journal subscriptions for 90 institutions in 30 countries.

Last but not least, the results of the studies supported by the Programme have been described in more than 6000 publications; the success of the institution-strengthening efforts of the Programme is reflected, for example, by the gradual increase in the proportion of publications authored by developing country scientists from approximately one-third (1972–1977) to one-half (1984–1987).

Collaboration and Coordination of Research

In its capacity as the main instrument of the WHO and of the entire United Nations system for conducting, promoting, evaluating and coordinating research on human reproduction, the Programme closely collaborates with the ministries of health of all member states. It also collaborates and coordinates its activities with a large number of intergovernmental and non-governmental international agencies and also with national and private agencies active in the area of human reproduction and related fields. For a detailed description, a previous review should be consulted (Diczfalusy 1986a).

Collaboration takes place in several ways, from simple exchange of information and mutual attendance at meetings to jointly organizing international symposia or launching major collaborative research projects. Examples of the latter are ongoing projects conducted in collaboration with the Center for Population Research at NIH (Bethesda, Maryland), the Population Council (New York), the

Ford Foundation (New York), the Family Health International (Triangle Park), the International Organization for Chemical Sciences in Development (Mexico, D.F.), and the Indian Council of Medical Research (New Delhi). Collaborative research projects are also carried out with other programmes within the WHO, for instance with the Special Programme on AIDS, the Division of Family Health, the Division of Microbiology and Immunology, and the Regional Offices.

Of special importance is the collaboration with industry in general and with the pharmaceutical industry in particular. The cornerstone of the Programme's relationship with industry is the promotion and protection of the interest of the public sector, with special emphasis on the needs of developing countries. Thus far, more than 60 drugs and devices from more than 30 companies and some 20 countries have been made available to the Programme for testing, and more than 30 agreements have been concluded or are under negotiation in countries such as Australia, the Federal Republic of Germany, Finland, France, Japan, Mexico, the Netherlands, Switzerland, the United Kingdom, and the United States.

With respect to coordinating functions the Programme regularly convenes coordination meetings with other agencies active in the field; these frequently involve the participation of active scientists.

Special Responsibilities

Among the special responsibilities of the Programme, brief mention should be made of the advisory function, ethical issues, patents, drug-regulatory issues and dissemination of information.

Advisory Function. The Programme's advisory function is an especially important one, since advice on a wide variety of technical aspects of family planning is frequently requested, not only by the ministries of health of many member states but also by international and national organizations and institutions and sometimes even by individual scientists.

Ethical Issues. The maintenance of uniformly high *ethical standards* in the conduct of clinical research in an area as sensitive as fertility regulation is a sine qua non for the Programme. The ethical aspects of each research project are reviewed in a sequential fashion by the Steering Committee of the relevant Task Force, the Toxicology Group, the Review Group, and finally by a special ethical review committee of the WHO, the Secreteriat Committee for Research Involving Human Subjects (SCRIHS). Furthermore, all project proposals must include evidence of approval by institutional and national ethical review mechanisms. Indeed, in institutions where it did not exist, the Programme has made it compulsory to create an ethical committee and has provided advice about its constitution and proper composition. In some developing countries these committees have formed a basis for a national system of ethical review. In fact, ethical concerns rank so high in the Programme that it requested the Council for International Organizations of Medical Sciences (CIOMS) to convene next year an International Conference on "Ethics and Human Values in Family Planning" with the subtitle of "An Inter-cultural (International) Dialogue on Rights and Responsibilities of Individuals and Societies Regarding Reproductive Decisions."

Patents. In 1982 the WHA decided that it should be the policy of the WHO to obtain *patent rights* (WHA 1982). Thus far there have been ten inventive efforts resulting in 16 patent applications; 14 of these have resulted from research sponsored by the Special Programme.

Drug-Regulatory Issues. Recommendation 69, adopted by consensus of the 146 member states represented at the 1984 International Conference on Population in Mexico City (United Nations 1984) called for an attempt to modernize and update the requirements for preclinical and clinical assessment of new fertility regulating agents. Therefore, in February 1987 the Programme organized a WHO Symposium on "Improving Safety Requirements for Contraceptive Steroids" with the participation of some 100 persons from 34 countries. Participants included basic and clinical scientists, representatives of drug-regulatory agencies, pharmaceutical companies and consumer groups, and those of national and international organizations interested in research on family planning. Based on a series of suggestions made by the Symposium and by subsequent consultations, the Programme is in the process of issuing a set of guidelines for the Toxicological and Clinical Assessment and Post-Registration Surveillance of Steroidal Contraceptive Drugs, which, together with the papers presented at the Symposium, will be published by the Programme.

Dissemination of Information. In addition to the more than 6000 scientific publications mentioned above and the large number of published Proceedings of the Symposia organized, the Programme regularly issues Annual Reports (from 1985, the Report will be issued biennially), and a newsletter entitled "Progress" every 3 months.

The Programme in the 1990s

Within a short time the Programme is expected to become an Inter-Agency Programme under the co-sponsorship of the United Nations Development Programme (UNDP), the United Nations Fund for Population Activities (UNFPA), the World Bank and the WHO. When this occurs, the WHO will be the Executing Agency and the Policy and Coordinating Committee (PCC) the governing body of the Programme. The PCC consists of representatives of the 11 largest financial contributor governments, 14 governments elected by the Regional Committees of the WHO, three governments elected by PCC, and three International Agencies collaborating with the Programme. Developing countries represent an absolute majority in PCC (at the present, 19 out of 31 members). This organization is expected to provide a closer contact with a large number of developing countries and a greater financial stability for the Programme during the coming years.

Many of the ongoing or recently initiated activities which are indicated in this review will be carried over to the early 1990s. In addition, there are still major needs to be met: a pill for men, a completely reversible method of male sterilization, several second-generation birth control vaccines, an efficient chemical method of female sterilization, long-acting systemic agents causing little or no bleeding irregularities, safe and inexpensive postcoital and anti-implantation agents, significantly improved barrier methods of contraception which also provide a high degree of protection against sexually transmitted diseases (including HIV). These represent only a few of the existing needs in the field of method development. Furthermore, present research efforts must be greatly expanded on the behavioural and social determinants of fertility regulation, and improved nation- or culture-specific approaches must be developed for the delivery of services.

Last but not least, since prevention and management of infertility is an integral part of family planning care, a great deal more must be learned about the principal causes of infertility in various cultures, and the impact upon this of sexually transmitted diseases. What is needed in this particular area is an intelligent collaboration with the inevitable.

Epilogue

This review started by pointing out that it took mankind a very long time, several hundreds of thousands of years, to reach the first billion in population, an event that happened less than 200 years ago. It took mankind a similarly long time to realize that – perhaps after all – it is not impossible to improve the human condition in global terms and to provide better health for all. Indeed – as pointed out by Arnold Toynbee – our times represent the first age since the dawn of civilization in which people have dared to think it practicable to make the benefits of civilization available to the whole human race. The Special Programme of Research, Development and Research Training in Human Reproduction is a humble attempt in this direction.

References

Demény P (1985) The World demographic situation. Center for Policy Studies, The Population Council, New York (Working paper no 121)

Diczfalusy E (1985) An international response to a global concern. Contraception 32:323–336

Diczfalusy E (1986a) The first fifteen years: a review. Contraception 34:3–119

Diczfalusy E (1986b) Has family planning a future? In: Diczfalusy E, Bygdeman M (eds) Fertility regulation today and tomorrow. Raven, New York, pp 3–19 (Serono symposia publications, vol 36)

Fathalla MF (1983) A synthesis of the various experiences and problems encountered with available methods of fertility regulation in developing countries. In: Diczfalusy E, Diczfalusy A (eds) Research on the regulation of human fertility. Scriptor, Copenhagen, pp 76–92

Kong YC, Cheng KF, Cambie RC, Waterman PG (1985) Yuehchukene, a novel indole alkaloid with anti-implantation activity. J Chem Soc Chem Commun 47–48

Mauldin WP, Segal SJ (1986) Prevalence of contraceptive use. Rockefeller, New York

Population Crisis Committee (1985) Issues in contraceptive development no 15

Qian S-Z (1986) Tripterygium Wilfordii, a new lead in male fertility regulation. In: Diczfalusy E, Bygdeman M (eds) Fertility regulation today and tomorrow. Raven, New York, pp 217–232 (Serono symposia publications, vol 36)
Swahn ML, Bygdeman M (1986) Interruption of early gestation with prostaglandins and antiprogestin. In: Diczfalusy E, Bygdeman M (eds) Fertility regulation today and tomorrow. Raven, New York, pp 109–118 (Serono symposia publications, vol 36)
United Nations (1968) Proclamation of Teheran. United Nations Publications E.70, I.1, pp 539–540
United Nations (1984) Report of the International Conference on Population, Mexico City, 6–14 August, 1984. E/Conf. 76/19, UN Publication, sales no E84.XIII.8
United Nations Department of International Economic and Social Affairs, Population Division (1981) Report on monitoring of population policies. UN Population Division, New York (Working papers no 69)
United Nations General Assembly (1962) Resolution 1838 (XVII), December 1962, cf Resolutions item 84 (A/05059)
United Nations Population Division (1984) World population prospects: estimates and projections assessed in 1982. Data reproduced in the Review and appraisal of the world population plan of action. Report of the Secretary General, United Nations International Conference on Population, Mexico City, August 1984; E/CONF. 76/4 Corr. 1–26 July, 1984, pp 29–30
United Nations Population Division (1986) Newsletter 40/41, December
World Development Report (1984) Oxford University Press, London
World Development Report (1986) Oxford University Press, London
World Health Assembly (1982) Resolution WHA35.14, May
World Health Organization (1971 a) Expanded programme of research, development and research training in human reproduction: report of a feasibility project. May, HR/71.4
World Health Organization (1971 b) Expanded programme of research, development and research training in human reproduction: report of a feasibility project – supplementary information. August, HR/71.4.add.1
World Health Organization (1985) World health statistics annual. WHO, Geneva
World Health Organization (1987) Evaluation of the strategy for health for all by the year 2000: Seventh report on the world health situation, vol 1: Global review. WHO, Geneva, p 94
World Health Organization Collaborative Study of Neoplasia and Steroid Contraceptives (1984) Breast cancer, cervical cancer and depot-medroxyprogesterone acetate. Lancet 2:1207
World Health Organization Collaborative Study of Neoplasia and Steroid Contraceptives (1985 a) Invasive cervical cancer and depot-medroxyprogesterone acetate. Bull WHO 63:505–511
World Health Organization Collaborative Study of Neoplasia and Steroid Contraceptives (1985 b) Breast cancer and depot-medroxyprogesterone acetate. Bull WHO 63:513–519
World Health Organization Collaborative Study of Neoplasia and Steroid Contraceptives (1985 c) Invasive cervical cancer and combined oral contraceptives. Br Med J 290:961–965
World Health Organization Special Programme of Research, Development and Research Training in Human Reproduction (1982) Sequelae of vasectomy. Contraception 25:119–123
World Health Organization Task Force on Female Sterilization (1982 a) Minilaparotomy or laparoscopy for sterilization: a multinational randomized study. Am J Obstet Gynecol 143:645–652
World Health Organization Task Force on Female Sterilization (1982 b) Randomized comparative study of culdoscopy and minilaparotomy for surgical contraception in women. Contraception 26:587–593
World Health Organization Task Force on Female Sterilization (1982 c) Mini-incision for post-partum sterilization of women: a multicentred, multinational prospective study. Contraception 26:495–503

World Health Organization Task Force on Intrauterine Devices (1985) A multinational case-control study of ectopic pregnancy. Clin Reprod Fertil 3:131–143
World Health Organization Task Force on Sequelae of Abortion (1979) Gestation, birth-weight and spontaneous abortion in pregnancy after induced abortion. Lancet 2:142–145
World Health Organization Task Force on Sequelae of Abortion (1984a) Comparison of rigid and flexible cannulae for early abortion without cervical dilatation. Stud Fam Plann 15:79–83
World Health Organization Task Force on Sequelae of Abortion (1984b) Secondary infertility following induced abortion. Stud Fam Plann 15:291–295
World Health Organization Task Force on Sequelae of Abortion (1986) Illegal abortion: an attempt to assess its costs to the health services and its incidence in the community. Int J Health Serv 16:375–389
Zhou BN, Ying BP, Song GQ, Chen ZX, Han J, Yan YF (1983) Pseudolaric acid from Pseudolarix kaempferi. Planta Med 47:35–38

Subject Index

W. Eicher, Mannheim; **G. Kockott, H.-J. Vogt,** Munich (Eds.)

Sexology

1988. 61 figures. Approx. 350 pages. Soft cover. ISBN 3-540-19400-2

Sexology as a discipline has had to fight for full-fledged recognition in the scientific community. Yet special knowledge of normal and disturbed sexual behavior is expected of medical professionals, psychologists and educators alike. Based on the papers given at the 8th World Congress for Sexology in 1987, this volume gives an up-to-date discussion of the most interesting and controversial topics, such as AIDS, in the field. Contributions have been grouped under the main headings: Family Planning, Sterility and Sexuality, Erectile Dysfunction, Sexuality in the Elderly and in Marriage, Transsexualism, Sexual Therapy, and Sexuality and Illness and include items of historical interest as well as trans-cultural comparisons.

Springer-Verlag
Berlin Heidelberg New York
London Paris Tokyo

Springer

MIX
Papier aus verantwortungsvollen Quellen
Paper from responsible sources
FSC® C105338

If you have any concerns about our products,
you can contact us on
ProductSafety@springernature.com

In case Publisher is established outside the EU,
the EU authorized representative is:
Springer Nature Customer Service Center GmbH
Europaplatz 3, 69115 Heidelberg, Germany

Printed by Libri Plureos GmbH
in Hamburg, Germany